Functional and Aesthetic Reconstruction of Burned Patients

Functional and Aesthetic Reconstruction of Burned Patients

Edited by

Robert L. McCauley, MD, FACS
University of Texas Medical Branch
Shriner's Hospital for Children—Galveston Unit
Galveston, Texas, U.S.A.

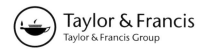

Taylor & Francis
Taylor & Francis Group

Boca Raton   London   New York   Singapore

Published in 2005 by
Taylor & Francis Group
6000 Broken Sound Parkway NW, Suite 300
Boca Raton, FL 33487-2742

No claim to original U.S. Government works
Printed in the United States of America on acid-free paper
10 9 8 7 6 5 4 3 2 1

International Standard Book Number-10: 0-8247-2583-2 (Hardcover)
International Standard Book Number-13: 978-0-8247-2583-9 (Hardcover)

Library of Congress Cataloging-in-Publication Data

Catalog record is available from the Library of Congress

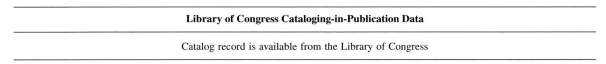

**Visit the Taylor & Francis Web site at
http://www.taylorandfrancis.com**

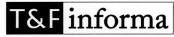

Taylor & Francis Group is the Academic Division of T&F Informa plc.

In Loving Memory
This book is dedicated to the memory of my mother and father, Hattie and Willie McCauley,
who built a well of inspiration and support so deep that I continue
to drink from it each and every day.

Preface

Over the past two decades, advances in the management of the acute burned patients have resulted in the routine survival of patients with 80–90% total body surface area burns. Needless to say, the reconstructive needs of these patients are numerous. This book addresses the reconstructive problems encountered in burn survivors by reviewing principles of wound healing, prioritizing their reconstructive needs and categorizing the multitude of techniques available to plastic surgeons for reconstruction. Surgical as well as non-surgical methods for improving the appearance and function are brought to the forefront.

This text, *Functional and Aesthetic Reconstruction of Burned Patients*, systematically dissects problems associated with burns of the head and neck, burns of the torso, perineum and upper extremity and burns of the lower extremities and feet. The indications for various reconstructive procedures such as grafts, flaps, tissue expansion, and microvascular free tissue transfers are incorporated throughout the text. The advantages and limitations of these techniques are thoroughly discussed. In addition, the application of certain principles of aesthetic surgery are applied to these patients. Regardless of the extent of the burn injury, wound closure is simply not enough. Today, as reconstructive surgeons, we must strive not only for function but also for the aesthetic restoration of our patients. The reintegration of burn patients back into society as productive members, in many ways, is dependent upon the restoration of form and function.

I would like to thank all the contributors to this book for their dedication and hard work. The secretaries in the Medical Staff Office, the Graphic Arts Department as well as the Medical Records Department at the Shriners Hospital for Children—Galveston Unit, all deserve a special thanks for their unyielding support in the completion of this project.

Robert L. McCauley

Contents

Contents

Contributors

Malachy E. Asuku, MD, FWACS   *Department of Plastic and Reconstructive Surgery, Ahmadu Bello University Teaching Hospital, Kaduna, Nigeria*

Alfonso Barrera, MD, FACS   *Department of Plastic Surgery, Baylor College of Medicine, Houston, Texas, USA*

John D. Bauer, MD   *Department of Surgery, University of Texas Medical Branch, Galveston, Texas, USA*

Debra Benjamin, RN   *Division of Clinical Research, Shriners Hospital for Children, Galveston, Texas, USA*

Kanika Bowen, BS   *University of Texas Medical Branch School of Medicine, Galveston, Texas, USA*

Steven T. Boyce, PhD   *Department of Surgery, University of Cincinnati, Cinicinnati, and Shriners Burn Hospital, Cincinnati, Ohio, USA*

Jason H. Calhoun, MD   *Department of Orthopedic Surgery, University of Missouri–Columbia, Columbia, Missouri, USA*

Angelo Capozzi, MD, FACS   *Division of Plastic and Reconstructive Surgery, Shriners Hospital for Children, Sacramento, and University of California, Davis, California, USA*

Kelly D. Carmichael, MD   *Department of Orthopedics and Rehabilitation, University of Texas Medical Branch, Galveston, Texas, USA*

Joaquin Cortiella, MD   *Department of Anesthesiology, Shriners Hospital for Children, Galveston, and University of Texas Medical Branch, Galveston, Texas, USA*

Prema Dhanraj, MD   *Department of Plastic Surgery, Christian Medical College & Hospital, Vellore, Tamil Nadu, India*

Marc Funke, MD   *Department of Plastic, Hand and Reconstructive Surgery, Medizinische Hochschule Hannover, Hannover, Germany*

Enrique Garavito, MD   *Department of Surgery, Shriners Hospital for Children, Mexico Unit and School of Medicine, Anahuac University, Mexico, Mexico*

Tewodros M. Gedebou, MD   *Department of Plastic and Reconstructive Surgery, Chang Gung University and Medical College, Taipei, Taiwan*

Aziz Ghahary, PhD   *Department of Surgery, University of Alberta, Edmonton, Alberta, Canada*

Lawrence J. Gottlieb, MD *Department of Surgery, University of Chicago, Chicago, Illinois, USA*

David G. Greenhalgh, MD *Department of Surgery, University of California, Davis, California, USA*

Mark A. Grevious, MD *Department of Plastic Surgery, University of Illinois, Chicago, Illinois, USA*

Mutaz B. Habal, MD, FAAP, FRCSC, FACS *Tampa Bay Craniofacial Center, Tampa, Florida, USA*

David N. Herndon, MD *Department of Surgery and Pediatrics, University of Texas Medical Branch and Shriners Burn Hospital, Galveston, Texas, USA*

Hazel Joseph, MD *Department of Surgery, Eastern Virginia Medical School, Norfolk, Virginia, USA*

Garry W. Killyon, MD, DDS *Department of Surgery, Division of Plastic Surgery, University of Texas Medical Branch and Section of Plastic and Reconstructive Surgery, Shriners Hospital for Children—Galveston Unit, Galveston, Texas, USA*

Suzanne L. Kilmer, MD *Shriners Hospital for Children, Sacramento, and Department of Surgery, University of California, Davis, California, USA*

W. John Kitzmiller, MD *Division of Plastic, Reconstructive and Hand Surgery, University of Cincinnati Medical Center, Cincinnati, Ohio, USA*

Robert L. McCauley, MD *Department of Surgery and Pediatrics, Division of Plastic Surgery, University of Texas Medical Branch and Section of Plastic and Reconstructive Surgery, Shriners Hospital for Children—Galveston Unit, Galveston, Texas, USA*

Alex McLaughlin, OTR *Department of Rehabilitation Services, Shriners Hospital for Children, Galveston, Texas, USA*

Michael K. Obeng, MD *Division of Plastic Surgery, University of Texas Medical Branch, Galveston, Texas, USA*

Albert K. Oh, MD *Shriners Hospital for Children, Sacramento, and University of California, Davis, California, USA*

Donald H. Parks, MD *Department of Plastic and Reconstructive Surgery, University of Texas—Houston Medical School, Houston, Texas, USA*

Lynn Peterson, CRNA *Department of Anesthesiology, Shriners Hospitals for Children, Galveston, and University of Texas Medical Branch, Galveston, Texas, USA*

Linda G. Phillips, MD *Department of Surgery, University of Texas Medical Branch, Galveston, Texas, USA*

Nelson Sarto Piccolo, MD *Instituto Nelson Picolo and Pronto Socorro para Queimaduras, Goiânia, Goiás, Brazil*

Rocco C. Piazza II, BS *University of Texas Medical Branch School of Medicine, Galveston, Texas, USA*

Evan Pickus, MD *Section of Plastic and Reconstructive Surgery, Shriners Hospital for Children—Galveston Unit, Galveston, Texas, USA*

Paul G. Scott, PhD *Department of Biochemistry, University of Alberta, Edmonton, Alberta, Canada*

Michael Serghiou, OTR *Department of Rehabilitation Services, Shriners Hospital for Children, Galveston, Texas, USA*

Robert L. Sheridan, MD *Shriners Hospital for Children and Department of Surgery, Massachusetts General Hospital, Boston, Massachusetts, USA*

Edward R. Sherwood, MD, PhD *Department of Anesthesiology, Shriners Hospital for Children, Galveston, and University of Texas Medical Branch, Galveston, Texas, USA*

Marcus Spies, MD *Department of Plastic, Hand and Reconstructive Surgery, Medizinische Hochschule Hannover, Hannover, Germany*

Dorothy M. Supp, PhD *Department of Surgery, University of Cincinnati, Cincinnati, and Shriners Burn Hospital, Cincinnati, Ohio, USA*

Edward E. Tredget, MD, MSc, FRCS *Department of Surgery, University of Alberta, Edmonton, Alberta, Canada*

Jacobo Verbitzky, MD *Division of Plastic Surgery, Shriners Hospital for Children, Mexico Unit, Mexico*

Peter M. Vogt, MD *Department of Plastic, Hand and Reconstructive Surgery, Medizinische Hochschule Hannover, Hannover, Germany*

Hugh L. Vu, MD, MPH *Shriners Hospital for Children, Sacramento, and University of California, Davis, California, USA*

David Wainwright, MD *Department of Plastic and Reconstructive Surgery, University of Texas—Houston Medical School, Houston, Texas, USA*

Fu-Chan Wei, MD, FACS *Department of Plastic and Reconstructive Surgery, Chang Gung University and Medical College, Taipei, Taiwan*

Lee C. Woodson, MD, PhD *Department of Anesthesiology, Shriners Hospital for Children, Galveston, and University of Texas Medical Branch, Galveston, Texas, USA*

Steven E. Wolf, MD *Department of Surgery, University of Texas Medical Branch and Shriners Burn Hospital, Galveston, Texas, USA*

Brian Wong, MD *Department of Ophthalmology, University of Texas Medical Branch, Galveston, Texas, USA*

Jui-Yung Yang, MD *Department of Plastic Surgery, Chang Gung Memorial Hospital, Taipei, Taiwan*

1

Properties of the Skin

JOHN D. BAUER

University of Texas Medical Branch, Galveston, Texas, USA

I. INTRODUCTION

Skin is the outer structural element, which contains an organism's component parts, thereby differentiating it from the surrounding environment. From the point of view of mammals, and other warm-blooded creatures, the skin acts in many other capacities beyond simple containment. In humans, it is the largest organ in the body, making up 16% of its weight. Grossly it is a major thermoregulatory organ along with its sensory, metabolic, immune, and protective qualities. Specifically, the acellular cornified exterior protects from abrasive and chemical trauma. Collagen confers resistance to mechanical force, and elastin allows skin to shrink, expand, and snap back. The resident immune system affords an effective barrier against assaults from bacteria, fungi, and viruses. Melanocytes allow for a response to solar radiation with a protective change in color. Sensory nerves allow withdrawal from extremes of heat and cold, and distinguish sharp and vibratory sensations. Skin has adapted to the various environments to which it is exposed. Hence, the glabrous skin of the hand lets a construction worker maintain a grip on a 9 lb hammer, while its more flexible counterpart over the leg will allow the muscles of a world-class sprinter to glide, expand, and contract. Sweat glands act like a swap cooler taking advantage of evaporation to help regulate the temperature of humans who have comparably little hair, as compared to fur-bearing creatures who thermoregulate through their pulmonary system.

As mentioned, skin has been described as an organ, which is essentially a group of differentiated cells acting in concert to carry out some identifiable function(s). The focus of this chapter will be to review the gross and molecular anatomy of skin; address biomechanics of aging and scarring; as well as explore iatrogenic alterations of skin like tissue expansion.

A.   Anatomy

1. Gross

As alluded to earlier, the skin acts as a protective covering to the body and is by weight the largest organ in the body. Its thickness and color vary by site. Whereas the skin on the back is thick, the skin on the eyelids can be as thin as 5/1000 of an inch. Clinically, these differences play a significant role in the planning of surgery from acquisition of skin grafts to the planning, placement, and effectiveness of flaps. Color variations over the surface of an individual, with progressive lightening from head to toe, make the proper choice of a donor site for the patient with an open wound essential.

As can be seen in Fig. 1.1, skin is bilayered with a thin, rapidly replicating outer layer (epidermis), containing keratinocytes, melanocytes, Langerhans cells, and Merkel cells. The much thicker dermis below contains structural components like collagen and elastin, as well as appendages like hair, sweat, eccrine, and sebaceous glands, as well as nerve endings.

2. Epidermis

The epidermis is the outer insensate, nonvascular layer with a rapidly dividing basal layer consisting mostly of mitotically active keratinocytes, which undergo a process of cornification. These cells progressively differentiate as they are carried through the spinous, granular, and cornified layers. Migration from the basal layer to the cornified layer takes about 28 days, and consists of a well-defined, genetically programmed series of steps. The process begins with rapid division of mitotically active basal keratinocytes followed by a cessation of division, production of keratin and other proteins involved in cross-linking, which leads to an increase in cell size. Next, a genetic and cellular reorganization occurs where intracellular organelles are lost and new proteins are produced in anticipation of apoptotic death and dehydration

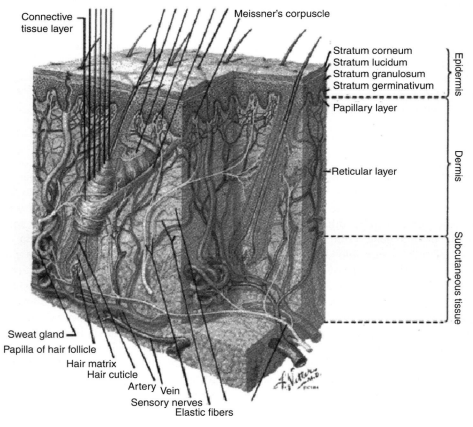

Figure 1.1   Normal skin anatomy. (With permission from Ross MH, Reith EJ, Romrell LJ. In: Kist K, ed. Histology: A Text and Atlas. 2nd ed. Baltimore: Williams & Wilkins, 1989:373.)

(1–3). The thickness of the cornified layer can vary drastically depending on its location. Whereas the entire thickness of the upper lid skin may be 5/1000 of an inch, the skin on the back can be 10 times thicker [Fig. 1.2(A) and (B)].

3. Basement Membrane

This process begins at the basement membrane. There are three distinct types of keratinocytes in this basal layer: stem cells, transit amplifying cells, and postmitotic cells. Stem cells comprise ~10% of the cells in this area, and can be identified by distinct $\beta 1$ integrins (4). As they divide, one stem cell is left behind and the second daughter begins the process of differentiation. Having this resident population of undifferentiated cells is of interest because these cells can accumulate mutations from assaults by solar radiation and chemicals, which can lead to uncontrolled division, and/or skin cancers like squamous cell, or basal cell. Through a chorus of signals by the dermis, several growth factors like epidermal growth factor (EGF), transforming growth factor alpha (TGF-α), and keratinocyte growth factor (KGF), as well as sterols like the retinoids, transit amplifying cells, are induced to go through a series of genetically programmed divisions. This provides an appropriate number of cells, which is followed up by the postmitotic phase where growth factors like TGF-β signal cellular differentiation. The keratin bundles in this layer are fine and flexible, which allows for cellular division. They are found in pairs, which are specific to this layer, K5/K14. The bundles and the cells themselves then undergo changes in shape, keratin type, as well as their interaction with desmosomes as they pass into the spinous layer.

4. Stratum Spinosum

The stratum spinosum is distinguished by its polyhedral shape, basophilic cytoplasm caused by high levels of RNA production, and large numbers of desmosomes. Though K5/K14 keratins persist, there is also a new form of keratin, K1/K10. These pairs are stretched between

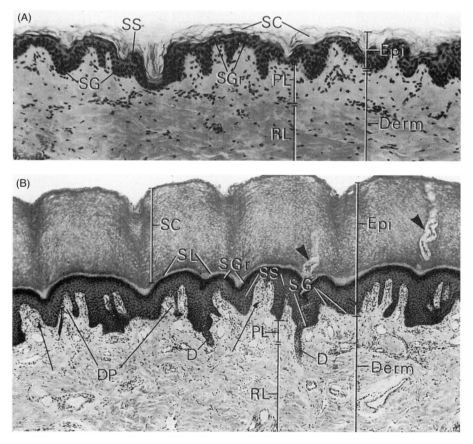

Figure 1.2 (A) Light micrograph showing the layers of thin human skin. (B) Light micrograph showing the layers of thick human skin. (With permission from Ross MH, Reith EJ, Romrell LJ. In: Kist K, ed. Histology: A Text and Atlas. 2nd ed. Baltimore: Williams & Wilkins, 1989:347–365.)

the nucleus and the desmosomes acting as intracellular bridges. As the keratinocytes move into the next transition, they enlarge and lamellar granules are formed in preparation for the next phase.

5. Stratum Granulosum

In the stratum granulosum both proteolysis and phosphorylation of K1/K10 keratin pairs occur with the production of new K2/K11 pairs. At the same time a series of proteins are produced which allow for the aggregation and cross-linking of keratin. Further, the aforementioned lamellar granules assemble in the cytoplasm and prepare to release a series of glycoproteins, glycolipids, phospholipids, which are acted upon by resident enzymes that will act to create a lipid barrier to skin permeation in the cornified layer.

6. Transitional Zone

Between the stratum granulosum and the stratum corneum lies a distinct transition zone. Here, the cells, which had been extremely metabolically active, now go through a programmed cell death called apoptosis. Here, degradative enzymes break down the cellular organelles, DNA fragmentation, and finally complete loss of the nucleus occurs. This leads us to the most superficial layer.

7. Stratum Corneum

The stratum corneum cells are anucleate, dead cells, which provide the majority of the barrier function attributed to the skin. As alluded to earlier, the keratin in these cellular remnants is cross-linked by strong disulfide bonds and their surfaces are protected by lipid rich lamellae. The thickness of this layer, unlike the other layers described, varies greatly and can go from only a few cell layers in the eyelid to tens of cells thick on the arms and legs. It gets even thicker on the back, and can be hundreds of cell layers thick in the palms and soles.

8. Cells of the Epidermis

Though the vast majority of the cells in the epidermis are keratinocytes, there are three other notable residents involved in such varied functions as skin pigmentation (melanocytes), antigen presentation (Langerhans cells), and neuroendocrine functions (Merkel cells). Melanocytes are the melanin producing cells, are of neural crest origin, and, in the skin, are interspersed among the basal keratinocytes. Their molecular, antibody signatures are S-100 and HMB-45. They transfer pigment via melanosomes to keratinocytes through dendritic processes, and are stimulated to do so, for instance, by ultraviolet radiation. It has been shown that melanosome regulation is intimately related to keratinocytes, and that the communication is through growth factors like basic fibroblast growth factor, endothelin-1, melanocyte stimulating hormone and stem cell factor (5,6). The density and activity of these cells varies not only across races, and individuals within these groups, but also within individuals. Importantly, three factors involved in the skin coloration are circulatory patterns, the number and activity of melanocytes, and the thickness of the epidermis. With these in mind, it makes sense that skin color becomes lighter when moving from cranial to caudal. This obviously also plays a role in the choice of skin graft donor sites, as well as the transfer of soft tissue from one area to another, when a choice exists. For instance, when transferring skin to the face, for color match, a donor site above the cavical is preferred.

Lagerhan or dendritic cells are antigen-presenting cells (Fig. 1.3), which exist in multiple tissues of the body including skin, mucous membranes, lymph nodes, thymus, and spleen. Their origin is the bone marrow, and they then migrate to the suprabasement membrane. TNF-α, IL-1β and the α6-integrin receptor are the induction signaling molecules (7). Transit through the basement membrane is accomplished with the expression of matrix metaloprotease-9 (8), which helps to disrupt intracellular adhesions and degrades collagen IV. Once in position in the dermis, the immature dendritic cells endocytose bacteria that they encounter, move through the lymphatic system, and in the maturing process, will present the bacterial cell antigens to T-cells in the local lymph node beds. This is accomplished through three surface receptors: MHC proteins which actually present antigens to the T-cell, costimulatory proteins involved in cell recognition, and adhesion molecules which maintain cell-to-cell contact. Like other cells formally known as clear cells, dendritic cells cannot be visualized on routine stains, but immunohistochemical visualization can be accomplished using the specific CD1a antibody (9).

Merkel cells (Fig. 1.4) are found both in the epidermis and the dermis, and act as mechanoreceptors in the skin. In the epidermis, through the production of nerve growth factor, they have been shown to function as mechanoreceptors (10). Though these cells appear to function in a neural capacity, studies on developing fetal skin have suggested an epidermal origin (11). Their unique antibody signature for the skin is cytokeratin-20. In the epidermis, Merkel cells are joined to the keratinocytes by desmosomes at epidermal ridges, and through microvilli at their cell surface respond to mechanical distortion. They are also localized around the arrector pili muscles in the hair follicles in the dermis, and probably play a role their activity (12). They have further been implicated in the development of eccrine sweat glands, the hair follicle, and nerves of the skin (13). Other neural elements exist and will be covered later in the chapter.

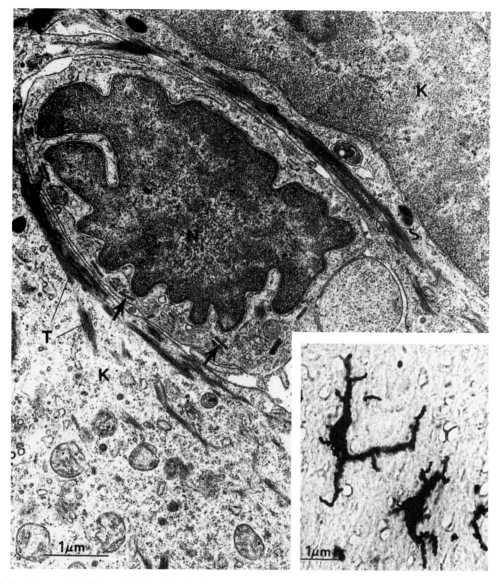

Figure 1.3 Light micrograph of Langerhan's cell (dendritic). (With permission from Ross MH, Reith EJ, Romrell LJ. In: Kist K, ed. Histology: A Text and Atlas. 2nd ed. Baltimore: Williams & Wilkins, 1989:347–365.)

9. Dermis

As described earlier, the dermis is a dynamic and variable structure which functions in a number of ways depending on the location and physical demands of the structures over which it lies. It needs to be very flexible and elastic over structures, which need to expand and contract like the thorax, or the joints. It requires durability and must maintain considerable tensile strength to survive the shearing forces inflicted on hands and feet with manipulation of objects, or ambulation. Thermoregulation, hydroregulation, sensation, and olfactory stimulation are but a few of the functions carried out by appendages found in the dermis.

10. Structure

Anatomically, the dermis has been divided into papillary and reticular portions, with a closely adjacent hypodermis. The papillary dermis is the most superficial and is distinguished by its dermal papillae which project upwardly and interdigitate with downwardly projecting rete pegs of the epidermis. It maintains small-diameter collagen, the immature and highly distensible form of elastin called oxytalan, has a large number of fibroblasts, and provides nutrition to the avascular epidermis through capillaries which extend from the subpapillary plexus to the edge of the basement membrane. Its most superficial

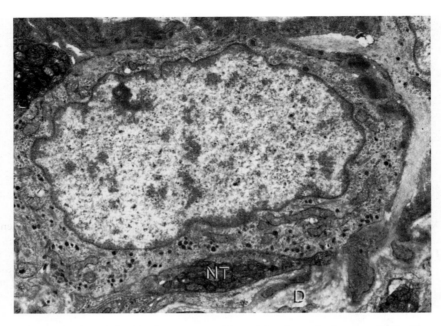

Figure 1.4 Electron micrograph of Merkel cell. Note contact with peripheral terminal neuron (NT). (Courtesy of Dr. B. Munger, 1984.) (With permission from Ross MH, Reith EJ, Romrell LJ. In: Kist K, ed. Histology: A Text and Atlas. 2nd ed. Baltimore: Williams & Wilkins, 1989:347–365.)

component is an area known as the compact zone or the sublamina densa. Along with an abundance of extracellular matrix adhesion molecules like tenacin, it also contains the ends of the anchoring fibrils of the epidermis made primarily of collagen VII. The reticular dermis is distinguished by much larger interdigitated bundles of collagen and elastin, giving the dermis its strength and resilience. The hypodermis is an adipose rich layer just deep to the dermis which fills several essential roles. It serves to insulate the body, provides a ready reserve of energy supply, and allows for mobility over structures like joints and most nonglabrous skin. It is mentioned here because it is intimately connected to the more fibrous reticular dermis by both vascular and neural tissues, and further contains many of the skin appendages like hair follicles and sweat glands.

11. Collagen

The major structural component of the dermis is collagen. It makes up 25% of the protein mass in animal, and a full 70% of the dry weight of skin. It has a triple helical structure, made of α chains rich in proline, lysine, and glycine, which together create a tightly packed rope-like structure. This compact structure is stabilized by interaction between glycine and the combination of both hydroxylated proline and lysine. Both tensile strength and elasticity are the hallmarks of this structural design, and as described above,

will vary depending on the structural needs. Though 25 distinct α chains have been identified, allowing for literally thousands of potential combinations, only 20 different collagen types have been identified (Table 1.1) (14).

The skin is composed primarily of the fibrillar form of collagens, namely I, III, IV, V, and VII. After secretion into the extracellular matrix, these fibrils assemble into strands between 10 and 300 nm in diameter, and up to hundreds of micrometers in length (Fig. 1.5). They then can aggregate into larger bundles, or collagen fibers. Types I and III are the dominant forms in the skin, with a ratio in normal skin of 4:1, though in injured skin this ratio can be temporarily decreased to 2:1. Interestingly, in scars this ratio tends never to return to normal in either skin or fascia and has therefore been implicated in the development of incisional hernias (15). Further, multiple studies have shown this decreased collagen I/III ratio in hypertrophic scarring (16). Type V collagen, is found primarily in the papillary dermis, the matrix of the basement membrane around blood vessels, nerves, and epidermal appendages, where it combines with types I and III collagen and is involved in regulating fibril diameter.

Collagen types IV and VII have been referred to as network-forming. Type IV assembles into sheets resembling a meshwork which makes up the majority of the basement membrane of the epithelium, and type VII forms into anchoring fibrils which act to secure the epithelial basement membrane to the dermis (17).

Table 1.1 Some Types of Collagen and Their Properties

	Type	Molecular formula	Polymerized form	Tissue distribution
Fibril-forming (fibrillar)	I	a1(I)$_2$α2 (I)	Fibril	Bone, skin, tendons, ligaments, cornea, internal organs (account for 90% of body collagen)
	II	[α1(II)]$_3$	Fibril	Cartilage, invertebral disk, notochord, vitreous humor of the eye
	III	[α1(III)]$_3$	Fibril	Skin, blood vessels, internal organs
	V	[α1(V)]$_2$α2(V) and α1(V)α2(V)α3(V)	Fibril (with type I)	As for type I
	XI	α1(XI)α2(IX)α3(XI)	Fibril (with type II)	As for type II
Fibril-associated	IX	α1(IX)α2(IX)α3(IX)	Lateral association with type II fibrils	Cartilage
	XII	[α1(XII)]$_3$	Lateral association with some type I fibrils	Tendons, ligaments, some other tissues
Network-forming	IV	[α1(IV)]$_2$α2(IV)	Sheetlike network	Basal lamina
	VII	[α1(VII)]$_3$	Anchoring fibrils	Beneath stratified squamous epithelia
Transmembrane	XVII	[α1(XVII)]$_3$	Not known	Hemidesmosomes
Others	XVIII	[α1(XVIII)]$_3$	Not known	Basal lamina around blood vessels

Note: Types I, IV, V, IX, and XI are each composed of two or three types of α chains, whereas types II, III, VII, XVII, and XVIII are composed of only one type of α chain each. Only 11 types of collagen are shown, but about 20 types of collagen and bout 25 types of α chains have been identified so far.
Source: With permission from Alberts B, Johnson A, Lewis J, Raff M, Roberts K, Walter P. Molecular Biology of the Cell. 4th ed. New York: Garland Science-Taylor & Francis Group, 2002:1065–1125.

12. Elastin

Elastin is the spring that allows skin which has been stretched or deformed to snap back into its original shape (Fig. 1.6). This 350 kDa molecule (18) is extremely distensible, though this capability is tempered by the relatively nondistensible collagen with which it is interwoven in the skin. Its precursor tropoelastin is secreted into the extracellular matrix, where it then is linked to a preexisting scaffold of glycoproteins called microfibrils, the most notable being fibrillin. It is assembled into sheets and then takes its position in the dermis where it extends from the lamina densa of the epidermal basement membrane, through the entire dermis, to the hypodermis.

Three forms of elstasic fibers have been defined. The first and most superficial is Oxytalan (19). It is mostly microfibrils coated with soluble elastin. They are vertically oriented, flexible, and are considered the least mature of the three forms. The second is Elaunin, considered the

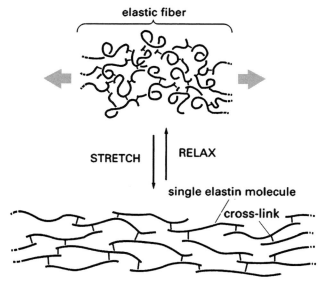

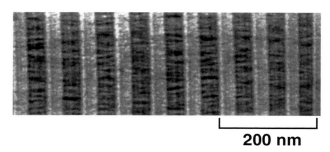

200 nm

Figure 1.5 Electron micrograph of collagen fibril note striated appearance. (Courtesy of Robert Horne.) (With permission from Alberts B, Johnson A, Lewis J, Raff M, Roberts K, Walter P. Molecular Biology of the Cell. 4th ed. New York: Garland Science-Taylor & Francis Group, 2002:1065–1125.)

Figure 1.6 Stretching a network of elastin molecules. Note cross-linking covalent bonds. (With permission from Alberts B, Johnson A, Lewis J, Raff M, Roberts K, Walter P. Molecular Biology of the Cell. 4th ed. New York: Garland Science-Taylor & Francis Group, 2002:1065–1125.)

intermediate form of the three with more cross-linked elastin fibrils. It is horizontally oriented and interdigitated with oxytalan in the deep papillary and reticular dermis. Finally, there is mature elastin, which lies deep in the reticular dermis. It is the least flexible and is also horizontally oriented. As a side note, the failure of the skin to snap back, seen so often in sun damaged skin, has been linked to abnormal elastin produced after exposure to UV radiation (20), and errors in elastin production are seen in diseases like Ehlers–Danlos syndrome (21). Further, breakdown of elastin has been shown to occur as skin ages, leading to laxity seen in the older population (22).

13.　Ground Substance

Along with the fibrous and flexible portions of the dermis are the skin's shock absorbers. These are glycoproteins, primarily glycosaminoglycans (GAGs), covalently linked to proteoglycans. They tend to attract water and surround the collagen and elastin, as a sort of gel or ground substance. Dermal occupants known as fibroblasts produce them, and they help protect against compression injury and dermal deformation.

GAGs are unbranched polysaccharide chains which are highly anionic and hydrophilic. They therefore attract positively charged ions like sodium, as well as large amounts of water, which helps produce the gel earlier. Some examples include hyaluronic acid, condroiton sulfate/dermatin sulfate, heparin sulfate, and keratin sulfate. Proteoglycans have a core polypeptide chain with multiple sugar side chains, one of which by definition is a GAG. Some examples include hyaluronic acid, condroiton sulfate/dermatin sulfate, heparin sulfate, and keratin sulfate. Other glycoproteins like fibronectin are intimately involved in cell–matrix adhesion through their interaction with the collagen, elastin, and integrins on the surface of fibroblasts.

14.　Cells of the Dermis

By far, the predominant cell of the dermis is the fibroblast, though other less numerous monocytes like macrophages, and dendritic cells, as well as mast cells, play a major role in the immune, inflammatory, and allergic activities of the skin. Other transient visitors include lymphocytes and granulocytes/neutrophils.

Fibroblasts, as stated, are the most populous cells in the dermis, and in uninjured skin exist in a senescent state. However, they are called into action after skin trauma, where they produce a variety of extracellular matrix proteins including collagen, elastin, and glycoproteins. They are also involved in the contraction of wounds and have been termed myofibroblasts or activated as illustrated by their production of smooth muscle actin-α (23). Transforming growth factor-β (TGF-β) has been identified as

a major regulatory factor. Other cytokines shown to play a role are IL-1 and IL-8. Interferon gamma has been identified as a potential downregulator (24). This is of particular interest especially as it relates to abnormal scarring, where fibroblast hyper-responsiveness to TGF-β has clearly been shown (23).

Macrophages, along with shorter-lived neutrophils, are the major phagocytic cells of the immune system. Both are able to engulf microorganisms, and destroy them with lysosomal derived superoxide free radicals, hypochlorite, and hydrolases. Unlike neutrophils, macrophages have a much more prominent role in the skin's immune system. They originate from bone marrow-derived monocytes, and convert to macrophages after entering the skin from the vascular system. Along with the aforementioned, lysosomes/phagasomes have a well-developed rough endoplasmic reticulum (Fig. 1.7), and Golgi apparatus for protein production and intermediate filament system for mobility. Besides phagocytosis and lysis of microorganisms, they process and present antigens to T- and B-cells. In addition, these cells are secretory with production of growth factors and other cytokines. They are involved in coagulation, as well as wound healing. Dermal dendritic cells, like the previously described Langerhans cells, are also phagocytic, but are more involved in the transport, processing, and presentation of antigens in the afferent loop of the immune system.

15.　Glands

Eccrine, apocrine, and sebaceous glands all reside in the dermis/hypodermis (Fig. 1.8). Eccrine or sweat glands have been described as the shower of the skin, and are found in great numbers over the entire skin surface. Apocrine glands are more localized to areas like the axilla and, groin. Compared to eccrine glands, they have a less well-defined physiological function, but are well known to be responsible for the odor caused when the fats produced by these glands are metabolized by resident bacteria. The physiologic function of the sebaceous gland is even less well defined, though phermonal and waterproofing roles have been suggested.

Eccrine sweat glands (Fig. 1.9) are thermoregulatory, and act to control elevations in body temperature. During extrinsic exposure to heat, intrinsic metabolic production of heat through exercise, and/or emotional stress, the release of water and electrolytes occur, producing evaporative heat loss. Humans have, by far, the most extensive eccrine sweat gland system in mammalian community. Interestingly, we are born with our full complement of sweat glands at birth, so none are added as we grow. So at birth we have an eightfold higher density of sweat glands compared to when we are adults. Further, one of the denser areas of distribution is on the palms of

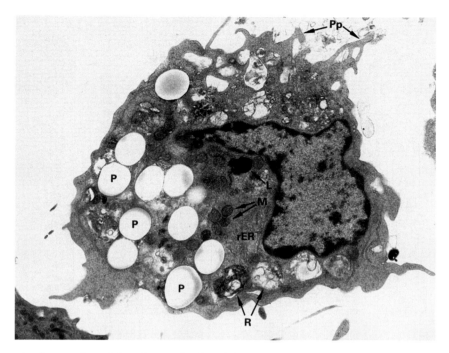

Figure 1.7 Micrograph of macrophage. Note phagocytized particles. (With permission from Wheater PR, Burkitt GH, Daniels VG. Connective tissue. In: Wheater PR, Burkitt GH, Daniels VG, eds. Functional Histology: A Text and Colour Atlas. New York: Churchill Livingstone, 1987:52–63.)

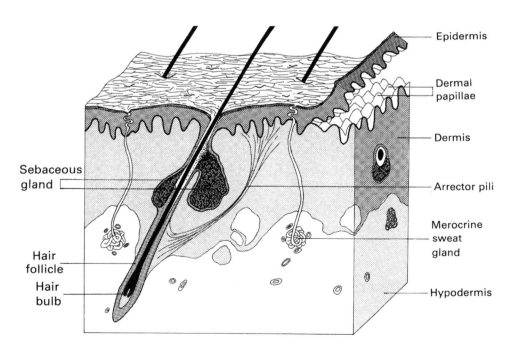

Figure 1.8 Skin and appendages. Note location of sebaceons and merocrine (eccrine) sweat glands. (With permission from Wheater PR, Burkitt GH, Daniels VG. Skin. In: Wheater PR, Burkitt GH, Daniels VG, eds. Functional Histology: A Text and Colour Atlas. New York: Churchill Livingstone, 1987:130–141.)

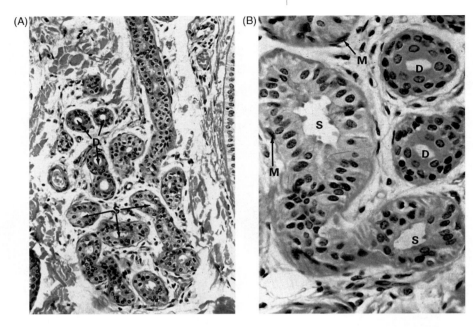

Figure 1.9 Merocrine (eccrine) sweat glands. Note pale string secretory cells. (With permission from Wheater PR, Burkitt GH, Daniels VG. Skin. In: Wheater PR, Burkitt GH, Daniels VG, eds. Functional Histology: A Text and Colour Atlas. New York: Churchill Livingstone, 1987:130–141.)

the hand, which provides a great benefit to us, since the grasping and holding of objects is facilitated by moist skin.

Numerically, there are between two and five million sweat glands on an average adult, and unlike apocrine glands, they are not associated with hair follicles. They are simple tubular glands with both ductal and secretory components. Eccrine sweat is clear and odorless and 99% water, the other 1% being electrolytes and organic material. Its release is an active secretory process via a sodium, potassium, and chloride cotransport system.

Apocrine glands are concentrated in the axillae, and perineal areas (Fig. 1.10). They are coiled glands embedded in the dermis, with a short duct, which empties into the hair follicle just superficial to the sebaceous duct in the pilo-sebaceous unit. Like sebaceous glands, they are under adrenergic control, and their output becomes active in adolescence, and decreases slowly with age. The exact composition is unclear since isolating this from eccrine sweat and sebum is difficult.

Finally, sebaceous glands are the sebum producing glands found over the entire skin surface, except the palms, soles, and dorsum of the feet (Fig. 1.11). Like hair, described later, they are unique to mammals. In humans, the density and size of these glands varies greatly with small single-celled glands on areas like the eyelids, all the way to huge cauliflower-shaped glands on the face, scalp, and ano-genital orifices. Most of the time they are associated with hair follicles, and the unit is referred to as a pilo-sebaceous gland, but they can

open directly onto the surface of the skin around the lips, from the buccal mucosa, the inner eyelids, labia minora, and around the nipple, where they are referred to as free glands. In the fetus, they tend to be quite prominent, secondary to maternal hormones, but they regress after birth until puberty, where they enlarge again secondary to intrinsic hormonal influences, and subsequently play a significant role in the development of acne.

Histologically, the sebum producing cells in the gland begin small with distinct lipid vacuoles, but they may increase to 100–150 times their original size as their vacuoles enlarge. In the latter stages, these lipid vacuoles may in fact fuse, as cytoplasmic organelles break down, and lysosomal enzymes ultimately produce cellular disruption as the apoptotic genetic program unfolds. Sebum containing triglycerides, wax esters, squalene, cholesterol esters, and cholesterol, are then released into the lumen of the gland along with keratinaceous squamae and bacteria. Hormonal activity is primarily from androgens (25), but influences, either through exogenous or endogenous exposure, by estrogens, progestins, glucocorticoids, as well as thyroid and pituitary hormones that are under investigation.

16. Hair

The topic of hair is as variable as hair itself. This keratin rich proteinaceous structure is peculiar to mammals. It protects the skin from solar radiation, provides insulation, sweeps foreign bodies from the eyes, and may become

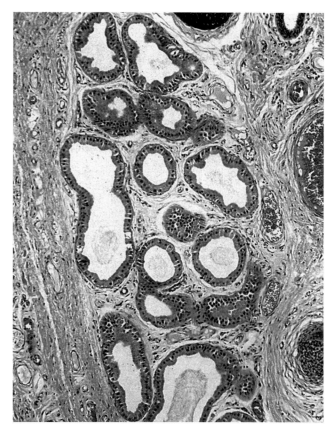

Figure 1.10 Apocrine sweat glands. Note their highest density in the axilla and groin. (With permission from Wheater PR, Burkitt GH, Daniels VG. Skin. In: Wheater PR, Burkitt GH, Daniels VG, eds. Functional Histology: A Text and Colour Atlas. New York: Churchill Livingstone, 1987:130–141.)

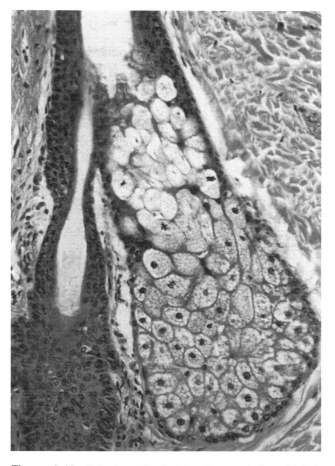

Figure 1.11 Sebacious glands. Note the association with hair follicles. (With permission from Wheater PR, Burkitt GH, Daniels VG. Skin. In: Wheater PR, Burkitt GH, Daniels VG, eds. Functional Histology: A Text and Colour Atlas. New York: Churchill Livingstone, 1987:130–141.)

erect in the face of fear or other types of arousal. The follicle contains sebaceous and apocrine glands, which bathe the skin with oils. Its color may be blond to black. Its length may be nearly unlimited on the scalp, yet short on the eyelids. Its texture can be coarse in the axilla and fine on the helical rim. The shape and architecture (curly or straight) varies across individuals as well as within an individual. Its phases of growth, involution, and quiescence provide a window into genetic cycling, stem cells, and apoptosis.

The anatomic structure of the hair follicle has been well studied (Fig. 1.12). Most of the time it is embedded in the dermis, although longer shafts can be located in the subcutaneous fat in areas like the scalp. The follicles exit the skin at an angle, which is significant when carrying out reconstructive or aesthetic hair transplantation. The lower portion, or the base, contains the bulb, which has a dermal papilla containing specialized fibroblasts intimately involved in hair growth signaling and follicle formation (26), dendritic melanocytes involved in color

formation, the papillary pore encasing the blood supply, as well as epithelial cells involved in the actual formation of both the sheaths and hair itself. More superficially is the permanent portion, which contains a bulge, to which the arrector pilori muscles attach. Within this bulge are stem cells believed to be involved in the regeneration of hair following the resting phase. The distalmost portion carries the hair to the surface, but also is home to the sebaceous and apocrine glands.

The cycle of hair growth has been broken into three distinct phases: antigen, catagen, and telogen. The period during which the hair producing cells are active is known as the antigen phase. The length of this phase is variable even within specific hair types like the scalp. The duration in the scalp is 2–5 years, with a growth rate of ∼0.35 mm per day. This variability is important, as it ensures scalp coverage as the individual hairs cycle. If each hair follicle's antigen phase ended simultaneously,

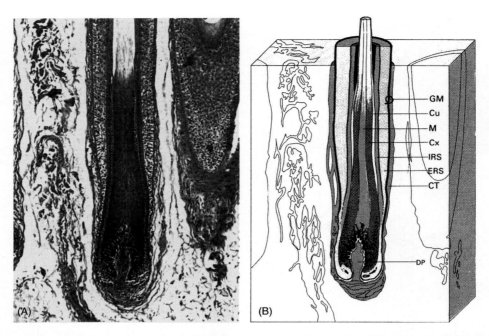

Figure 1.12 Hair follicle. (With permission from Wheater PR, Burkitt GH, Daniels VG. Skin. In: Wheater PR, Burkitt GH, Daniels VG, eds. Functional Histology: A Text and Colour Atlas. New York: Churchill Livingstone, 1987:130–141.)

areas of baldness would result. This can, and in fact, does happen when follicles are traumatized. A good example is hair transplantation, where a transient loss of all transplanted hair shafts often occurs, which must be carefully explained to patients. Other examples include fever stress, and some types of drugs.

The catagen phase last only a few days. During this phase, mitotic activity ceases, the hair bulb and the proximal, transient portion of the shaft involute, and the hair dies, though it may remain in place. The telogen phase is the time when no hair is produced by the follicle. The remaining hair may remain in the shaft, but does not grow. It may also be sluffed if appropriate mechanical stress is applied. On the scalp, under normal circumstances, ~10% of hairs are in telogen phase, at any one time.

The regulation of these phases is under active investigation, and along with the specialized fibroblasts of the dermal papilla described earlier, cytokines including PDGF, TGF-B, and EGF have been implicated in both stimulatory and inhibitory functions (27–29). The apoptotic transition of the follicle from antigen to catagen and finally to telogen appears to be at least partially regulated by protooncogenes blc-2, c-myc, c-myb, and c-jun (27,30).

17. Blood Supply

The blood supply to the skin, along with the obvious function of providing nutritional and metabolic transport, carries

out many other functions. Vasoconstriction/dilation of the vasculature assists in thermoregulation. Endothelial cells in the walls of blood vessels are a source and a target for inflammatory cytokines, as well as the source of vasoactive molecules like nitric oxide. They are vital in activating the clotting cascade (31). The upregulation of selections, integrins, and I-cams allows for cellular adhesion, demargination, and transmigration of leukocytes and monocytes, which is critical in the response to injury and wound healing (32,33). Further, understanding the gross and microscopic anatomy is essential in addressing tissue loss and reconstruction, especially as it relates to flap design.

As classically described, the blood supply to the skin begins with segmental vessels, originating from the aorta, which then branch into perforating vessels, which connects to the cutaneous vasculature (Fig. 1.13). The cutaneous vasculature is then broken into two critical subgroups: the musculocutaneous perforators and the direct cutaneous vessels. These two subgroups then supply two horizontally oriented plexuses, one at the junction of the dermis and the subcutaneous fat, and another at the papillary dermis, just deep to the epidermis. These two systems are connected through multiple anastomoses. Finally, the superficial plexus gives off dermal papillary loops, which are located in the dermal papillae, directly opposed to the epidermal rete pegs. Papillary loops approach as close as 1 μm to the basement membrane of the epidermis. This is where nutrient and metabolic exchange occurs, for the otherwise nonvascularized epidermis.

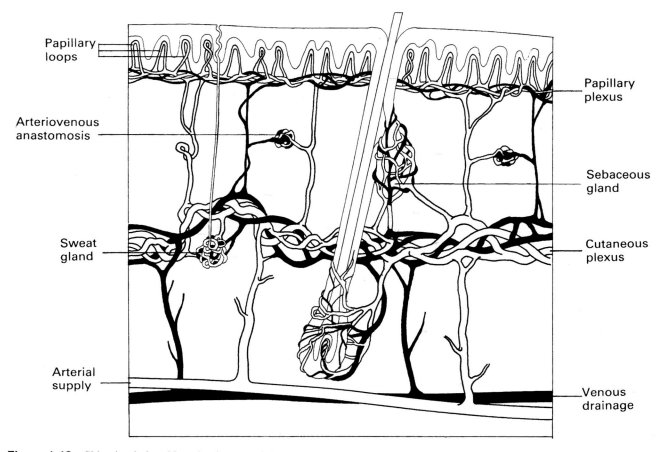

Figure 1.13 Skin circulation. Note the deep arterial and venous vessels giving way to branches progressing superficially to the two superficial plexes. (With permission from Wheater PR, Burkitt GH, Daniels VG. Skin. In: Wheater PR, Burkitt GH, Daniels VG, eds. Functional Histology: A Text and Colour Atlas. New York: Churchill Livingstone, 1987:130–141.)

The subgroups of the cutaneous vasculature mentioned earlier, musculocutaneous perforators and direct cutaneous vessels require special consideration as they relate to flap reconstruction. Prior to the development of the concept of angiosomes, which supply an axial blood supply to an area of skin through direct cutaneous vessels, flaps were designed with the thought that the blood supply was random. In other words, it was thought that skin was supplied through the musculocutaneous perforators, which were perpendicularly oriented to the horizontally oriented deep and superficial plexuses. So, as one elevated a skin flap, the perpendicular connections were divided, and the only blood supply to the tip of the flap was the nearest perpendicular perforators at the base. So, length-to-width ratios and tube flap strategies were devised for random flaps, which would provide the distalmost portion of the flap adequate musculocutaneous perforators at the base to survive. This limited the flexibility of skin flaps, and often led to multi staged procedures. Unfortunately, flap morbidity was also all too common.

When it was discovered that there were areas of the skin, which were supplied by direct cutaneous or axial vessels, entire new flap strategies could be devised. This concept of angiosomes (34) allowed not only for much longer, thinner rotation, advancement, and interpolated skin flaps, but also for the development of island flaps. This is where an area of skin can be elevated with its axial vessels attached, completely free from its surrounding skin, and be moved and inset to an adjacent, but separate, area.

When it comes to injuries to the skin, whether traumatic or iatrogenic, the vascular tree plays an important role in healing. The process of re-establishing blood flow to the injured tissue is referred to as angiogenesis. When blood vessels are disrupted, the normally quiescent endothelial cells are activated and begin both dividing and migrating. The mechanisms by which these occur are under investigation, and several key cytokines have been identified. Vascular endothelial growth factor (VEGF) is produced locally by keratinocytes and several other cell types, and has been shown to bind with tyrosine kinase receptors on the surface of endothelial cells initiating cellular division (35). Proteolytic enzymes then begin to degrade the surrounding basement membrane and extracellular matrix releasing basic bFGF, and upregulating integrins and selectins, and VCAM-1, thereby allowing the endothelial cells to migrate toward the stimulus and carry out capillary tube formation. Actual vessel formation is accomplished also by the activation of resident pericytes, which form chords. These chords then develop gaps through which the sprouting endothelial cells migrate to form a lumen. The newly formed vessels then extend into the injured tissue and merge with established blood vessels as well as with other newly formed vessels. Ultimately, this results in the development of a patent vascular system with capillary loops, microvessels, and anastomoses between larger vessels, thus providing a blood supply for the healing wound.

18. Nerves

In its capacity as a sense organ, this skin acts to protect us through the sensations of heat, cold, and pain, may stimulate us with sensations of light touch to irritating itch, as well as response to cold or fear, and goose bumps. All this is accomplished through a ubiquitous neural network carrying incoming and outgoing signals. Afferent sensory nerves carry sensations of pain, touch, temperature, and pressure to the CNS, where voluntary and involuntary responses are formulated and effected. The efferent autonomic system, on the other hand, responds to environmental stimuli with reactions like vasoconstriction/dilation, sweating, and inflammation. The organization of this system is varied and the density and type of innervation is commensurate with the requirements of the tissue.

Grossly, the sensory innervation to the skin is laid out in strips known as dermatomes. These come from the dorsal and ventral rami of each spinal nerve. In the head and neck, cranial nerves provide sensation, primarily through the trigeminal nerve. In the hands, sensation is carried through the brachial plexus (C5–T1), to the radial, median, and unlar nerves. Specifically, cutaneous braches of musculocutaneous nerves enter the subcutaneous fat and then separate into a deep plexus which innervates vascular and adnexal structures, and a superficial plexus which ascends to a plexus in the papillary dermis. The skin also has autonomic nerve fibers which travel initially with the sensory fibers, but then branch off to supply innervation to glands, blood vessels, and the tiny arrector pili muscles.

Microscopically, sensation to the skin is divided into free and corpuscular components. Free nerve endings are primarily nonmylenated C-fibers, which are widely distributed throughout the papillary dermis, skin appendages, and hair follicles. Interestingly, in areas where fine discrimination is required, for example, in the fingertips, each nerve fiber may innervate a single dermal papilla. This leads to an axonal density as high as 1000 axons per 1 square centimeter of skin surface, and represents rapidly adapting receptors (36). These C-fibers account for the sensation of touch and temperature, and to some degree, pain and itch. But there is a group of mylinated sensory fibers, namely Aδ-fibers which may play a significant role in pain and itch (37).

There are several specialized structures in the skin involved in various aspects of sensation which merit mention at this point. Merkel cells, as discussed earlier, are structurally consistent with a neuroendocrine origin and form cell–axon complexes with C-fibers mostly among the basal keratinocytes in the fingertips, lips, and nailbeds. They form so called "touch spots," and have been implicated to function mostly as the slow adapting mechanoreceptors of the skin. This slow response is responsible for both changing and static conditions and these continue to fire after the stimulus has ceased. Pacinian corpuscles are encapsulated receptors which are multilayered and have an onion layered appearance and consist of an outer perineural layer, and an inner structure with an axon surrounded by Schwann cells collagen, elastin, and fibroblasts. Their greatest concentration is in the palms and soles, and they have been shown to act as a rapidly adapting mechanoreceptor and respond to pressure while the skin is being indented. In other words, they only respond when the skin is being deformed. Meisner's corpuscles are located at the dermal epidermal junction, and like the other specialized cells listed, are primarily located on the palmar and plantar skin. They are cylindrical in shape and have supporting structures consisting of modified Schwann cells, and an unmylinated afferent terminal, which responds to touch.

Finally, along with peptides like histamine, the nervous system of the skin has been shown to be intimately involved in the inflammatory process, as exemplified by the Triple response of Lewis. So, not only are the afferent C-fibers responsible for responding to noxious stimuli with sensation of pain, itch, warm, and cold, but they also can initiate a local inflammatory reaction. As the action potentials are carried toward the CNS, upon arriving in the spinal chord, an additional pathway is initiated whereby retrograde antidromic impulses cause the release of neuropeptides stored along the peripheral nerve. This produces local erythema, followed by a wave of arterial vasodilation extending beyond the area of injury (flare). Finally, increased permeability of venules results in plasma extravasation, influx of inflammatory cells, and wheal formation.

19. Skin as a Flexible Organ

Though technology like electron microscopes, molecular biology, and protein specific stains did not exist at the time Karl Langer did his classic experiments on skin tension and extensibility, simple observation of incised skin gave clues to the structures which we now know exist. An awl is not required to understand that these properties of the skin are urgently important, especially to the plastic surgeon faced with traumatic soft tissue defects requiring closure, or with iatrogenically produced defects in the process of tumor excision. It is easy to see the difference between the rapid snap of the cheek of a baby encountering the first contact with an overzealous aunt, and the sluggish return to position of the lower lid of that elderly aunt as she is examined for her first blepharoplasty. It is also clear that the inelastic, tension resistant skin that we depend upon to help us grasp that valuable, flower filled antique crystal vase, would not be very useful situated on the elbow which we will flex to have a satisfying floral whiff. So differences exist not only between the skin of different individuals, but also between the skin of a single individual. Further, these properties can change when aging, exposure, trauma and scarring, as well as location on the body vary. Finally, these properties can be exploited when innovators like Radovan, Argenta, and Austad see the opportunity to stretch the skin when the scalp of a burned child needs resurfacing.

20. Extensibility vs. Elasticity

Skin is not a rigid structure. It is flexible, albeit variably between different areas in any one individual and between individuals, as described earlier. Skin's ability to respond to acute stress has two well-defined components: extensibility, or the ability to resist tension, and elasticity, or its ability to return to its original shape when tension is released. As described earlier, collagen is abundant in the skin, and it is this, which is responsible for extensibility. Normally, this cross-linked, triple helical structure appears relaxed, loose, and convoluted [Fig. 1.14(A)]. But as tension is applied the fibers tend to take on a more parallel pattern [Fig. 1.14(B)], and a classic stress–strain curve occurs (Fig. 1.15). This extensibility has limits as any surgeon who closes soft tissue defects can easily attest. Elastin, on the other hand, gives skin the ability to snap back after being stretched. Like collagen, it is rich in proline, glycine, and hydroxyproline. But, unlike collagen, it has no hydroxylysine, and is not glycosylated. Its α-helical segments are cross-linked through covalent bonds and coated with a sheath of glycoproteins known as fibrillin. Elastin is not distinct from collagen, but instead forms a loose network within the collagen framework. Interestingly, mutations in fibrillin

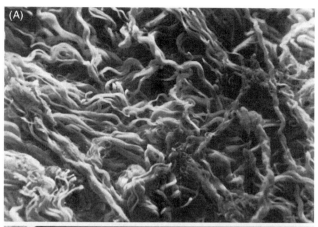

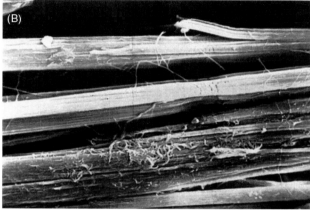

Figure 1.14 (A) Typical stress–strain curve of human skin in tension. (With permission from Gibson T, Kenedi RM.) (B) The stress relaxation that occurs in skin increases with the applied load. (With permission from Gibson T, Kenedi RM. The structural components of the dermis. In: Montagna W, Bentley JP, Dobson RL, eds. The Dermis, 1970. Courtesy of Appleton-Century-Crofts, Publishing Division of Prentice-Hall, Inc., Englewood Cliffs, NJ.)

lead to a structural instability in elastin, and result in Marfan's syndrome.

Finally, it is important to understand that collagen and elastin do not exist in a vacuum. This network is lubricated with a mucopolysaccharide rich ground substance, which insulates individual fibers and allows for optimal function. The dermis is also interspersed with blood vessels, nerves, and lymphatics, each of which may be affected by skin deformation, and may ultimately, though not necessarily directly, affect the flexibility of skin. Vascular plexes may be obstructed by deformational forces, and lead to congestion, ischemia, necrosis, and ultimately tissue loss and/or scarring. Nerves can be stretched and cause pain and lymphatics can be obstructed causing either acute or chronic edema.

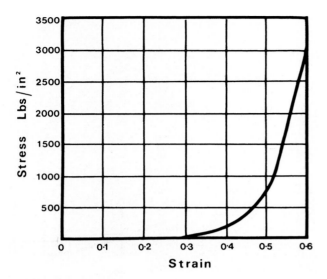

Figure 1.15 Scanning electron microscope (SEM) photograph of the collagen fibers of relaxed human dermis. (With permission from Gibson T, Kenedi RM. The structural components of the dermis. In: Montagna W, Bentley JP, Dobson RL, eds. The Dermis, 1970. Courtesy of Appleton-Century-Crofts, Publishing Division of Prentice-Hall, Inc., Englewood Cliffs, NJ.)

21. *Viscoelasticity*

The fact that skin has the ability to stretch is one that presents itself in everyday life in both acute and chronic venues. The concept of viscoelasticity deals with the former, and the two terms are classically applied to describe the skin's immediate response to an applied force. These are creep and stress relaxation, and as you will see, they are basically a way of describing a single phenomenon from two different points of view. With creep, we observe that skin tends to extend when a constant force is applied over time. Stress relaxation is the observation that when the skin is stretched to a given length, the force required to hold it there decreases over time. Obviously, the strain curves derived from these experiments are not linear and flatten as the dermis reaches its expandable limits. These limits, as one might surmise, are related to the ability of the resident collagen and elastin to "give" by unwinding and becoming more parallel. Further, it is also dependent on the viscous molecules, which surround and cushion the structural components, to "move out of the way" as the skin stretches and thins, namely, the aforementioned mucopolysaccharide rich, ground substance.

Clinically, these phenomena are vitally important, especially when one endeavors to plan the orientation of an incision (Fig. 1.16), or recruit adjacent tissue to close soft tissue defects with local flaps like Z-plasties (Fig. 1.17). In the 1970s, Gibson and Kendi presented the concept of "load cycling," pointing out that skin

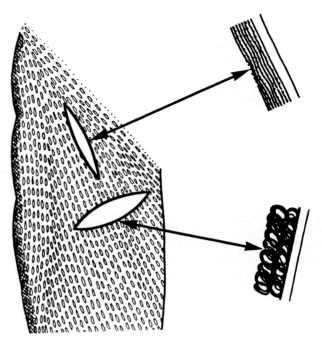

Figure 1.16 When skin is stretched, many of the fibers become aligned in a straight manner in the direction of stretch, thus imposing a limit on extensibility in that direction. (With permission from Brown IA. Structural and Mechanic Skin. Ph.D. Thesis, University of Strathclyde, Glasgow, 1971.)

could be stretched to a greater extent if the load were applied then relaxed a number of times, thereby better displacing the ground substance and getting that sometime crucial few millimeters of length (Fig. 1.18). Similarly, "immediate tissue expansion" proponents (38), have observed that increased tissue length can be obtained with load cycling, but that little true increase in skin length actually occurs. This though, is not the case with chronic or true tissue expansion as described in the following text.

22. *Tissue Expansion*

The idea that skin can stretch when force is applied over a long period of time can easily be observed, for instance, in the obese patient. Even better, an apparent increase in skin area seems to occur when this obese patient loses significant weight and an empty hanging pannus results. The question arises, is this increase in area a result of actual skin growth, or simply the realigning of collagen, elastin, and ground substance with a measure of dermal tearing that occurs with "stretch marks"? Though in the patient described earlier, it is probably a combination of both of these, it has been clearly shown that chronic force applied to skin can make it grow, and that this growth can be clinically advantageous when a need to

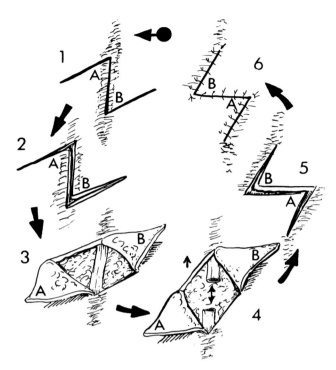

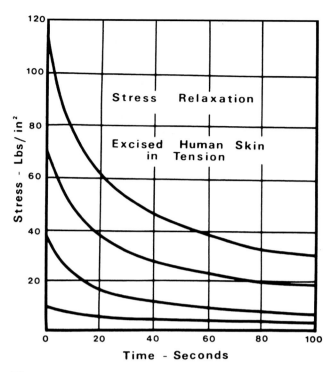

Figure 1.17 Langer lines on the leg. When the skin on the front of the thigh was cut along the cleavage lines, most of the fibers on the cut edge could be seen running parallel to the lines. When it was incised at right angles to the lines, most of the fibers had been cut transversely or obliquely. (With permission from Gibson T. Physical properties of skin. In: McCarthy JG, ed. Plastic Surgery. Vol. 1. General Principles. Philadelphia: W.B. Saunders Co., 1990:207–220).

Figure 1.18 Z-plasty technique. (With permission from McCarthy JG. Introduction to plastic surgery. In: McCarthy JG, ed. Plastic Surgery. Vol. 1. General Principles. Philadelphia: W.B. Saunders Co., 1990:1–68.)

resurface large areas of the body arises (Fig. 1.19). Further, experimentation has made it clear that this force can be applied, with the placement of silicone rubber expanders under normal skin, adjacent to the area to be resurfaced. This balloon can then be sequentially filled, initiating the growth of normal skin, ultimately allowing the excision of the abnormal or scarred tissue and advancement of normal skin over the area.

Though Dr. Charles Neumann has been credited with first the use of a latex balloon to expand the skin in a ear reconstruction in 1956, the major developments and scientific investigation came some 20 years later with the work of Dr. Chedomir Radovan and Dr. Eric Austad in the 1970s. Radovan (personal communication) developed the closed system silicone balloon expander, and Austad (39) was credited with the development of an osmotically driven, self-inflating expander. Along with these two innovators, Dr. Gordon Sasaki and Dr. Argenta can also be credited with early work leading to the widespread use of this technology in the reconstructive arena (Fig. 1.20). The clinical details of tissue expansion are discussed elsewhere in this text, but it is important to note the physical

changes to tissue-expanded skin that make this procedure possible.

In the epidermis, a quantitative increase in thickness occurs over the typical expansion period of 6–12 weeks. This is the result of division of the resident keratinocytes. Histologically, the increase in thickness is in the stratum spinosum, and notably, a significant flattening of the rete pegs occurs. These changes have been shown to regress over the next several years. Dermal changes tend to occur most prominently in the reticular portion, and include an overall thinning which persists for several years following expansion, a thickening of the collagen bundles with a predictable more parallel arrangement, and fragmentation of the elastin which tends not to present as striae. The number and distribution of resident cells like fibroblasts, mast cells, and macrophages do not appreciably change, though presumably the activity of the fibroblasts is altered during the expansion phase. The dermal appendages like hair follicles, sebaceous and eccrine glands do not increase in number and have been shown to atrophy, depending on the aggressiveness of the expansion. Though tissue expansion has been used with great effectiveness in addressing scalp alopecia as with type I and some type IIs as in the scale proposed by McCauley (39a), the failure of the hair follicles to

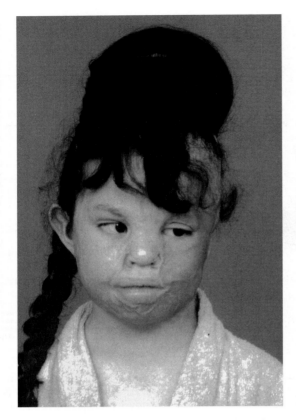

Figure 1.19 Burn child undergoing scalp expansion for coverage of burn alopecia. (Courtesy R. L. McCauley, MD, Shriners Hospitals for Children, Galveston, TX.)

divide, explains its limited usefulness in large and/or patchy hair loss as with some type II and type III alopecia. With large losses, the hair becomes noticeably thinner with an increased interfollicular distance. Vascularity has been shown to transiently increase, and the neural network shows few changes with expansion.

Finally, over the past decade, extensive work has been paid to the issue of tissue expansion and the use of postoperative radiation in patients with breast cancer. A significantly higher rate of complications like capsular contracture and implant exposure, have been identified, and tissue expansion, if not contraindicated, has classically been discouraged (40,41). The histological explanations have revolved around the irreversible dermal injury, which occurs with subsequent fibrosis, though the histological explanation has remained unexplained.

23. Scar

Normally, after skin is injured, it goes through a series of phases, namely the inflammatory, proliferative, and remodeling. Early in the inflammatory phase, platelets and leukocytes release a host of inflammatory mediators like

TGFβ, FGF, PDGF, which act to allow for hemostasis, and chemotaxis. As the inflammatory phase gives way to the proliferative phase, these and other growth factors stimulate keratinocytes and fibroblasts to divide and migrate into the wound leading to angiogenesis, epithelialization, contraction, and collagen production. In the remodeling phase, as the name suggests, components of the healing wound like fibronectin, proteoglycans, and collagen are converted from a disorganized array to a stable healed wound or scar through interactions with matrix metalloproteinase (MMPs) (42) and tissue inhibitor metalloproteinase (TIMPs) (43).

The final outcome of this process, the scar or cicatrix, is defined in medical dictionaries as a mark left over after the healing of a wound. Interestingly, this phenomenon does not occur in early fetal life (44,45), but begins at about the fifth month of gestation. The fact that it exists after this point suggests that it provides a survival advantage, and although even at its strongest, it only provides ~80% of the strength of normal skin, scarring allows us to heal wounds quickly, thereby allowing us to re-establish a protective, occlusive, and sturdy barrier (46). Just as wounds heal by epithelization and contraction, once closed, the resulting scar goes through phases of maturation.

As can be observed in many clinical scenarios, scarring begins with an immature phase (Fig. 1.21). Commonly these scars are red and raised. As the scar matures, it softens, flattens, and takes on a color closer to the surrounding skin. The length of time that this takes is variable, but most authorities agree that scars mature over a 1- to 2-year period.

A number of attempts to classify this progression have been made, most notably the Vancouver Scar Scale. It relies on a subjective rating, where an observer assigns points based on the size, shape, texture, and pliability of the scar over time. The reliability and validity of such a system have been questioned and attempts to create a more objective evaluation continue (47,48).

Scar maturation may be altered by aging, genetic predisposition, or environmental circumstances, and can also result in abnormal outcomes like keloid, hypertrophic (49), widened, atrophic, or contracted scars. The mechanisms of both normal and abnormal wound healing, as well as the best way to treat scarring as a phenomenon, is under intense investigation.

Hypertrophic and keloid scars represent good examples of abnormal scarring. Hypertrophic scars tend to remain within the boundaries of the original injury, and often begin to regress spontaneously after about a year post-injury. They are red, raised, inflamed, and often display symptoms of itching and pain. They are often located around joints after burn injury and can lead to scar contractures. A cytokine based etiology for this condition

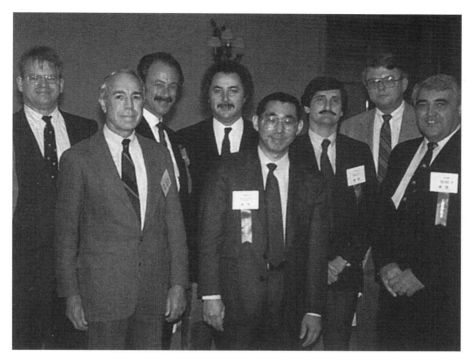

Figure 1.20 The 5th National Tissue Expansion Symposium, under the auspices of the Plastic Surgery Educational Foundation, was held at the Century Plaza Hotel in Century City, CA, in 1989. Left to right: Drs. Ernest Manders, Armand Versaci, Alan Gold, Hilton Becker, the author, Jacic Fisher, Eric Austad, and John Gibney. (With permission from Sasaki GH. History and evolution of tissue expansion. In: Tissue Expansion in Reconstructive and Aesthetic Surgery. Mosby, 1998:2–7.)

has been suggested by *in vivo* experiments showing alterations in the type I:III collagen ratios, elevated serum TGFβ1 levels, as well as *in vitro* experiments showing alterations in MMP/TIMP ratios (50,51). Keloids may also be inflamed raised areas displaying similar itchy, painful symptoms, but they differ in that they extend beyond the boundaries of the original injury and do not regress. Though no etiology has been clearly elucidated, alterations in keloid fibroblast TGFβ1 sensitivity (52), and alterations in cytokines like IL-6 have been shown *in vitro* (53). Ultimately, both lead to an abnormal abundance of collagen, resulting in skin with thickened, inelastic properties.

24. Special Cases

There are multiple factors that can affect the properties of "normal" skin. These may include extrinsic factors like sun exposure along with intrinsic factors like aging. Though these processes occur simultaneously in any one individual, they are not the same. The dark, thickened, leathery, skin on the face of the aging sun worshiper is very different from the lighter less wrinkled skin on the bathing suite covered areas. Further, scarred skin appears very different from normal skin whether it is "normal," hypertrophied, or keloid. Neither does it function the

same as is exemplified by the need for scar releases so often required around the contracted joints of the burn patient.

25. Photodamage

Classically, the UV-B wavelengths (290–320 nm) have been blamed for the majority of the injury (54,55), but more recent work has also implicated UV-A (320–400 nm) (56,57). The term solar elastosis has been used to describe this thickened, nodular, darkened skin. The changes include a thickening of the epidermis with increased atypia and loss of keratinocyte polarity, an increased density of melanocytes, and thickening/hyperplasia of the elastic fibers. This accumulation of elastin along with collagens I and III, microfibullar proteins, and fibronectin eventually degrades leaving a basophilic, amorphous layer in the papillary dermis (58). Interestingly, and unlike elastin, collagen production is decreased in sun-damaged skin. Specifically, types I and III, the predominant form in skin, are decreased from 20% to 30% in the papillary dermis (59). Collagen cross-linking has been shown to be decreased (60), and there is an increase in metaloprotease activity (61–63). Finally, chronic inflammation (64) occurs, and all of these together lead to a total loss of visoelastic flexibility of the skin.

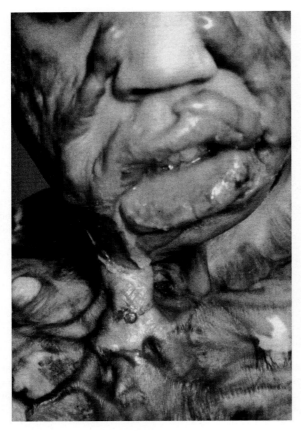

Figure 1.21 A young child with untreated immature burns with neck contractures and immature hypertrophic scars. (Courtesy of R. L. McCauley, Shriners Hospitals for Children, Galveston, TX.)

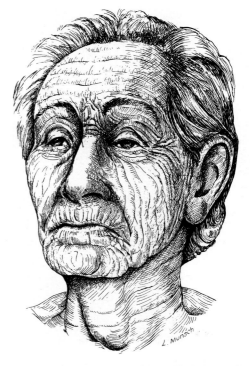

Figure 1.22 The lines of minimal tension of the face and neck. (With permission from McCarthy JG. Introduction to plastic surgery. In: McCarthy JG, ed. Plastic Surgery. Vol. 1. General Principles. Philadelphia: W.B. Saunders Co., 1990:1–68.)

26. Intrinsic Aging

Any intern who has been called to the bedside of an elderly patient and asked to place an IV, has personal experience with the clinical changes that occur in the skin as we age (Fig. 1.22). It usually appears thin with a mottled appearance. It is loose and has poor elasticity. It often feels dry with a decreased hair density, and once injured, it takes longer to heal than young skin. These phenomena are explained by the significant alterations in both the epidermis and the dermis.

Thinning of the epidermis has been described, but is more related to a flattening of the rete pegs. For the most part there is little alteration in the stratum corneum, spinus, or granular layers. The basal layer is altered in that there is a loss of the convoluted interface between the epidermis and dermis caused by a decrease in microvillar projections between the epidermal basal cells and the dermis (65). This flattening leads to an overall decrease in the shared dermal–epidermal surface area (66), and with the decrease in the villous cytoplasmic projections, which help to sustain the dermal–epidermal adherence,

an increased risk of shearing and overall skin fragility develops. There is a 6–8% decrease in the number of melanocytes in each decade after 30 (67), leading to the mottling alluded to earlier, and Gilchrest also showed a decrease in the number of Langerhans cells in aged skin affecting the immune response.

Notable dermal changes also occur. There is a decrease in total density, collagen content, ground substance, and vascularity. The overall number of fibroblasts decreases and the elastin degrades over time leading to the thinning, laxity, and fine wrinkling characterizing aged skin (22). Further, fibroblasts have a limited ability to divide (50–100 population doublings in culture). This correlates to their activity *in vivo* and as skin ages, fibroblasts become senescent and their ability to respond to injury decreases. Their synthetic capacity decreases, and thus, there is a decreased ability to respond to injury with procollagen production (68). They overexpress collagenases (69), and underexpress TIMPs (70). Ground substance molecules like dermatan sulfate and hyaluronic acid also decrease leading to a loss of hydration. The number of skin appendages changes with a loss of eccrine sweat glands, but there is an increase in the size and number of sebaceous glands (although there is a decrease in their activity). Finally, hair follicles decrease in number, size, and activity leading to fewer, thinner less pigmented hairs.

REFERENCES

1. Gandarillas A. Epidermal differentiation, apoptosis, and senescence: common pathways? Exp Gerontol 2000; 35:53–62.
2. Weisfelner ME, Gottlieb AB. The role of apoptosis in human epidermal keratinocytes. J Drugs Dermatol 2003; 2:385–391.
3. Sayama K, Hanakawa Y, Shirakata Y, Yamasaki K, Sawada Y, Sun L, Yamanishi K, Ichijo H, Hashimoto K. Apoptosis signal-regulating kinase 1 (ASK1) is an intracellular inducer of keratinocyte differentiation. J Biol Chem 2001; 276:999–1004.
4. Jones PH. Isolation and characterization of human epidermal stem cells. Clin Sci (Lond.) 1996; 91:141–146.
5. Halaban R, Funasaka Y, Lee P, Rubin J, Ron D, Birnbaum D. Fibroblast growth factors in normal and malignant melanocytes. Ann N Y Acad Sci 1991; 638:232–243.
6. Abdel-Malek Z, Swope VB, Suzuki I, Akcali C, Harriger MD, Boyce ST, Urabe K, Hearing VJ. Mitogenic and melanogenic stimulation of normal human melanocytes by melanotropic peptides. Proc Natl Acad Sci USA 1995; 92:1789–1793.
7. Cumberbatch M, Dearman RJ, Kimber I. Langerhans cells require signals from both tumour necrosis factor alpha and interleukin 1 beta for migration. Adv Exp Med Biol 1997; 417:125–128.
8. Uchi H, Imayama S, Kobayashi Y, Furue M. Langerhans cells express matrix metalloproteinase-9 in the human epidermis. J Invest Dermatol 1998; 111:1232–1233.
9. Rowden G, Lewis MG, Sullivan AK. Ia antigen expression on human epidermal Langerhans cells. Nature 1977; 268:247–248.
10. Ogawa H. The Merkel cell as a possible mechanoreceptor cell. Prog Neurobiol 1996; 49:317–334.
11. Moll I, Moll R, Franke WW. Formation of epidermal and dermal Merkel cells during human fetal skin development. J Invest Dermatol 1986; 87:779–787.
12. Narisawa Y, Hashimoto K, Kohda H. Merkel cells participate in the induction and alignment of epidermal ends of arrector pili muscles of human fetal skin. Br J Dermatol 1996; 134:494–498.
13. Kim DK, Holbrook KA. The appearance, density, and distribution of Merkel cells in human embryonic and fetal skin: their relation to sweat gland and hair follicle development. J Invest Dermatol 1995; 104:411–416.
14. Kadler KE, Holmes DF, Trotter JA, Chapman JA. Collagen fibril formation. Biochem J 1996; 316(Pt 1):1–11.
15. Klinge U, Si ZY, Zheng H, Schumpelick V, Bhardwaj RS, Klosterhalfen B. Abnormal collagen I to III distribution in the skin of patients with incisional hernia. Eur Surg Res 2000; 32:43–48.
16. Phan TT, Lim IJ, Bay BH, Qi R, Huynh HT, Lee ST, Longaker MT. Differences in collagen production between normal and keloid-derived fibroblasts in serum-media co-culture with keloid-derived keratinocytes. J Dermatol Sci 2002; 29:26–34.
17. Sakai LY, Keene DR, Engvall E. Fibrillin, a new 350-kD glycoprotein, is a component of extracellular microfibrils. J Cell Biol 1986; 103:2499–2509.
18. Sakai LY, Keene DR, Morris NP, Burgeson RE. Type VII collagen is a major structural component of anchoring fibrils. J Cell Biol 1986; 103:1577–1586.
19. Ushiki T. Collagen fibers, reticular fibers and elastic fibers. A comprehensive understanding from a morphological viewpoint. Arch Histol Cytol 2002; 65:109–126.
20. Uitto J. Understanding premature skin aging. N Engl J Med 1997; 337:1463–1465.
21. Pope FM, Burrows NP. Ehlers–Danlos syndrome has varied molecular mechanisms. J Med Genet 1997; 34:400–410.
22. Montagna W, Carlisle K. Structural changes in aging human skin. J Invest Dermatol 1979; 73:47–53.
23. Desmouliere A, Geinoz A, Gabbiani F, Gabbiani G. Transforming growth factor-β 1 induces α-smooth muscle actin expression in granulation tissue myofibroblasts and in quiescent and growing cultured fibroblasts. J Cell Biol 1993; 122:103–111.
24. Pittet B, Rubbia-Brandt L, Desmouliere A, Sappino AP, Roggero P, Guerret S, Grimaud JA, Lacher R, Montandon D, Gabbiani G. Effect of γ-interferon on the clinical and biologic evolution of hypertrophic scars and Dupuytren's disease: an open pilot study. Plast Reconstr Surg 1994; 93:1224–1235.
25. Thody AJ, Shuster S. Control and function of sebaceous glands. Physiol Rev 1989; 69:383–416.
26. Jahoda CA, Oliver RF, Reynolds AJ, Forrester JC, Gillespie JW, Cserhalmi-Friedman PB, Christiano AM, Horne KA. Trans-species hair growth induction by human hair follicle dermal papillae. Exp Dermatol 2001; 10:229–237.
27. Stenn KS, Lawrence L, Veis D, Korsmeyer S, Seiberg M. Expression of the bcl-2 protooncogene in the cycling adult mouse hair follicle. J Invest Dermatol 1994; 103:107–111.
28. Takakura N, Yoshida H, Kunisada T, Nishikawa S, Nishikawa SI. Involvement of platelet-derived growth factor receptor-α in hair canal formation. J Invest Dermatol 1996; 107:770–777.
29. Blessing M, Nanney LB, King LE, Jones CM, Hogan BL. Transgenic mice as a model to study the role of TGF-β-related molecules in hair follicles. Genes Dev 1993; 7:204–215.
30. Stenn KS, Eilertsen K. Molecular basis of hair growth control. J Invest Dermatol 1996; 107:669–670.
31. Gerlach H, Esposito C, Stern DM. Modulation of endothelial hemostatic properties: an active role in the host response. Annu Rev Med 1990; 41:15–24.
32. Winn R, Vedder N, Ramamoorthy C, Sharar S, Harlan J. Endothelial and leukocyte adhesion molecules in inflammation and disease. Blood Coagul Fibrinolysis 1998; 9(suppl 2):S17–S23.
33. Salas A, Shimaoka M, Chen S, Carman CV, Springer T. Transition from rolling to firm adhesion is regulated by the conformation of the I domain of the integrin lymphocyte function-associated antigen-1. J Biol Chem 2002; 277:50255–50262.
34. Taylor GI, Palmer JH. The vascular territories (angiosomes) of the body: experimental study and clinical applications. Br J Plast Surg 1987; 40:113–141.
35. Risau W. Mechanisms of angiogenesis. Nature 1997; 386:671–674.
36. Cauna N. Fine morphological characteristics and microtopography of the free nerve endings of the human digital skin. Anat Rec 1980; 198:643–656.

37. Lynn B. Cutaneous sensation. In: Goldsmith LA, ed. Physiology, Biochemistry, and Molecular Biology of the Skin. New York: Oxford University Press, 1991:779–815.

38. Machida BK, Liu-Shindo M, Sasaki GH, Rice DH, Chandrasoma P. Immediate versus chronic tissue expansion. Ann Plast Surg 1991; 26:227–232.

39. Austad ED, Rose GL. A self-inflating tissue expander. Plast Reconstr Surg 1982; 70:588–594.

39a. McCauley RL, Oliphant JR, Robson MC. Tissue expansion in the correction of burn alopecia: classification and methods of correction. Ann Plast Surg 1990; 25:103–115.

40. Spear SL, Onyewu C. Staged breast reconstruction with saline-filled implants in the irradiated breast: recent trends and therapeutic implications. Plast Reconstr Surg 2000; 105:930–942.

41. Evans GR, Schusterman MA, Kroll SS, Miller MJ, Reece GP, Robb GL, Ainslie N. Reconstruction and the radiated breast: is there a role for implants? Plast Reconstr Surg 1995; 96:1111–1115; discussion, 1116–1118.

42. Ravanti L, Kahari VM. Matrix metalloproteinases in wound repair (review). Int J Mol Med 2000; 6:391–407.

43. Reynolds JJ. Collagenases and tissue inhibitors of metalloproteinases: a functional balance in tissue degradation. Oral Dis 1996; 2:70–76.

44. Dang C, Ting K, Soo C, Longaker MT, Lorenz HP. Fetal wound healing current perspectives. Clin Plast Surg 2003; 30:13–23.

45. Ferguson MW, Whitby DJ, Shah M, Armstrong J, Siebert JW, Longaker MT. Scar formation: the spectral nature of fetal and adult wound repair. Plast Reconstr Surg 1996; 97:854–860.

46. Bayat A, McGrouther DA, Ferguson MW. Skin scarring. Br Med J 2003; 326:88–92.

47. Nedelec B, Shankowsky HA, Tredget EE. Rating the resolving hypertrophic scar: comparison of the Vancouver Scar Scale and scar volume. J Burn Care Rehabil 2000; 21:205–212.

48. Powers PS, Sarkar S, Goldgof DB, Cruse CW, Tsap LV. Scar assessment: current problems and future solutions. J Burn Care Rehabil 1999; 20:54–60.

49. Niessen FB, Spauwen PH, Schalkwijk J, Kon M. On the nature of hypertrophic scars and keloids: a review. Plast Reconstr Surg 1999; 104:1435–1458.

50. Tredget EE, Shankowsky HA, Pannu R, Nedelec B, Iwashina T, Ghahary A, Taerum TV, Scott PG. Transforming growth factor-β in thermally injured patients with hypertrophic scars: effects of interferon α-2b. Plast Reconstr Surg 1998; 102:1317–1330.

51. Tredget EE, Nedelec B, Scott PG, Ghahary A. Hypertrophic scars, keloids, and contractures. The cellular and molecular basis for therapy. Surg Clin North Am 1997; 77:701–730.

52. Bettinger DA, Yager DR, Diegelmann RF, Cohen IK. The effect of TGF-β on keloid fibroblast proliferation and collagen synthesis. Plast Reconstr Surg 1996; 98:827–833.

53. Xue H, McCauley RL, Zhang W. Elevated interleukin-6 expression in keloid fibroblasts. J Surg Res 2000; 89:74–77.

54. Ley RD, Sedita A, Grube DD, Fry RJ. Induction and persistence of pyrimidine dimers in the epidermal DNA of two strains of hairless mice. Cancer Res 1977; 37:3243–3248.

55. Ananthaswamy HN, Loughlin SM, Cox P, Evans RL, Ullrich SE, Kripke ML. Sunlight and skin cancer: inhibition of p53 mutations in UV-irradiated mouse skin by sunscreens. Nat Med 1997; 3:510–514.

56. Cavarra E, Fimiani M, Lungarella G, Andreassi L, de Santi M, Mazzatenta C, Ciccoli L. UVA light stimulates the production of cathepsin G and elastase-like enzymes by dermal fibroblasts: a possible contribution to the remodeling of elastotic areas in sun-damaged skin. Biol Chem 2002; 383:199–206.

57. Erden Inal M, Kahraman A, Koken T. Beneficial effects of quercetin on oxidative stress induced by ultraviolet A. Clin Exp Dermatol 2001; 26:536–539.

58. Chen VL, Fleischmajer R, Schwartz E, Palaia M, Timpl R. Immunochemistry of elastotic material in sun-damaged skin. J Invest Dermatol 1986; 87:334–337.

59. Bernstein EF, Chen YQ, Kopp JB, Fisher L, Brown DB, Hahn PJ, Robey FA, Lakkakorpi J, Uitto J. Long-term sun exposure alters the collagen of the papillary dermis. Comparison of sun-protected and photoaged skin by northern analysis, immunohistochemical staining, and confocal laser scanning microscopy. J Am Acad Dermatol 1996; 34:209–218.

60. Yamauchi M, Prisayanh P, Haque Z, Woodley DT. Collagen cross-linking in sun-exposed and unexposed sites of aged human skin. J Invest Dermatol 1991; 97:938–941.

61. Fisher GJ, Choi HC, Bata-Csorgo Z, Shao Y, Datta S, Wang ZQ, Kang S, Voorhees JJ. Ultraviolet irradiation increases matrix metalloproteinase-8 protein in human skin *in vivo*. J Invest Dermatol 2001; 117:219–226.

62. Fisher GJ, Wang ZQ, Datta SC, Varani J, Kang S, Voorhees JJ. Pathophysiology of premature skin aging induced by ultraviolet light. N Engl J Med 1997; 337:1419–1428.

63. Varani J, Spearman D, Perone P, Fligiel SE, Datta SC, Wang ZQ, Shao Y, Kang S, Fisher GJ, Voorhees JJ. Inhibition of type I procollagen synthesis by damaged collagen in photoaged skin and by collagenase-degraded collagen *in vitro*. Am J Pathol 2001; 158:931–942.

64. Kligman AM, Baker TJ, Gordon HL. Long-term histologic follow-up of phenol face peels. Plast Reconstr Surg 1985; 75:652–659.

65. Lavker RM. Structural alterations in exposed and unexposed aged skin. J Invest Dermatol 1979; 73:59–66.

66. Katzberg A. The area of the dermo-epidermal junction in human skin. Anat Rec 1958; 131:717–723.

67. Gilchrest BA, Blog FB, Szabo G. Effects of aging and chronic sun exposure on melanocytes in human skin. J Invest Dermatol 1979; 73:141–143.

68. Furth JJ. The steady-state levels of type I collagen mRNA are reduced in senescent fibroblasts. J Gerontol 1991; 46:B122–B124.

69. West MD, Pereira-Smith OM, Smith JR. Replicative senescence of human skin fibroblasts correlates with a loss of regulation and overexpression of collagenase activity. Exp Cell Res 1989; 184:138–147.

70. Millis AJ, Hoyle M, McCue HM, Martini H. Differential expression of metalloproteinase and tissue inhibitor of metalloproteinase genes in aged human fibroblasts. Exp Cell Res 1992; 201:373–379.

2

Wound Healing

MICHAEL K. OBENG, LINDA G. PHILLIPS

University of Texas Medical Branch, Galveston, Texas, USA

I. INTRODUCTION

Plastic and reconstructive surgeons are expected to heal wounds with minimal or no scarring. However, burn wounds and wounds that are created in burned areas of the skin possess a heightened challenge to even the most astute reconstructive surgeon. The ultimate goal is to get these specialized wounds to heal in a timely fashion with very little scarring, good cosmesis, and most importantly excellent functional outcome. To achieve these goals, we need to understand how these wounds heal and what we can do to optimize this process. In this modern era of molecular biologic technique, these wounds can be manipulated to some extent with good clinical outcome. The last two decades have witnessed more advances in the art of wound care than what was available 100 years ago (1–3). The goals of this chapter are to briefly describe the pathophysiology of the burn wound, the reparative process of the wound, factors affecting wound healing, and cytokine manipulation of the wound.

II. PATHOPHYSIOLOGY OF THE BURN WOUND

Functional and cosmetic outcomes of the reconstructed burned skin depend in large part on how the initial burn wounds are managed. The acute burn wound that heals in <2 weeks presents with minimal scarring, possibly eliminating future reconstructive efforts.

The acute burn wound causes both local and systemic effects mediated by host responses that can sometimes be very devastating. Early excision and grafting of burn wounds can eliminate some of the systemic response and improve healing. The burn wound can be divided into three zones based on histological findings as proposed by Jackson (4) in the early 1950s (Fig. 2.1).

The part of the skin where the initial contact is made is known as the zone of coagulation (necrosis). This zone is characterized by tissue destruction and necrosis usually starting at the point of contact in the epidermis and extending downward into the dermis. This is created as a result of

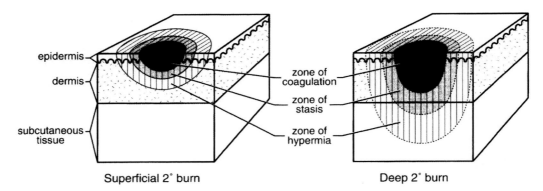

Figure 2.1   Diagrammatic rendition of Jackson's three zones of burn injury. Superficial 2° injury on left, deeper 2° injury on right. (In deep 2° burn note potential for conversion to full-thickness tissue loss if zone of stasis progresses to necrosis.) (With permission from Williams WG. Pathophysiology of the burn wound. In: Herndon DN, ed. Total Burn Care. 2nd ed. Philadelphia: W.B. Saunders Company, 2002:514–521.)

denaturing of proteins beyond repair caused by the high thermal energy (5). Protein denaturation with subsequent tissue necrosis depends mainly on the temperature to which tissues are exposed and the duration of contact. This phenomenon has been well proven by Moritz and Henriquez (5) in their classical paper in 1947.

Surrounding the zone of coagulation peripherally and extending into the dermis is the zone of stasis (ischemia). This is the zone of lesser injury. Initially the cells are viable, but can progress clinically to skin necrosis. This occurs because the circulation in this zone is significantly impaired (6). The decreased circulation results from events in the microvasculature in a well-concerted effort, orchestrated by platelets and its derived factors leading to vasoconstriction (7). In addition, thermally injured erythrocytes lose their ability to conform to the microvessels, with concomitant reduction in oxygen delivery (8). Blood flow impairment continues for up to 24 h with cessation in about 48 h after sustaining the burn injury (9). It is believed that under favorable conditions, stasis and ischemia may be reversed with cell recovery within a week (9). The cells in this zone are very susceptible to further insult during recovery (10). Infection, changes in pressure as in hypovolemia and overresuscitation, and even electrolyte abnormalities such as hypernatremia can cause further necrosis during the recovery phase (10). Robson and others have extensively studied the pathophysiology of this zone, and the ischemic effects of prostaglandin $F_{2\alpha}$ and thromboxane A_2 (6,8,11,12). Specific thromboxane inhibitors and more generalized inhibitors of prostanoids have been used experimentally with some success in improving dermal perfusion after thermal injury (9,11,12).

The zone of hyperemia surrounds the zone of stasis. There is increased vascular permeability secondary to pronounced vasodilation. Edema ensues from extravasation of fluid from the intravascular space to the interstitial

space. Sometimes this can be overwhelming, leading to hypovolemic shock. Cellular recovery in this zone can proceed to total recovery.

Edema in burn wounds can be more pronounced in comparison to other wounds. This produces harmful effects on nutrient and oxygen delivery, as well as causing significant decreases in intravascular volume (13–15). In addition, large quantities of protein leak through the burn-induced endothelial cell gap (16,17). Chemical mediators such as histamine, bradykinin, sensory neuropeptides, and oxygen-free radicals can cause some of the increases in vascular permeability due to their own vasodilatory effects (17–19). Prostanoids found in burn fluid may also account for some of the edema formation. Some studies have demonstrated that the inhibitors of prostaglandin production such as ibuprofen and indomethacin can be of use with some success to reduce edema formation (20–23). Other causes of edema include elevated capillary filtration pressures from impaired outflow in the venous system, secondary to sludging and agglutination of erythrocytes in the postcapillary venules (24). Serotonin mediated venular constriction also serve to elevate capillary filtration pressure and subsequent increased edema. Hydrostatic pressure reduction occurs in the interstitium in the early postburn period (25). There continues to be efflux of intravascular fluid, since the interstitial pressures are too low to counteract this effect. The time course for edema formation is very important. The formation of edema is rapid, occurring within the first 3 h after injury. A biphasic pattern explains this phenomenon with a transient phase lasting ~15 min followed by a sustained phase. The edema is maximized within 24 h postinjury and can persist for up to 3 days. The severity of the burn injury determines the extent to which and how rapidly the edema forms. Subsequently, the edema resolves, but slowly, depending on the physiologic condition of the wound and overall health status of

Healing Responses

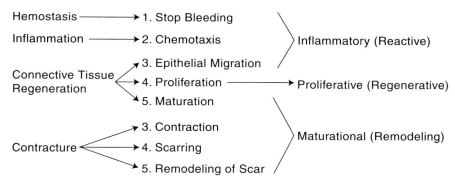

Figure 2.2 Schematic of wound healing continuum. [With permission from Phillips (26).]

the patient. The pathophysiology of the burn wound continues to be uncovered leading to better management of the acute phase of burn injury. It is only when this process is maximally controlled that early wound closure is possible. Subsequently, our reconstructive efforts may be more fruitful, yielding better cosmesis and function.

III. REPARATIVE PROCESS OF WOUNDS

Wound healing is a complex, dynamic, and interactive process that progresses in an orderly and predictable fashion, unless interrupted. This cascade involves soluble mediators, different cell types and elements, and the extracellular matrix (ECM). The healing cascade for wounds differs among different tissue types. In this discussion, we will focus on the broad spectrum of the wound healing process. This cascade involves three main phases: inflammatory (coagulation and inflammation), proliferative (cell proliferation and matrix repair), and remodeling of the scar tissue. These phases are a continuum and overlap, and can last up to several months (Fig. 2.2). For simplicity and clarity purposes, the phases of wound healing will be described in a linear fashion.

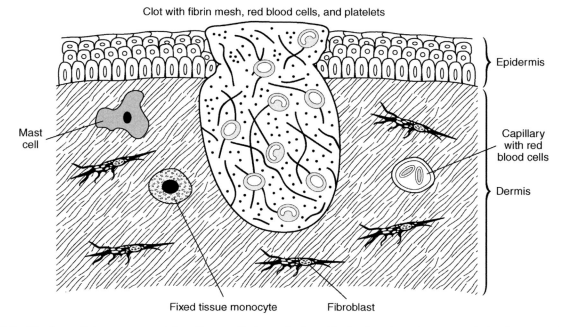

Figure 2.3 The immediate response to injury forms a fibrin mesh clot with platelets that release coagulation factors and cytokines, initiating healing. [With permission from Phillips (26).]

A.   Inflammatory Phase

The inflammatory phase of wound healing is the immediate response to the injury characterized and heralded by hemostasis and inflammation. John Hunter first described the characteristics of inflammation in 1794 (27). The four characteristics of inflammation are erythema (rubor), edema (tumor), heat (calor), and pain (dolor). The wound healing process cannot continue, until hemostasis is achieved. Clot, a conglomerate of fibrin mesh, aggregated platelets, and blood cells, signals the end of the hemostatic stage (Fig. 2.3) (28). The principal cell type during this phase is the platelet. The events leading to hemostasis include platelet aggregation, vasoconstriction, and deposition of fibrin from the clotting cascade (Fig. 2.4). Platelets initiate this phase of wound healing after the injury by releasing a number of soluble factors, including platelet derived growth factor (PDGF), insulin-like growth factor-1

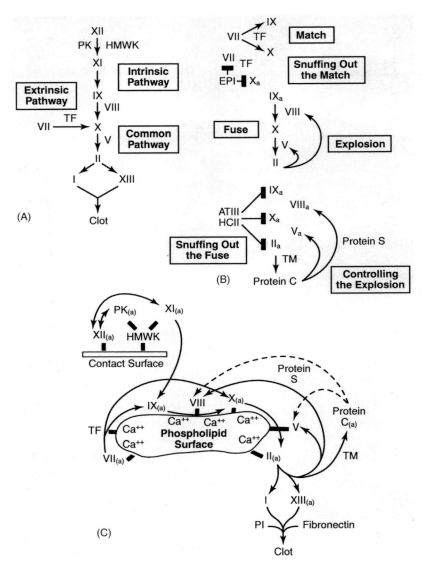

Figure 2.4   Diagrams of interactions among coagulation factors. (A) The intrinsic, extrinsic, and common pathways in their simplest forms. (B) Critical stages in activation and control of blood coagulation. (C) This diagram is organized around the contact surface and the phospholipids surface. Solid lines with arrows indicate proteolytic activation. Broken lines with arrows indicate proteolytic inactivation. Solid lines with bars indicate complex formation and inactivation. The stippled patches indicate binding of proteins to surfaces or to one another. The subscript a indicates proteins that are zymogens and can be converted to active enzymes. PK = prekallikrein; HMWK = high molecular weight kininogen; TF = tissue factors; PI = alpha$_2$-antiplasmin; TM = thrombommodulin; EPI = extrinsic pathway inhibitor; ATIII = antithrombin III; HCII = heparin cofactor II. (With permission from Mosher DF. Disorders of blood coagulation. In: Wyngaarden JB, Smith LH Jr, Bennett JC, eds. Cecil Textbook of Medicine. 19th ed. Philadelphia: W.B. Saunders Company, 1992:999–1017.)

(IGF-1), epidermal growth factor (EGF), fibroblast growth factor (FGF), and transforming growth factor-β (TGF-β).

1. Hemostasis

The hemostatic stage is the cornerstone of the inflammatory phase. Tissue injury causes damage to blood vessels, disrupting the lining of the vessels. Platelets bind to the exposed collagen types IV and V in the subendothelium and become activated in the process (26,29). The activated platelets in turn release a host of biologically active soluble factors from storage organelles: alpha granules, dense bodies, and lysosomes within their cytoplasm (Table 2.1) (30–32). The contents of the alpha granules are mainly immunoregulatory and procoagulation factors and participate in the early as well as the late phase of wound healing. The contents of the dense bodies are mainly energy providing factors, while that of the lysosomes are degradative enzymes. PDGF, TGF-β and FGF-2 are some of the most important factors.

As the subendothelium is exposed and the platelets become activated, both the intrinsic and the extrinsic pathways of the clotting cascade are initiated. While the extrinsic cascade is essential for normal wound healing, the intrinsic cascade is not required (33). The extrinsic pathway is initiated by exposure of blood and platelets to a factor in the subendothelium named "tissue factor" that binds factor VIII activating it to f-VIIIa. Factor XII activates the intrinsic pathway after exposure of blood and platelets to the subendothelial layer. Activated factors VII and XII, orchestrated by soluble factors derived from complex interactions result in the production of thrombin that serves as a catalyst for the formation of fibrin from fibrinogen (Fig. 2.4).

In addition to converting fibrinogen to fibrin, thrombin also stimulates increased vascular permeability and aids in the extravascular migration of inflammatory cells (34). The fibrin strands ensnare red cells, aggregated platelets, and other harmless debris to form a clot (28). The formed clot seals the wound preventing contamination from the outside environment as well as fluid and electrolyte losses. The lattice meshwork formed by fibrin and the trapped cells, becomes the scaffold for the key players of the wound-healing cascade. Vitronectin, derived from the alpha granules of platelets and serum, coats fibrin. This interaction produces "glue-like" material that binds fibronectins, produced by fibroblast and epithelial cells (35). The fibrin–vitronectin–fibronectin complex is also an important matrix framework, with over a dozen binding sites on the fibronectin molecule for cellular attachments and migration along the matrix (27). This matrix selectively traps circulating cytokines for use in the later stages of the cascade (36). Any process that interferes with fibrin formation disrupts the matrix scaffold and ultimately impairs wound healing (37–39).

2. Inflammation

The arachidonic acid cascade (Fig. 2.5) also plays a significant role in the inflammatory phase. Thromboxane A_2 (TXA$_2$) and prostaglandin (PG) F-2α (PGF-2α) aid in platelet aggregation and vasoconstriction (26). While the role of the products of the arachidonic acid cascade is to regulate the amount of injury, localized ischemia can ensue causing further damage to cell membranes and elaboration of the cascade with more release of PGF-2α and TXA$_2$.

The inflammation stage is characterized by increased vascular permeability and leukocyte migration mediated by chemoattractants into the extravascular space (26). The purpose is to deliver inflammatory cells to the injured site to kill bacteria and eliminate debris. These inflammatory cells include leukocytes, lymphocytes, and macrophages.

The signs of inflammation are evident shortly after the initial vasoconstrictive episode which reverses in 15 min (29). Vasodilatation occurs causing erythema and heat. The edema formation that follows, in large part, contributes to the sensation of tightness and pain. This edema formation is a result of gaps developing in the endothelial cells lining the capillaries in the area of insult with concomitant leakage of plasma and other factor into the extravascular space (17). The vasodilitory effect seen is mediated by a host of factors derived from plasma endothelial products and mast cells (40–42). These factors

Table 2.1 Released Factors from Platelets Storage Granules

I. Alpha 1 granules	II. Dense bodies
1. Platelet-derived growth factor (PDGF)	1. Vasoactive amines (serotonin)
2. Transforming growth factor-β (TGF-β)	2. Calcium
3. Insulin-like growth factor-1 (IGF-1)	3. ADP
4. Fibronectin	4. ATP
5. Fibrinogen	
6. Thrombospondin	III. Lysosomes
7. Von Willebrand's factor (vWF)	1. Hydrolase
8. Albumin	2. Protease
9. IgG	
10. Coagulation factors V and VIII	
11. Fibroblast growth factor-2 (FGF-2)	
12. Platelet-derived epidermal growth factor (EGFs)	
13. Endothelial cell growth factors	

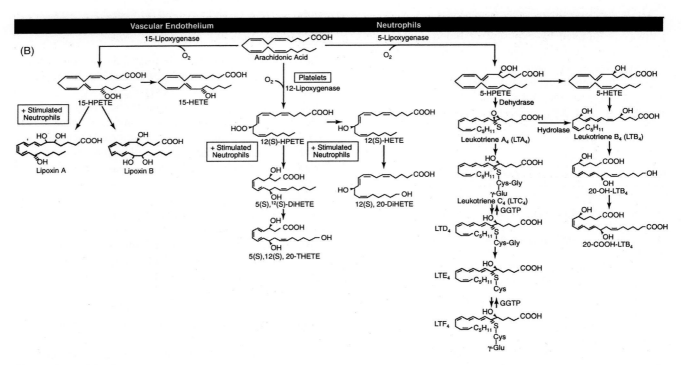

Figure 2.5 (A) Metabolism of arachidonic acid by cyclo-oxygenase. The major tissues of origin of the eicosanoids. (B) Metabolism of arachidonic acid by lipoxygenase enzymes. (With permission from FitzGerald GA. Prostaglandins and related compounds. In: Wyngaarden JB, Smith LH Jr, Bennett JC, eds. Cecil Textbook of Medicine. 19th ed. Philadelphia: W.B. Saunders Company, 1992:1206–1212.)

include, but are not limited to, leukotrienes (LT), PGs, histamine, serotonin, and kinins. Complement factors C3a and C5a, in addition to playing a major role in capillary leak, also serves as a chemoattractant for neutrophils and monocytes (26).

3. Leukocytes

Leukocytes are chemoattracted to the area of injury by a vast array of soluble factors. TGF-β, TNF-α, IL-1, PDGF, LTB4, platelet factor IV, complement factors C3a and C5a, collagen and elastin breakdown products, and bacterial products such as N-formyl-methionyl-leucyl-phenylalanine (FMLP) are among the chemoattractants responsible for leukocyte migration (26,43–46). Neutrophils begin diapedesis into the wounded area between endothelial cells when signaled by these chemotactic factors (Fig. 2.6). A process known as margination precedes diapedesis. This process is facilitated by integrins and intracellular adhesion molecule (ICAM) expressed on the surface of leukocytes and endothelial cells, respectively. Diapedesis is also hastened by the expression of CD11/CD18 on the surface of neutrophils whose expression is stimulated by platelet activating factor (PAF) and platelet factor IV (47).

Once in the wounded area, neutrophils scavenge bacteria, necrotic tissue, and foreign material. This is made possible because of surface receptors that allow neutrophils to identify, attach, engulf, and process or destroy any foreign material. Once debris and bacteria are phagocytosed, they are digested by hydrolytic enzymes and oxygen-free radicals are generated within the neutrophils. This oxidative burst can be both extracellular and intracellular and, if not regulated, it can be detrimental to the surrounding tissue. The activated neutrophils generate free-oxygen radicals via donated electrons from nicotinamide adenine dinucleotide (NADPH) (26). These electrons are transported into the lysosomes and aid in the formation of superoxide anion. Hydrogen peroxide (H_2O_2) can be formed by two superoxide anions, catalyzed by the enzyme superoxide dismutase (SOD). Myeloperoxidase, contained in the azurophilic granules of leukocyte, can degrade H_2O_2, generating by-products such as hypochlorous acid (HOCl) and hydroxyl radicals (26). These generated hydroxyl radicals are both bactericidal and toxic to the neutrophils themselves and the surrounding tissue.

Neutrophils also have the capability of killing bacteria with proteins such as Cathepsin-G that disrupts the outer lipopolysaccharide (LPS) membrane layer (26). Cathepsin-G is effective against both gram-positive and gram-negative organisms.

In light of how activated neutrophils can be destructive to the surrounding tissue, early intervention to debride a wound and rid it of debris and bacteria is paramount. Once the neutrophils are done with their work, they become senescent and undergo programmed cell death (48). The trapped neutrophils in the clots slough off (49). Neutrophils are the first among the inflammatory cells to undergo apoptosis, and it is characterized by the activation

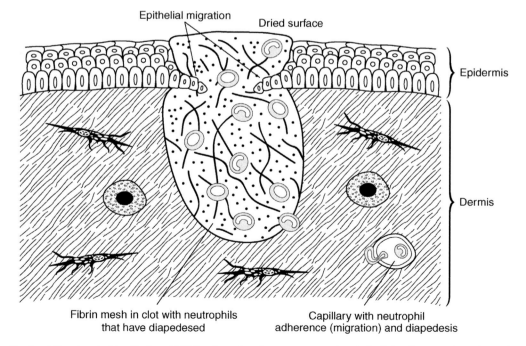

Epithelial migration Dried surface

Epidermis

Dermis

Fibrin mesh in clot with neutrophils
that have diapedesed

Capillary with neutrophil
adherence (migration) and diapedesis

Figure 2.6 Neutrophils, signaled by IL-1 and TNF-α from local monocytes and endothelial cells, marginate in capillaries and diapedeses. They enter the fibrin clot as do the endothelial cells from the wound edges. [With permission from Phillips (26).]

of endogenous endonucleases that are calcium dependent (29). Once these proteases are activated, the nuclear chromatin cleaves into oligonucleosome DNA fragments indicating irreversible cell death.

Basophils and eosinophils do not play a specific role in the wound healing cascade. Their role in the inflammation phase is yet to be unraveled but, if they are allowed to accumulate, host tissue damage is inevitable as evidenced by eosinophil-mediated systemic necrotizing vasculitis (50). Within 48 h after injury, these cells are at their peak concentrations with the ability to produce TGF-α (51). Like neutrophils, the ones caught in clots die (49).

4. *Macrophage*

The macrophage is the single most important cell in the wound-healing cascade. It serves as the principal orchestrator, coordinating the different cell types and cytokines in the various stages of wound healing (Fig. 2.7). Macrophages are derived from circulating monocytes. As monocytes enter the extravascular space they become macrophages. This transformation is stimulated by many factors including elastin derived from damaged matrix, enzymatically active thrombin, fibronectin, TGF-β, complement factors C3a and C5a, IL-2, and IFN-γ derived from T-lymphocytes (37,52). Before performing their respective duties in the wound, all leukocytes require activation.

Activated macrophages continue the work of the neutrophils, phagocytosing necrotic debris and bacteria (53). Like neutrophils, macrophages have binding receptors including the CD11b/CD18 $\alpha\beta$-integrins and the immunoglobulin-type adhesion molecule CD14 that binds LPS (47,54).

Once the bacteria and foreign material are bound and engulfed, they are digested by hydrolytic enzymes and oxygen radicals in the cytoplasm of the macrophage. There is an increased release of free radicals in the presence of IL-2 as well as increased bactericidal activity (26). Macrophages can cause digestion of debris extracellularly by the release of matrix metalloproteinases (MMPs) in the wound when activated by bacterial degradation by-products such as LPS or activated lymphocytes dependent on the cyclic-AMP pathway (55). Nonsteroidal anti-inflammatory drugs (NSAIDs) or glucocorticoids can block this process (56). Activated macrophages also induce phospholipase with resultant degradation of the cell membrane phospholipids (57). The release of TXA$_2$, PGF$_{2\alpha}$, leukotrienes B$_4$ and C$_4$ (LTB$_4$ and LTC$_4$), 5-HETE, and 15-HETE potentially causes further damage (57). LTB$_4$ induces suppressor cells and inhibits peripheral lymphocyte proliferation and mixed lymphocyte response.

One of the attributes that make macrophages critically important is their ability to generate cytokines that play a key role downstream in the wound-healing cascade. Without macrophages, wound healing is delayed secondary to ineffective debridement and decreased proliferation of fibroblast and endothelial cells (58). While early removal of neutrophils from the wound can limit the amount of damage and increase the rate of wound infections, removal of macrophages will compromise the healing process (59).

The cytokines generated by activated macrophages play an instrumental role in angiogenesis, fibroblast

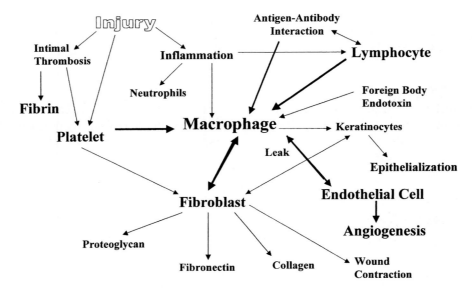

Figure 2.7 Cell interactions. Acute wound healing is dependent on a complex interplay of various inflammatory markers and cell types. Macrophages are crucial to the various phases of acute wound healing and serve as a central stimulator for several different cell types involved in wound healing. [With permission from Monaco and Lawrence (29).]

activation and proliferation, and collagen production and maturation (59). The many different cytokines produced by macrophages include IL-1, TGF-α, TGF-β, IGF-1, FGF-2, TNF-α, PDGF and nitric oxide (59–61).

5. Lymphocytes

Lymphocytes play a critical role in heavily contaminated wounds, and their removal from the wound, especially T-lymphocytes, impedes the wound-healing process (51). T-lymphocytes account for 70–80% of the circulating lymphocytes, while B-lymphocytes make up the remaining percentage (50). Within 5–7 days postinjury, CD4-positive and CD8-positive T-lymphocytes are present in large numbers, under the direction of IL-2 and other cytokines (50,62). After the macrophage binds, engulfs, debrides, and processes bacteria and foreign material, it presents it to the lymphocytes. The lymphocyte in turn proliferates and releases cytokines. IL-1, IL-2, TNF-α, fibroblast activating factor, EGF, TGF-β, IFN-γ are among the cytokines produced by T-lymphocytes (63–66). These cytokines modulate T-cell proliferation and differentiation in an autocrine fashion.

T-cells can further mature into killer cells with the ability to destroy foreign cells and cells infected with viruses (51). The number of lymphocytes remain low until a harmful stimulant or further inflammation occurs.

6. Cytokines

Virtually every cell involved in wound-healing produces cytokines. The more important sources of cytokine production include macrophages, platelets, neutrophils, endothelial cells, and fibroblasts. These cytokines as mentioned previously are produced in an orderly fashion, and they regulate activation of genes that control cellular activation, migration, proliferation, and synthetic activity.

Cytokine production may be autocrine or paracrine in nature, and may also be dictated by the milieu of the wound, such as hypoxia (28,64,66,67). Tissue hypoxia has been shown to fuel macrophages, endothelial cells, and fibroblasts to produce and release TNF-α, TGF-β, VEGF, and IL-8 (64,66,67). The reasons why cytokines work in such concerted efforts is the fact that different cell types have receptors for the same cytokine and vice versa. This duplication inherent to wound healing allows one cytokine to stimulate as many cells as possible either at the same time or at different times. Also, one particular cytokine can stimulate different cellular functions of the same cell. Multiple cytokines can stimulate the same function of one cell, making this process highly interdigitated. For most of these properties, the concentration of the cytokine dictates the cytokine function. For instance, at low concentrations, PDGF chemoattracts fibroblasts and stimulates fibroblast proliferation at 100-

fold greater concentration (68,69). Similarly, TGF-β chemoattracts macrophages in the fentomolar range, and stimulates fibroblasts to produce collagen in the nanomolar range (29). Some cytokines work synergistically, while others work in an antagonistic manner.

TGF-β regulates its own production by macrophages in an autocrine fashion. It stimulates the secretion of PDGF, FGF-2, TNF-α, and IL-1 by macrophages by binding the EGF receptors (43). TGF-β is the most powerful stimulant of fibroplasia and it is released by activated monocytes. It can stimulate monocytes to express TGF-α, IL-1, and PDGF (26). It also serves as a chemotactic factor for monocytes. At increased concentration, it stimulates fibroblast to produce collagen and fibronectin (26,70). TGF-α is released by activated monocytes and it stimulates epidermal growth and angiogenesis (26,29). Nitric oxide is released by macrophages. Its role in wound healing is not completely understood, but may play a role as an antimicrobial agent, and its inhibition has been shown to hamper wound healing in a mouse model (59,71).

IL-1 is a macrophage-derived endogenous acute-phase pyrogen. It activates lymphocytes and stimulates the hypothalamus to induce the febrile response. It also affects hemostasis by stimulating platelet activating factor (PAF) and causing the release of vasodilators (29). In the presence of endotoxin and TNF, endothelial cells produce IL-1. It also stimulates cartilage degradation and bone resorption, and augments collagenase production (28). IL-2 is also synthesized by T-cells; it promotes IFN-γ synthesis. It also has antimicrobial activity (26,29).

Produced by T-cell, IFN-γ stimulates monocytes to release TNF-α and IL-1, before destroying the monocyte. It has also been shown to decrease the synthesis of prostaglandins. It inhibits monocyte migration, thereby keeping the cells at the site of injury. It aids in the synthesis of glycosaminoglycans (GAGs) and suppresses the synthesis of collagen (26,31). These functions set up the hypothesis of IFN-γ being an important mediator of chronic wounds (72).

TNF-α (cachectin) is released by macrophages after induction by microbial by-products. It also induces fever. It serves to amplify the effects of IL-1 by working synergistically with it. Like IL-1, it increases bone and cartilage resorption, and increased procoagulant activity (29). It can also cause the release of PDGF and IL-1 (73).

IL-6 induces T-cell proliferation, fever, and other acute phase protein. It works synergistically with IL-1 (26).

B. Proliferative Phase

The proliferative phase of wound healing follows the inflammatory phase, although in reality these two phases overlap and there is no clear demarcation. This phase is characterized by granulation tissue formation consisting of a capillary bed, fibroblast, macrophages, collagen, fibronecting, hyaluronic acid, and bacteria (Table 2.2).

The processes of angiogenesis, fibroplasia, and epithelialization, regulated by a complex network of cytokines, predominate this phase. The fibrin–fibronectin matrix serves as a scaffold for further construction of the complex interdigitated structure of this phase of the wound-healing cascade.

1. Angiogenesis

Angiogenesis begins approximately 2 days after the initial injury (74). This process is highly regulated by cytokines. It is also affected by local factors such as the pH of the surrounding milieu. Several cytokines regulate this process, but the two important cytokines are VEGF and FGF-2 (75,76). Heparin can stimulate the migration of capillary endothelial cells. Heparin in the basement membrane (BM) extracellular matrix binds to bFGF-2 (77). The BM is degraded as a result, releasing FGF to initiate angiogenesis. Capillary tube formation is mediated by TNF-α, a chemotactic agent for endothelial cells (29).

VEGF is predominantly produced by epithelial cells. It is endothelial cell specific, and both mitogenic and chemotactic. Hypoxia is also a potent stimulator of VEGF. The complex interaction of endothelial cells, ECM, BM, local factors and cytokines initiates angiogenesis. Intact capillaries at the wound edges give rise to endothelial

Table 2.2 Cytokines at Affect Wound Healing

Cytokine	Symbol	Source	Functions
Platelet-derived growth factor	PDGF	Platelets, macrophages, endothelial cells, keratinocytes	Chemotactic for PMNs, macrophages, fibroblasts, and smooth muscle cells; activates PMNs, macrophages, and fibroblasts; mitogenic for fibroblasts, endothelial cells; stimulates production of MMPs, fibronectin, and HA; stimulates angiogenesis and wound contraction; remodeling
Transforming growth factor beta (including isoforms b1, b2, and b3)	TGF-β	Platelets, T-lymphocytes, macrophages, endothelial cells, keratinocytes, fibroblasts	Chemotactic for PMNs, macrophages, lymphocytes, fibroblasts; stimulates TIMP synthesis, keratinocyte migration, angiogenesis, and fibroplasias; inhibits production of MMPs and keratinocyte proliferation; induces TBF-β production
Epidermal growth factor	EGF	Platelets, macrophages	Mitogenic for keratinocytes and fibroblasts; stimulates keratinocyte migration
Transforming growth factor alpha	TGF-α	Macrophages, T-lymphocytes, keratinocytes	Similar to EGF
Fibroblast growth factor-1 and -2 family	FGF	Macrophages, mast cells, T-lymphocytes, endothelial cells, fibroblasts	Chemotactic for fibroblasts; mitogenic for fibroblasts and keratinocytes; stimulates keratinocyte migration, angiogenesis, wound contraction, and matrix deposition
Keratinocyte growth factor (also called FGF-7)	KGF	Fibroblasts	Stimulates keratinocyte migration, proliferation, and differentiation
Insulin-like growth factor	IGF-1	Macrophages, fibroblasts	Stimulates synthesis of sulfated proteoglycans, collagen, keratinocyte migration, and fibroblast proliferation; endocrine effects similar to growth hormone
Vascular endothelial cell growth factor	VEGF	Keratinocytes	Increases vasopermeability; mitogenic for endothelial cells
Tumor necrosis factor	TNF	Macrophages, mast cells, T-lymphocytes	Activates macrophages; mitogenic for fibroblasts; stimulates angiogenesis; regulates other cytokines
Interleukins	IL-1, etc	Macrophages, mast cells, keratinocytes, lymphocytes	Chemotactic for PMNs (IL-1) and fibroblasts (IL-4); stimulates MMP-1 synthesis (IL-1), angiogenesis (IL-8), TIMP synthesis (IL-6); regulates other cytokines
Interleukins	IFN-α, etc.	Lymphocytes and fibroblasts	Activates macrophages, inhibits fibroblast proliferation and synthesis of MMPs; regulates other cytokines

Note: PMNS = polymorphonuclear leukocytes; MMPs = matrix metalloproteinases; HA = hyaluronic acid; TIMP = tissue inhibitor of matrix metalloproteinase.
Source: Modified with permission from Schwartz SI. Principles of Surgery. 7th ed. New York: McGraw-Hill, 1999, Chapter 8, 269.

sprouts that grow through cellular migration and proliferation (74,75,77). The endothelial cells eventually develop a curvature and a lumen is produced as a chain of elongated endothelial cell (29). The sprouts come into contact and interconnect generating a new capillary. Integrins and MMPs play a major role in the migration of endothelial cells during angiogenesis. Upregulation of $\alpha\beta$-3 integrins is necessary for angiogenesis (29). Degradation of BM collagen by MMPs facilitates migration of endothelial cells. As the injured area becomes revascularized, the dynamics of the cytokines change, and the vascular system eventually matures. The process of angiogenesis is permanent for the cascade to continue harmoniously.

2. Fibroplasia

The principle cell type during this process is the fibroblast. Fibroblasts are chemoattracted to the inflammatory site where they amplify and produce the components of the ECM. Under the influence of cytokines, undifferentiated cells in the vicinity of the wound may be transformed into fibroblasts (78). The arrested fibroblast in the Go phase is stimulated by PDGF or bFGF to advance to the G1 phase of the cell cycle (68). The progression through the subsequent phases (S2, G2, and M) of the cell cycle is facilitated by IGF, which is derived primarily from fibroblast and hepatocytes (66). PDGF works in concert with IGF to facilitate fibroblast proliferation (69). PDGF and TGF-β remain the two most important cytokines during fibroplasia. They stimulate fibroblast migration as well as proliferation (69,78). Other factors that stimulate fibroblast migration include epidermal growth factor (EGF) and fibronectin (42,79).

Integrins play a central role in fibroblast migration. The upregulation of integrin receptors that bind fibronectin and fibrin in the provisional wound matrix is required for migration to occur (80,81). This alteration of the receptors is stimulated by PDGF and TGF-β (82,83). Cellular migration requires cell membrane-bound integrin to be bonded to fibronectin in the ECM (84). A migrating cell then develops "lamellopodia" that extends outward until another binding site is detected in the ECM (85). Using the new site as an anchor, the cell migrates by "pulling" itself toward this second site and releases its primary binding site (41). This migratory process is stimulated by fibronectin fragments (42). Cellular migration also depends on the direction of the fibers in the ECM with migration forming in the orientation of the fibers rather than being across fibers. Also, MMP-1, MMP-2 (gelatinase), and MMP-3 (stromelysin) individually facilitate migration by enzymatically lysing debris, in order for migrating cells to move with much ease (84). These enzymatic debriders are themselves produced by fibroblast after stimulation by TGF-β (86).

Proteoglycans are proteins synthesized by fibroblast after injury. They contribute to the dermal matrix. Like collagen, proteoglycan synthesis is unregulated in response to injury and their concentration increases over time. They consist of a central core made up of proteins that is covalently bonded to a GAG (87).

Proteoglycans have the ability to change their orientation after binding to other proteins and their activity can be subsequently affected. For instance, dermatan sulfate has the ability to orient collagen to facilitate fibril formation (26).

GAGs are found on the surface of virtually all vertebrate cells. They aid in cellular support, provide tissue turgor, and make possible cell-to-cell interaction. Proteoglycans have the ability to resist compression as a result of their accompanying hydration shells. Higher concentrations are found because of an increase in vascular permeability. Granulation tissue contains increased levels of dermatan sulfate. Proteoglycans are acidic in nature and are highly ionized, making them able to bind water and different cations (87).

Hyaluronan, a potent modulator of cellular migration, contributes to the visoelastic properties of skin (87). It has a large hydration shell which enhances cell migration.

C. Maturational and Remodeling Phase

All wounds will eventually contract. Beginning postinjury day 5, to about day 14, wound contraction becomes evident as normal surrounding tissue is seen in the vicinity of the wound (29). This contraction rate differs depending on the location of the wound but averages about 0.6–0.7 mm/day (29). The wound contraction rate can often be envisaged by the extent of skin laxity at the wound site. While a gluteal wound will contract in a significantly short period of time, a scalp wound will contract much slower. The rate of wound contraction depends on the time, type of tissue, degree of laxity of the tissue surrounding the wound, and shape of the wounds.

Square wounds contract faster than circular wounds (29). The contraction of the wound is less apparent in incisional-type wounds, but more apparent in open and skin-grafted wounds. In a grafted or open wound, the wound edges are seen pulling towards a vector directed toward the center of the wound, while wound contraction causes shortening of the scar in incisional-type wounds, and is less apparent.

Since the 1970s, wound contraction has been mainly attributed to myofibroblasts, but more recent work is placing fibroblast as the "motor" behind wound contraction (88,89). Paul Ehrlich (89) demonstrated that aborted cell locomotion appears to cause bunching and contraction of collagen fibers by using a fibroblast-populated collagen lattice (FPCL). He attributed these tractional forces to fibroblasts.

The contraction process seems to occur by a complex interplay between the extracellular matrix and the fibroblast. Myofibroblasts have been witnessed to be in abundance at the periphery of wounds (88). Gabbiani and colleagues were the first to describe myofibroblast in 1971 as the "motor" behind contracting wounds. Myofibroblasts in essence are stimulated fibroblasts with a multilobulated nucleus, profuse rough endoplastic reticulum, and cytoplasmic microfilaments, rich in actin and myosin. Myofibroblast becomes evident 4–6 days postinjury and lingers on for about 2–3 weeks, and later disappears by apoptosis (88). These cells have both function and structure in common between the fibroblast and the smooth muscle cell (Fig. 2.8) (26). Their contractile ability seems to be related to the contractile activities of their rich cytoplasmic actin-myosin microfilaments. *In vitro* studies have shown that when colchicine, a microtubule inhibitor, or cytochalasin-D, a microfilament inhibitor, is added to tissue culture, minimal contraction of the collagen gels is witnessed (90).

MMPs recently have been shown to be vital in wound contraction. Bullard et al. (91), using a knock-out mice model, have shown impaired contraction in stromelysin-1 (MMP-3)-deficient fibroblast (91). MMPs are involved with the breakdown of proteoglycans, laminin, fibronectin, and collagen. It is possible that MMP-3 and other MMPs influence the extracellular matrix in a variety of ways, modifying attachment sites between collagen fibrils and fibroblast via β-1 integrins. Therefore, one might speculate that the stromelysin-1-deficient fibroblast lacks the ability to come in contact with its surrounding matrix due to this mechanism.

A myriad of cytokines including TGF-β1, IGF-1, and PDGF play a role in the wound contraction process (69,84,92). The contraction process is cell mediated and no new collagen is synthesized. These cytokines impact this process by complex interaction with the existing cells and structures in the ECM through their activation of β-1 integrins.

In burned patients, the end result of wound contraction is scar contracture. Here, contractures limit function and the culprit is usually a hypertrophic scar. These scars are more common across joints (including the neck) and prevent both flexion and extension. Scar contractures can also involve the axilla and eyelid causing abduction difficulties and ectropions, respectively. By limiting wound contraction, closing wounds as quickly as possible with an adequate amount of dermis, we can limit or even prevent contractures.

After the wound heals through contraction, the remodeling process begins. Theoretically, the remodeling process commences ~21 days postinjury, and is a balance between collagen synthesis and degradation. Collagen synthesis plateaus and diminishes and reaches

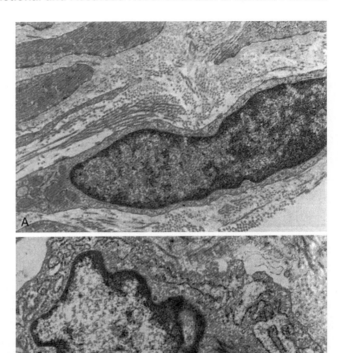

Figure 2.8 (A) Normal resting fibroblast from human connective tissue. Note the large, smooth oval nucleus; normal mitochondria; and a small amount of rough endoplasmic reticulum. The cell is surrounded by collagen fibrils cut in longitudinal and cross-section. The cell fragments seen in the upper left are typical smooth muscle cells. Electron micrograph, ×22,000. (B) Myofibroblast from a patient with plantar fascitis. Compared with the fibroblast, note the highly irregular nucleus, the large amount of rough endoplasmic reticulum, and the dense collection of myofilaments. No basal lamina is seen, and the cell is surrounded by numerous collagen fibrils. This cell has ultrastructural features typical of both a fibroblast and a smooth muscle cell. Electron micrograph, ×25,000. (Courtesy of Edward C. Carlson, PhD.) (From Sabiston DC Jr. Textbook of Surgery. 15th ed. Chapter 12, fig. 12-3, p. 210.)

equilibrium with collagen breakdown. This decrease in collagen synthesis is regulated and mediated by the collagen matrix itself, IFN-γ and TNF-α (60,93,94). MMPs and tissue inhibitors of metalloproteinases (TIMPs) are very instrumental during this phase of the healing process. MMPs, as alluded to earlier, consist of at least 25 enzymes that degrade different components in the ECM, while TIMPs, with its four different isoforms, control in part, the activity of the MMPs (84,95). TGF-β, IL-1, and PDGF regulate the equilibrium between MMPs and TIMPs (61,86,95). MMPs are elevated in chronic wounds; MMP-3-deficient mice have shown to have problems with wound contraction (96,97).

The remodeling process can continue up to 2 years as the wound heals. The scar continues to mature as evident by the replacement of disorganized thin collagen fibers by thicker fibers that parallels skin tension lines. Cross-linking of collagen is upregulated thereby increasing the tensile strength of the scar. The cross-linking results in a more fragile and less resilient scar. The tensile strength of a wounded skin never approximates that of the unwounded skin. Wound tensile strength increases in a rapid manner for the first 6 weeks and levels in the ensuing weeks that follow (Fig. 2.9). The tensile strength of the healed and remodeled scar eventually will attain about 80% of the tensile strength of the un-wounded skin. In addition to cross-linking, the amount of water decreases, thereby changing the proteoglycans, and the ratio of type I to type III collagen (26).

D. Factors Affecting Wound Healing

Several factors affect the healing wound and can impede or disrupt the wound-healing cascade. These factors can be intrinsic or extrinsic and can be further categorized as

local vs. systemic (Table 2.3). Some of these factors are inherent like aging and very little can be done about it, while others like infection can be controlled to positively reflect on the outcome of the healed wound.

Infection is probably the most common cause of delayed wound healing. Robson et al. (98) have demonstrated that if the bacterial count in a wound exceeds 10 to the fifth organism per gram of tissue, the wound will not heal. In addition, if any amount of beta-hemolytic streptococcus or clostridium is present, impairment in the healing process will occur. Infections prolong the inflammatory phase and further interfere with epithelialization, contraction, and deposition of collagen. Collagen degradation is upregulated by endotoxins released by the bacteria.

Hypoxia impedes wound healing, even though angiogenesis is upregulated (99–101). The wound-healing cascade will not proceed effectively with tissue oxygen levels <35 mmHg (102). When the tissue oxygen levels fall below this critical value, the replication of fibroblast is impaired, resulting in impaired collagen production. Disorders including occlusive arterial disease, vasospastic disease, vasculitis, and hematologic disorders such as polycythemia vera cause tissue hypoxia and delayed wound healing (Table 2.4) (100). External factors such

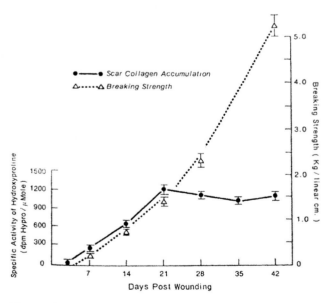

Figure 2.9 Comparison of scar collagen accumulation and breaking strength of rat skin wounds. Note that over the first 3 weeks, strength and collagen content correlate. After 21 days, strength increases with no change in wound collagen, reflecting scar remodeling. There is no correlation between collagen content and strength after 3 weeks. (With permission from Madden JW, Peacock EE Jr. Studies on the biology of collagen during wound healing III. Dynamic metabolism of scare collagen and remodeling in dermal wounds. Ann Surg 1971; 174:511.)

Table 2.3 Factors that Interfere with Wound Healing

Local
Infection
Foreign bodies
Ischemia
Smoking
Radiation
Trauma
Cancer
Local toxins
Arterial insufficiency
Venous insufficiency
Hyperthermia
Systemic
Inherited disorders affecting collagen formation
Nutritional deficiencies
Aging
Diabetes
Liver disease
Alcoholism
Uremia
Medications
Blood transfusions
Jaundice

Source: Modified from Lawrence WT. In: Cohen IK, Diegelmann RF, Lindblad WJ, eds. Wound Healing: Biochemical and Clinical Aspects. Philadelphia: W.B. Saunders Company, 1992.

Table 2.4 Disorders Associated with Impaired Blood Flow

Occlusive arterial disease
Arteriosclerosis obliterans
Microembolism
Thromboangiitis obliterans (Buerger disease)
Vasopastic disease
Cold sensitivity (Raynaud type)
Erythromelagia
Livedo reticularis (severe forms)
Vasculitis
Scleroderma
Systemic lupus erythematosus
Periateritis nodosa
Hematologic disorders
Cryoglobulinemia
Polycythemia vera
Hypertensive ulcers

Source: From Stadelmann WK, Digenis AG, Tobin GR. Impediments to wound healing. Am J Surg 1998; 176(suppl 2A):39S–47S; with permission.

as tension on closure of wounds or too much pressure on wounds from the dressing can undermine the critical level of tissue oxygen tension. Anemia was once thought to retard the wound-healing cascade, but this has been refuted in studies of hypoperfusion and immediate resuscitation (103–105). It now stands that hypoperfusion is more of a risk factor of impaired wound healing than anemia (99–103). Elderly patients heal slower compared to younger patients. In addition, the same person heals slower as he or she ages. All phases of the healing cascade are affected as one ages and this stems from the effects of aging on macrophages (106,107).

Diabetes mellitus deserves a special mention, as people with this disease have been witnessed to heal slowly with many complications often leading to limb loss. The relationship between diabetes and impaired wound healing is complex, and continues to evolve. Many factors contribute to the altered wound healing seen in diabetics. These include, but are not limited to, predisposition to other systemic diseases such as atherosclerosis, renal failure with concomitant uremia, peripheral arterial disease, and coagulopathy. Another contributing factor seen in diabetics is a thickened capillary perivascular membrane which decreases perfusion in the microenvironment (108).

Glycemic control has been the focus of many investigators and has been proven to adversely affect wound healing (109). Goodson and Hunt (110) demonstrated improved wound healing in animals with destroyed islets of Langerhans cells by preventing hyperglycemia in these animals. Three hypotheses seem to explain this phenomenon. The first hypothesis is the alteration of Na^+/K^+ ATPase activity at the cellular level (110–112).

Hyperglycemia upregulates the enzyme aldose reductase that converts glucose to sorbitol via the polyol pathway. In this pathway, sorbitol is then converted to fructose generating NADH. Two things happen. First, the conversion of sorbitol to fructose by sorbitol dehydrogenase is slow, thereby causing a buildup of sorbitol. The increased concentration of sorbitol causes an increase in the osmotic load of cells. The cells eventually swell as water enters, to equilibrate the concentration of sorbitol. In addition, sorbitol inhibits the uptake of myo-inositol that consequently alters the Na^+/K^+ ATPase activity. The increased conversion of sorbitol to fructose eventually causes diminution in NADPH levels, which in turn increases the risk of oxidative stress. Tesfamariam (113) has shown some improvement of the effects of hyperglycemia on endothelial cells in wound healing using inhibitors of aldose reductase.

The second hypothesis on the impaired wound healing noted in diabetics is the activation of protein kinase C (PKC) by hyperglycemia (114). Diacyl–glycerol synthesis is elevated by hyperglycemia, which in turn causes PKC activity to increase. PKC is an important signaling molecule, and many cellular activities use the PKC signaling pathway. Cellular proliferation and calcium metabolism utilize this pathway.

The third mechanism is hyperglycemia induced "advanced glycosylation end products" (AGEs) (115). AGEs are large aggregates of aldoses bound to reactive amino groups by covalent bonds. AGEs may activate nuclear factor-κB (NF-κB) a key transcription factor involved in many cytokine-related cell responses (116). AGEs may induce PDGF, TNF-α, and IL-1α and inhibit normal collagen degradation (117–119). The antidiabetic drug aminoguanidine may be used to suppress the production of AGEs (120,121).

Hyperglycemia also causes impairment in leukocyte and lymphocytic function and immune function suppression as a whole. Many investigators have shown that reduction in growth factor production and increased proteoglycans in the ECM contribute to some of the impairment in the diabetic wound (117–119). There is a decreased expression of mRNA and production of IGF-1, IGF-II, KGF, and many others (122–124). Many investigators have shown increased re-epithelialization of burn wounds using IGF-1 liposomal gene transfer in animal models (125,126). MMP levels are increased in diabetic wounds.

Malnutrition adversely affects wound healing. Inadequate calorie intake and nutritional balance impair wound healing (Table 2.5) (118). Proteins play a major role in the synthesis of collagen (Fig. 2.10). While most agree that the normal wound-healing process cannot proceed with albumin levels <2 g/dL, deficiencies in the cascade have been reported with albumin level <3 g/dL (127). Protein replacement and supplementation can

Table 2.5 Nutritional Deficiencies Associated with Delayed Wound Healing

Decreased proteins levels
Carbohydrate depletion
Decreased levels of amino acids
    Arginine
    Glutamine
Vitamins
    Decreased vitamin C
    Decreased vitamin A
    Excess vitamin E
Trace element deficiencies
    Zinc
    Iron
    Copper
    Magnesium

Source: Burns et al. (129).

reverse this process (128), hence the importance of early enteral feeds rich in protein.

Vitamin deficiencies have been noted to impact wound healing due to the role of vitamins as cofactors in several pathways. The key vitamins are vitamins A, C, E, and K. Vitamin A has been shown to improve wounds retarded by steroids (130). Vitamin A deficiency impairs the activation of monocytes and deposition of fibronectin, which in turn affects cellular adhesion and TGF-B receptor impairment (131–133). Freiman et al. (133) demonstrated in the early 1970s that decreased tensile strength ensued from decreased vitamin A levels. Vitamin A plays a role in lysosomal enzyme stabilization in wounds and functions in cell mediated response and cytotoxity, antibody response, and production of cytokines (134). Vitamin A deficiency is usually rare and almost every food source contains vitamin A.

Vitamin C (ascorbic acid) deficiency results in faulty collagen synthesis. As mentioned in the production of collagen, vitamin C serves as a cofactor in the hydroxylation of proline and lysine. Even in as little as 3 months of deprivation of vitamin C can delay wound healing. Severe vitamin C deficiency can even cause dehiscence of previously healed wounds (135). Vitamin C also plays a role in leukocyte recruitment into a wound and contributes to the formation of superoxides that aids in the killing of bacteria. Its deficiency in this sense causes an immune compromise. As an antioxidant, vitamin C has been shown to improve healing (135). Supplementation of vitamin C can be done at doses of up to 1000 mg/day. It is a water-soluble vitamin and as such has a better safety profile unlike vitamins A, E, and K, which are lipid soluble. Renal dysfunction can occur due to the formation of oxalate crystals in the renal tubules.

Vitamin K plays a major role in the clotting cascade and individually affects wound healing. Deficiencies in vitamin K result in decreased synthesis of factors II, VII, IX, and X, and impede the rate of the initial "plug" formation (129).

Trace elements are overlooked when it comes to abnormalities in wound healing. These elements are important, as they serve as cofactors in the wound-healing cascade. Zinc, iron, copper, and magnesium are the key trace elements in wound healing. Zinc is an important cofactor in over 100 different enzymatic pathways (26). It serves as a cofactor for DNA polymerase and superoxide dismutase and helps in cellular proliferation and

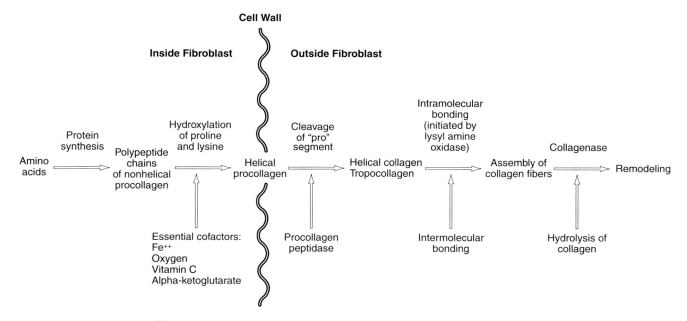

Figure 2.10 Collagen synthesis. [With permission from Burns et al. (129).]

epithelialization (136). Zinc deficiency has been shown to cause decrease tensile strength in a rat model (136). Zinc deficiency is rare except in large burns, chronic alcoholism, and cirrhosis of the liver (129). Ferrous iron serves as a cofactor in collagen synthesis; therefore, a deficiency can cause faulty collagen synthesis. In addition to ascorbic acid serving as a cofactor in collagen synthesis, the hydroxylation of proline and lysine requires iron as a cofactor. There has been no conclusive study linking iron deficiency anemia to impaired healing (105). Recent studies depict iron as detrimental to wound healing (137). These studies propose that increase of iron causes increased reactive oxygen species that causes increased connective tissue destruction, persistent inflammation, and lipid peroxidation leading to chronic wounds (137).

1. Drugs

Many drugs impair the wound-healing process (Table 2.6). While the list continues to increase, chemotherapeutic agents, steroids, and NSAIDs are among the widely studied drugs that affect wound healing (26,129).

Steroids impair wound healing by directly dampening the cellular response. Fibroblast proliferation is affected, which in turn affects collagen production. The ECM content is scanty in steroid-treated animals and granulation tissue formation is decreased (29). By stabilizing lysosomal membranes, steroids block the release of intracellular contents (29). Consequently, steroids decrease wound tensile strength in a time- and dose-dependent fashion. Vitamin A reverses this action of steroids (138).

NSAIDs play a controversial role in wound healing. Several studies implicate NSAIDs in delayed wound healing, even in low does, but a group of Scandinavian scientists have demonstrated the limitation of necrosis in ischemic wounds with the use of NSAIDs (139).

Table 2.6 Drugs Associated with Wound-Healing Delays

Anticoagulants	Phenytoin
Antihistamines	Glucocorticoids
Antimicrobials (some)	Immunosuppressive agents
Aspirin	Lathyrogens
Azathioprine	Nonsteroidal anti-inflammatory agents
B-aminoproprionitrile (BAPN)	
Povidone-iodine	Papaverine
Chemotherapeutic agents	Penicillamine
Chlorhexidine	Phenylbutazone
Colchicine	Quinoline sulfate
Cyclosporine	Retinoids
Dakin's solution (sodium hypochlorite 0.25%)	Thiphenamil hydrochloride

Source: Burns et al. (129).

As physicians, we expect wounds to heal in a timely fashion, but have witnessed that this is not always the case. In the last several decades, it was thought that optimal wound closure could be achieved by accurate tissue approximation, control of infection, and protection of the wound from excessive pressure. Current research in the last two decades has been focusing on wound manipulation using recombinant technology at the molecular level. Several cytokines exist today that have all impacted wound healing in a positive manner. While most of these are experimental, only PDGF-BB has been approved by the FDA for diabetic foot ulcers (2). These agents are used topically and include PDGF, bFGF, KGF, EGF, TGF-B, granulocyte-macrophage colony-stimulating factors (GM-CSF), IGF family of proteins, IL-1β, and a combination of these agents (2). All these agents have shown promise in the improvement of chronic wounds. However, their role in the management of burn wounds is uncertain. The only remaining factor is FDA approval for some of the more promising ones. Cost is another issue, as these agents are very expensive to produce.

Attempts are being made to manipulate acute wounds. The cytokines mentioned above have been used to speed up surgical incisions as well (140). Fu et al. (141) recently reported the role of topical recombinant bovine fibroblast growth factor for second-degree burns. This study was a multicenter clinical trial with a total of 600 patients from 32 hospitals. The authors further divided the wounds into superficial and deep second-degree burns. The treated group healed their wounds in 9.9 $\pm$ 2.5 days for the superficial wounds and 17.0 $\pm$ 4.6 days for the deep wounds compared with the nontreated groups [12.4 $\pm$ 2.7 days (superficial) and 21.2 $\pm$ 4.9 days (deep)]. The remarkable impact of these agents in wound healing can only be underscored by the rate of their approval by the FDA.

The pathophysiology of the burn wound continues to be uncovered leading to better management of the acute phase of burn injury. It is only when this is maximally controlled that our reconstructive efforts will be more fruitful, yielding better cosmesis and function.

ACKNOWLEDGMENTS

Special thanks are given to Seunghee Oh, Steve Schuenke, and Eileen Figueroa for their contributions to the chapter.

REFERENCES

1. Miller MJ, Patrick CW Jr. Tissue engineering. Clin Plast Surg 2003; 30:91–103.
2. Robson MC. Cytokine manipulation of the wound. Clin Plast Surg 2003; 30:57–65.

3. Yamaguchi Y, Yoshikawa K. Cutaneous wound healing: an update. J Dermatol 2001; 28:521–534.

4. Jackson DM. The diagnosis of the depth of burning. Br J Surg 1953; 40:588–596.

5. Moritz AR, Henriquez FC. Studies of thermal injury II. The relative importance of time and surface temperature in the causation of cutaneous burns. Am J Pathol 1947; 23:695–720.

6. Robson MC, DelBeccaro EJ, Heggers JP, Loy GL. Increasing dermal perfusion after burning by decreasing thromboxane production. J Trauma 1980; 20:722–725.

7. Boykin JV, Eriksoon E, Pittman RN. Microcirculation of scald burn: an *in vivo* experimental study of the hairless mouse ear. Burns 1980; 7:335–338.

8. Johnson CE, Granstrom E, Hamburg M. Prostaglandins and thromboxane in burn injury in man. Scand J Plast Reconstr Surg 1979; 13:45.

9. Zawacki BE. Reversal of capillary stasis and prevention of necrosis in burns. Ann Surg 1974; 180:98–102.

10. Harada T, Izaki S, Tsutsumi H, Kobayashi M, Kitamura K. Apoptosis of hair follicle cells in the second-degree burn wound unders hypernatremic conditions. Burns 1998; 24:464–469.

11. DelBeccaro EJ, Robson MC, Heggers JP, Swaminathan R. The use of specific thromboxane inhibitors to preserve the dermal microcirculation after burning. Surgery 1980; 87:137–141.

12. Robson MC, Del Beccaro EJ, Heggers JP. The effect of prostaglandins on the dermal microcirculation after burning, and the inhibition of the effect by specific pharmacological agents. Plast Reconstr Surg 1979; 63:781–787.

13. Remensnyder JP. Topography of tissue oxygen tension changes in acute burn edema. Arch Surg 1972; 105:477–482.

14. Arturson G. Microvascular permeability to macromolecules in thermal injury. Acta Physiol Scand Suppl 1979; 463:111–122.

15. Arturson G, Soeda S. Changes in transcapillary leakage during healing of experimental burns. Acta Chir Scand 1967; 133:609–614.

16. Brouhard BH, Carvajal HF, Linares HA. Burn edema and protein leakage in the rat. I. Relationship to time of injury. Microvasc Res 1978; 15:221–228.

17. Cotran RS. The delayed and prolonged vascular leakage in inflammation. II. an electron microscopic study of the vascular response after thermal injury. Am J Pathol 1965; 46:589–620.

18. Hatherill JR, Till GO, Bruner LH, Ward PA. Thermal injury, intravascular hemolysis, and toxic oxygen products. J Clin Invest 1986; 78:629–636.

19. Siney L, Brain SD. Involvement of sensory neuropeptides in the development of plasma extravasation in rat dorsal skin following thermal injury. Br J Pharmacol 1996; 117:1065–1070.

20. Anggard E, Arturson G, Jonsson CE. Efflux of prostaglandins in lymph from scalded tissues. Acta Physiol Scand 1970; 80:46A–47A.

21. Arturson G, Hamberg M, Jonsson CE. Prostaglandins in human burn blister fluid. Acta Physiol Scand 1973; 87:270–276.

22. Heggers JP, Loy GL, Robson MC, Del Beccaro EJ. Histological demonstration of prostaglandins and thromboxanes in burned tissue. J Surg Res 1980; 28:110–117.

23. Demling RH, Lalonde C. Topical ibuprofen decreases early postburn edema. Surgery 1987; 102:857–861.

24. Robb HJ. Dynamics of the microcirculation during a burn. Arch Surg 1967; 94:776–780.

25. Lund T, Wiig H, Reed RK. Acute postburn edema: role of strongly negative interstitial fluid pressure. Am J Physiol 1988; 255:H1069–H1074.

26. Phillips LG. Wound healing. In: Townsend CM Jr, ed. Sabiston Textbook of Surgery. 16th ed. Philadelphia: W.B. Saunders, 2001:131–144.

27. Grinnell F. Fibronectin and wound healing. J Cell Biochem 1984; 26:107–116.

28. Lawrence WT. Physiology of the acute wound. Clin Plast Surg 1998; 25:321–340.

29. Monaco JL, Lawrence WT. Acute wound healing an overview. Clin Plast Surg 2003; 30:1–12.

30. Weksler B. Platelets. New York: Raven Press, 1988.

31. White JG, Gerrard JM. Ultrastructural features of abnormal blood platelets. A review. Am J Pathol 1976; 83:589–632.

32. Deuel TF, Senior RM, Huang JS, Griffin GL. Chemotaxis of monocytes and neutrophils to platelet-derived growth factor. J Clin Invest 1982; 69:1046–1049.

33. Dahlback B. Blood coagulation. Lancet 2000; 355:1627–1632.

34. Stiernberg J, Redin WR, Warner WS, Carney DH. The role of thrombin and thrombin receptor activating peptide (TRAP-508) in initiation of tissue repair. Thromb Haemost 1993; 70:158–162.

35. Hynes RO. Fibronectins. Sci Am 1986; 254:42–51.

36. Blatti SP, Foster DN, Ranganathan G, Moses HL, Getz MJ. Induction of fibronectin gene transcription and mRNA is a primary response to growth-factor stimulation of AKR-2B cells. Proc Natl Acad Sci USA 1988; 85:1119–1123.

37. Fukai F, Suzuki H, Suzuki K, Tsugita A, Katayama T. Rat plasma fibronectin contains two distinct chemotactic domains for fibroblastic cells. J Biol Chem 1991; 266:8807–8813.

38. Clark RA, Lanigan JM, DellaPelle P, Manseau E, Dvorak HF, Colvin RB. Fibronectin and fibrin provide a provisional matrix for epidermal cell migration during wound reepithelialization. J Invest Dermatol 1982; 79:264–269.

39. Wysocki AB, Grinnell F. Fibronectin profiles in normal and chronic wound fluid. Lab Invest 1990; 63:825–831.

40. Majno G, Shea SM, Leventhal M. Endothelial contraction induced by histamine-type mediators: an electron microscopic study. J Cell Biol 1969; 42:647–672.

41. Carter SB. Cell movement and cell spreading: a passive or an active process? Nature 1970; 225:858–859.

42. Postlethwaite AE, Keski-Oja J, Balian G, Kang AH. Induction of fibroblast chemotaxis by fibronectin. Localization of the chemotactic region to a 140,000-molecular weight non-gelatin-binding fragment. J Exp Med 1981; 153:494–499.

43. Wahl SM, Hunt DA, Wakefield LM, McCartney-Francis N, Wahl LM, Roberts AB, Sporn MB. Transforming growth factor type beta induces monocyte chemotaxis and

growth factor production. Proc Natl Acad Sci USA 1987; 84:5788–5792.

44. Pohlman TH, Stanness KA, Beatty PG, Ochs HD, Harlan JM. An endothelial cell surface factor(s) induced *in vitro* by lipopolysaccharide, interleukin 1, and tumor necrosis factor-alpha increases neutrophil adherence by a CDw18-dependent mechanism. J Immunol 1986; 136:4548–4553.

45. Sklar LA, Jesaitis AJ, Painter RG. The neutrophil N-formyl peptide receptor: dynamics of ligand-receptor interactions and their relationship to cellular responses. Contemp Top Immunobiol 1984; 14:29–82.

46. McIntyre TM, Zimmerman GA, Prescott SM. Leukotrienes C4 and D4 stimulate human endothelial cells to synthesize platelet-activating factor and bind neutrophils. Proc Natl Acad Sci USA 1986; 83:2204–2208.

47. Hynes RO. Integrins: a family of cell surface receptors. Cell 1987; 48:549–554.

48. Simpson DM, Ross R. The neutrophilic leukocyte in wound repair a study with antineutrophil serum. J Clin Invest 1972; 51:2009–2023.

49. Gailit J, Clark RA. Wound repair in the context of extracellular matrix. Curr Opin Cell Biol 1994; 6:717–725.

50. Martin CW, Muir IF. The role of lymphocytes in wound healing. Br J Plast Surg 1990; 43:655–662.

51. Peterson JM, Barbul A, Breslin RJ, Wasserkrug HL, Efron G. Significance of T-lymphocytes in wound healing. Surgery 1987; 102:300–305.

52. Ono I. Roles of cytokines in wound healing processes. Nippon Geka Gakkai Zasshi 1999; 100:522–528.

53. Newman SL, Henson JE, Henson PM. Phagocytosis of senescent neutrophils by human monocyte-derived macrophages and rabbit inflammatory macrophages. J Exp Med 1982; 156:430–442.

54. Wright SD, Ramos RA, Tobias PS, Ulevitch RJ, Mathison JC. CD14, a receptor for complexes of lipopolysaccharide (LPS) and LPS binding protein. Science 1990; 249:1431–1433.

55. Werb Z, Banda MJ, Jones PA. Degradation of connective tissue matrices by macrophages. I. Proteolysis of elastin, glycoproteins, and collagen by proteinases isolated from macrophages. J Exp Med 1980; 152:1340–1357.

56. Wahl LM, Winter CC. Regulation of guinea pig macrophage collagenase production by dexamethasone and colchicine. Arch Biochem Biophys 1984; 230:661–667.

57. Parker C. Fundamental immunology. In: Paul W, ed. Mediators: Release and Function. New York: Raven Press, 1984:697–747.

58. Leibovich SJ, Ross R. The role of the macrophage in wound repair. A study with hydrocortisone and antimacrophage serum. Am J Pathol 1975; 78:71–100.

59. Malawista SE, Montgomery RR, van Blaricom G. Evidence for reactive nitrogen intermediates in killing of staphylococci by human neutrophil cytoplasts. A new microbicidal pathway for polymorphonuclear leukocytes. J Clin Invest 1992; 90:631–636.

60. Madden JW, Peacock EE Jr. Studies on the biology of collagen during wound healing. I. Rate of collagen synthesis and deposition in cutaneous wounds of the rat. Surgery 1968; 64:288–294.

61. Circolo A, Welgus HG, Pierce GF, Kramer J, Strunk RC. Differential regulation of the expression of proteinases/antiproteinases in fibroblasts. Effects of interleukin-1 and platelet-derived growth factor. J Biol Chem 1991; 266:12283–12288.

62. Nielson EG, Phillips SM, Jimenez S. Lymphokine modulation of fibroblast proliferation. J Immunol 1982; 128:1484–1486.

63. Schreiber AB, Winkler ME, Derynck R. Transforming growth factor-alpha: a more potent angiogenic mediator than epidermal growth factor. Science 1986; 232:1250–1253.

64. Minchenko A, Salceda S, Bauer T, Caro J. Hypoxia regulatory elements of the human vascular endothelial growth factor gene. Cell Mol Biol Res 1994; 40:35–39.

65. Dore-Duffy P, Perry W, Kuo HH. Interferon-mediated inhibition of prostaglandin synthesis in human mononuclear leukocytes. Cell Immunol 1983; 79:232–239.

66. Patel B, Khaliq A, Jarvis-Evans J, McLeod D, Mackness M, Boulton M. Oxygen regulation of TGF-beta 1 mRNA in human hepatoma (Hep G2) cells. Biochem Mol Biol Int 1994; 34:639–644.

67. Scannell G, Waxman K, Kaml GJ, Ioli G, Gatanaga T, Yamamoto R, Granger GA. Hypoxia induces a human macrophage cell line to release tumor necrosis factor-alpha and its soluble receptors *in vitro*. J Surg Res 1993; 54:281–285.

68. Ross R. Platelet-derived growth factor. Annu Rev Med 1987; 38:71–79.

69. Seppa H, Grotendorst G, Seppa S, Schiffmann E, Martin GR. Platelet-derived growth factor in chemotactic for fibroblasts. J Cell Biol 1982; 92:584–588.

70. Wahl SM, Hunt DA, Wong HL, Dougherty S, McCartney-Francis N, Wahl LM, Ellingsworth L, Schmidt JA, Hall G, Roberts AB et al. Transforming growth factor-beta is a potent immunosuppressive agent that inhibits IL-1-dependent lymphocyte proliferation. J Immunol 1988; 140:3026–3032.

71. Schaffer MR, Tantry U, Gross SS, Wasserburg HL, Barbul A. Nitric oxide regulates wound healing. J Surg Res 1996; 63:237–240.

72. Jimenez SA, Freundlich B, Rosenbloom J. Selective inhibition of human diploid fibroblast collagen synthesis by interferons. J Clin Invest 1984; 74:1112–1116.

73. Bachwich PR, Chensue SW, Larrick JW, Kunkel SL. Tumor necrosis factor stimulates interleukin-1 and prostaglandin E2 production in resting macrophages. Biochem Biophys Res Commun 1986; 136:94–101.

74. Grotendorst GR, Pencev D, Martin GR et al. Molecular mediators of tissue repair. New York: Praeger, 1984.

75. Gospodarowicz D, Neufeld G, Schweigerer L. Fibroblast growth factor: structural and biological properties. J Cell Physiol Suppl 1987; (suppl 5):15–26.

76. Gospodarowicz D, Abraham JA, Schilling J. Isolation and characterization of a vascular endothelial cell mitogen produced by pituitary-derived folliculo stellate cells. Proc Natl Acad Sci USA 1989; 86:7311–7315.

77. Shing Y, Folkman J, Sullivan R, Butterfield C, Murray J, Klagsbrun M. Heparin affinity: purification of a tumor-derived capillary endothelial cell growth factor. Science 1984; 223:1296–1299.

78. Postlethwaite AE, Keski-Oja J, Moses HL, Kang AH. Stimulation of the chemotactic migration of human fibroblasts by transforming growth factor beta. J Exp Med 1987; 165:251–256.

79. Westermark B, Blomquist E. Stimulation of fibroblast migration by epidermal growth factor. Cell Biol Int Rep 1980; 4:649–654.

80. Singer II, Scott S, Kawka DW, Kazazis DM, Gailit J, Ruoslahti E. Cell surface distribution of fibronectin and vitronectin receptors depends on substrate composition and extracellular matrix accumulation. J Cell Biol 1988; 106:2171–2182.

81. Hynes RO. Integrins: versatility, modulation, and signaling in cell adhesion. Cell 1992; 69:11–25.

82. Ahlen K, Rubin K. Platelet-derived growth factor-BB stimulates synthesis of the integrin alpha 2-subunit in human diploid fibroblasts. Exp Cell Res 1994; 215:347–353.

83. Gailit J, Xu J, Bueller H, Clark RA. Platelet-derived growth factor and inflammatory cytokines have differential effects on the expression of integrins alpha 1 beta 1 and alpha 5 beta 1 by human dermal fibroblasts in vitro. J Cell Physiol 1996; 169:281–289.

84. Parks WC. Matrix metalloproteinases in repair. Wound Repair Regen 1999; 7:423–432.

85. Reed MJ, Puolakkainen P, Lane TF, Dickerson D, Bornstein P, Sage EH. Differential expression of SPARC and thrombospondin 1 in wound repair: immunolocalization and in situ hybridization. J Histochem Cytochem 1993; 41:1467–1477.

86. Werb Z, Tremble P, Damsky CH. Regulation of extracellular matrix degradation by cell-extracellular matrix interactions. Cell Differ Dev 1990; 32:299–306.

87. Hassell JR, Kimura JH, Hascall VC. Proteoglycan core protein families. Annu Rev Biochem 1986; 55:539–567.

88. Gabbiani G, Ryan GB, Majne G. Presence of modified fibroblasts in granulation tissue and their possible role in wound contraction. Experientia 1971; 27:549–550.

89. Ehrlich HP. Wound closure: evidence of cooperation between fibroblasts and collagen matrix. Eye 1988; 2(Pt 2):149–157.

90. Bellows CG, Melcher AH, Aubin JE. Association between tension and orientation of periodontal ligament fibroblasts and exogenous collagen fibres in collagen gels in vitro. J Cell Sci 1982; 58:125–138.

91. Bullard KM, Sylvester K, Yang E, Sheppard D, Herlyn M, Adzick N. Epithelial integrin expression is rapidly upregulated in human fetal wound repair. Surg Res 1999; 84:31–34.

92. Gharaee-Kermani M, Phan SH. Role of cytokines and cytokine therapy in wound healing and fibrotic diseases. Curr Pharm Des 2001; 7:1083–1103.

93. Granstein RD, Murphy GF, Margolis RJ, Byrne MH, Amento EP. Gamma-interferon inhibits collagen synthesis in vivo in the mouse. J Clin Invest 1987; 79:1254–1258.

94. Buck M, Houglum K, Chojkier M. Tumor necrosis factor-alpha inhibits collagen alpha1(I) gene expression and wound healing in a murine model of cachexia. Am J Pathol 1996; 149:195–204.

95. Brew K, Dinakarpandian D, Nagase H. Tissue inhibitors of metalloproteinases: evolution, structure and function. Biochim Biophys Acta 2000; 1477:267–283.

96. Fahey TJ III, Sadaty A, Jones WG II, Barber A, Smoller B, Shires GT. Diabetes impairs the late inflammatory response to wound healing. J Surg Res 1991; 50:308–313.

97. Bullard KM, Lund L, Mudgett JS, Mellin TN, Hunt TK, Murphy B, Ronan J, Werb Z, Banda MJ. Impaired wound contraction in stromelysin-1-deficient mice. Ann Surg 1999; 230:260–265.

98. Robson MC, Heggers J. Eicosanoids, cytokines and free radicals. In: Diegelmann R, Lindblad W, eds. Wound Healing: Biochemical and Clinical Aspects. Philadelphia: W.B. Saunders Company, 1992:292–304.

99. Hunt TK, Zederfeldt B, Goldstick TK. Oxygen and healing. Am J Surg 1969; 118:521–525.

100. Stadelmann WK, Digenis AG, Tobin GR. Impediments to wound healing. Am J Surg 1998; 176:39S–47S.

101. Xia YP, Zhao Y, Tyrone JW, Chen A, Mustoe TA. Differential activation of migration by hypoxia in keratinocytes isolated from donors of increasing age: implication for chronic wounds in the elderly. J Invest Dermatol 2001; 116:50–56.

102. Knighton DR, Hunt TK, Scheuenstuhl H, Halliday BJ, Werb Z, Banda MJ. Oxygen tension regulates the expression of angiogenesis factor by macrophages. Science 1983; 221:1283–1285.

103. Jurkiewicz MJ, Garrett LP. Studies on the influence of anemia on wound healing. Am Surg 1964; 30:23–25.

104. Macon WL, Pories WJ. The effect of iron deficiency anemia on wound healing. Surgery 1971; 69:792–796.

105. Bains JW, Crawford DT, Ketcham AS. Effect of chronic anemia on wound tensile strength: correlation with blood volume, total red blood cell volume and proteins. Ann Surg 1966; 164:243–246.

106. Chvapil M, Koopmann CF Jr. Age and other factors regulating wound healing. Otolaryngol Clin North Am 1982; 15:259–270.

107. Danon D, Kowatch MA, Roth GS. Promotion of wound repair in old mice by local injection of macrophages. Proc Natl Acad Sci USA 1989; 86:2018–2020.

108. Shimomura H, Spiro RG. Studies on macromolecular components of human glomerular basement membrane and alterations in diabetes. Decreased levels of heparan sulfate proteoglycan and laminin. Diabetes 1987; 36:374–381.

109. Goodson WH III, Hunt TK. Wound healing and the diabetic patient. Surg Gynecol Obstet 1979; 149:600–608.

110. Kamal K, Powell RJ, Sumpio BE. The pathobiology of diabetes mellitus: implications for surgeons. J Am Coll Surg 1996; 183:271–289.

111. Greene DA, Lattimer SA, Sima AA. Sorbitol, phosphoinositides, and sodium-potassium-ATPase in the pathogenesis of diabetic complications. N Engl J Med 1987; 316:599–606.

112. Winegrad AI. Banting lecture 1986. Does a common mechanism induce the diverse complications of diabetes? Diabetes 1987; 36:396–406.

113. Tesfamariam B. Role of sorbitol and myoinositol in the endothelial cells dysfunction caused by elevated glucose. In: Fed Proc; 1990:A867.

114. Lee TS, Saltsman KA, Ohashi H, King GL. Activation of protein kinase C by elevation of glucose concentration: proposal for a mechanism in the development of diabetic vascular complications. Proc Natl Acad Sci USA 1989; 86:5141–5145.

115. Brownlee M, Cerami A, Vlassara H. Advanced glycosylation end products in tissue and the biochemical basis of diabetic complications. N Engl J Med 1988; 318:1315–1321.

116. Yan SD, Schmidt AM, Anderson GM, Zhang J, Brett J, Zou YS, Pinsky D, Stern D. Enhanced cellular oxidant stress by the interaction of advanced glycation end products with their receptors/binding proteins. J Biol Chem 1994; 269:9889–9897.

117. Kirstein M, Brett J, Radoff S, Ogawa S, Stern D, Vlassara H. Advanced protein glycosylation induces transendothelial human monocyte chemotaxis and secretion of platelet-derived growth factor: role in vascular disease of diabetes and aging. Proc Natl Acad Sci USA 1990; 87:9010–9014.

118. Vlassara H, Brownlee M, Manogue KR, Dinarello CA, Pasagian A. Cachectin/TNF and IL-1 induced by glucose-modified proteins: role in normal tissue remodeling. Science 1988; 240:1546–1548.

119. Lubec G, Pollak A. Reduced susceptibility of nonenzymatically glucosylated glomerular basement membrane to proteases: is thickening of diabetic glomerular basement membranes due to reduced proteolytic degradation? Ren Physiol 1980; 3:4–8.

120. Hammes HP, Martin S, Federlin K, Geisen K, Brownlee M. Aminoguanidine treatment inhibits the development of experimental diabetic retinopathy. Proc Natl Acad Sci USA 1991; 88:11555–11558.

121. Soulis-Liparota T, Cooper M, Papazoglou D, Clarke B, Jerums G. Retardation by aminoguanidine of development of albuminuria, mesangial expansion, and tissue fluorescence in streptozocin-induced diabetic rat. Diabetes 1991; 40:1328–1334.

122. Brown DL, Kane CD, Chernausek SD, Greenhalgh DG. Differential expression and localization of insulin-like growth factors I and II in cutaneous wounds of diabetic and nondiabetic mice. Am J Pathol 1997; 151:715–724.

123. Frank S, Hubner G, Breier G, Longaker MT, Greenhalgh DG, Werner S. Regulation of vascular endothelial growth factor expression in cultured keratinocytes. Implications for normal and impaired wound healing. J Biol Chem 1995; 270:12607–12613.

124. Werner S, Breeden M, Hubner G, Greenhalgh DG, Longaker MT. Induction of keratinocyte growth factor expression is reduced and delayed during wound healing in the genetically diabetic mouse. J Invest Dermatol 1994; 103:469–473.

125. Meyer NA, Barrow RE, Herndon DN. Combined insulin-like growth factor-1 and growth hormone improves weight loss and wound healing in burned rats. J Trauma 1996; 41:1008–1012.

126. Pierre EJ, Perez-Polo JR, Mitchell AT, Matin S, Foyt HL, Herndon DN. Insulin-like growth factor-I liposomal gene transfer and systemic growth hormone stimulate wound healing. J Burn Care Rehabil 1997; 18:287–291.

127. Dempsey DT, Mullen JL, Buzby GP. The link between nutritional status and clinical outcome: can nutritional intervention modify it? Am J Clin Nutr 1988; 47:352–356.

128. Jeschke MG, Herndon DN, Ebener C, Barrow RE, Jauch KW. Nutritional intervention high in vitamins, protein, amino acids, and omega3 fatty acids improves protein metabolism during the hypermetabolic state after thermal injury. Arch Surg 2001; 136:1301–1306.

129. Burns JL, Mancoll JS, Phillips LG. Impairments to wound healing. Clin Plast Surg 2003; 30:47–56.

130. Ehrlich HP, Hunt TK. Effects of cortisone and vitamin A on wound healing. Ann Surg 1968; 167:324–328.

131. Hunt TK. Disorders of wound healing. World J Surg 1980; 4:271–277.

132. Hayashi K, Frangieh G, Wolf G, Kenyon KR. Expression of transforming growth factor-beta in wound healing of vitamin A-deficient rat corneas. Invest Ophthalmol Vis Sci 1989; 30:239–247.

133. Freiman M, Seifter E, Connerton C, Levenson SM. Vitamin A deficiency and surgical stress. Surg Forum 1970; 21:81–82.

134. Ross AC. Vitamin A and protective immunity. Nutr Today 1992; 27:18.

135. Hunt A. The role of vitamin C in wound healing. Br J Surg 1940; 28:436.

136. Prasad ÀS, Oberleas D. Changes in activities of zinc-dependent enzymes in zinc-deficient tissues of rats. J Appl Physiol 1971; 31:842–846.

137. Wenk J, Foitzik A, Achterberg V, Sabiwalsky A, Dissemond J, Meewes C, Reitz A, Brenneisen P, Wlaschek M, Meyer-Ingold W, Scharffetter-Kochanek K. Selective pick-up of increased iron by deferoxamine-coupled cellulose abrogates the iron-driven induction of matrix-degrading metalloproteinase 1 and lipid peroxidation in human dermal fibroblasts *in vitro*: a new dressing concept. J Invest Dermatol 2001; 116:833–839.

138. Ehrlich HP, Hunt TK. The effects of cortisone and anabolic steroids on the tensile strength of healing wounds. Ann Surg 1969; 170:203–206.

139. Riley GP, Cox M, Harrall RL, Clements S, Hazleman BL. Inhibition of tendon cell proliferation and matrix glycosaminoglycan synthesis by non-steroidal anti-inflammatory drugs *in vitro*. J Hand Surg (Br) 2001; 26:224–228.

140. Lazarus GS, Cooper DM, Knighton DR, Margolis DJ, Pecoraro RE, Rodeheaver G, Robson MC. Definitions and guidelines for assessment of wounds and evaluation of healing. Arch Dermatol 1994; 130:489–493.

141. Fu X, Shen Z, Chen Y, Xie J, Guo Z, Zhang M, Sheng Z. Randomised placebo-controlled trial of use of topical recombinant bovine basic fibroblast growth factor for second-degree burns. Lancet 1998; 352:1661–1664.

3

Principles in Management of Acute Burns

STEVEN E. WOLF, DAVID N. HERNDON

University of Texas Medical Branch and Shriners Burn Hospital, Galveston, Texas, USA

I. INTRODUCTION

Mortality due to major burn has improved, so much so that most young patients who are burned without significant comorbidities should be expected to survive, regardless of burn severity (1). These improvements were probably due to prevention strategies resulting in fewer burns of lesser severity, as well as significant progress in treatment techniques. Probably the most significant advance in patient care was the institution of excision and grafting to remove the inflammatory nidus of eschar and to accelerate recovery.

Dr. Cope and others first espoused early excision and grafting for treatment of the acutely burned in the 1940s (2), initially as a means of accelerating time to healing (3). Oftentimes, this required application of a temporary biological dressing such as cadaveric skin (4). These initial efforts led to the practice followed by most burn centers, which is to excise the majority of the wound within the first week after injury. Coverage of the wound after excision is with a mixture of available autograft and/or cadaver skin or a synthetic skin substitute. This chapter is devoted to the description of techniques of wound closure with considerations for survival first, followed by function, and last, cosmesis. Of course, survival, function, and cosmesis all enter into decisions regarding the choice of wound closure, recognizing that the appearance of the scar in survivors will be present for the rest of his or her life. Knowledge of the effects, appearance, and functionality of different wound closure techniques is then paramount for the surgeon.

II. BURN MORTALITY

Over one million people suffer from burn injuries in the United States each year, most of which are minor and treated in the outpatient ward. Almost all of these people

43

are treated as outpatients, and do not require operative treatment. However, ~60,000 burns per year are more severe and require hospitalization, and roughly 3000 of these patients die (5). Most of these will require operations for timely burn wound closure to prevent infection as well as allow for timely return to normal function.

Improved patient care in the severely burned, including operative strategy and techniques, has undoubtedly improved survival, particularly in children. Bull and Fisher first reported in 1952 the expected 50% mortality rate for burn sizes in several age groups based on data from their unit. They reported that approximately one-half of children aged 0–14 with burns of 49% total body surface area (TBSA) would die, 46% TBSA for patients aged 15–44, 27% TBSA for those of age 45 and 64, and 10% TBSA for those aged ≥65 years (6). These dismal statistics have drastically improved, with the latest reports indicating 50% mortality for 98% TBSA burns in children under 15, and 75% TBSA burns in other young age groups (7,8). Therefore, a healthy young patient with a burn of any size might be expected to survive (9). The same cannot be said, however, for those aged ≥45 years, where the improvements have been much more modest, especially in the elderly (10). Between 1971 and 1991, burn deaths in the United States decreased by 40%, with a concomitant 12% decrease in deaths associated with inhalation injury (11). Since 1991, burn deaths per capita have decreased another 25% according to Centers for Disease Control statistics (www.cdc.gov/ncipc/wisqars).

Reasons for these dramatic improvements in mortality after burn that are related to treatment include increased understanding of resuscitation, better support of the hypermetabolic response to injury, and probably, most important, control of wound complications through aggressive operative excision and closure of the burn wound. Recently, it was found that total excision and grafting of the burn wound within 72 h of injury decreased wound complications, sepsis, and hospital length of stay (12). The dramatic effect of the practice of early wound excision on burn mortality cannot be overemphasized. Further improvements of this magnitude in the future are likely to be in the area of faster and better return of function, and improved cosmetic outcomes.

III. RESUSCITATION AND INITIAL ASSESSMENT

Before wound closure can be entertained, resuscitation from burn shock must commence to support the patient through the ravages of fluid shifts, edema formation, and organ dyshomeostasis. Before undergoing specific treatment, burned patients must be removed from the source of injury and the burning process stopped. Inhalation

injury should always be suspected and 100% oxygen should be given by facemask. Burning clothing should be extinguished and removed as soon as possible to prevent further injury. All rings, watches, jewelry, and belts should be removed as they retain heat and can produce a tourniquet-like effect. Water at room temperature can be poured on the wound within 15 min of injury to decrease the depth of the wound, but any subsequent measures to cool the wound should be avoided to prevent hypothermia during resuscitation.

After arrival at the hospital, attention should be first drawn to the airway. Exposure to heated gases and smoke may result in damage to the upper respiratory tract with direct injury to the upper airway causing edema and obstruction to the passage of air. Loss of the airway is the most common cause of death in the early phases of burn assessment and resuscitation. Harbingers of airway injury include facial burns, singed nasal hairs, carbonaceous sputum, and tachypnea.

Progressive hoarseness is a sign of impending airway obstruction, and endotracheal intubation should be instituted early before edema distorts the upper airway anatomy. This is especially important in patients with massive burns, who may appear to breathe without problems early in the resuscitation period until several liters of volume are given resulting in significant airway edema. If any question is raised regarding the security of the airway, the patient should be intubated.

A. Initial Wound Care

Prehospital care of the burn wound is basic and simple because it requires only protection from the environment with application of a clean dry dressing or sheet to cover the involved part. Damp dressings should not be used. The patient should be wrapped in a blanket to minimize heat loss and for temperature control during transport. The first step in diminishing pain is to cover the wounds to prevent contact with exposed nerve endings. Intramuscular or subcutaneous narcotic injections for pain should never be used because drug absorption is decreased as a result of the peripheral vasoconstriction. This might become a problem later when the patient is resuscitated, and vasodilation increases absorption of the narcotic depot with resulting apnea. Small doses of intravenous morphine may be given after complete assessment of the patient and after it is determined to be safe by an experienced practitioner. Application of salves or other treatments should be withheld at this point, as infection will not ensue in the few hours until definitive care is provided, and such treatments may actually obscure the wound such that those responsible for the final care of the wound are unable to make a correct assessment.

B. Resuscitation

Adequate resuscitation of the burned patient depends on the establishment and maintenance of reliable intravenous access. Increased times to beginning resuscitation of burned patients result in poorer outcomes, and delays should be minimized. Venous access is best attained through short peripheral catheters in unburned skin; however, veins in burned skin can be used and are preferable to no intravenous access. Superficial veins are often thrombosed in full-thickness injuries and, therefore, are not suitable for cannulation. Saphenous vein cutdowns are useful in cases of difficult access and are used in preference to central vein cannulation because of lower complication rates. In children <6 years of age, experienced practitioners can use intramedullary access in the proximal tibia until intravenous access is accomplished. Lactated Ringer's solution without dextrose is the fluid of choice except in children <2 years, who should receive 5% dextrose Ringer's lactate. The initial rate can be rapidly estimated by multiplying the TBSA burned by the patient's weight in kilograms and then dividing by 8. Thus, the rate of infusion for an 80 kg man with a 40% TBSA burn would be 80 kg $\times$ 40% TBSA/8 = 400 mL/h. This rate should be continued until a formal calculation of resuscitation needs to be performed.

Many formulas have been devised to determine the proper amount of fluid to give a burned patient, all originating from experimental studies on the pathophysiology of burn shock. Baxter (13) established the basis for modern fluid resuscitation protocols culminating in the Parkland formula for burn resuscitation that is now used around the world as an estimate for intravenous fluid needs after severe burn. This formula is $2-4 \text{ cm}^3/\text{kg}$ per %TBSA burned with half to be given in the first 8 h after injury, and the rest in the subsequent 16 h. Because of differences in weight per body surface area in children, different formulas have been devised for them based on body surface area. Suggested intravenous resuscitation for children is $5000 \text{ cm}^3/\text{m}^2$ burned plus an additional $1500 \text{ cm}^3/\text{m}^2$ TBSA for maintenance needs. Again, one-half of the volume should be given in the first 8 h from burn and the rest in the ensuing 16 h. These estimates are guidelines for the amount of volume that may be required. Monitoring of urine output with a urinary catheter should be done, with hourly modifications made in the infusion rate to attain a goal of $1-2 \text{ cm}^3/\text{kg}$ per hour assuming normal renal function. In the absence of normal renal function, central monitoring of venous pressures can assist in volume estimates.

Some elect to use albumin during resuscitation to decrease volumes; however, recently the use of albumin during intravenous resuscitation has come under criticism. The Cochrane group showed in a meta-analysis of 31 trials that the risk of death was higher in burned patients receiving albumin than in those receiving crystalloid, with a relative risk of death at 2.40 (95% confidence interval 1.11–5.19 (14). Another meta-analysis of all critically ill patients refuted this finding, showing no differences in relative risk between albumin-treated and crystalloid-treated groups (15). In fact, as quality of the trials improved, the relative risks were reduced. Recent evidence suggests that albumin supplementation even after resuscitation does not affect the distribution of fluid among the intracellular/extracellular compartments (16). What we can conclude from these trials and meta-analyses is that albumin used during resuscitation is at best equal to crystalloid, and at worst detrimental to the outcome of burned patients. For these reasons, we cannot recommend the use of albumin during resuscitation.

To combat any regurgitation with an intestinal ileus, a nasogastric tube should be inserted in all patients with major burns to decompress the stomach. This is especially important for all patients being transported in aircraft at high altitudes. Additionally, all patients should be restricted from taking anything by mouth until the transfer has been completed. Decompression of the stomach is usually necessary because the apprehensive patient will swallow considerable amounts of air and distend the stomach.

Recommendations for tetanus prophylaxis are based on the condition of the wound and the patient's immunization history. All patients with burns of $>10\%$ TBSA should receive 0.5 mL tetanus toxoid. If prior immunization is absent or unclear, or the last booster dose was >10 years ago, 250 units of tetanus immunoglobulin is also given.

C. Escharotomies

When deep second- and third-degree burn wounds encompass the circumference of an extremity, peripheral circulation to the limb can be compromised. Development of generalized edema beneath a nonyielding eschar impedes venous outflow and eventually affects arterial inflow to the distal beds. This can be recognized by numbness and tingling in the limb and increased pain in the digits. Arterial flow can be assessed by determination of Doppler signals in the digital arteries and the palmar and plantar arches in affected extremities. It should be noted, however, that presence of a Doppler signal does not mean the extremity is not at risk for ischemic complications. Capillary refill can also be assessed. Extremities at risk are identified either on clinical examination or on measurement of tissue pressures >40 mmHg. These extremities require escharotomies, which are releases of the burn eschar performed at the bedside by incising the lateral and medial aspects of the extremity with a scalpel or electrocautery unit. The entire constricting eschar must be incised longitudinally to completely relieve the impediment to blood flow. The incisions are carried down onto the thenar and hypothenar eminences, and along the dorsolateral sides of the digits to completely open the hand if it is involved (Fig. 3.1). If it is clear that the wound will require excision and grafting because of its depth, escharotomies are safest to restore perfusion to the underlying nonburned tissues until formal excision. If vascular compromise has been prolonged, reperfusion after an escharotomy may cause reactive hyperemia and further edema formation in the muscle, making continued surveillance of the distal extremities necessary. Increased muscle compartment pressures may necessitate fasciotomies. The most common complications associated with these procedures are blood loss and the release of anaerobic metabolites, causing transient

hypotension. If distal perfusion does not improve with these measures, central hypotension from hypovolemia should be suspected and treated.

A constricting truncal eschar can cause a similar phenomenon, except that the effect is to decrease ventilation by limiting chest excursion. Any decrease in ventilation of a burn patient should be followed by inspection of the chest with appropriate escharotomies to relieve the constriction and allow adequate tidal volumes. This need becomes evident in a patient on a volume control ventilator whose peak airway pressures increase. In some cases, abdominal constriction and bowel edema may result in abdominal compartment syndrome, requiring laparotomy to restore central organ perfusion. Measurement of bladder pressures >30 mmHg is a reasonable indication for this treatment. A word of caution should be mentioned, in that our experience dictates that excision

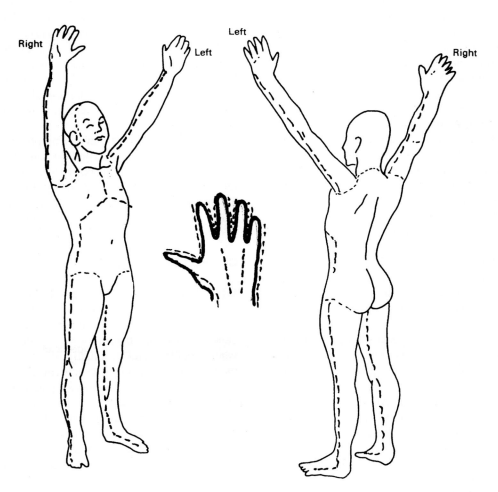

Figure 3.1 Placement of escharotomies. Incisions should be made in the eschar on the medial and lateral aspects of the extremities, hands, and fingers in those areas with significant constriction and tissue ischemia. In the presence of clear circumferential full-thickness wounds, escharotomy should be done with little provocation as the wounds will be excised after resuscitation, and thus no risk of additional scarring is present.

of the burn wound often decreases bladder pressure in this situation, obviating the need for open laparotomy and its attendant complications.

D. Initial Wound Assessment

Once efforts at resuscitation are successful, definitive care of the wound can commence. Burn wounds can be roughly categorized into two classes, partial thickness and full thickness. Partial-thickness wounds will generally heal by local treatment with skin substitutes or topical antimicrobials, and therefore do not require operative treatment. Full-thickness and very deep partial-thickness wounds, however, will require other treatments to garner timely wound healing. Since all the elements of the epidermis have been obliterated in full-thickness wounds, healing can occur only through wound contraction and/or spreading of epithelialization from the wound edges. In a wound >3 cm, this process will take weeks to months to years to complete. In order to accelerate this process, the technique of skin grafting with the necessary keratinocytes from other parts of the body can be used.

The depth of burn varies depending on the degree of tissue damage. Burn depth is classified into degree of injury in the epidermis, dermis, subcutaneous fat, and underlying structures (Fig. 3.2). First-degree burns are, by definition, injury confined to the epidermis. These burns are painful, erythematous, and blanch to the touch with an intact epidermal barrier. Examples include

sunburn or a minor scald from a kitchen accident. These burns do not result in scarring, and treatment is aimed at comfort with the use of topical soothing salves with or without aloe and oral nonsteroidal anti-inflammatory agents. Generally, no long-term sequelae or scarring is expected from these injuries, and therefore no specific treatments are required.

Second-degree burns are partial-thickness burns divided into two types, superficial and deep. All second-degree burns have some degree of dermal damage, and the division is based on the depth of injury into this structure. Superficial dermal burns are erythematous, painful, blanch to touch, and often blister. Examples include scald injuries from overheated bathtub water and flash flame burns from open carburetors. These wounds spontaneously re-epithelialize from retained epidermal structures in the rete ridges, hair follicles, and sweat glands in 7–14 days. After healing, these burns may have some slight skin discoloration over the long term. Deep dermal burns into the reticular dermis appear more pale and mottled, do not blanch to touch, but remain painful to pinprick. These burns heal in 14–35 days by re-epithelialization from hair follicles and sweat gland keratinocytes, often with severe scarring as a result of the loss of significant portions of the dermis.

Third-degree burns are full thickness through the epidermis and dermis, and are characterized by a hard leathery eschar that is painless and black, white, or cherry red in color. No epidermal or dermal appendages remain; thus,

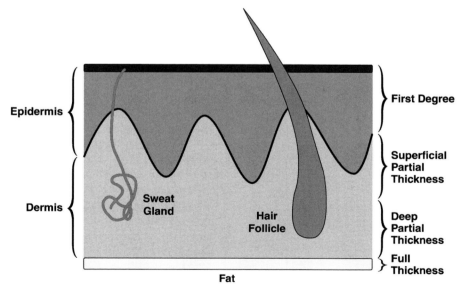

Figure 3.2 Burn depth. Burns cause tissue damage that can be classified based on the depth of that damage. First-degree burns are limited to the epidermis. Superficial partial thickness burns are limited to the epidermis and superficial dermis. Deep partial thickness wounds extend into the deep reticular dermis. Full-thickness burns extend through the dermis, leaving no viable skin appendages and thus no keratinocyte rests.

these wounds must heal by re-epithelialization from the wound edges. Deep dermal and full-thickness burns require excision with skin grafting from the patient in order to heal the wounds in a timely fashion. Fourth-degree burns involve other organs beneath the skin, such as muscle, bone, and brain.

Currently, burn depth is most accurately assessed by judgment of experienced practitioners. Accurate determination of depth is critical because wounds that will heal with local treatment are treated differently from those requiring operative intervention. Examination of the entire wound by the physicians ultimately responsible for their management then is the "gold standard" used to guide further treatment decisions. New technologies, such as the multisensor heatable laser Doppler flowmeter, hold promise for quantitatively determining burn depth. Several recent reports claim superiority of this method over clinical judgment in the determination of wounds requiring skin grafting for timely healing (Fig. 3.3), which may lead to a change in the standard of care in the near future (17–19).

E. Burn Size

Determination of burn size estimates the extent of injury. Burn size is generally assessed by the "rule of nines" (Fig. 3.4). In adults, each upper extremity and the head and neck are 9% of the TBSA, the lower extremities and

the anterior and posterior trunk are 18% each, and the perineum and genitalia are assumed to be 1% of the TBSA. Another method of estimating smaller burns is to equate the area of the open hand (including the palm and the extended fingers) of the patient to be ~1% TBSA and then to transpose that measurement visually onto the wound for a determination of its size. This method is helpful when evaluating splash burns and other burns of mixed distribution.

Children have a relatively larger portion of the body surface area in the head and neck, which is compensated for by a relatively smaller surface area in the lower extremities. Infants have 21% of the TBSA in the head and neck and 13% in each leg, which incrementally approaches the adult proportions with increasing age. The Berkow formula is used to accurately determine burn size in children (Table 3.1).

IV. INITIAL WOUND MANAGEMENT AND OPERATIVE PLANNING

Once resuscitation is under way and the patient is physiologically settled, wound care can begin. Each patient will have burns differing in their distribution and depth, necessitating individualized planning for wound treatment. The most important initial assessment is whether the burns are partial or full thickness and the extent of the injury as the considerations for survival, function, and cosmesis differ.

Partial thickness burns in general will heal spontaneously from retained cellular elements with a minimum of contracture. However, changes in skin contour and color are common, which may be addressed in the reconstructive period after complete healing. The initial treatment of partial-thickness burns is usually accomplished by dressing changes with antimicrobial salves such as Silvadene® or Bacitracin® or new silver impregnated dressings until epithelialization is complete. Alternatively, partial-thickness burns can be treated with artificial skin coverings such as Biobrane® (Bertek, East Amherst, NY), or TransCyte® (Smith and Nephew, Largo, FL) to diminish pain and dressing changes (20,21).

In partial-thickness burns over 40% of the TBSA, some follow the practice of taking the patient to the operating theater for sharp debridement and coverage with cadaveric skin. This treatment has the inherent advantages of immediate coverage of the wound with an immunologically active substance, thus providing a potential advantage in terms of resistance to infection. The disadvantage to this treatment is the incorporation of cadaver dermis into the skin after epithelialization resulting in cosmetically distasteful contour abnormalities, particularly if meshed cadaveric skin is used. To avoid this, a skin substitute such as Biobrane could be used. Second, sharp

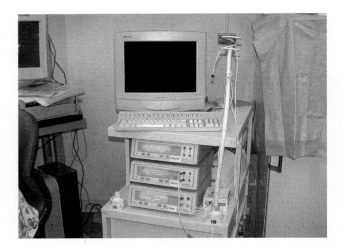

Figure 3.3 Laser Doppler. This machine consists of a monitor, software/hardware, and a heatable laser probe that uses Doppler technology to estimate blood flow in a tissue. The probe used for the skin has seven separate sensors that are integrated with a heat source that stabilizes skin temperature to reduce variability in measurements. The probe is placed lightly on the skin while the measurements are being made. Partial-thickness wounds will have higher blood flows, and full-thickness injuries lower blood flows compared to normal skin.

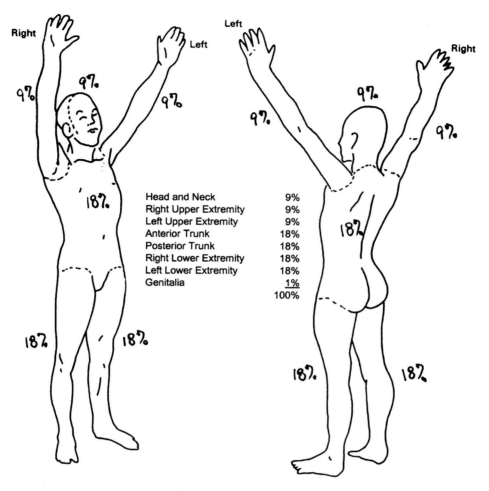

Head and Neck 9%
Right Upper Extremity 9%
Left Upper Extremity 9%
Anterior Trunk 18%
Posterior Trunk 18%
Right Lower Extremity 18%
Left Lower Extremity 18%
Genitalia .... <u>1%</u>
100%

Figure 3.4   Rule of nines.

debridement in the operating room will remove some viable dermal elements, thus putting the wound at greater risk for scarring. Regardless, this treatment should be considered in those at risk of death, such as those with significant comorbidities to diminish mortality risk.

The other extreme is the finding of full-thickness burns throughout. These wounds do not heal in a timely fashion without autografting, which must be done in the operating theater. In fact, the practice of leaving these dead tissues only serves as a nidus for inflammation and infection that could lead to the patient's death. Most burn surgeons currently practice early excision and grafting of these wounds within the first week of injury. The technique of early excision and grafting has made conservative treatment of full-thickness wounds a practice to be used only in the elderly and in the infrequent cases in which anesthesia and surgery are contraindicated.

When autografting is entertained, consideration must be given for donor sites. Optimally, donor sites are taken from "hidden" areas that are not normally visible with clothing. Such sites include the buttocks, upper thighs, lower trunk, and scalp. Another consideration is for color match of the donor skin and the area to graft. Generally, skin above the clavicles has less pigment than that below; therefore, efforts should be made to graft areas on the head and neck with donor sites above the clavicle (scalp or posterior auricular skin).

Once donor sites have been identified, plans for taking the skin should be made. It was found long ago that wound closure with full-thickness skin grafts containing a complete epidermis and dermis provide for the best outcomes in terms of wound contraction, appearance, and pliability. Unfortunately, full-thickness grafts are limited in acute wound closure because the donor site must be closed primarily and is only available for one-time use. The corollary of this finding as a general principle is that a split-thickness graft with increasing levels of dermis should provide the best functional and cosmetic outcomes. Split-thickness donor sites will heal spontaneously from retained rete ridges and hair follicles, and

Table 3.1 Berkow Diagram to Estimate Burn Size Based on Area of Burn in an Isolated Body Part

Area	0–1 years	1–4 years	5–9 years	10–14 years	15–18 years	Adult
Head	19	17	13	11	9	7
Neck	2	2	2	2	2	2
Anterior trunk	13	13	13	13	13	13
Posterior trunk	13	13	13	13	13	13
Right buttock	2.5	2.5	2.5	2.5	2.5	2.5
Left buttock	2.5	2.5	2.5	2.5	2.5	2.5
Genitalia	1	1	1	1	1	1
Right upper arm	4	4	4	4	4	4
Left upper arm	4	4	4	4	4	4
Right lower arm	3	3	3	3	3	3
Left lower arm	3	3	3	3	3	3
Right hand	2.5	2.5	2.5	2.5	2.5	2.5
Left hand	2.5	2.5	2.5	2.5	2.5	2.5
Right thigh	5.5	6.5	8	9	9	9.5
Left thigh	5.5	6.5	8	9	9	9.5
Right leg	5	5	5.5	3.5	6.5	7
Left leg	5	5	5.5	6.5	6.5	7
Right foot	3.5	3.5	3.5	3.5	3.5	3.5
Left foot	3.5	3.5	3.5	3.5	3.5	3.5

Note: Estimates are made and recorded, then summed to gain an accurate estimate of the body surface area burned.

so can be used over much greater donor site areas, and can be used repeatedly after re-epithelialization. These grafts can be taken at many depths, the deeper of which contain more dermis, and therefore when these are used as autografts will presumably have decreased scarring at the wound site. This concept, however, has recently been called into question. A study comparing standard thickness grafts (0.015 in.) to thick grafts (0.025 in.) applied to full-thickness hand wounds revealed no differences in range of motion, appearance, or patient satisfaction (22), making more research necessary to define the relevance of donor site depth.

The extent of donor sites to be taken is the next consideration. In general, only the required amount of donor site skin should be taken so as to minimize donor site scarring. Donor site skin will contract somewhat after harvesting because of the elastic properties of skin. Therefore, donor site and wound cannot be matched one to one. Donor site skin can be expanded with meshing in various degrees (1:1, 2:1, 4:1, and 9:1) using commercially available devices. A benefit of this management is the ability to expand the donor site to minimize donor site in small wounds, or expand the donor site when large burns limit it. Another benefit is the presence of interstices in the grafted skin that allows for drainage of wound exudate to improve graft take. The risk of meshing donor sites lies in functional and cosmetic deficits from greater contracture to close the interstices and the persistence of a meshed pattern on the skin, which the patient will wear for the rest of his or her life. This may not be a

problem in cosmetically less important areas such as the thighs or back, but in cosmetically important areas such as the face and hands it is not satisfactory. Choosing donor site location, amount, and treatment then cannot be readily standardized but must conform to the needs of the individual patient.

Wounds covering <20% TBSA can usually be closed at one operation with autograft split-thickness skin taken from the patient's available donor sites. In these operations, the skin grafts are not meshed, or they are meshed with a narrow ratio (2:1 or less), to maximize cosmetic outcome. Survival is generally not in question in the minor to moderate burns, therefore cosmesis should receive more emphasis. Consideration should be given in preoperative planning to donor site morbidity. These sites will also scar, usually with just some skin discoloration and/or minor contour deficits; therefore, consideration might be given toward staging closure into two operations where hidden donor sites can be maximized by repeat harvesting.

In major burns, reasonable amounts of autograft skin may be limited to the extent that the wound cannot be completely closed. Second, mortality risk is real in this population regardless of age, which can presumably be minimized with rapid wound closure. The availability of cadaver allograft skin has changed the course of modern burn treatment for these massive wounds. A typical method of treatment is to use widely expanded autografts (4:1 or greater) covered with cadaver allograft to completely close the wounds for which autograft is available. The 4:1 skin heals underneath the cadaver skin in ~21 days, and the cadaver skin falls off (Fig. 3.5). The portions of the wound that cannot be covered with even widely meshed autograft are covered with allograft skin in preparation for autografting when donor sites are healed. Ideally, areas with less cosmetic importance are covered with the widely meshed skin to close most of the wound before using nonmeshed grafts at later operations for the cosmetically important areas, such as the hands and face.

Once in the operating room, donor sites are taken first based on operative planning. As these are being laid out and/or meshed, the burn wound is excised. Attempts should be made to excise tangentially to optimize cosmetic outcome. A number of instruments are commonly used to perform these excisions (Fig. 3.6). Rarely, excision to the level of fascia is necessary to remove all nonviable tissue, or it may become necessary at subsequent operations for infectious complications. These excisions can be performed with tourniquet control, or with application of topical epinephrine and thrombin to minimize blood loss.

Most surgeons excise the burn wound in the first week, sometimes in serial operations by removing 20% of the burn wound per operation on subsequent days. Others remove the whole of the burn wound in one operative procedure; however, this can be limited by the development of hypothermia or continuing massive blood loss. It is our practice to perform the excision immediately after stabilization of the patient after injury, because blood loss diminishes if the operation can be done the first day. This finding may be due to the relative predominance of vasoconstrictive substances such as thromboxane and

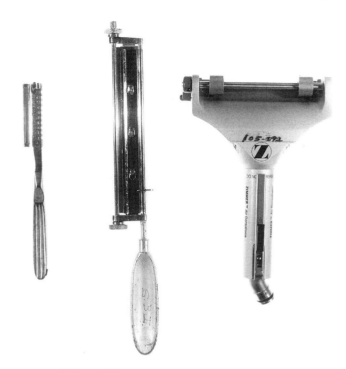

Figure 3.6 Knives used for eschar excision.

catecholamines, and the natural edema planes that develop immediately after the injury. When the wound becomes hyperemic after 2 days, blood loss can be a considerable problem.

Early excision should be reserved for full-thickness wounds. A deep partial-thickness burn can appear to be a third-degree wound at 48 h after injury, particularly if it has been treated with topical antimicrobials, which combine with wound fluid to form a dense pseudo eschar. A randomized prospective study comparing early excision vs. conservative therapy with late grafting of deep second-degree wounds showed that those excised early had more wound excised, more blood loss, and more time in the operating room. No difference in hospital length of stay or infection rate was seen (23). Long-term scarring and functional outcome, however, have not been examined in detail.

The intent of burn wound operations is to (1) remove devitalized tissue and (2) restore skin continuity. These are the only two things that must be accomplished. The techniques that can be used to achieve these goals are numerous, the choice of which is the challenge and art of burn surgery.

Once the technique for excision and closure of the wound is chosen, care must be taken to provide a technically sound result. Although in small burns, the use of local flaps for wound closure can be entertained, most significant burn wounds will require closure with skin grafts. These skin grafts are applied to wound beds where the cells

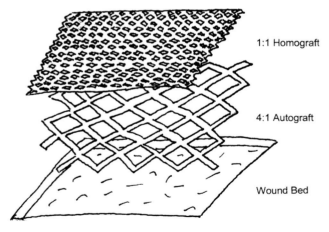

1:1 Homograft

4:1 Autograft

Wound Bed

Figure 3.5 4:1 Skin grafting technique. An excised wound bed (bottom) can be covered with autograft skin meshed 4:1 applied directly to the wound base. Wide interstices are then closed with overlying cadaveric homograft that will engraft and eventually separate with normal rejection.

of the graft are kept alive by nutrients in the serum produced by the wound bed until vascularization takes place 1–4 days after application. For this process to take place and for the skin graft to "take", four things are required:

- a viable wound bed
- no accumulation of fluid between the graft and the wound bed
- no shear stresses on the wound
- avoidance of massive microorganism proliferation

So, the performance of the selected technique must be reliable to ensure adequate outcome. Emphasis must be placed on adequate excision to a viable wound bed, then meticulous attention should be paid to placement of the grafts and adhering them to the wound bed. Lastly, selection and application of the dressing is more than just an exercise, as the dressing should be one that applies pressure to the wound to minimize dead space under the graft, minimizes shear stress, and provides antimicrobial properties. This portion of the operation is often overlooked, and if performed inadequately will lead to poor results.

Full-thickness wounds are optimally covered with autograft. In planning autograft coverage, the smaller the mesh ratio, the better the cosmetic outcome (sheets >1:1 > 2:1 > 4:1 > 9:1). However, this must be weighed against how much autograft is available and how much wound is present. Generally, if the amount of autograft is insufficient to close the wound if applied in sheets or 1:1 mesh ratio, a 2:1 ratio should be considered. If even this is insufficient, 4:1 or 9:1 ratios should be considered. We usually try to limit 4:1 or 9:1 ratios to coverage of the trunk, thighs, and upper arms for cosmetic reasons. An estimate can be made of how much autograft skin will be required for 4:1 closure of the trunk, thighs, and upper arms. This amount of autograft is then meshed in that fashion. The rest of the autograft skin is then meshed in a smaller ratio and applied to other areas. If even widely expanded autografts are insufficient to close the wounds, the remaining open areas should be treated with application of homografts. These can be removed at subsequent operations with application of autograft taken from the available donor sites that have healed. When donor sites have been taken at 10/1000ths of an inch, the donor sites usually heal within a week, and are ready to be reharvested.

Application of autografts to excised wound beds assumes that hemostasis has been obtained. As stated previously, one of the reasons for graft loss is development of hematoma under the grafts, thus depriving the transplanted cells of nutrients and the ability to vascularize. If a wide mesh is used (4:1 ratio), this is of less concern. Placement of autografts should be designed so that the lines inherent in the graft from seams and the mesh pattern follow the lines of Langer when possible. In our practice, autograft skin is placed dermal side up on a fine mesh gauze

backing after it is meshed to facilitate placement on the wound bed. Natural curling of the autograft toward the dermal side can be obviated by gentle irrigation with a bulb syringe to completely expand the graft while it is on the mesh. The autograft is then applied to the wound bed and the fine mesh gauze removed. At this point, we usually affix one side of the graft with staples and maximally expand the graft in the other directions. Grafts can then be applied adjacent to this as required for wound closure.

When using 4:1 or 9:1 mesh ratios, the wound will still be mostly open after application of the autograft. At this point, we advise that the wound be completely closed by application of cadaveric homograft over the autograft. When using this technique, staples are not applied until all layers of the skin are in place. With successful graft take using this technique, the autograft and homograft become adherent and vascularized. With time, the homograft cells reject while the autograft cells expand, thus completing wound healing.

Selection of the donor sites, mesh ratio, and placement of the grafts comprises the majority of the art of burn surgery. The wound bed can be viewed as a puzzle, and the autograft as pieces to it. The advantage of this model over that of a cardboard puzzle is that the pieces can be cut to fit the puzzle. However, efforts should be made to keep the pieces whole to minimize seams.

Recently, the use of vacuum assisted closure of wounds has been reported. These vacuum assisted devices have been used successfully for closure of complicated decubitus ulcers, among other uses, and have now been tried in burn wounds to secure skin grafts and improve take rates (24). Those treated with vacuum assisted devices compared to standard bolster securement of skin grafts had significantly improved rates of reoperation for failed skin grafts without differences in complications.

In review, the principles of burn surgery are to provide timely burn wound excision to a viable wound bed. At that point, the wound is closed using either local flaps or, more likely, skin grafts. These flaps and skin grafts should be chosen in a way to minimize scarring. This is done by selecting donor sites, which are cosmetically acceptable, and including as much dermal layer as is reasonable. Attention must be paid to how the skin grafts are meshed, and how they are placed on the wound bed to minimize unsightly lines and mesh pattern. Lastly, careful consideration must be paid to placing the dressings and postoperative care to maximize graft takes.

V. SPECIAL AREAS

Particular anatomic regions require specific treatments. These issues should be considered and incorporated into the operative plan. For instance, the hands and face are probably the most important in terms of function and cosmesis; therefore, these areas should be given priority for nonmeshed grafts. Alternatively, the back is not of as much importance, and rapid closure with widely meshed grafts early in the operative course should be considered to decrease incidence of infection, graft loss, and length of hospital stay. In this section, we will go through suggested approaches to anatomic areas beginning in the cephalad regions.

The head and neck has an ample blood supply which enables it to resist invasive infection better than other parts of the body. It is also probably the most important area in terms of cosmesis and function (eyes, mouth). Lastly, the color of the skin in this area is relatively specific to the head and neck. For these reasons, it is treated differently from other areas. Since the face is so important cosmetically, sharp excision of eschar is not recommended in order to preserve any dermal and epidermal structures that may survive. This practice is tolerated because of the excellent blood supply to the area that resists infection. Once the eschar separates in 10–14 days, the underlying wound can be grafted. Because of the unique skin coloration in this area, autograft skin should be obtained from donor sites above the clavicles. We generally use donor skin taken from the scalp for this purpose. Lastly, the autograft skin should be applied in sheets to minimize scarring. Since it is almost always necessary to have seams in the grafts, the autograft skin pieces should be applied in cosmetic units, which are designed to hide the seams in natural lines on the face (Fig. 3.7). The neck can be treated similarly.

Common reconstructive problems occurring in the head and neck outside of scar contour and color are eyelid contractures and ectropion, nasolabial fold hypertrophic scarring, nasal alar contracture, nasal tip projection loss, microstomia, and lip ectropion. These can be minimized by sheet grafting in cosmetic units and postoperative pressure with face masks for up to 2 years after injury.

Treatment of the scalp also deserves mention. Generally, excision of the wound should be avoided in all but those that are clearly full thickness to maximize retention of hair follicles. After separation, the remaining open areas can be grafted with meshed graft for wound closure. After 2–3 weeks, if unhealed areas are present, these should be grafted to decrease the risk of folliculitis with spontaneous healing, which can be very troublesome. Resulting areas of alopecia can be reconstructed later with flaps or tissue expansion.

The trunk is generally not of great cosmetic importance with the exception of the upper chest, which may be visually exposed, particularly in women wearing low-cut v-neck shirts. If this area is unburned, we try to avoid using it as a donor site for this reason. For the rest of the

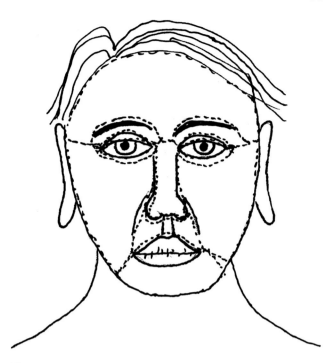

Figure 3.7 Cosmetic units. Skin grafts should be applied to open areas on the face in cosmetic units, so as to hide graft seams in normal facial depressions and lines. Dotted lines indicate suggested placement of seams.

trunk, meshed grafts can be used for rapid wound closure. The nipple/areolar complex is also a specialized area. Because of the nature of the mammary ducts, oftentimes keratinocytes are found deep beneath the skin, and these will proliferate and affect wound closure in this area if left in place. The coloration of the areola is also very specific, and not easily reconstructed. For these reasons, the nipple areolar complex should not be excised even if it appears to have eschar and all the surrounding skin is lost.

Common reconstructive problems developing in the trunk involve mostly the axilla. These generally cannot be avoided by skin graft technique, but can be minimized with postoperative splinting. Breast contour deformities can also develop in the breast regardless of acute closure method, and can be dealt with in the reconstructive period.

The buttock and perineum occupy a very difficult position for skin grafts to take, as the dressings applied are often soiled from excrement, and cleaning the result often shears the grafts. For this reason, we always try to graft this region first before loose stools ensue, usually 1–2 weeks into treatment. If this is unsuccessful, it may be necessary to leave the patient in the prone position at later operations after application of grafts to this area while they adhere. This is also an area of less cosmetic importance, so widely meshed grafts can be used. The only caveat is that narrower mesh ratios tend to take more quickly before shearing forces in the area are necessary for hygiene, and if possible should be used.

The penis and scrotum in the male has an excellent blood supply, so they will heal usually in a timely fashion. The skin in this region also occupies a highly important function. So, in general, excision of this area is avoided. In the case of a small burn to the shaft of the penis, an excision and primary closure akin to a circumcision will often suffice. The scrotum is also a very good donor site because it heals well, is relatively hidden, and can be vastly expanded to provide a surprising amount of donor site skin.

The hands occupy a very important anatomic area in terms of function and cosmesis. Most of the time, burns of the hand are limited to the dorsal surface as the hand is clenched during injury.

Unfortunately, sometimes the digits receive a second injury associated with diminished perfusion during resuscitation. Therefore, it is not uncommon for some parts of the digits to be lost. We usually allow the necrotic part to clearly demarcate prior to amputation in an attempt to preserve as much length as possible, as even a few millimeters will contribute greatly to function. Once a viable wound bed is achieved on the hand, grafts should be placed that are either not meshed or meshed tightly at a 1:1 ratio to improve cosmesis. Because of the anatomic structure on the dorsum of the digits, burns through to the extensor tendons can result in development of boutonnière deformities even with complete wound closure due to sliding of tendons medial and lateral around the proximal interphalangeal joint. Extension contractures at the metacarpophalangeal joint are also common because the burn and subsequent scarring are limited to the dorsal surface. For these two reasons, consideration should be given to fixing the digits in extension at the proximal interphalangeal joint and flexion at the metacarpophalangeal joint by insertion of threaded Kirschner wires. These can be removed after complete wound healing. Alternatively, position can be maintained with splints. Early mobilization of the hand will also decrease these contractures.

The skin on the palm of the hand is specialized in that it is very thick and highly keratinized to withstand the significant shearing forces. Burns to the palm of the hand are uncommon, but when they occur, should be treated with debridement and spontaneous separation, as they will often heal spontaneously because of the depth of the skin. Allowing this to happen preserves the skin type and, thus, function. Should the palm of the hand sustain a full-thickness burn, the autograft skin should come from the sole of the foot to match the keratinocyte function.

The arms and, in particular, the forearms also have cosmetic and functional importance. For this reason, narrow meshed grafts or skin grafts are preferred. Flexion contractures of the elbow do occur, which can be minimized by splinting in extension, especially at night.

The foot has two specialized surfaces, the sole and the dorsum. The sole is very thick with both keratin and layers of keratinocytes; therefore, it often will heal spontaneously, similar to the palm of the hand. The dorsum of the foot, however, has a thin layer of skin that has a different pliability from other areas of skin. For this reason, it does not make a good donor site. Great care must also be taken with excision of full-thickness eschar in this area, as the extensor tendons are in very close proximity to the skin. Lastly, autograft skin applied to this area should be of a narrow mesh to avoid hypertrophic scarring, which can make it difficult to fit shoes. The toes of the foot also have the same considerations as the fingers, in that portions of them can become necrotic both from the burn itself and due to the vagaries of resuscitation. We treat all the regions of the foot in a fashion similar to the hand except for the use of Kirschner wires.

The thighs rarely have any problems with contracture and scarring, therefore meshed grafts are appropriate. The lower legs can be visually exposed, therefore narrow meshed grafts or sheet grafts are preferable when possible.

VI. DERMAL EQUIVALENTS IN PRIMARY CLOSURE

It is known that scarring can be minimized with the use of full-thickness grafts that have a complete layer of epidermis and dermis. Most of the techniques described above with partial-thickness skin grafts provide for epidermal coverage, but do not address the loss of dermis, leading to significant scarring. An extrapolation of the finding of decreased scarring with full-thickness grafts has led to the search for a dermal replacement to be used with partial-thickness skin grafts. Two products are currently available which hold this promise, Integra® and Alloderm®. These two products have different properties, and are thus used differently. These products are currently being widely used in many centers based on the hope that they will improve outcomes. These improvements, however, have not yet been firmly established. Their use is also associated with significant increases in monetary cost.

A. Integra

This product is a skin substitute that has a dermal equivalent layer consisting of collagen and other matrix proteins that vascularizes and functions as a neodermis (Fig. 3.8). With good take, this neodermis is reported to improve the pliability and appearance of the scar. Integra also has an epidermal component of a silicone layer that functions as a barrier while the underlying neodermal layer vascularizes. After this takes place over 10–14 days after application, the silicone layer can be removed and replaced

Integra

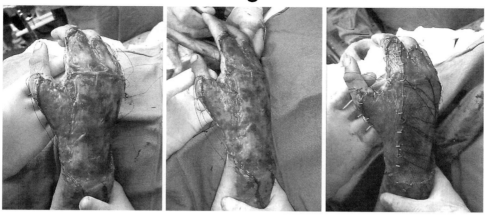

Figure 3.8 Integra. This is a series of photos taken after excision of a densely hypertrophic scar on the dorsum of the hand and placement of Integra for wound closure. The first photo on the left is taken 3 weeks after placement with the silicone layer still in place. The next photo is with the silicone layer removed, and the last is with split-thickness autograft in place.

with thin, split-thickness autografts. In the interim, the wound is completely closed.

Integra is applied and treated postoperatively in a similar fashion to autograft or homograft skin. Some apply it in sheets, while others mesh it at a 1:1 ratio to minimize underlying fluid accumulations. Securing staples are generally not placed between sheets of Integra, but instead the staples are applied to single sheets to minimize losses due to shearing, as the sheets of Integra are not as pliable as skin because of the silicone layer. The Integra will progressively vascularize over 10–21 days, which is signified by increasing redness upon inspection. When the silicone layer begins to spontaneously separate, it must be replaced with autograft in a staged procedure. This is one of the drawbacks of this product in that it requires more than one procedure to be used. Recent reports on the use of Integra purport acceptable take rates and infection rates (25). One of the potential advantages of this product is the limitation of scarring because of the presence of the dermal substitute; however, this has not been borne out in the initial reports (26,27). Further studies with larger numbers of patients will be required to test whether decreased scarring is an additional benefit with the use of this product.

B. Alloderm

Alloderm is a substance obtained from cadaveric homograft skin, which is treated in such a way as to remove all the cells, leaving only the dermal matrix (Fig. 3.9). This process removes all the allogenic properties from the dermis, so that it does not reject. So, this product is a dermal replacement that does not have an epidermal

component, which must be provided with autograft. Use of this product, then, is predicated on the availability of autograft skin to close the wound. It is generally applied to the wound bed directly followed by application of autograft on top of this in a sandwich fashion. All of this then vascularizes, leaving wound coverage with both a dermal layer and an epidermal layer in one procedure. This product also holds the reported advantage of decreases in scarring; however, this concept too has not been rigorously tested.

VII. METABOLISM AND WOUND HEALING ADJUNCTS

The use of anabolic agents to accelerate wound healing has been investigated. The most effective agent to date has been systemic administration of recombinant human growth hormone (28). The use of growth hormone has stimulated donor sites to heal faster, allowing more frequent donor site harvest and thus less time between operations. Growth hormone decreased donor site healing time by an average of 2 days with therapy that was associated with a reduction in length of hospital stay from 0.8 to 0.54 days/%TBSA burn. This improved healing time was associated with a cost saving of 23% for a typical 80% TBSA burn, including the cost of the growth hormone. This effect is thought to be due to stimulation of insulin-like growth factor 1 release as well as upregulation of insulin-like growth factor 1 receptors in the wound (29). It has recently been shown that insulin in pharmacologic doses may have similar effects on wound healing. Insulin given at 30 μU/kg per minute for 7 days decreased donor site healing time from 6.5 ± 0.9 days to 4.7 ± 2.3

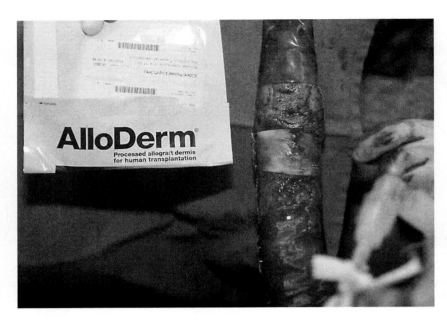

Figure 3.9 Alloderm. The piece of Alloderm is seen lying in the antecubital fossa sandwiched between pieces of Integra in a clinical trial. Autograft skin was placed immediately over the open areas and the Alloderm, while the Integra areas required return to the operating theater for staged grafting.

days (30). In this study, the caloric intake necessary to maintain euglycemia during the insulin infusion was double that of the placebo time period. The effects of insulin on wound healing also seem to be potentiated with additional amino acids (31). Studies are under way using much lower doses to determine whether a significant effect is still present at doses that would be clinically safer to use.

VIII. CULTURED EPITHELIAL AUTOGRAFTS

One alternative to split-thickness autografts typically used for skin grafting is cultured keratinocytes from the patient's own skin. Keratinocytes can be cultured in sheets from full-thickness skin biopsies, which are used as autografts. This technology has been used to greatly expand the capacity of a donor site, such that most of the body can be covered with grafts from a single small full-thickness biopsy sample. Cultured epithelial autografts are of use in truly massive burns (>80% TBSA) because of their limited donor sites. The disadvantages of cultured epithelial autografts are the length of time required to grow the autografts (2–3 weeks), a 50–75% take rate of the grafts after initial application, the low resistance to mechanical trauma over the long term, and a proposed increase in scarring potential associated with the lack of dermis. These grafts are also very expensive to produce. When a group of patients with >80% TBSA burns receiving cultured epithelial autografts was

compared with a group receiving conventional treatment, the acute hospitalization length of stay and the number of subsequent reconstructive operations was lower in the conventional group (32). These results demonstrate that more research and experience are needed to further optimize this technique.

In the future, it might be reasonable to predict that skin culture technologies will progress to the point that both epidermis (cultured epithelial autografts) and dermis (like Integra or Alloderm) will be available from sources other than the patient or can be procured from a very small biopsy site. If this were to be developed, wound closure could potentially be performed at a single setting with minimal donor sites and very minimal scarring, thus providing a dramatic benefit for survival, function, and cosmesis. We in the burn community anxiously await this day.

IX. CONCLUSIONS

Techniques of burn management today call for institution of resuscitation and prevention of further injury prior to definitive wound care. Once stabilization has been performed, operations are planned which seek to use available resources to first ensure survival with an eye toward function and cosmesis in the long term. Many techniques are available, and all should be in the armamentarium of the practicing burn surgeon treating the acutely burned.

REFERENCES

1. Spies M, Herndon DN, Rosenblatt JI, Sanford AP, Wolf SE. Prediction of mortality from catastrophic burns in children. Lancet 2003; 361:989–994.
2. Cope O, Langohr JL, Moore FD, Webster RC. Expeditious care of full thickness burn wounds by surgical excision and grafting. Ann Surg 1947; 125:1–22.
3. Burke JF, Bondoc CC, Quinby WC. Primary burn excision and immediate grafting: a method shortening illness. J Trauma 1974; 14:389–395.
4. Burke JF, May JW Jr, Albright N, Quinby WC, Russell PS. Temporary skin transplantation and immunosuppression for extensive burns. N Engl J Med 1974; 290:269–271.
5. Pruitt BA, Goodwin CW, Mason AD Jr. Epidemiologic, demographic, and outcome characteristics of burn injury. In: Herndon DN, ed. Total Burn Care. London: W.B. Saunders, 2002:16–30.
6. Bull JP, Fisher AJ. A study in mortality in a burn unit: standards for the evaluation for alternative methods of treatment. Ann Surg 1949; 130:160–173.
7. Herndon DN, Gore D, Cole M, Desai MH, Linares H, Abston S, Rutan T, Van Osten T, Barrow RE. Determinants of mortality in pediatric patients with greater than 70% full-thickness total body surface area thermal injury treated by early total excision and grafting. J Trauma 1987; 27:208–212.
8. McDonald WS, Sharp CW Jr, Deitch EA. Immediate enteral feeding in burn patients is safe and effective. Ann Surg 1991; 213:177–183.
9. Sheridan RL, Remensnyder JP, Schnitzer JJ, Schulz JT, Ryan CM, Tompkins RG. Current expectations for survival in pediatric burns. Arch Pediatr Adolesc Med 2000; 154:245–249.
10. Stassen NA, Lukan JK, Mizuguchi NN, Spain DA, Carrillo EH, Polk HC Jr. Thermal injury in the elderly: when is comfort care the right choice? Am Surg 2001; 67:704–708.
11. Brigham PA, McLoughlin E. Burn incidence and medical care use in the United States: estimates, trends, and data sources. J Burn Care Rehabil 1996; 17:95–107.
12. Xiao-Wu W, Herndon DN, Spies M, Sanford AP, Wolf SE. Effects of delayed wound excision and grafting in severely burned children. Arch Surg 2002; 137:1049–1054.
13. Baxter CR. Fluid volume and electrolyte changes of the early postburn period. Clin Plast Surg 1974; 1:693–703.
14. Alderson P, Bunn F, Lefebvre C, Li WP, Li L, Robrts I, Schierhout G. Human albumin solution for resuscitation and volume expansion in critically ill patients. Cochrane Database Syst Rev 2002:CD001208.
15. Wilkes MM, Navickis RJ. Patient survival after human albumin administration. A meta-analysis of randomized, controlled trials. Ann Intern Med 2001; 135:149–164.
16. Zdolsek HJ, Lisander B, Jones AW, Sjoberg F. Albumin supplementation during the first week after a burn does not mobilise tissue oedema in humans. Intensive Care Med 2001; 27:844–852.
17. Atiles L, Mileski W, Spann K, Purdue G, Hunt J, Baxter C. Early assessment of pediatric burn wounds by laser Doppler flowmetry. J Burn Care Rehabil 1995; 16:596–601.
18. Holland AJ, Martin HC, Cass DT. Laser Doppler imaging prediction of burn wound outcome in children. Burns 2002; 28:11–17.
19. Kloppenberg FW, Beerthuizen GI, ten Duis HJ. Perfusion of burn wounds assessed by laser doppler imaging is related to burn depth and healing time. Burns 2001; 27:359–363.
20. Lal S, Barrow RE, Wolf SE, Chinkes DL, Hart DW, Heggers JP, Herndon DN. Biobrane improves wound healing in burned children without increased risk of infection. Shock 2000; 14:314–319.
21. Lukish JR, Eichelberger MR, Newman KD et al. The use of a bioactive skin substitute decreases length of stay for pediatric burn patients. J Pediatr Surg 2001; 36:1118–1121.
22. Mann R, Gibran NS, Engrav LH, Foster KN, Meyer NA, Honari S, Costa BA, Heimbach DM. Prospective trial of thick vs standard split-thickness skin grafts in burns of the hand. J Burn Care Rehabil 2001; 22:390–392.
23. Desai MH, Rutan RL, Herndon DN. Conservative treatment of scald burns is superior to early excision. J Burn Care Rehabil 1991; 12:482–484.
24. Scherer LA, Shiver S, Chang M, Meredith JW, Owings JT. The vacuum assisted closure device: a method of securing skin grafts and improving graft survival. Arch Surg 2002; 137:930–934.
25. Heimbach DM, Warden GD, Luterman A, Jordan MH, Ozobia N, Ryan CM, Voigt DW, Hickerson WL, Saffle JR, DeClement FA, Sheridan RL, Dimick AR. Multicenter postapproval clinical trial of Integra dermal regeneration template for burn treatment. J Burn Care Rehabil 2003; 24:42–48.
26. Dantzer E, Braye FM. Reconstructive surgery using an artificial dermis (Integra): results with 39 grafts. Br J Plast Surg 2001; 54:659–664.
27. van Zuijlen PP, Vloemans JF, van Trier AJ, Suijker MH, vanUnen E, Groenevelt F, Kreis RW, Middelkoop E. Dermal substitution in acute burns and reconstructive surgery: a subjective and objective long-term follow-up. Plast Reconstr Surg 2001; 108:1938–1946.
28. Herndon DN, Barrow RE, Kunkel KR, Broemeling L, Rutan RL. Effects of recombinant human growth hormone on donor-site healing in severely burned children. Ann Surg 1990; 212:424–431.
29. Herndon DN, Hawkins HK, Nguyen TT, Pierre E, Cox R, Barrow RE. Characterization of growth hormone enhanced donor site healing in patients with large cutaneous burns. Ann Surg 1995; 221:649–659.
30. Pierre EJ, Barrow RE, Hawkins HK, Nguyen TT, Sakurai Y, Desai M, Wolfe RR, Herndon DN. Effects of insulin on wound healing. J Trauma 1998; 44:342–345.
31. Zhang XJ, Chinkes DL, Irtun O, Wolfe RR. Anabolic action of insulin on skin wound protein is augmented by exogenous amino acids. Am J Physiol Endocrinol Metab 2002; 282:E1308–E1315.
32. Barret JP, Wolf SE, Desai MH, Herndon DN. Cost-efficacy of cultured epidermal autografts in massive pediatric burns. Ann Surg 2000; 231:869–876.

4

Management of Electrical Injuries

HAZEL JOSEPH
Eastern Virginia Medical School, Norfolk, Virginia, USA

ROBERT L. McCAULEY
University of Texas Medical Branch and Shriners Hospital for Children—Galveston Unit, Galveston, Texas, USA

I. INTRODUCTION

The National Center for Health and the Centers for Disease Control have estimated that 52,000 trauma admissions per year are due to electrical injuries (1). Pediatric patients make up a significant proportion of this number (1,2) and account for more than 2000 pediatric emergency room visits (3). In both the pediatric and adult population, the number of males affected with this type of injury is greater than the number of females (4,5). The Census of Fatal Occupational Injuries (CFOI) and the Survey of Occupational Injuries and Illnesses (SOII) data revealed that 32,807 U.S. workers spent days away from work due to electrical shock or electrical burn injuries between 1992 and 1998 (6). Electrical injuries are responsible for more than 500 deaths per year (3). The mortality rate for electrical injuries is between 2% and 15% (7–9), although the morbidity is significantly higher than for burns from other causes.

Electrical injuries were reported as early as 1879 (10). Our knowledge of the optimal management of these injuries continues to expand since the earliest reports (11–14). A review of the literature on electrical injuries over the past 50 years has revealed that we have increased our understanding of the epidemiology, types of injuries, pathology of the burn wound, acute management, and surgical options in these patients. In this chapter, an overview of the management of patients with electrical trauma is presented with emphasis placed on new data supporting trends in the care of these complex injuries, including the reconstructive challenges.

The opinions or assertions contained herein are the private views of the author(s) and do not represent the views of the Department of the Army or the Department of Defense.

II. PATHOPHYSIOLOGY OF ELECTRICAL INJURY

Electricity may cause injury by arc, flame, flash, or current (1,3,15). Arc injuries occur when the current passes external to the body. Arcs from high-voltage electrical sources can generate a significant amount of heat (16) and can result in flash burns and deep thermal burns (3). When the source is not in close proximity to the victim and the current grounds external to the body, flash burns may be encountered (17). Flame burns are not uncommon and may result when clothing ignites; these burns are often full-thickness (15,17). "True" current injury occurs when electricity passes through the body from an entry point to an exit point. The current produces heat as it passes through tissues of different resistances and cross-sectional areas (12,15).

Resistance of various tissues to current increases in the following order: nerve, blood, muscle, skin, tendon, fat, and bone (12). Skin resistance is $\sim$40,000 ohm but varies with thickness, surface area, and moisture content. Areas of thick skin offer greater resistance to current. The digits and distal extremities have a smaller cross-sectional area and are more vulnerable to damage. Sweat can reduce the resistance of the skin to $<$1000 ohm. Mucous membranes offer little resistance to current (3). Recent animal studies suggest that the body conducts current as a composite of all of the tissues of the body, acting as a single uniform resistance, rather than as individual resistances as previously thought (18,19).

Heat is generated as it passes through the body and is described by the following equation:

$$J = I^2R$$

where J is the heat in joules, I the current, and R the resistance. Current is directly proportional to voltage (V) and inversely proportional to resistance (15). Electrical burns are traditionally classified as either low-voltage injuries ($<$1000 V) or high-voltage injuries ($>$1000 V) (19). Low-voltage injuries are more common in younger children and high-voltage injuries are more common in older children and adults (20). Orofacial burns and extremity burns in the home make up the majority of low-voltage injuries (120 and 240 V) that occur in children (1). Orofacial burns remain the most common type of electrical burns in infants and young children (21–23).

The extent of injuries from high-voltage electrical injuries is much greater. Complications include extremity amputation, fasciotomy, deep muscle loss, cardiac arrest, sepsis, renal failure, and permanent neurological damage (9,24). One notable exception is cardiac arrythmias, which may result from low-voltage injuries (3). Data on intermediate voltage electrical injuries (200–1000 V) are not as clear. Sheridan provides a comprehensive review

of 16 cases of 600 V direct current injuries. The injuries and outcome of this subset of patients appear to be unique; the morbidity rate from intermediate-voltage injuries is higher than that from low-voltage injuries. The mortality rate in this series is 18.7% (25).

The mechanism of tissue damage may be thermal or cellular (by strong electrical fields or biochemical changes) (26–28). It was thought that injury from electrical trauma was due to joule heating. In the last two decades, data have revealed that the mechanism of tissue damage in electrical injury also includes membrane permeability and denaturation of cellular macromolecules and proteins (29). If the contact time is brief, cellular damage is secondary to the effects on the membrane. If the contact time is longer, damage due to thermal effects occurs, which affects the entire cell. Lee used a geometric model of an elongated cell to demonstrate the importance of orientation and cell size: larger cells, such as muscle and nerve cells, are more vulnerable to injury from electricity (30). Data support the theory that cells can survive membrane injury if proper therapy is initiated (31).

III. ACUTE CARE

The initial assessment of patient with electrical injury is guided by the principles and practices of Advanced Burn Life Support (ABLS) and Advanced Trauma Life Support (ATLS). Patients with electrical injury meet the American Burn Association criteria for referral to a burn unit and providers caring for these patients should seek early consultation. The primary survey includes the A, B, and C. The patient's airway, oxygenation, ventilation, and circulation are the first priorities. Cervical immobilization and spinal precautions should be maintained until spinal injury is excluded. Tetanic muscle contractions and falls from heights make these patients vulnerable to spinal trauma. All clothing should cut away from the patient to be able to determine the extent of any other injuries. Surface burns may be present and care should be taken to prevent hypothermia. A urinary catheter should be in place to monitor urine output and the color. Darkened urine signals the possibility of myoglobinuria or hemoglobinuria, which require urgent intervention in order to prevent renal complications. Urine output should be maintained at 1–1.5 mL/kg per hour and vital signs should be continuously monitored. A 12-lead ECG is done and appropriate x-rays should be ordered.

The secondary survey will include a complete history and physical examination. Additional studies to be considered in these patients include x-rays of the entire spine and computed tomography of the head, especially in patients with documented loss of consciousness. The history and physical examination will guide the trauma workup. Particular attention should be given to the ophthalmologic and neurological examinations. The ears should be examined for tempanic membrane perforation. The scalp and torso should be carefully examined to look for contact points. Contact wounds on the torso should signal the possibility of underlying lung injury or intra-abdominal visceral injury. Full-thickness abdominal burns should be explored and if the posterior fascia is necrotic then exploratory celiotomy is indicated. The percentage of total body surface area burn and the depth of the burns should be documented. Visible skin burns may grossly underestimate the underlying injury; therefore, the calculation of fluid requirement in the first 24 h should be taken as the minimum fluid needed. Patients with associated large deep burns will require more fluid. Pulses in all four extremities should be documented and the vascular status must be continuously reassessed. Fasciotomy or amputation may be warranted within hours of admission. Wounds should be cleansed with an antiseptic soap such as chlorhexidine gluconate and a topical agent such as sulfamylon (for full-thickness burns, which provides good penetration) or silvidine (for partial-thickness burns) should be applied (32).

IV. GENERAL MANAGEMENT

A. Ocular Injuries

Ocular injuries such as macular holes, iritis, and cataracts have an incidence rate of 6–10% in several series (33,34). Gradual loss of visual acuity and blurred vision are the presenting complaints (35,36). Retinal lesions and extraocular movement abnormalities may occur and resolve without long-term sequelae. Cataracts may occur years after injury (17). A careful eye examination should be done with follow-up occurring soon after, in patients at risk of ocular complications. Any reports of visual changes must be evaluated. These patients usually respond well to surgical intervention and visual rehabilitation (35,37,38).

B. Renal Complications

Major risk factors for renal failure associated with burn trauma are well described and include high-voltage electrical injury, cardiac arrest, compartment syndrome, and full-thickness burns. However, the incidence of renal failure in patients with electrical injuries is low despite the fact that myoglobinuria is a major risk factor for acute tubular necrosis (38), partly due to early identification of myoglobinuria and hemoglobinuria and the initiation of therapy in most emergency rooms.

The presence of discolored (often tea-colored) urine suggests the possibility of significant muscle damage. Volume expansion is indicated and intravenous fluid (Ringer's lactate) can be administered at a rate to give a

urine output of 1–1.5 cm³/kg per hour allowing for prompt clearance of the urine pigment. Serial urine specimens should be collected and visually inspected at the bedside to ensure an appropriate response to therapy. Purdue reports zero incidence of acute renal failure using a protocol that includes mannitol and sodium bicarbonate in addition to Ringer's lactate (39).

C. Cardiac Arrhythmias

Cardiac arrhythmias occur more commonly in the acute phase and are seen in 10–15% of patients with electrical injuries (7,40,41). Electrical current can also cause dysrythmias or direct damage to the myocardium (42,43). Ventricular fibrillation and asystole may cause cardiac arrest at the scene. Dysrhythmias commonly reported in patients treated in the emergency room include sinus tachycardia, supraventricular tachycardia, and atrial fibrillation. Nonspecific ST-segment changes and prolonged QT intervals are also common (44). Patients who present with these cardiac problems usually respond well to medical management. When one looks at complications arising from low-voltage electrical injury, cardiac arrhythmias are usually the most serious problem. Wound problems tend to be minor. A 12-lead ECG should be done on admission. When the initial ECG is normal, subsequent cardiac problems are not common. Because of associated skeletal muscle trauma, creatinine kinase and creatinine kinase-MB levels are poor indicators of myocardial damage in these patients (42,45). If an abnormality is documented in the field or on admission, if loss of consciousness occurred (45,46), or when electrical injuries occur in the pediatric age group, an extended period of monitoring is warranted. Prolonged monitoring of patients with contact injuries on the chest wall or when current has transversed the chest wall may be indicated (although this is a matter of current controversy) (47,48). Late dysrhytmias have been reported and may be due to focal areas of myocardial necrosis (42,43,49).

V. WOUND CARE

Low-voltage electrical injuries may range from erythema to full-thickness burns (3,50). Partial- and full-thickness injuries are treated in the same manner as thermal burns. Low-voltage contact points can be excised. Skin grafts (and less commonly, local flaps) are required to provide adequate coverage. Morbidity is limited in low-voltage injuries; however, orofacial burns sustained when a child bites an electrical cord can result in severe microstomia necessitating staged reconstruction and prolonged rehabilitation (50,51). Determining the full extent of underlying tissue and deep muscle injury is of critical importance in dealing with high-voltage injuries. Unlike thermal burns, the severity of an internal injury is not evident based on the external burns. Delayed necrosectomy may result in refractory acidosis, abscess formation, and overwhelming sepsis. To date, there are no diagnostic tools widely used to assess the extent of tissue damage. MRI, muscle perfusion scintigraphy, and arteriography are among the modalities being studied. Physical examination is critical in the assessment. Routine fasciotomies are not recommended and are in fact associated with increased amputation rates. Selective fasciotomies are the rule and are indicated when there is evidence of progressive diminution of perfusion (51).

Currently there are two schools of thought regarding wound management of high-voltage electrical injuries. The traditional method errs on the side of early debridement with preservation of questionably viable tissue. Wounds are covered with xenograft or homograft. Subsequent re-explorations are done at 48–72 h intervals to remove nonviable tissue. When a healthy wound is identified, definitive coverage is done (17,52,53). This treatment paradigm supports the observed changes of the wound over time in the days following injury. New data indicate that these changes may be due to

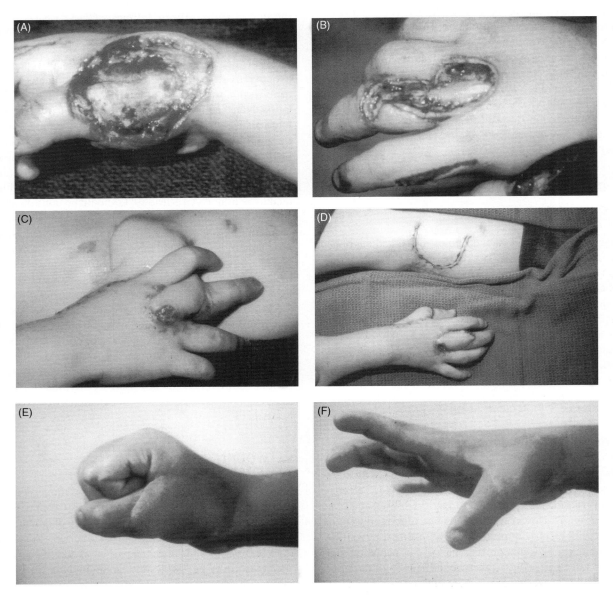

Figure 4.1   (A) Electrical injury with full-thickness burns of the radial aspect of the thumb. (B) Full-thickness burns of the dorsal aspect of the third finger with exposure of the extensor tendon and proximal interphalangeal joint. (C) Coverage with a groin flap, split longitudinally to cover both defects. (D) Flap division and insetting. (E) Final outcome, demonstrating extension. (F) Final outcome, demonstrating flexion.

ischemia-reperfusion injury rather than progressive ischemia from endothelial damage at the time of the electrical injury (18,34,54).

In contrast to this approach, over the last two decades, enthusiasm has increased for early debridement and coverage (18,34,55). This approach has two caveats: considerable surgical experience is necessary to avoid removal of potentially viable tissue that would compromise functional limb length; moreover, the surgeon must not leave nonviable tissue behind that is a nidus for infection when skin graft and flap survival is critical. Outstanding results have been obtained by Chick, Lister, and Sowder, who applied their protocol for early flap coverage of traumatic wounds to electrical injuries of the extremities (Fig. 4.1). Patients

underwent "early" debridement of nonviable and questionably nonviable tissue. Skin was excised to bleeding dermis and nerves, bones and tendons were left intact. Closure was obtained with free flaps; all of the flaps survived and none required re-exploration. Chick et al. (56) purported that good initial debridement and early coverage minimizes desiccation, saves skin, and prevents nerve injuries. Their data suggest that although the need for escharotomies and fasciotomies is not reduced, morbidity and outcome is improved. Three of the five patients returned to work; one has returned to activities of daily living; one has a forequarter amputation and latissimus dorsi flap coverage to his lower extremity and ambulates with the full range of motion (56). Zhu (57) reported his experiences with

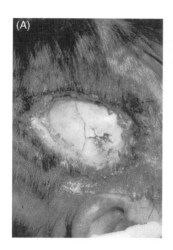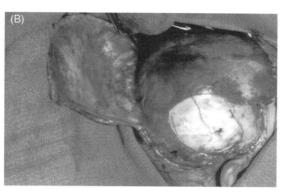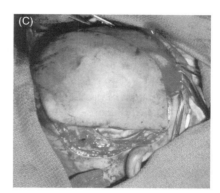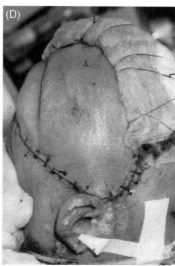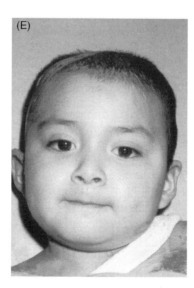

Figure 4.2 (A) Four-year-old girl with a 45% total body surface area burn after coming in contact with a transformer box. Full-thickness calvarial burn with an open linear skull fracture with epidural air and a cerebral spinal fluid leak in the right parietoccipital area. (B) A large transposition scalp flap is elevated for coverage within 20 h after transfer to hospital. (C) Coverage of defect with the scalp flap providing a watertight seal. (D) Scalp flap sutured in place; donor site covered with a split-thickness skin graft (STSG). (E) Postoperative frontal view 1 month later.

emergency reconstruction of electrical injuries over a 14-year period and showed similar favorable outcomes.

Others have adopted the idea of early *definitive* debridement, ideally performed within several hours of admission, after resuscitation is well under way and hemodynamic stability is achieved (5,24). A "second-look" operation is then performed in 48 h. During the first 48 h, xenografts or allografts provide biological coverage and the dressing is not changed. Definitive closure is usually done at 48 h (24). A study by Hussman (5) reports that 87% of patients in his series were ready to be closed by the second or third visit to the operating room (day 5 after injury). Amputations were done at the first or second operation when clearly indicated. This study asserts that excessive delay between injury and the first debridement or subsequent debridements and coverage leads to desiccation, colonization, and tissue loss (5).

A. Injuries to the Scalp and Skull

Treatment of injuries to the skull depends on the depth of injury and extent of damage to the bone. Partial-thickness injury to the skull can be treated by debridement (tangential removal of the necrotic bone) and delayed or immediate autografting (58–60). The use of soft tissue expanders followed by reconstruction with the expanded vascularized skin has also been reported (61). Full-thickness injuries of the skull can be managed by removal of the bone, use of autogenous omentum, and skin grafting or flap coverage (62). Options for flap closure include both free flaps and rotational flaps (59,60,63,64). Regardless of the method of closure, delays from injury to debridement and definitive closure should be avoided to prevent colonization and osteomyelitis (Fig. 4.2).

B. Oral Commissure Burns

Children <5 years of age are at highest risk for oral commissure burns (1) which may be full-thickness. Eschar formation occurs early and usually falls off in 2–3 weeks and may result in a significant deformity (Fig. 4.3) (Table 4.1). If the labial artery is exposed, significant bleeding may occur and this should be discussed with the parents (3). Oral commissure burns usually result in microstomia, which may be treated by early surgery or conservative management including oral stenting and elective surgery after scar maturation.

C. Injuries to the Torso

Electrical burns to the torso should alert one to the possibility of underlying visceral injury. Focal injuries to the lung including pleural effusion, hemothorax, pneumonitis,

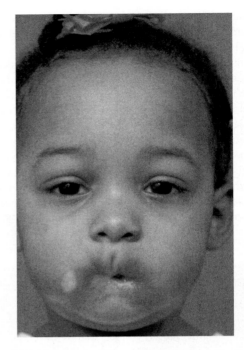

Figure 4.3 Three-year-old female referred 6 months after injury secondary to biting on an electric cord with severe microstomia.

and lung infarction have been reported as well as intra-abdominal viscera injury (small intestine, stomach, and colon) (65–69) (Fig. 4.4). In the former, ventilatory support may be required. Abdominal visceral injury should always be considered, especially when a contact injury is noted on the anterior abdominal wall. If full-thickness excision of the eschar reveals that the posterior fascia is necrotic, an exploratory celiotomy should be performed. If necrotic bowel is resected, a "second-look" celiotomy should be done in 48–72 h. Failure to diagnose

Table 4.1 Electric Burns of the Lip

Degree	Acute (0–4 days) and subacute (4 days to 2 months)	Sequela (>2 months)
Light	Up to one-third upper or lower lip or up to one-sixth of both lips without commissure involvement	Esthetic impairment
Moderate	Over one-third upper or lower lip or both without commissure involvement	Esthetic and functional impairment
Severe	Over one-third of both lips with commissure over two-third upper or lower lip; local tissue involvement (tongue, gingivolabial, gutter, etc.)	Severe esthetic and functional impairment

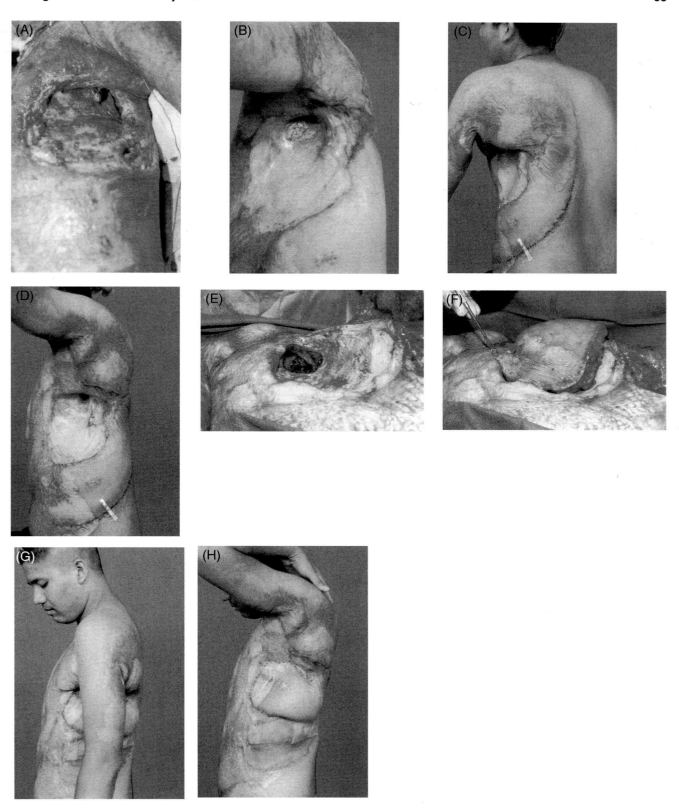

Figure 4.4 (A) Referred electrical burn to the lateral chest wall with destruction of lattisimus dorsi muscle and ribs with exposure of lung. (B) Early coverage with STSG. (C) Patient subsequently developed a bronchopleural cutaneous fistula. (D–F) Excision of skin graft and closure of wound with delayed thororacoabdominal flap. (G, H) Results with complete closure at 3 weeks.

an occult visceral injury may result in delayed perforation with a mortality rate >50% (67).

D. Genital Injuries

Genital and perineal burns may occur as a result of electrical injuries and may be severe. Partial- and full-thickness burns may occur as well as loss of the testicles and the penis. Conservative management of these types of injuries includes debridement and topical antibiotics. Edelman (70) reports good outcome of these complex injuries after evaluation, which includes local wound exploration, cystourethroscopy, and proctoscopy followed by early serial debridements and wound closure. Operative procedures in patients with electrical injuries may range from debridement and grafting to penile amputation (70,71). Both microsurgical and nonmicrosurgical options exist for the creation of a neopenis (72). With rare exceptions, foley catheterization is appropriate and does not increase morbidity rates due to perineal and genital burns except in children <1 year old (71).

VI. LIGHTNING INJURIES

Lightning injuries are rare, but associated burns are not uncommon, reportedly occurring in 89% of the cases in one series. Due to the short duration and "flash-over" effect of a lightning strike, deep burns fortunately occur in only 5% of victims (73). The pathognomonic sign of the injury is an erythmatous branching pattern on the skin, which is transient. This may be the only evidence of the "true" mechanism of injury in the unconscious patient. There is no characteristic pattern of the cutaneous burns, which may be minimal. Reverse triage should be done because patients in cardiopulmonary arrest benefit from aggressive resuscitative measures (74,75). Victims may suffer from sudden cardiac and pulmonary arrest. Loss of consciousness, paralysis, and seizures are common. As in patients with high-voltage electrical injury secondary to other sources, spinal cord injury can present early or late, and imaging studies may be normal. Injury can occur from the electrical current in the absence of bone fracture or dislocation. The prognosis of neurological complications in these patients, however, tends to be better than in those with other mechanisms of trauma injury (76).

VII. PREGNANT PATIENTS

Electrical shock in pregnancy is not common. There are no set patterns of fetoplacental injury in this setting and fetal outcome ranges from no apparent affect to oligohydramnios, placental abruption, and growth retardation may

occur later. Fetal death may occur early or late (77). Electrical injuries in pregnant women range from a feeling of a minor shock to passage of current from head to foot (78–81). All pregnant women who suffer electrical shock should be evaluated and a careful fetal assessment should be done.

REFERENCES

1. Rai J. Electrical injuries: a 30-year review. J Trauma 1999; 46(5):933–936.
2. Celik A, Ergun O, Ozok G. Pediatric electrical injuries: a review of 38 consecutive patients. J Pediatr Surg 2004; 39(8):1233–1237.
3. Koumbourlis AC. Electrical injuries. Crit Care Med 2002; 30(suppl 11):424–430.
4. Haberal M. Electrical burns: a five-year experience—1985 Evans lecture. J Trauma 1986; 26(2):103–109.
5. Hussmann J. Electrical injuries—morbidity, outcome and treatment rationale. Burns 1995; 21(7):530–535.
6. Cawley JC, Homce GT. Occupational electrical injuries in the United States, 1992–1998, and recommendations for safety research. J Safety Res 2003; 34(3):241–248.
7. Solem L, Fischer RP, Strate RG. The natural history of electrical injury. J Trauma 1977; 17(7):487–492.
8. Grube BJ. Neurologic consequences of electrical burns. J Trauma 1990; 30(3):254–258.
9. Ferreiro I. Factors influencing the sequelae of high tension electrical injuries. Burns 1998; 24(7):649–653.
10. Jex-Blake AJ. Death by electrical currents and by lightening. Br Med J 1913; 1:425.
11. Moncrief JA, Pruitt BA Jr. Hidden damage from electrical injury. Geriatrics 1971; 26(4):84–85.
12. DiVincenti FC, Moncrief JA, Pruitt BA Jr. Electrical injuries: a review of 65 cases. J Trauma 1969; 9(6):497–507.
13. Artz CP. Electrical injury simulates crush injury. Surg Gynecol Obstet 1967; 125(6):1316–1317.
14. Dale RH. Electrical accidents. Br J Plast Surg 1954; 7:44.
15. Parshley PF. Aggressive approach to the extremity damaged by electric current. Am J Surg 1985; 150(1):78–82.
16. Bernstein T. Electrical injury: electrical engineer's perspective and an historical review. Ann NY Acad Sci 1994; 720:1–10.
17. Baxter CR. Present concepts in the management of major electrical injury. Surg Clin North Am 1970; 50(6):1401–1418.
18. Hunt JL. Electrical injuries of the upper extremity. Major Probl Clin Surg 1976; 19:72–83.
19. Lee RC, Gottlieb LJ, Kriezek T. The pathophysiology and clinical management of electrical injury. In: Lee RC, Cravalho EG, Burke JF, eds. Electrical Trauma: The Pathophysiology, Manifestations, and Clinical Management. London: Cambridge University Press, 1992.
20. Zubair M, Besner GE. Pediatric electrical burns: management strategies. Burns 1997; 23(5):413–420.

21. Al-Qattan MM, Gillett D, Thomson HG. Electrical burns to the oral commissure: does splinting obviate the need for commissuroplasty? Burns 1996; 22(7):555–556.

22. Leake JE, Curtin JW. Electrical burns of the mouth in children. Clin Plast Surg, 1984; 11(4):669–683.

23. Thompson HG, Juckes AW, Farmer AW. Electrical burns of the mouth in children. Plast Reconstr Surg 1965; 35:466–477.

24. Luce EA. Electrical burns. Clin Plast Surg 2000; 27(1):133–143.

25. Sheridan RL et al. Noncontact electrosurgical grounding is useful in burn surgery. J Burn Care Rehabil 2003: 24(6):400–401.

26. Lee RC, Canaday DJ, Hammer SM. Transient and stable ionic permeabilization of isolated skeletal muscle cells after electrical shock. J Burn Care Rehabil 1993; 14(5):528–540.

27. Lee RC, Canaday DJ, Doong H. A review of the biophysical basis for the clinical application of electric fields in soft-tissue repair. J Burn Care Rehabil 1993; 14(3):319–335.

28. Robson MC, Murphy RC, Heggers JP. A new explanation for the progressive tissue loss in electrical injuries. Plast Reconstr Surg 1984; 73(3):431–437.

29. Lee RC, Zhang D, Hannig J. Biophysical injury mechanisms in electrical shock trauma. Annu Rev Biomed Eng 2000; 2:477–509.

30. Lee RC, Kolodney MS. Electrical injury mechanisms: electrical breakdown of cell membranes. Plast Reconstr Surg 1987; 80(5):672–679.

31. Lee RC. Injury by electrical forces: pathophysiology, manifestations, and therapy. Curr Probl Surg 1997; 34(9):677–764.

32. Joseph HL. The first 48 hours. In: Joseph HL et al., eds. Interns and Residents on Call, Pocket Handbook of Burn Care. Philadelphia, PA: CN International Medical Publishing, Inc., 2003.

33. Boozalis GT. Ocular changes from electrical burn injuries. A literature review and report of cases. J Burn Care Rehabil 1991; 12(5):458–462.

34. Luce EA, Gottlieb SE. "True" high-tension electrical injuries. Ann Plast Surg 1984; 12(4):321–326.

35. Chaudhuri Z, Pandey PK, Bhatia A. Electrical cataract: a case study. Ophthalmic Surg Lasers 2002; 33(2):166–168.

36. Saffle JR, Crandall A, Warden GD. Cataracts: a long-term complication of electrical injury. J Trauma 1985; 25(1):17–21.

37. Reddy SC. Electric cataract: a case report and review of the literature. Eur J Ophthalmol 1999; 9(2):134–138.

38. Rosen CL. Early predictors of myoglobinuria and acute renal failure following electrical injury. J Emerg Med 1999; 17(5):783–789.

39. Purdue GF, Hunt JL. Electrical injuries. In: Herndon DN, ed. Total Burn Care. London: Harcourt Publishers Limited, 2002.

40. Arturson G, Hedlund A. Primary treatment of 50 patients with high-tension electrical injuries. I. Fluid resuscitation. Scand J Plast Reconstr Surg 1984; 18(1):111–118.

41. Burke JF. Patterns of high tension electrical injury in children and adolescents and their management. Am J Surg 1977; 133(4):492–497.

42. Housinger TA. A prospective study of myocardial damage in electrical injuries. J Trauma 1985; 25(2):122–124.

43. Carleton SC. Cardiac problems associated with electrical injury. Cardiol Clin 1995; 13(2):263–266.

44. Ku CS. Myocardial damage associated with electrical injury. Am Heart J 1989; 118(3):621–624.

45. Arrowsmith J, Usgaocar RP, Dickson WA. Electrical injury and the frequency of cardiac complications. Burns 1997; 23(7–8):576–578.

46. Purdue GF, Hunt JL. Electrocardiographic monitoring after electrical injury: necessity or luxury. J Trauma 1986; 26(2):166–167.

47. Guinard JP et al. Myocardial injury after electrical burns: short and long term study. Scand J Plast Reconstr Surg Hand Surg 1987; 21(3):301–302.

48. Jensen PJ et al. Electrical injury causing ventricular arrhythmias. Br Heart J 1987; 57(3):279–283.

49. Chandra NC, Siu CO, Munster AM. Clinical predictors of myocardial damage after high voltage electrical injury. Crit Care Med 1990; 18(3):293–297.

50. Pensler JM, Rosenthal A. Reconstruction of the oral commissure after an electrical burn. J Burn Care Rehabil 1990; 11(1):50–53.

51. Mann R. Is immediate decompression of high voltage electrical injuries to the upper extremity always necessary? J Trauma 1996; 40(4):584–587; discussion 587–589.

52. Skoog T. Electrical injuries. J Trauma 1970; 10(10):816–830.

53. Bingham H. Electrical burns. Clin Plast Surg 1986; 13(1):75–85.

54. Zelt RG. High-voltage electrical injury: chronic wound evolution. Plast Reconstr Surg 1988; 82(6):1027–1041.

55. Quinby WC. The use of microscopy as a guide to primary excision of high-tension electrical burns. J Trauma 1978; 18(6):423–431.

56. Chick LR, Lister GD, Sowder L. Early free-flap coverage of electrical and thermal burns. Plast Reconstr Surg 1992; 89(6):1013–1019; discussion 1020–1021.

57. Zhu ZX. Experience of 14 years of emergency reconstruction of electrical injuries. Burns 2003; 29(1):65–72.

58. Paletta FX. Surgical management of the burned scalp. Clin Plast Surg 1982; 9(2):167–177.

59. Caffee HH. Scalp and skull reconstruction after electrical burn. J Trauma 1980; 20(1):87–89.

60. Spies M. Management of acute calvarial burns in children. J Trauma 2003; 54(4):765–769.

61. Wang NZ, Shen ZY, Ma CX. Application of skin and soft tissue expansion in treatment of burn injury. Zhongguo Xiu Fu Chong Jian Wai Ke Za Zhi 2000; 14(5):286–289.

62. Sun YH. Use of autogenous omentum for grafting electrical injury affecting the scalp and skull. Burns Incl Therm Inj 1985; 11(4):289–292.

63. Ebihara H, Maruyama Y. Free abdominal flaps: variations in design and application to soft tissue defects of the head. J Reconstr Microsurg 1989; 5(3):193–201.

64. Fried M. Electrical burn injury of the scalp—bone regrowth following application of latissimus dorsi free flap to the area. Burns 1991; 17(4):338–339.

65. Goldenberg DC. Pulmonary lesion in electric injury: report of a case. Rev Hosp Clin Fac Med Sao Paulo 1996; 51(1):15–17.

66. Masanes MJ et al. A high voltage electrical burn of lung parenchyma. Burns 2000; 26(7):659–663.

67. Haberal M. Visceral injuries, wound infection and sepsis following electrical injuries. Burns 1996; 22(2):158–161.

68. Yang JY, Tsai YC, Noordhoff MS. Electrical burn with visceral injury. Burns Incl Therm Inj 1985; 11(3):207–712.

69. Zhu ZX. Successful treatment of a severe electrical injury involving the stomach. Burns 1993; 19(1):80–82.

70. Edelman GC. Treatment of severe electrical burns of the genitalia and perineum by early excision and grafting. Burns 1991; 17(6):506–509.

71. Angel C. Genital and perineal burns in children: 10 years of experience at a major burn center. J Pediatr Surg 2002; 37(1):99–103.

72. Mutaf M. Nonmicrosurgical use of the radial forearm flap for penile reconstruction. Plast Reconstr Surg 2001; 107(1):80–86.

73. Cooper MA. Electrical and lightning injuries. Emerg Med Clin North Am 1984; 2(3):489–501.

74. O'Keefe Gatewood M, Zane RD. Lightning injuries. Emerg Med Clin North Am 2004; 22(2):369–403.

75. Jain S, Bandi V. Electrical and lightning injuries. Crit Care Clin 1999; 15(2):319–331.

76. Arevalo JM, Lorente JA, Balseiro-Gomez J. Spinal cord injury after electrical trauma treated in a burn unit. Burns 1999; 25(5):449–452.

77. Steer RG. Delayed fetal death following electrical injury in the first trimester. Aust NZ J Obstet Gynaecol 1992; 32(4):377–378.

78. Yoong AF. Electrical shock sustained in pregnancy followed by placental abruption. Postgrad Med J 1990; 66(777):563–564.

79. Mazor M, Leiberman JR. Abortion caused by electrical current. Arch Gynecol Obstet 1987; 241(1):71–72.

80. Leiberman JR et al. Electrical accidents during pregnancy. Obstet Gynecol 1986; 67(6):861–863.

81. Goldman RD, Einarson A, Koren G. Electric shock during pregnancy. Can Fam Physician 2003; 49:297–298.

5

Chemical Burns: Small Burns with Severe Consequences

DAVID G. GREENHALGH

University of California, Davis, California, USA

I. INTRODUCTION

Chemical burns tend to be small but often disfiguring burns. The most common site of injury is the face or hands. The resultant scarring is often severe and lifelong. To make matters worse, the injuries are frequently a result of an assault with the intent to disfigure. This review will site examples of typical chemical burns to demonstrate the typical problems that the burn caregiver must deal with to optimize the cosmetic and functional outcome.

There are several types of chemical burns that can lead to different types of burns (1). Classically, acid burns lead to coagulation of the surface and are often characterized as leading to less severe burns. The alkali burns are more insidious in that the agent tends to cause damage for a more protracted period of time. Petroleum products tend to dissolve the cell membrane, so their immediate appearance may change with time. There are specific types of chemical burns that all burn caregivers have familiarity with. The chemical burn that causes the most concern is from hydrofluoric acid (2,3), which progresses until consumed by calcium. These burns require treatment with a calcium-containing antidote in order to stop the process. These injuries progress over many hours, so the surgeon may not know the extent of injury until later.

While there is a great deal written to describe the different forms of injury that occur from the various forms of chemicals, the actual care that is required does not vary that much. All chemical burns need extensive irrigation as the first line of treatment. The ultimate extent of injury may not be known for at least a day or so. The principle that all burns that heal within 2 weeks usually do not scar, while those that require more time to close will tend to scar still applies. For this reason, the burns should initially be treated with a topical antimicrobial agent to minimize the chance of infection. The next decision to be made is to decide whether the area should be grafted or not. If the burn is obviously full-thickness or if it has failed to heal within 2 weeks, then grafting should be considered. One problem with chemical burns is that there frequently are "splash marks" that lead to multiple small wounds. These "splash mark" burns are difficult to manage because they are too small to graft but heal with either altered pigmentation (Fig. 5.1) or multiple small hypertrophic scars. Otherwise, grafts tend to do as well as for other types of burns.

The scarring problems and reconstructive needs of chemical burns are a special problem because of the areas of the body that are affected. Chemical burns tend to involve the face, hands, and genitalia. Clothing, at

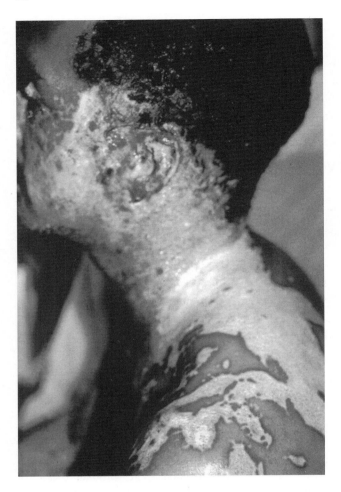

Figure 5.1 Typical pigment changes that occur after a chemical burn to the face and chest.

least for a short while, will protect the skin from chemical exposure. The exposed areas (face or hands), then, are at the highest risk. In addition, chemical agents are used for assaults (4). The face is a target, because there is intent to disfigure. The genitalia are involved because the person was caught "in the act." The other risk of exposure is while at work. The classical hydrofluoric acid burn involves the hands while someone is using the agent to etch glass or clean items. For instance, hydrofluoric acid is used to clean the outside of "semi" trucks. Workers use protective gear but the gloves leave gaps or are torn to expose the hands. All of these principles will be illustrated in the chapter.

II. CASE 1: CHEMICAL BURN BY CONTACT

This case illustrates the insidious nature of chemical burns. A middle-aged woman used a cleaning agent to "strip" the

wax off the floor. She was kneeling on the floor while she was performing this task. She did not realize that the agent was soaking through her pants and onto her knees. She presented the next day to the burn unit with black, leathery burns over her knees. The burns were insensate and palpably thick (Fig. 5.2). She was treated with silver sulfadiazine until the day of surgery. When the excision was performed the surgeons were surprised to fine that the burns extended well into the fat and left only a thin layer of viable tissue over the patella. Small sheet grafts were placed over the areas without a problem. The ultimate scarring was minimal.

III. CASE 2: HYDROFLUORIC ACID BURN TO THE FINGERS

This case illustrates the typical burn that people suffer from hydrofluoric acid. A 45-year-old man was working with hydrofluoric acid as a cleaner when the agent spilled and at the same time, his right index and middle fingers suffered crush injuries and exposure to the agent. He complained of severe pain to the two fingers. The initial examination revealed a subungual hematoma and slight erythema of the fingers. The burn appeared to look like a first-degree burn. His x-rays were negative. His fingers were placed in a calcium gluconate gel to treat the hydrofluoric acid burn. Because of the persistent pain, the subungual hematoma was drained but he had only mild relief. The fingers started to swell significantly but the burn did not appear to be that "deep." Because of the persistent pain, there was a discussion on whether to inject the fingers with calcium gluconate. It was our decision to avoid injection because of the risk of finger compartment pressure. The patient was discharged the next day with the calcium gluconate gel and oxycodone for pain. He was followed in the outpatient clinic where the edema and pain were noted to persist for 3–4 weeks. He was instructed on range of motion exercises. The nails eventually fell off and skin never appeared to change much. After several weeks, the pain resolved and he returned to work.

This case illustrates several of the classic findings with hydrofluoric burns. Fortunately, the extent of burn is often quite small but, unfortunately, involves the hands. Hydrofluoric acid burns that are only moderately larger (>10–15% TBSA) may be fatal (5,6). The involved area frequently has mild erythema that resembles a first-degree burn. It is not uncommon, especially with more dilute (<20%) solutions, for symptoms to develop hours after contact. Deeper burns tend to develop central gray areas that indicate full-thickness injury. The main symptom is severe pain and swelling, and treatment is focused on resolving the pain. The persistent pain indicates the

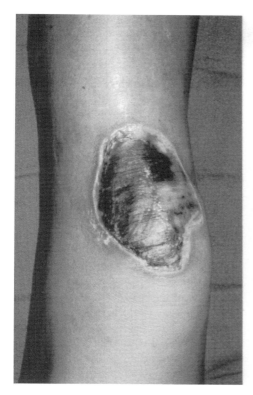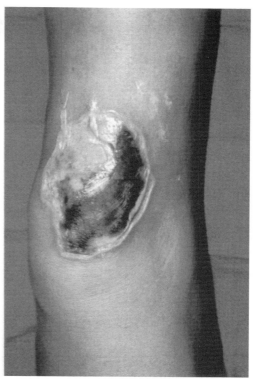

Figure 5.2 Third-degree burns to the knees that resulted from the patient kneeling on a floor stripper.

ongoing diffusion of the fluoride ion. Neutralization should lead to the reduction of pain. The main debate, however, is whether to treat with the topical calcium agent or to treat the area with local subcutaneous or arterial calcium injections (2). There are problems with either treatment option. Fluoride diffuses rapidly through the tissues so one may ask whether the topical application of calcium-containing gels plays a role once the agent enters the tissues. Studies do suggest, however, that they are effective. Some even suggest combining calcium gluconate gels with DMSO to improve diffusion, but most avoid that treatment because of potential toxicities of the solvent. Fortunately, topical agents seem to work quite well.

The reasoning behind injecting calcium-containing solutions into the involved tissues is that the fluoride ions rapidly diffuse into the tissues and cause continuing damage until neutralized. One has to wonder whether topical calcium can reach these areas. Because of this reasoning, clinicians have suggested injecting calcium gluconate into the subcutaneous tissues if pain persists for hours after topical treatment. The recommended dose is 0.5 mL of 10% calcium gluconate solution per square centimeter. Studies suggest that there are benefits but one must also worry about inducing compartment syndromes in the fingers. Those that favor injection suggest

that the volume injected per area should be limited to 0.5 mL per finger, which does not produce the volume recommended above. In addition, calcium salts, themselves are toxic to tissues, so one must be careful. Extravasation of calcium chloride is especially toxic and should never be used. Others have suggested the use of arterial injections for relief of pain with good results. The complication rate has also been quite high so its use should be restricted to severe cases. In our case, the minor burn led to delayed but persistent pain that eventually resolved with conservative care.

IV. CASE 3: ASSAULT TO THE PENIS BY ACID

The next case involved a man who was discovered by his partner to be involved with another person. An acid was thrown onto his genitalia as a revengeful punishment. The resulting burn involved approximately one-third of the shaft of the penis (Fig. 5.3). The initial burn developed a thick, leathery eshcar that was initially treated with silver sulfadiazine. Although the burn required 3 weeks to heal, it did so mostly by contraction. Due to the small size of the burn, the penis was not grafted. The end result was quite satisfactory.

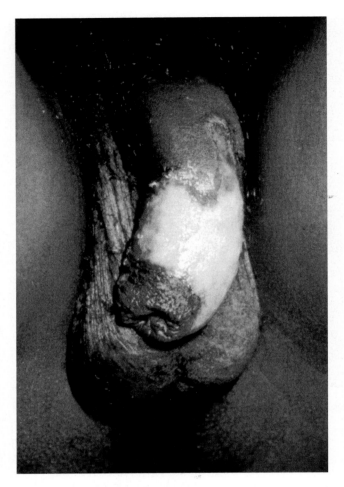

Figure 5.3 A chemical burn to the penis that was the result of an assault with a chemical.

The genitalia are a relatively common target of burn-related abuse. The major reason is that the assailant feels that the victim has been unfaithful or has been actually caught in the "act." Being "caught" exposes the genitalia to attack. In addition, genitalia are targets because of the importance our culture places on the (especially male) genitalia. Due to obvious anatomic reasons, the female genitalia are rarely burned to the point of needing reconstructive surgery. The penis and scrotum, being exposed, tolerate burn injury quite well. Due to the looseness of the skin, even deep burns on relatively small amounts of the penis will contract without major deformities. The scrotum is even more forgiving due to the looseness of its skin. Experience with necrotizing fasciitis has also led to the conservative treatment of these burns. I have covered exposed testicles when only one-third of the scrotum remains.

Grafting of the penis is not very difficult. The penis is grafted if a large portion of the skin is involved or if

there is a sizeable circumferential burn. The nonviable tissue needs to be debrided, with care to protect the underlying corpora and urethra. Sheet skin can be applied and I use "Rest-on Foam" as a circumferential splint. The grafts are then treated like any other part of the body. The results are quite good. Direct injury to the glans is a different problem that is usually treated conservatively. I have no experience with reconstruction of the glans.

V. CASE 4: ASSAULT TO THE FACE WITH AN UNKNOWN CHEMICAL

A 28-year-old man was walking out of a bar when an unknown assailant threw a chemical onto his face. He experienced immediate pain to the face but, fortunately, the eyes were not involved. He sustained indeterminant depth burns to the forehead, eyelids, cheeks, and left mandible. The burn also dripped onto his neck [Fig. 5.4(A) and (B)]. He was initially treated with bacitracin and followed for 10 days when he was noted to have obvious granulation tissue on areas of the face. He underwent sheet grafting from the scalp to the involved areas of the face. Since the burn did not cover aesthetic units, no attempt was used to excise and graft these units. He had excellent graft take and was discharged with instructions for massage and with a clear plastic facemask.

Unfortunately, he returned to the clinic with obvious bilateral upper and a left lower eyelid ectropia [(Fig. 5.4(C)]. Attempts at adjusting the mask and increasing massage were not successful in improving the ectropia. Due to ongoing exposure that was only partially improved with optical lubricants, he underwent sequential bilateral upper and then left lower eyelid releases with full-thickness skin grafts. The ectropia improved after the releases [Fig. 5.4(D)]. Ultimately, he developed significantly hypertrophic scars over bilateral zygomatic regions, the left maxilla, and the left neck. These areas were excised and regrafted. The ultimate result was only fair since there were significant color and texture changes in the grafted skin, despite using skin from above the clavicle. At this point, the patient opted to hold on further surgery until he could "get his head together." He currently is relatively well adjusted but has persistent obvious disfiguring scars.

This case illustrates several principles that are common to chemical burns to the face. The philosophy that wounds that heal within 2 weeks usually do not scar is important. No one knows why there is a tendency to scar after a wound is exposed for a set period but, for some reason, the prolonged inflammatory stimulus leads to an imbalance in collagen deposition/degradation. A great deal of research is needed to answer this difficult question. The

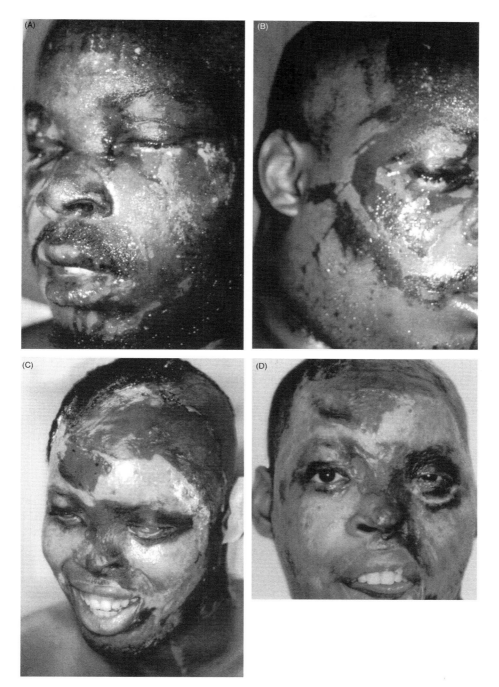

Figure 5.4 An unidentified chemical was thrown on this patient's face just as he exited a bar (A, B). Even though a small area was affected, the consequences were severe. He developed ectropia of both upper and the left lower eyelids (C). The surgical releases improved the exposure to the eyes but the ultimate outcome was only fair (D).

insidious nature of chemical injuries is illustrated with this case. The initial burn did not appear to be very deep but healing still took too long to prevent scarring. In addition, small but isolated "splash" areas frequently heal quickly but leave an alteration of pigment. The burn surgeon then is left with a relatively small burn in a cosmetically important area.

What does one do with a relatively small burn in the middle of the face? The debate is whether to allow the area to close over time and then plan to deal with the scar later vs. grafting the area when one knows that the 2-week time period will not be met. Unfortunately, none of the options are optimal. Either technique will lead to a noticeable scar. The goal is to minimize the ultimate scar. Frequently, small scars result in areas that are relatively easy to deal with. For instance, a small burn just anterior to the ear may be easily handled by excision and primarily closure to create a scar in a similar fashion as for a facelift. Similar incisions can be made to go at the edges of aesthetic units. Incisions along the nasolabial fold or at the mandibular line also turn out quite well. I have also found that creating little z-plasties in the incisions tend to help pulling along the line of the incision. Primary excision and closure of scars in the middle of aesthetic units (such as the middle of the cheek or forehead) do not lead to a great result. The ultimate scar, no matter how good, will always be noticeable. Primary excision and closure is also not possible with many burn scars on the face.

The other option is to perform skin grafts to the involved area. This option is more essential for larger burns such as for the case discussed earlier. I find that grafting of the face is more difficult for chemical burns than flame burns because such localized areas are involved. Flame burns tend to originate from the burning clothes and thus the lower face is frequently involved. The lower face and neck are frequently involved so that grafting to the neck is frequently all that is necessary. Neck contractures tend to be more of the problem than facial reconstruction. The other type of face flame burn involves the entire face. I find that grafting of the entire face by using large pieces of skin from the back to minimize seams tends to lead to better results than treating smaller and localized chemical burns.

With the localized face burns, two issues are important: matching the color and making a decision about replacing an entire aesthetic unit. The donor site should be harvested from an area above the clavicles in order to best match the color. Skin harvested from below the clavicles is almost always more yellow or darker. The color match is not as much of a problem for the grafting of the entire face since the graft dictates the entire color. Full-thickness skin should be used for the small areas. The skin from behind the ear or just above the clavicles can be used. Split-thickness skin should be harvested from the scalp. Scalp donors are more difficult to take and are extremely vascular. The use of an injectable solution containing epinephrine (and local anesthetic, if possible) is very helpful. The goal is to get the donor as thick as possible to prevent shrinkage. The thicker the skin, the more hair is transferred. Very thick donor sites can lead to alopecia and a hairy graft. I scrape the hair-bearing side to eliminate as much hair as possible but the transfer of some hair may still occur. The use of a laser may be helpful to eliminate the hair.

The other question is whether to graft just the affected area or replace an entire aesthetic unit. The smaller the graft, the more it tends to wrinkle so that is one argument for replacing an entire aesthetic unit. In addition, there will be no seam in the middle of the unit. I still have problems with replacing large uninjured areas so I tend to just graft the area. The wrinkling requires aggressive massage and a pressure device such as a cloth or plastic facemask. This technique can lead to adequate results. Another reason to save as much normal skin as possible is because that normal skin might be used for tissue expansion during future reconstructive surgery. Tissue expansion of the uninvolved cheek, forehead, or neck can produce enough skin to excise large areas of the face. The expansion can be designed with seams to fit aesthetic units in many cases.

The case described above also exemplifies the types of complications that result from these localized burns to the face. Despite aggressive grafting, the patient's graft still contracted significantly and led to eyelid ectropions. The treatment of the ectropions cannot be delayed because exposure can lead to opacification of the cornea and blindness. The eyelids need releases with full-thickness or split-thickness grafts. The releases improve the exposure but the ectropions often recur. The new grafts also leave noticeable scars in many cases. Ectropions can also occur on the lips. The releases of these scars are never similar to the original tissue. The recreation of the "Cupid's bow" is never satisfactory so the lip deformities are permanent.

The other classic problem involves contractures of the lateral oral commissures. These scars must be dealt with by stretching during exercises or with devices. We frequently have the patient place as many tongue depressors as possible in order to stretch the area. In addition, there are devices that will stretch the commissures. These devices supply lateral stretch, which some state will lead to the out-turning of the lips. These patients will frequently need operative commissure releases.

The other area to be adversely affected is the ear. These burns are often severely disfiguring. The classic teaching has been to allow ears to heal spontaneously. The deformity can be reconstructed later. I have become much more aggressive with covering exposed areas on the ear. Frequently, granulation tissue will develop in the exposed areas. During the grafting of the face, there are frequently strips of skin remaining, so I started placing them on areas of exposed ear. I even place grafts on areas of exposed cartilage. I debride the area of obviously necrotic skin or cartilage and then place skin with staples. My rationale is that, at the very least, the graft is a biologic dressing that will make the patient more comfortable. I have been pleasantly surprised that the grafts frequently "take" and accelerate the healing of the ear. I have not proven that the ultimate scar is better but I suspect that it may be improved. The reconstruction of the ear is an entire chapter in itself and will not be covered here.

Overall, the cosmetic outcomes for chemical burns to the face are only fair. The patient is left with a scar that is noticeable, no matter how well the wounds are treated. I suppose that was the original intent of the assailant. These patients need a great deal of emotional and social support, despite suffering what burn surgeons would categorize as a "minor" burn. These injuries illustrate why even small burns in difficult areas are still devastating injuries. Chemical burns, since they tend to target the functionally and cosmetically important areas, require the expertise of burn specialists. Despite this expertise, the results still have a great deal of room for improvement.

REFERENCES

1. Mozingo DW, Smith AA, McManus WF, Pruitt BA, Mason AD Jr. Chemical burns. J Trauma 1988; 28:642–647.
2. Kirkpatrick JJR, Enion DS, Burn DAR. Hydrofluoric acid burns: a review. Burns 1995; 21:483–493.
3. Kirkpatrick JJR, Burd DAR. An algorithmic approach to the treatment of hydrofluoric acid burns. Burns 1995; 21:495–499.
4. Yeong EK, Chen MT, Mann R, Lin T-W, Engrav LH. Facial mutilation after an assault with chemicals: 15 cases and literature review. J Burn Care Rehabil 1997; 18:234–237.
5. Mayer TG, Gross PL. Fatal systemic fluorosis due to hydrofluoric acid burns. Ann Emerg Med 1985; 14:149–153.
6. Tepperman PB. Fatality due to acute systemic fluoride poisoning following a hydrofluoric acid skin burn. J Occup Med 1980; 22:691–692.

6

Reconstructive Needs of the Burn Patient

W. JOHN KITZMILLER
University of Cincinnati Medical Center, Cincinnati, Ohio, USA

ROBERT L. McCAULEY
University of Texas Medical Branch and Shriners Hospital for Children—Galveston Unit, Galveston, Texas, USA

I. INTRODUCTION

The goal of reconstructive surgery after serious thermal injury is to preserve and restore functional appearance to the highest possible level. The approach is that of total patient care. After a thorough assessment of the physical, psychological, and social needs of the patient, a comprehensive treatment plan should be devised with input from all burn team members. The process continues whereby the patient and the family is educated about the possibilities and limitations available through both operative and nonoperative treatment for burn scars. The events from the date of injury until the individual reaches their maximal level of improvement is a continuum, often with several significant milestones. Ideally, the rehabilitative treatment plan begins the day of burn injury. Early comprehensive burn treatment includes burn wound management to achieve optimal closure (including the use of allograft); priorities for autograft placement and donor site selection are obviously critical to outcome. Brou and others have outlined a very logical inventory of

reconstruction needs in patients with a 75% total body surface area burn (1,2) (Figs. 6.1–6.4). An inventory of potential reconstructive needs are identified anatomically into these categories: head/neck, torso, and upper and lower extremities. Prioritization in addressing these needs includes the location and severity of the areas injured in the burn accident. In addition, analysis of potential donor sites for reconstruction is crucial. This chapter will focus on management of burn scars and complications related to burn scar contractures.

The priority during the acute burn hospitalization includes resuscitation, control of the hypermetabolic response, prevention of infection, and an early wound closure. Advances in all of these areas allows for increased survival of patients with large total body surface area burns. Prior to discharge, a comprehensive plan is made for occupational therapy and physical therapy. The fundamental principles that seem to result in the best possible outcome include vigorous massage of burn scars with moisturizers, the application of pressure garments, and the use of splints to resist physiologic contraction during

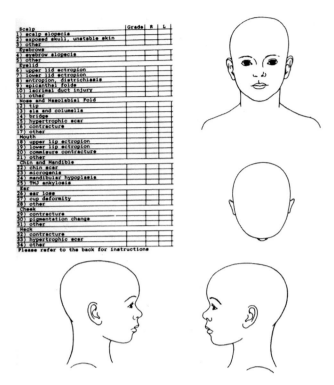

Scalp	Grade	R	L
1) scalp alopecia			
2) exposed skull, unstable skin			
3) other			
Eyebrows			
4) eyebrow alopecia			
5) other			
Eyelid			
6) upper lid ectropion			
7) lower lid ectropion			
8) entropion, districhiasis			
9) epicanthal folds			
10) lacrimal duct injury			
11) other			
Nose and Nasolabial Fold			
12) tip			
13) ala and columella			
14) bridge			
15) hypertrophic scar			
16) contracture			
17) other			
Mouth			
18) upper lip ectropion			
19) lower lip ectropion			
20) commissure contracture			
21) other			
Chin and Mandible			
22) chin scar			
23) microgenia			
24) mandibular hypoplasia			
25) TMJ ankylosis			
Ear			
26) ear loss			
27) cup deformity			
28) other			
Cheek			
29) contracture			
30) pigmentation change			
31) other			
Neck			
32) contracture			
33) hypertrophic scar			
34) other			
Please refer to the back for instructions			

Figure 6.1 Head and neck inventory diagram. [Reprinted with permission from Brou et al. (1).]

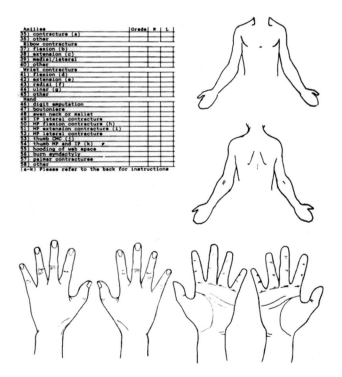

Axilla	Grade	R	L
35) contracture (a)			
36) other			
Elbow contracture			
37) flexion (b)			
38) extension (c)			
39) medial/lateral			
40) other			
Wrist contracture			
41) flexion (d)			
42) extension (e)			
43) radial (f)			
44) ulnar (g)			
45) other			
Hand			
46) digit amputation			
47) boutoniere			
48) swan neck or mallet			
49) IP lateral contracture			
50) MP flexion contracture (h)			
51) MP extension contracture (i)			
52) MP lateral contracture			
53) thumb CMC (j)			
54) thumb MP and IP (k)			
55) hooding of web space			
56) burn syndactyly			
57) palmar contractures			
58) other			
(a-k) Please refer to the back for instructions			

Figure 6.2 Upper extremity inventory diagram. [Reprinted with permission from Brou et al. (1).]

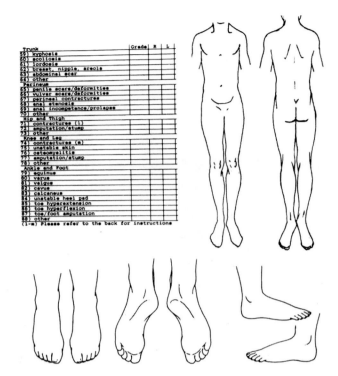

Trunk	Grade	R	L
59) kyphosis			
60) scoliosis			
61) lordosis			
62) breast, nipple, areola			
63) abdominal scar			
64) other			
Perineum			
65) penile scars/deformities			
66) vulvar scars/deformities			
67) perineal contractures			
68) anal stenosis			
69) anal incompetance/prolapse			
70) other			
Hip and Thigh			
71) contractures (l)			
72) amputation/stump			
73) other			
Knee and Leg			
74) contractures (m)			
75) unstable skin			
76) osteomyelitis			
77) amputation/stump			
78) other			
Ankle and Foot			
79) equinus			
80) varus			
81) valgus			
82) cavus			
83) calcaneus			
84) unstable heel pad			
85) toe hyperextension			
86) toe hyperflexion			
87) toe/foot amputation			
88) other			
(l-m) Please refer to the back for instructions			

Figure 6.3 Torso and lower-extremity diagram. [Reprinted with permission from Brou et al. (1).]

the early maturation process (3). In patients with partial-thickness wounds, especially in the face, healing can occur in a satisfactory manner (Fig. 6.5). The wound healing process involves three stages; stage I, the inflammation stage; stage II, the proliferation stage which occurs from weeks to months; and stage III, the scar maturation phase (4). Over the 3-week to 3-month period, the priorities are to maintain range of motion while facilitating the scars that are soft and flat to become as close as possible to the original aesthetic color. The management of hypertrophic scars continues to be a topic of intense discussion. Various treatment modes exist without any showing 100% uniformity of results. Topical silicone gel sheeting has, in limited series, shown to be promising to facilitate scar maturation (5), even though the mechanism of action is still not fully understood. Laser photocoagulation in the range of oxyhemoglobin seems to lessen erythema and may facilitate more rapid scar maturation (6). However, the experience among surgeons using laser photocoagulation is variable.

The early stages of rehabilitation can be difficult. The initial steps toward reintegration of patients back into society are filled with anxiety and uncertainty. The patient and family require social support and education as they return to the community, school, or workplace. A burn support network greatly facilitates these transitions. Recovering from the hardship of extensive

INSTRUCTIONS

I) Identify the patient's abnormality and check the appropriate box [R] for right and [L] for left or both for single or midline structures. Use the empty space in each line to write additional information.
II) Use the diagrams to draw the observed abnormality when needed for more detailed information.
III) Signal each abnormality in the diagram by writing the corresponding number.
IV) Grade each observed abnormality as [S] for severe, [Mo] for moderate, and [Mi] for mild.
V) Some items have specific grading criteria such as:

  (a) Shoulder abduction (normal ROM 0 to 180 degrees)
      Severe: 0 to 60 degrees
      Moderate: 0 to 120 degrees
      Mild: 0 to 180 degrees
  (b) Elbow flexion (normal ROM 0 to 150 degrees)
      Severe: 100 to 150 degrees
      Moderate: 50 to 100 degrees
      Mild: ,0 to 50 degrees
  (c) Elbow extension (normal ROM 150 to 0 degrees)
      Severe: 0 to 50 degrees
      Moderate: 0 to 100 degrees
      Mild: 0 to 150 degrees
  (d) Wrist flexion (normal ROM 0 to 70 degrees)
      Severe: 60 degrees or more
      Moderate: 60 to 20 degrees
      Mild: 20 to -20 degrees
  (e) Wrist extension (normal ROM 0 to -60 degrees)
      Severe: -60 degrees or more
      Moderate: -60 to -40 degrees
      Mild: -40 to -20 degrees
  (f) Wrist ulnar deviation (normal ROM 0 to 30 degrees)
      Severe: 30 degrees or more
  (g) Wrist radial deviation (normal ROM 0 to 20 degrees)
      Severe: 20 degrees or more
  (h) MP flexion (normal ROM 0 to 90 degrees)
      Severe: 90 degrees or more
      Moderate: 90 to 45 degrees
      Mild: 45 to 0 degrees
  (i) MP extension (normal ROM 90 to 0 degrees)
      Severe: less than 0 degrees
  (j) Thumb CMC
      Severe: no opposition or pinch possible
      Moderate: lateral pinch only
      Mild: opposition present
  (k) Thumb MP and IP
      Severe: no opposition or pinch possible
      Moderate: lateral pinch only
      Mild: opposition present
  (l) Hip
      Severe: affects gait and posture
      Moderate: affects sporting activity
      Mild: no functional impairment
  (m) Knee
      Severe: affects gait and posture
      Moderate: affects sporting activity
      Mild: no functional impairment

Figure 6.4 Instructions for completing inventory diagram. [Reprinted with permission from Brou et al. (1).]

scarring after burn injury can be a significant test of the support network (7). Ultimately, these measures of support are equally as important as surgical intervention for the final outcome of our burn patients. Certainly, no secondary reconstructive procedure should be considered without completely taking into account the patient's social context. Recuperation from extensive and multiple reconstructive efforts requires added attention from family members as well as adjustments in the workplace or school. Without these support systems working together, the results of reconstruction may be compromised.

II. OPERATIVE INTERVENTION FOR RECONSTRUCTION

By definition, late reconstruction involves the period after 3 months during the maturation phase of wound healing. The early priorities are to maintain an adequate airway through the prevention of perioral contractures and to maintain full range of motion for the neck. Protection of the cornea in extensive facial burns is an early concern and remains so throughout the reconstructive process. Maintaining range of motion of the extremities and monitoring growth in pediatric patients is also a common concern. The timing of reconstruction is a function of the severity of the deformity, the degree of limitation in range of motion, as well as the anatomic location of the problem. Priority is usually given to concerns in the head/neck region. Certainly, every nonoperative measure should be taken to maintain range of motion and protect the airway and eye. An early neck release is probably the most common early reconstructive need. Priority of the neck release not only facilitates anesthesia for subsequent procedures, but also lessens the extrinsic distortion on facial features which is often seen (8). The principles for neck release involve making a transverse incision from midlateral axis to the contra midlateral axis through the platysma (8). A wide release is performed with the patient in hyperextension. Split thickness skin grafts, usually 0.018 in. or greater, offer the first choice alternative for these patients. Alternatively, full-thickness skin grafts, if available, can provide excellent coverage. However, here, a two-stage approach may be required with allograft placement at the initial operation. A period of hyerextension over the next 5–7 days in bed subsequently treated by acute pressure using heart cervical collars allows for excellent release. Commonly, inadequate releases are performed. This in combination with poor compliance can lead to poor results and frequent relapses.

III. RECONSTRUCTION OF FACIAL BURNS

Extensive thermal burns of the face can result in corneal exposure (8). A high index of suspicion will lessen the morbidity of corneal exposure which ultimately may produce permanent visual impairment. Lubrication and temporary tarsorrhaphy sutures are commonly done during the early phase of healing (8). However, their widespread use has been limited in recent years because of further destruction of the eyelids. A lower eyelid release should be considered in patients with adequate corneal protection. During the operation, a frost suture is placed through the gray line and used for retraction of the lower lid. Some surgeons, however, do not recommend the use of this suture. The release is performed below the ciliary margin and commonly extends through the orbicularis muscle. A full-thickness skin graft harvested from the retro-auricular area may be chosen for subsequent resurfacing. The donor site is closed primarily. Thick split-thickness grafts from the scalp or full-thickness

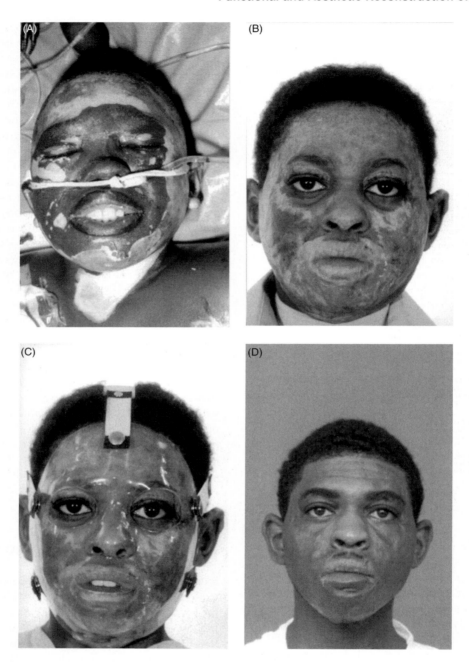

Figure 6.5 (A) Fifteen-year-old black male with partial thickness facial burns. (B) Wounds re-epithelialized with areas of hypopigmentation after 3 weeks. (C) The use of the U-Vex mask to present hypertrophic scar formation. (D) Follow-up 3 years later after correction of lower lip ectropion.

skin grafts from the upper inner arm or the supraclavicular region, if available, are also acceptable donor sites. If possible, the graft should be taken above the collarbone to have the best chance of facial color match. The grafts are sutured in place and quilting sutures will help adherence to the underlying bed and lessen the likelihood of seroma formation and partial graft loss. Tie-over bolsters are commonly used to help facilitate graft healing.

Alternatively, the grafts may be rolled. The patients may have significant obstruction of their visual axis during the early healing period. In such cases, patients require some assistance in the perioperative period. The stents are removed in 1 week.

Aside from maintaining the airway and protection of the cornea, facial burns cause loss or distortion of facial features that include the eyebrows, nose, lips, oral commissure, cheeks, scalp, and ears (Fig. 6.6). There are significant options for restoration of these in anatomic structures through a series of reconstructive operations after the acute period. Burn reconstruction of the scalp, particularly in scalp burns, has been quite satisfactory using tissue expansion (9). In general, if the burn involves up to 40% of the scalp, a highly satisfactory result can be obtained (Fig. 6.7). Tissue expansion may require some adjustments when multiple scalp scars exist. In patients with calvarial burns it is important to determine if care must be taken to ascertain whether or not the underlying skull is intact when scalp expansion is being considered.

Gonzalez-Ulloa (10) has improved our approach to the reconstruction of facial burn scars. In general, the resurfacing of burn scars is performed in specific aesthetic units using skin grafts (Fig. 6.8). If possible, thick split-thickness autografts are taken. Hemostasis is critical to optimize graft take. The grafts may be treated by rolling the edges or tie-over bolster dressings. The lower lip unit is described by Neale et al. (8) is a common priority after the release of the neck contractures. Lateral darts diminish the likelihood of recurrent contraction when there is extensive burn scar of the face. When both the upper and lower lip are burned, the lower may be addressed first and then the upper lip (8). One should avoid the tendency toward ectropions of the lower lip and intropions of the upper lip. No uniformly satisfactory

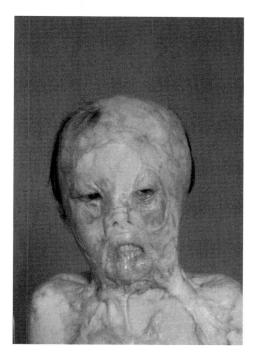

Figure 6.6 Severe distortion of facial burns after deep partial-thickness and full-thickness wounds are allowed to heal, secondary. Note intrinsic and extrinsic ectropions, encasement of the nose is burn scar, severe upper and lower lip ectropions, and a severely constructed neck.

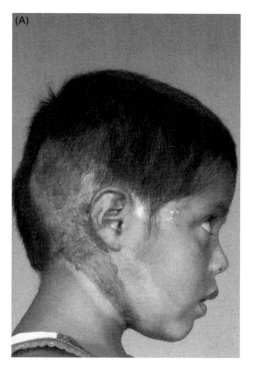

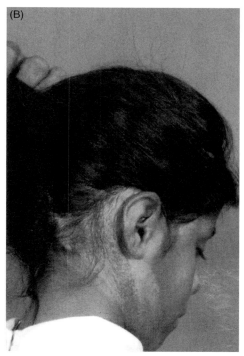

Figure 6.7 (A) Seven-year-old female referred for correction of type 1A right occipital alopecia. (B) Two years after closure of the scalp alopecia with tissue expansion.

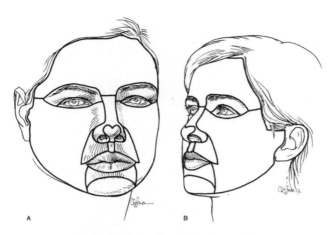

Figure 6.8 Diagram of facial aesthetic units. (With permission from Feldman JJ. Facial burns in plastic surgery. In: McCarthy J, eds. St. Louis, MO: W.B. Saunders, 2000.)

approach is available for reconstruction of the philtrum dimple. Previous attempts at reconstruction using composite grafts have not been ideal aesthetically. Oral commissure contractures are treated by mucosal advancement flaps or the ventral tongue flap. After operative correction, stomal appliances may diminish the likelihood of recurrence.

Nasal deformities after burn injury are quite varied. Although the boney pyramid is rarely destroyed, the lower lateral cartilage is quite susceptible to injury. Deformities can range from alar notching to alar retraction to total loss of the nasal cartilaginous vault. Total nasal reconstruction is accomplished, ideally, with mobilization of local tissue to restore nasal lining and the placement of the cartilaginous unit using bone and cartilage grafts. Subsequent resurfacing of the nasal unit can be accomplished using the forehead flap as described by Menick and Burget (11). Delay of the forehead flap may be necessary to capture skin territories that may be compromised from previous scars. However, its use in burn patients may be contraindicated if the frontalis muscle is destroyed and skin grafts are placed on periosteum for forehead wound closure.

Eyebrow reconstruction may significantly enhance facial burn reconstruction. The alternative surgical approaches include the use of composite grafts or pedicle flaps. Composite grafts are preferred in women who have relatively thin eyebrows. Success with this procedure depends on the blood supply of the underlying recipient site and the quality of the harvested scalp graft. In males, the creation of thicker eyebrows is desired. The use of pedicled scalp flap using the superficial temporal artery as either an external pedicle or island flap is desired. The grafts should be harvested meticulously with the hair growth in the preferred alignment. Currently, the use of

micrografts and minigrafts has become the preferred method for the reconstruction of eyebrows (12).

The development of auricular deformities is a common sequela after severe burns. A spectrum of deformities are seen. A number of techniques exist for the correction of small helical rim defects. However, correction of major cartilaginous defects requires carefully planned procedures with the harvesting of cartilage grafts either from the ear or from the rib. Once the new framework is reconstructed, it then requires a vascularized flap for coverage. The postauricular skin or the superficial temporoparietal fascial flap is typically selected. If scar tissue is present in the postauricular region, caution should be used when raising the postauricular skin since the blood supply to this flap may be precarious.

IV. RECONSTRUCTION OF BREAST BURNS

In children, reconstruction of the burned breast is delayed until the scar restricts breast development. Wide infra- and intramammary releases with thick split-thickness autografts followed by postoperative pressure garment have produced satisfactory results (13). Occasionally, recurrent complex scarring may require excisional treatment of the hypertrophic scar. However, in this case, the requirements for skin grafts increases significantly. Clearly, loss of the nipple areolar complex (NAC) in girls does not mean that the breast bud is injured. Many patients will proceed with breast development with subsequent reconstruction of the NAC. In cases where the breast bud is involved in the burn injury, the breast mound is reconstructed using the techniques that have been described for reconstruction of the breast after mastectomy. The latissimus dorsi myocutaneous flap with or without implants or transverse rectus abdominus myocutaneous has been used (9). In thin individuals in whom the donor site has not been harvested, gluteal flaps may provide an alternative course. However, this flap can be technically challenging with prolonged healing of the donor area (14).

V. RECONSTRUCTION OF EXTREMITY BURNS

Extremity tightness is a particularly common problem in children who have undergone extensive burn injury. The tightness across joints may not only limit active and passive range of motion but also affect skeletal growth (3). Correction of contractures in the axilla and antecubital fossa is common. Local flaps are the initial choices for correction followed by skin grafts. When skin grafts are chosen the donor site selection should be such that high-quality skin is available for resurfacing. A thickness of at least 0.0175 in. on average is recommended.

Alternatively, full-thickness skin grafts are also satisfactory. Stenting and postoperative pressure are the keys of long-term success. The use of pressure postoperatively and splinting in the early perioperative period can make a significant difference. In electrical injuries, the exposure of joints, bare tendons, or bare bone is commonly seen after debridement. Flap reconstruction is particularly indicated for these cases. The choice of local flaps vs. free-tissue transfer is a function of the extent of the injury and the availability of flap donor sites for coverage of these complex defects.

VI. OTHER ISSUES

Extensive abdominal burns which require resurfacing with skin grafts do not interfere, in general, with the ability of the abdominal wall to accommodate pregnancy. Releases are generally not necessary. The unburned abdominal wall seems to adjust. Even in patients with circumferential truncal burns, pregnancy proceeds uninterrupted (15,16).

Local scar revision is occasionally performed when a wound has been allowed to heal secondarily since hypertrophic scars may result. With suitable pliable tissue and adjuvant scar management, occasionally scars may improve. Z-plasties across tethered scars which transverse across joints can result in relief of tethering contractures without the need for skin grafts. The basic principle of the operation is to perform a complete release of the burn scar. One should not sacrifice the quality of the release to avoid closure using a graft. Frequently, reconstructive procedures can be combined when multiple areas need to be addressed. One needs to consider donor site harvesting and postoperative positioning in choosing combined procedures. Surgical options include local scar release and resurfacing with grafts, release and coverage with pedicled flaps, the use of tissue expansion, free flaps, and lasers.

Incisional or excisional release of burn scars and resurfacing with skin grafts are the mainstay of surgery for the correction of burn scar contractures. After re-creation of the defect, the underlying base is usually highly vascular. Thick split-thickness skin grafts, full-thickness skin grafts, or local flaps are the best option. Recently, Alloderm® and Integra® have been proposed to allow one to obtain comparable results with much thinner grafts (17). However, results have been variable. The use of these products may involve significant delays, increase in expenses, and multiple procedures. Again, the results are variable. Yet these modalities certainly are an alternative in extensively burned individuals who have very limited donor sites.

Scar release and resurfacing with pedicled flaps are most commonly employed for reconstruction of facial structures such as the nose, ears, eyebrows, and lips. The concept of facial aesthetic units as described by Gonzalez-Ulloa, Menick, and Burget is followed to obtain the best functional and cosmetic results. In general, reconstruction is best accomplished by replacing tissue with tissue of identical color and texture. In planning reconstruction procedures, the skin above the collarbone should be used for facial reconstruction where color match is crucial and pigmentation changes are less acceptable. The workhorse flaps in this area have been the paramedian forehead flap for nasal reconstruction, the Abbe flap for upper lip reconstruction, and the superficial temporoparietal facial flap for ear reconstruction.

Tissue expansion is the first choice for correction of significant burn scar alopecia. The technique is also helpful in reconstruction in facial defects. The pitfalls of tissue expansion in head and neck reconstruction have been previously described. In general, facial defects of skin above the cheek should be expanded to replace facial scars. However, when advancing across the mandibular borders, a delayed interior pull of the expanded flap can cause secondary distortion. Yet, some surgeons have shown success in the use of expanders for facial resurfacing (18).

Free-flap reconstruction is a part of the armentarium of procedures utilized by plastic surgeons when the magnitude of the defects is large and local tissue is inadequate. Common applications for free-flap reconstruction have been for extensive full-thickness scalp defects, composite facial defects, electrical burns to the extremities, and salvage of joints and preservation of amputation lengths.

Lasers are currently being employed, selectively, as an adjunct to lessen some of the erythema and hypertrophy of thick scars that result in burn injury. We have used lasers to debilitate scalp grafts and undesirable hair growth. We have empirically tried treating hyperpigmentation with lasers with variable results. Capozzi et al. seem to have had better success in the use of the laser for hyperpigmentation of burn scars.

VII. SUMMARY

The evolution of techniques and principles in burn reconstruction continues. As patients continue to survive increasingly large total body surface area burns, the reconstruction needs will continue to increase exponentially (1). Not only is an inventory of potential reconstructive needs outlined but prioritization of these needs is crucial. The surgical plan must be embraced by both the patient and the surgeon. Our success is only measured by minimizing complication rates and maximizing both aesthetic and functional outcomes.

REFERENCES

1. Brou JA, Robson MC, McCauley RL, Herndon DN, Phillips LG, Ortega M, Evans EB, Alvarado MI. Inventory of potential reconstructive needs in the patient with burns. J Burn Care Rehabil 1989; 10(6):555–560.

2. Burns BF, McCauley RL, Murphy FL, Robson MC. Reconstructive management of patients with >80% TBSA burns. Burns 1993; 19(5):429–433.

3. Larson DL, Abston S, Evans EB. Techniques for decreasing scar formation and contractures in the burn patient. J Trauma 1971; 11:807.

4. Rohrich RJ, Robinson JB. Selected readings in plastic surgery. Wound Healing 1999; 9(3):1–32.

5. Quinn KJ. Silicone gel in scar treatment. Burns 1987; 13:S33.

6. Alster TS, Nanni CA. Pulsed dye laser treatment of hypertrophic burn scars. Plast Reconstr Surg 1998; 102:2190–2195.

7. Abar R, Ross IS. Selected readings in plastic surgery. Postburn Reconstr 2000; 9:10–25.

8. Neale HW, Billmire DA, Carey JP. Reconstruction following head and neck burns. Clin Plast Surg 1986; 13:119–136.

9. MacLennan SE, Corcoran JF, Neale HW. Tissue expansion in head and neck burn reconstruction. Clin Plast Surg 2000; 27:121–132.

10. Gonzalez-Ulloa M. Restoration of the face covering by means of selected skin in regional aesthetic units. Br J Plast Surg 1956; 9:212.

11. Burget GC, Menick MF. Nasal support and lining the marriage of beauty and blood-supply. Plast Reconstr Surg 1989; 84:189–203.

12. Barerra A. Use of micrografts and minigrafts in functional. In: McCauley RL, ed. Functional and Aesthetic Reconstruction of Burns. New York: Marcel Dekker, 2004.

13. Neale HW. Reconstruction of burns of the trunk and breast. In: Marsh J, ed. Current Therapy in Plastic and Reconstructive Surgery. New York: Marcel Dekker, 1989.

14. Codner MA, Nahai F. The gluteal free flap breast reconstruction. Making it work. Clin Plast Surg 1994; 21(2):289–296.

15. Kitzmiller WJ, Neale HW, Warden GD, Smith D. The effect of full thickness abdominal wall burns during childhood on subsequent childbearing. Ann Plast Surg 1999; 40(2):111–113.

16. McCauley RL, Stenberg BA, Phillips LG, Blackwell SJ, Robson MC. Long-term assessment of the effects of circumferential truncal burns in pediatric patients on subsequent pregnancies. J Burn Care Rehabil 1991; 12(1):51–53.

17. Heimbach DM, Warden GD, Luterman A, Jordan MH, Ozobia N, Ryan CM, Voigt DW, Hickerson WL, Saffle JR, DeClement FA, Sheridan RL, Dimick AR. Multicenter postapproval clinical trial of Integra dermal regeneration template for burn treatment. J Burn Care Rehabil 2003; 24(1):42–48.

18. McCauley RL, Oweisy F. Aesthetic reconstruction of facial burns with expanded cervicofacial flaps. Proc Am Burn Assoc 2001; 29:91.

7

Anesthesia for Reconstructive Burn Surgery

LEE C. WOODSON, EDWARD R. SHERWOOD, JOAQUIN CORTIELLA, LYNN PETERSON

Shriners Hospital for Children, Galveston, and University of Texas Medical Branch, Galveston, Texas, USA

I. INTRODUCTION

Over the last 20 years, survival from large total body surface area burns has steadily improved. With early admission to a specialized burn center, survival from these major injuries is now often the rule rather than the exception (1–3). As a consequence, an increasing number of patients with extensive burn-associated deformities will present for reconstructive surgery.

Cutaneous burn injuries produce cosmetic and functional defects that require surgical correction. The sequelae of burn injuries also create unique challenges for anesthetic management. Among the most visible changes are the burn scars that distort airway anatomy and limit range of motion, making airway management difficult. Thick scars can also obliterate peripheral vascular access. Less obvious effects of burn injury are an increased metabolic rate and dramatically altered drug responses. Increased oxygen consumption speeds hemoglobin desaturation during periods of apnea and altered drug effects include decreased sensitivity to intravenous induction agents (4), decreased sensitivity to nondepolarizing muscle relaxants (5), and potentially lethal exaggerated hyperkalemic responses to succinylcholine (6).

Severe burn injuries also may leave psychological scars. Traumatic events associated with the initial injury along with intense pain associated with the postburn sequelae and subsequent therapy have profound and long-lasting psychological effects. These include a reduced pain threshold as well as increased anxiety, especially in the perioperative period (7). Increased anxiety can make induction of general anesthesia stormy and increase the incidence of postoperative nausea, vomiting, and delirium. Decreased pain tolerance requires more attention to analgesia.

From these considerations it is clear that patients for reconstructive surgery after burn injuries present the anesthetist with unique challenges involving every phase of perioperative care. From the preoperative evaluation through the postoperative period each phase of anesthetic care for these patients involves considerations specific to this particular group of patients.

Rather than outline general principles of anesthetic management, this chapter will focus on unique features of the perioperative care of burn reconstruction patients that require extra attention or special procedures. Our practice involves primarily pediatric burn patients (up to 20 years of age). However, we will also discuss problems presented by adults who may be more cooperative than children but more commonly present with serious comorbidities such as long-standing diabetes mellitus, coronary artery disease, or chronic obstructive pulmonary disease.

II. PREOPERATIVE EVALUATION

The recent Practice Advisory by the American Society of Anesthesiologists (ASA) Task Force on Preanesthesia Evaluation outlines current expert opinion regarding preanesthetic evaluation (8). Decisions regarding the timing and scope of preanesthetic assessment depend on the severity of the patient's disease and the invasiveness of planned surgical procedures. Preoperative evaluation of patients with low severity of disease for minimally invasive procedures can usually be performed on the same day of surgery. As a general rule reconstructive burn surgery is only mildly invasive. Surgical trauma is usually limited to cutaneous tissues. In some cases rib cartilage or iliac bone may be harvested as donor material for grafting. In general, body cavities are not entered. Postoperative pain can be significant, however, and this can be an important source of physiological stress. Patients with high severity of disease (ASA III or IV) may require evaluation before the day of surgery if additional diagnostic studies or consultation might be expected to affect outcome by optimizing medical condition or significantly influencing decisions.

Planning anesthetic care for postburn patients requires specific information about the patient's burn injury. Knowledge of the extent (total body surface area of full thickness burns) and distribution of injuries is necessary for planning vascular access and airway management. This information is available in the form of burn diagrams included with the patient's medical records from the acute period of burn treatment (Fig. 7.1). The presence and distribution of hypertrophic scars and contractures is

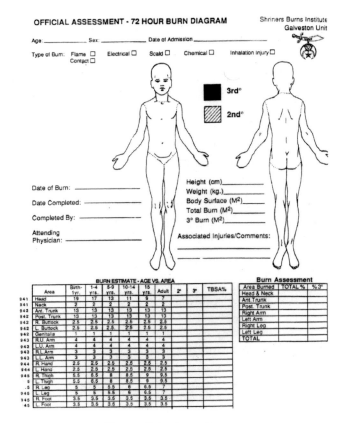

Figure 7.1 Burn diagram.

important in this respect. The time interval from the initial burn injury as well as the time since healing of acute burn wounds must be known in order to assess the metabolic state and response to drugs such as muscle relaxants.

Previous anesthetic records are a valuable source of information for the preoperative evaluation. This is especially relevant for burn reconstruction patients. After extensive burn injuries, scar contracture deformities often continue to develop and these patients will require many surgical interventions over a long period of time. Review of the medical record allows the anesthetic management to be individualized to each patient's unique needs. Specific issues for burn reconstructive patients include airway management, intravenous access, effectiveness of preoperative medication, and susceptibility to postoperative nausea and vomiting. Knowledge of previous experience with each of these management issues for an individual patient can have a major impact on care decisions.

A. Airway Evaluation

Burn scar contractures can make airway management with conventional techniques very difficult, if not impossible.

Scars from deep facial and neck burns can produce a variety of defects each of which is associated with a unique airway management problem. Information gained from a thorough airway evaluation (including careful review of the medical record) is critical to adequate planning for airway management.

Dense scars over the lower face and neck can displace the mandible posteriorly as well as restrict its mobility (Fig. 7.2) making exposure of laryngeal structures difficult during direct laryngoscopy. In young patients mandibular growth can be retarded by overlying scars producing, in effect, an acquired micrognathia, which further impairs direct laryngoscopy (Fig. 7.3). Microstomia due to scar contractures can prevent insertion of a laryngoscope blade into the mouth (Fig. 7.4). Nasal scars can make it difficult to introduce a nasal endotracheal tube (Fig. 7.5). When these conditions coexist (Fig. 7.6) the challenge is doubly difficult. Traumatic injuries associated with burns can cause tissue loss and scar contractures and deformities that make recognition of airway structures difficult, even by flexible fiberoptic laryngoscopy (Fig. 7.7).

With such a broad range of deformities, it is clear that the preoperative airway evaluation requires more than a Mallampati classification exam. The size of the mouth opening should be examined to determine if it is large enough to allow direct laryngoscopy. The nares should also be examined to determine whether or not passage of an endotracheal tube is possible or if mask ventilation is possible while the mouth is closed. Cervical spine mobility should be evaluated because limited motion of the neck may preclude the "sniffing position" and alignment of the airway axes. Posterior displacement of the mandible can be evaluated by measuring the thyromental distance.

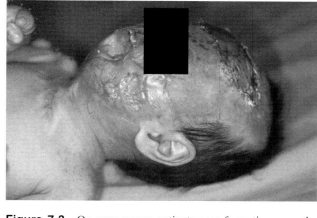

Figure 7.3 On very young patients scar formation over the lower face can limit mandibular growth resulting in a form of acquired micrognathia.

The deformities described above can not only make direct laryngoscopy impossible, but limited mandibular mobility may also make it difficult or impossible to accomplish mask ventilation of the patient after induction of general anesthesia.

Most anesthetics and sedatives cause relaxation of pharyngeal muscles. As a result, obstruction of the upper airway often occurs during induction of anesthesia. This obstruction can be relieved in most patients by lifting the chin and advancing the mandible. When the mandible is immobile due to thick overlying scar tissue the airway cannot be opened by these maneuvers and airway obstruction cannot be relieved. Safe and effective management of these patients requires examination of mandibular

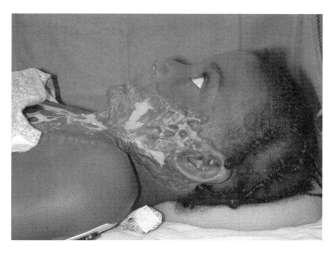

Figure 7.2 Direct laryngoscopy is made difficult by the presence of dense scar tissue over the face and neck which can displace the mandible posteriorly and restrict mandibular motion.

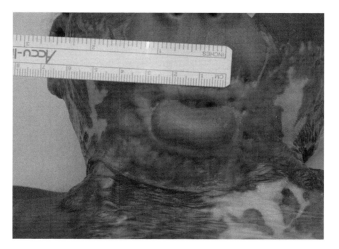

Figure 7.4 Burn scar contractions involving the mouth can cause microstomia, which can preclude insertion of a laryngoscope blade.

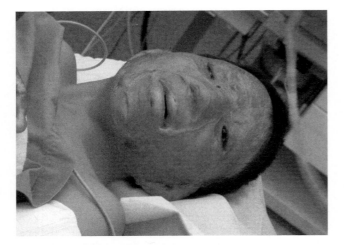

Figure 7.5 Burn scars involving the nose can reduce nares dimensions making nasotracheal intubation difficult or impossible.

mobility to predict ease of mask ventilation after induction of general anesthesia. When dense scar tissue impairs mandibular mobility, the anesthetic plan must provide a means to keep the airway patent until the trachea is intubated. Specialized techniques other than conventional direct laryngoscopy are often required.

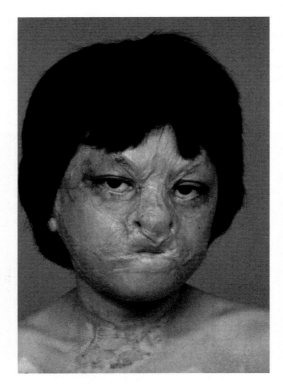

Figure 7.6 Endotracheal intubation can be especially challenging when both microstomia and small nares occur together.

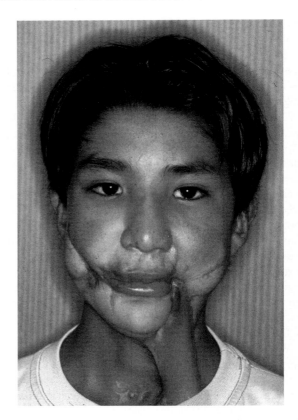

Figure 7.7 Burns occasionally are accompanied by traumatic injury resulting in mandibular and soft tissue loss that causes anatomic distortion that can make fiberoptic intubation difficult.

B. Pulmonary Evaluation

Patients suffering massive burns are subject to a variety of insults to the respiratory system (9). At the time of injury there may be inhalation of hot gases and smoke that damage the larynx, respiratory epithelium of the airways, or pulmonary parenchyma. Epithelial injury can impair ciliary function and result in retained mucous or other materials. During the acute phase of injury there is a high risk of pneumonia and adult respiratory diotress syndrome (ARDS) in patients with inhalation injury. Prolonged ventilation with high volumes and pressures can contribute to parenchymal damage. Laryngeal injury from heat and irritation from an endotracheal tube can produce long-term complications such as laryngeal stenosis or motor dysfunction. These can impair vocal cord function and lead to chronic aspiration. These insults can result in chronic pulmonary pathology including pulmonary fibrosis, reduced pulmonary capillary volume, bronchilolitis obliterans, chronic bronchitis, and bronchiectasis (10–13). These conditions can lead to a variety of associated pulmonary function problems including reactive airway disease, altered compliance, increased dead space and closing volume, and limitation of diffusion. Additional mechanical deficiencies also may impair pulmonary function. Prolonged ventilation and immobilization can cause muscle atrophy and weakness of respiratory muscles. Thoracic burn scars (especially when circumferential) may contribute to a restrictive respiratory defect. Spinal deformities due to burn scar contractures can also cause a severe restrictive respiratory defect. Long-term follow-up of pulmonary function among ARDS survivors has revealed a large degree of heterogeneity. Function may be near normal in those who were young and did not smoke at the time of injury. However, respiratory function may be significantly impaired in older patients and in those who had additional comorbidities at the time of injury (14). The most common abnormalities seen have been reduced diffusing capacity and easy fatigability. The observation that poor exercise tolerance did not correlate with the decrease in diffusion capacity suggests that the early fatigue seen in these patients is unrelated to pulmonary pathology (14).

General anesthesia produces a variety of effects that may be associated with perioperative pulmonary complications. These effects include depressed respiratory drive, respiratory muscle dysfunction, decreased functional residual capacity, and atelectasis (15,16). In patients with pre-existing pulmonary dysfunction, these effects are more likely to lead to perioperative pulmonary complications such as bronchospasm, pneumonia, or respiratory failure requiring mechanical ventilation. These complications are also more likely in patients with chronic sequelae of burn and inhalation injury.

In order to assess risk of perioperative pulmonary complications, review of the medical records is required. The record should be examined for evidence of smoke inhalation injury or aspiration as well as complications resulting from that initial injury. Knowledge of the hospital course is also critical for assessment of risk and planning anesthetic management. A history of prolonged mechanical ventilation indicates risk of serious pulmonary complications. The indications for mechanical ventilation should be sought, along with evidence of pneumonia, tracheostomy, and ARDS.

Patient history should include questions regarding more recent pulmonary symptoms of decreased exercise tolerance, bronchospasm, shortness of breath, and sputum production. This information may prove helpful in planning anesthetic management to minimize perioperative pulmonary complications.

In asymptomatic patients preoperative pulmonary function tests have been found to be ineffective in predicting perioperative pulmonary complications (17). Pulmonary function tests are a clinically and economically inefficient screen for clinically occult pulmonary dysfunction. However, these tests may be valuable as a management tool to optimize pulmonary function and, in patients with marginal function, the information derived from these tests may help guide separation from mechanical support postoperatively.

C. Preoperative Diagnostic Tests

In the past some preoperative tests were performed routinely, meaning that they were used to identify a disease or disorder in asymptomatic persons. Evidence-based considerations have discredited this practice. For example, it is no longer considered necessary to order preoperative hemoglobin determinations or urinalysis without specific indications. A report of the ASA Task Force on Preanesthesia Evaluation recommends that preanesthetic tests should not be ordered routinely (8). These recommendations are appropriate for burn reconstruction patients. It is unusual for these patients to bleed sufficiently to require intraoperative transfusion. This means that unless the patient appears clinically anemic or when extensive blood loss is expected, it is unnecessary to order hemoglobin levels preoperatively. Diagnostic tests should not be ordered routinely, but should be based on indications revealed during the preoperative evaluation. One exception is the routine pregnancy testing of all premenopausal menstruating females. In five studies, the results were positive in 0.3–2.2% of cases. This information led to alterations in management or cancellation in 100% of cases where the patient was found to be pregnant (8).

III. MANAGEMENT OF ANESTHESIA

In the absence of significant coexisting disease, airway management, and vascular access are the major considerations for the anesthetic management of patients presenting for reconstructive surgery after extensive burn injuries. Problems relating to airway management in these patients are not only technically challenging but may also create life-threatening situations where it is difficult or impossible to ventilate, intubate, or even to establish a surgical airway. Extensive scaring can obscure all peripheral veins so that central venous access is required and this may be very difficult in some patients. Patient age or cooperativity is another important consideration in this patient population because it can restrict treatment options. Awake procedures are safest and are possible with sedation combined with local or topical anesthesia in adults, but pediatric patients or anxious adults often require deep sedation or general anesthesia for central venous cannulation or airway management. Deep sedation or general anesthesia in these patients prior to establishing vascular access or securing the airway creates a period of vulnerability. Under these conditions safe and effective care requires thorough planning and preparation.

It is always important that patients are made comfortable and free of anxiety, but for the burn reconstruction patient this consideration takes on added significance. These patients often require multiple procedures under anesthesia. A stressful or unpleasant experience in the operating room can make subsequent inductions even more challenging especially in pediatric patients. This makes it more important to review the records and question the patient and family regarding which premedications and induction techniques were most effective.

A final specific issue to consider for anesthetic management of burn reconstruction patients is the metabolic consequences of large burns. For a variable period of time following healing of major burn wounds, metabolic changes persist. These changes include hypermetabolic and hyperdynamic circulatory states in addition, drug responses are altered enough to affect anesthetic management.

A. Preoperative Preparation

Preoperative anxiety is a major concern for any patient who has sustained a burn and presents for reconstructive surgery. Many postburn patients do not exhibit long-term major psychiatric or psychosocial impairment (18). However, individuals who have sustained significant burn injury are at risk for a variety of psychiatric disorders such as posttraumatic stress disorder, phobias and other anxiety disorders (7). The incidence of psychiatric disorders in burned children has been compared with the incidence in survivors of other traumatic events. Burned children had significantly more phobic disorders, anxiety disorders, and posttraumatic stress disorders (19). Many postburn patients continue to have intermittent periods of increased anxiety. Return to the hospital for reconstructive surgery is an especially strong stimulus for return of anxiety (7).

Preoperative anxiety is not only unpleasant for the patient and complicates induction of general anesthesia, but it can contribute to adverse psychological and physiological outcomes. Preoperative anxiety has been found to be an independent predictor in children of postoperative maladaptive behavior such as nightmares, separation anxiety, eating problems, and increased fear of doctors at follow-up visits (20).

Preparation of a patient for surgery begins with the preoperative visit. In a now classic study, Egbert et al. (21) found that patients were less anxious after a preoperative visit by the anesthesiologist than after a sedative premedication. In the case of pediatric patients, parental fear and anxiety have an important effect on the child's level of preoperative anxiety. Confidence from a reassuring visit with an opportunity to ask questions and relate concerns can

significantly reduce the parents' anxiety and help calm the patient. As stated earlier, because burn patients often require many reconstructive operations it is very important to review the medical record. Information about the effectiveness of premedications in the past can be very helpful. It is also important to ask the patient about previous anesthetics with regard to unpleasant experiences and what premedications or induction techniques worked best. In this way the care can be individualized for the patient.

A frequent problem for pediatric patients returning for repeat procedures is fear of the anesthetic mask. This can be discovered at the time of preoperative visit and plans can be made to deal with the issue. One helpful strategy is to give the patient a mask to play with before induction. A patient-selected flavor can be applied to the mask to facilitate acceptance and disguise the scent of the inhalation agent. Other children prefer mask induction but fear placement of intravenous catheters. Therefore, it is important to discuss the plan for anesthetic induction with the patient. The sense of participation by the patient provides more confidence and reduces fear.

Benzodiazepines are the first-line drug class for perioperative pharmacological anxiolysis. They produce not only anxiolysis but amnesia and sedation as well. Benzodiazepines have a wide therapeutic index and little toxicity. They are not analgesics, however, and some patients respond with a paradoxical excitement rather than sedation. Benzodiazepine selection is guided primarily by pharmacokinetic considerations (Table 7.1). Not only is the onset of action for orally administered diazepam and lorazepam slower than for midazolam, but their duration of action are also much longer lasting. There are also pharmacodynamic differences; amnesia is most profound with lorazepam. This may be an advantage or a disadvantage depending on the patient's expectations and planned procedures.

Table 7.1 Pharmacological Comparison of Benzodiazepines

	Diazepam	Lorazepam	Midazolam
Dose equivalent (mg/kg)	0.3–0.5	0.05	0.15–0.5 (20 mg max)
Volume of Distribution (L/kg)	1–1.5	0.8–1.3	1–1.5
Protein binding (%)	96–98	96–98	96–98
Time to peak effect (oral dose/h)	1–1.5	2–4	0.5–1
Elimination half-time (h)	20–40	10–20	1–4

McCall and colleagues (22) examined the effectiveness of preoperative sedatives in postburn pediatric patients scheduled for reconstructive surgery. They hypothesized that administration of the long-acting lorazepam in conjunction with conventional preoperative medication would be more effective in reducing perioperative anxiety. They found that patients who received lorazepam the night before surgery were less anxious than patients who only received sedation the day of surgery.

Midazolam is the most commonly used benzodiazepine used for preoperative sedation. McGraw et al. (23) evaluated the effect of midazolam (0.5 mg/kg given orally) as a preoperative sedative in healthy nonburned pediatric patients. Children given oral midazolam were less likely to cry and fight and had a smoother induction. An oral dose of 0.5 mg/kg of midazolam up to a maximum of 20 mg is effective. Midazolam has also been found effective for pediatric patients when administered intranasally in a dose of 0.2–0.3 mg/kg.

Ketamine has also been found to be an effective preoperative medication in children. Ketamine differs from the benzodiazepines in that it is a very potent analgesic. Gutstein and colleagues (24) evaluated oral ketamine given preoperatively to facilitate induction of anesthesia. In children aged 1–7 years ketamine improved separation from parents and induction of anesthesia. A dose of 6 mg/kg was found superior to 3 mg/kg. In this study oral ketamine was not associated with prolonged recovery time or increased emergence phenomena. Children are much less susceptible to emergence delirium than adults (25).

In extremely anxious and combative pediatric patients, ketamine administered intramuscularly is effective. A needleless air gun delivery system (Bioject®) (Fig. 7.8) can be less traumatic for the patient and less dangerous for operating room personnel than using a needle and syringe. The volume injected with this system is limited to 1 mL, however. A dose of 4 mg/kg of ketamine usually produces acceptable sedation. An alternative use of the needleless system is to use it for injection of lidocaine into the planned site for ketamine injection. This reduces pain and improves patient acceptance of intramuscular injection of a volume of ketamine that could not be delivered with the needleless system. Since these patients often require multiple procedures, these extra steps often become worthwhile by making future inductions less difficult.

α-2 Adrenergic agonists are another class of drugs that have shown promise as preoperative medications (26). These drugs have sedative and analgesic effects that can be very helpful in the perioperative period. In addition these drugs potentiate the anesthetic action of other agents and reduce anesthetic requirements during surgery. Clonidine is the first drug in this class to be used as a preoperative medication. Clonidine is well tolerated and has a wide margin of safety.

Adverse effects of clonidine are a dose-related extension of its pharmacologic profile (sedation, bradycardia, hypotension, and dry mouth). Bradycardia and hypotension can be treated with a vagolytic drug such as atropine. It has been suggested that clonidine possess cardioprotective effects for elderly patients with coronary artery disease (26). Clonidine also attenuated the sympathomimetic effect of ketamine (27). Clonidine is rapidly and almost completely absorbed after oral administration and is effective in a dose of 5 μg/kg either orally or intravenously (26).

Dexmedetomidine is a more recently released α-2 adrenergic agonist with clinically significant sedative and analgesic properties (28). Dexmedetomidine is the pharmacologically active dextroisomer of medetomidine. It is eight times more specific for α-2-adrenoceptors than clonidine. Clinical experience with dexmedetomidine mainly involves sedation of intubated postoperative patients. However, because it does not cause respiratory depression dexmedetomidine does not have to be discontinued at the time of extubation and it has also been found effective in postoperative patients after extubation. Dexmedetomidine may also find use as a premedicant in the future.

Another nonpharmacological anxiolytic technique for pediatric patients is parental presence during induction. In some pediatric patients separation anxiety is so intense that preoperative sedation may be ineffective. The patient may refuse medication or the patient may be so anxious that very large doses of sedation are required. In selected patients we have found that parental presence in the operating room during induction offers advantages. Avoidance of separation from parents before induction can

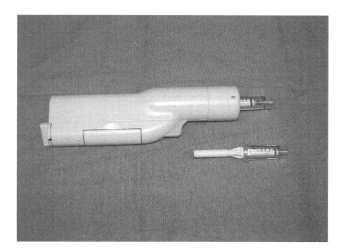

Figure 7.8 In some cases a needless drug delivery device (e.g., Bioject®) can provide a safer and less traumatic means of intramuscular injection.

reduce anxiety. Parent satisfaction is also improved if the parent is present and participates in some way. Parental acceptance of this technique is high (29) and it has been adopted by many anesthesiologists (30). Parents must be instructed ahead of time that they must leave as soon as the child is unconscious. Personnel should be designated to escort the parent from the operating room (OR) so that the anesthesia team is not distracted from the patient. Little outcome data are available for parental presence during induction of general anesthesia, but this practice is commonly used and considered by most practitioners to be beneficial in selected cases.

B. Airway Management

Airway issues are often the primary consideration in planning anesthetic management for reconstructive surgery for burn patients. As described earlier, burn scar contractures can make tracheal intubation impossible by conventional direct laryngoscopy. Airway management options are even more limited when mandibular immobility makes mask ventilation difficult. It may be impossible to open the airway when it becomes obstructed during sedation or general anesthesia. These two conditions, difficult laryngoscopy and difficult mask ventilation, should be recognized as separate problems each requiring specific management techniques.

Management of the difficult airway is a very large topic. Much has been written and many techniques described. Some of these techniques are not effective in all burn reconstructive patients. For example, extensive neck scars can preclude the use of a retrograde technique or a light wand. Microstomia can make it impossible to use specialized laryngoscope blades such as the Bullard laryngoscope. A comprehensive review of difficult airway management is beyond the scope of this chapter. We will focus on techniques specifically described for burn reconstruction surgery and techniques that have been found safe and effective in our pediatric burn hospital.

Although many techniques and devices have been described (31), under difficult conditions, it is generally accepted that the most effective technique for tracheal intubation is with a flexible fiberoptic bronchoscope (32). In fact, fiberoptic intubation has become the technique of choice for management of the difficult airway under most circumstances (33). Improvements in equipment have provided instruments that are small enough to be effective in neonates (34).

When tracheal intubation is considered difficult, an awake technique is safest. In almost all circumstances an awake patient with an unimpaired respiratory drive can maintain airway patency better than any technique available for the anesthetized patient. Techniques of awake

fiberoptic intubation have been thoroughly reviewed recently (32).

With sedation and topical or regional anesthesia, awake intubation with a flexible fiberoptic bronchoscope can usually be performed in cooperative patients without undue stress. A number of studies have examined the cardiovascular response to awake fiberoptic intubation (33). When compared with direct laryngoscopy and intubation the hemodynamic changes associated with fiberoptic intubation vary with technique and pharmacological management. In some cases fiberoptic intubation caused more hypertension and tachycardia than with conventional direct laryngoscopy (35). Cardiac ischemia has been observed during fiberoptic bronchoscopy in patients with documented coronary artery disease (36) and in patients over 60 years of age but with no documented coronary artery disease (37). It is not unreasonable to assume that similar changes may occur in susceptible patients during fiberoptic intubation. For elderly patients and patients at risk for coronary artery disease it is important to use adequate monitoring and appropriate pharmacologic therapy to blunt the hemodynamic response and limit myocardial ischemia.

In contrast to adults who will cooperate with awake procedures, deep sedation or general anesthesia is required for intubation of pediatric patients or adults who are combative or highly anxious. Since deep sedation and most anesthetics cause collapse of pharyngeal tissues and airway obstruction (38) they are unsuitable for fiberoptic intubation in patients whose airway would be difficult to manage with a mask. Ketamine, however, is unique among anesthetic drugs because it maintains spontaneous ventilation and airway patency (39,40). Wrigley et al. (41) evaluated the use of halothane for fiberoptic intubation of pediatric patients. In this series of 40 patients several complications were experienced including laryngospasm and failure to achieve intubation with the fiberscope. This is in contrast to numerous reports of safe and effective airway management with ketamine in a variety of difficult airway situations (see following text).

When mandibular mobility is preserved and mask ventilation appears possible, administration of N_2O or even inhalation induction of general anesthesia can be used to facilitate peripheral vein cannulation. Once venous access is obtained, ketamine can be given and the inhalation agent discontinued. To avoid laryngospasm, it is important not to instrument the airway until the inhalation agent has been eliminated. A drying agent such as glycopyrrolate or scopolamine administered as soon as possible will reduce the amount of secretions. During fiberoptic intubation, secretions not only obscure the view but also impair the action of local anesthetics applied topically to the airway. If the epiglottis falls back near the posterior pharyngeal wall an assistant can open the airway by lifting the mandible anteriorly. Occasionally it also may be helpful to grasp the tongue with a gauze sponge or McGill forceps to pull it forward and create more space.

When mandibular mobility is not preserved, mask ventilation under deep sedation or general anesthesia is often difficult or impossible. Under these conditions, collapse of pharyngeal tissues and obstruction of the upper airway cannot be relieved by manipulation of the jaw when the mandible is immobilized by dense scar. In this situation ketamine has been reported safe and effective by many clinicians (39–47). If venous access is available, 2 mg/kg of ketamine usually is adequate for flexible fiberoptic intubation. Additional ketamine can be given as needed. If vascular access is not available 10 mg/kg of ketamine given intramuscularly provides conditions suitable for fiberoptic intubation. Pain of ketamine injection can be minimized in pediatric patients by first injecting 2 mL of 2% lidocaine then without removing the needle replacing the syringe with another one containing the ketamine dose. Pain of injection is much reduced by slow injection of the ketamine into the area infiltrated with lidocaine.

When patients present with both difficult vascular access and an airway that is difficult to ventilate with a mask, the safest and most effective sequence is to secure the airway before obtaining vascular access. Extensive scarring can obscure landmarks including peripheral pulses and displace soft tissues including blood vessels. Under these circumstances vascular cannulation can require a significant amount of time. During this time a patient sedated with ketamine may accumulate secretions and the sedation may begin to wear off. These conditions are less than optimal for fiberoptic intubation and titrating sedation with additional intramuscular ketamine injections is imprecise and difficult. When intubation is performed first, an inhalation agent can then be administered to facilitate vascular cannulation.

An additional challenge occurs in patients with tissue expanders placed in the neck. Anecdotally, our experience is that these tissue expanders can lead to airway obstruction after ketamine administration. This is especially true when the expanders are placed bilaterally (Fig. 7.9). The airway obstruction can be relieved when an assistant lifts on the tissue expander to reduce the force exerted on the larynx.

For patients with difficult airways, ketamine produces conditions not available during deep sedation or general anesthesia with other agents. Magnetic resonance images of the upper airway were used by Lang et al. (48) to compare the effects of ketamine and propofol on airway patentcy. As in a previous study (38), propofol consistently caused obstruction at the level of the soft palate. With ketamine, however, airway dimensions were not altered from the awake state (48). Airway protective reflexes are also preserved and although protection

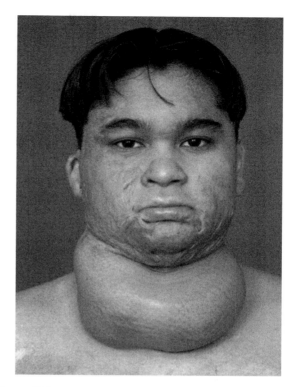

Figure 7.9 Presence of large bilateral neck tissue expanders increase the risk of airway obstruction after induction of general anesthesia even when ketamine is used. When this occurs the airway can be opened by lifting on the tissue expanders.

against aspiration is not absolute, aspiration is rare during sedation or anesthesia with ketamine (49). Green and others reported that in 1022 emergency department cases of ketamine administration to pediatric patients, the incidence of emesis was 6.7% but there was no clinical evidence of aspiration (50).

In our institution ketamine has been used extensively for stressful procedures as well as burn surgery since its opening in 1966 (39). Ketamine alone without tracheal intubation has been described as safe and effective for major burn surgery (39,40,51,52). The unique ability of ketamine to produce profound analgesia, amnesia, and insensibility yet preserve airway patency and respiratory drive has especially been found useful in patients with severe neck scar contractures (44–47). Ketamine has also been reported effective for bronchoscopy in children (53) and blind nasal intubation in adults (43). In addition, because it preserves airway patency and respiratory drive, ketamine has been found safe and effective in pediatric interventional cardiac procedures (54) during procedures in emergency departments (50), as a preoperative anxiolytic (24), and for total intravenous anesthesia in office based surgery (55).

The pharmacology of ketamine has been reviewed several times (25,56–58). In addition to preserving airway reflexes ketamine does not depress respiratory drive. CO_2 sensitivity is not depressed (59) and, in fact, minute ventilation is usually increased by ketamine (39). Mild respiratory depression has been reported with ketamine (60), but this is uncommon unless a large dose is given rapidly or in combination with large doses of benzodiazepines.

A side effect that has limited the use of ketamine is the behavioral changes that have been reported in up to 30% of patients during emergence from sedation or anesthesia with ketamine (25). These changes have been described as floating sensations, vivid dreams, illusions, or hallucinations. These sensations may be either pleasant or disturbing and possibly frightening. The incidence and intensity of these emergence reactions are less in pediatric patients (50). Postoperative emergence reactions including delirium, however, are not uncommon among pediatric patients, even in the absence of ketamine administration. There is no evidence that emergence reactions after ketamine administration have any long-lasting behavioral effects in children or adults (61–63).

Benzodiazepines have been found to reduce the incidence of ketamine-induced emergence reactions in adults (64). However, in recent randomized, double blind studies, midazolam did not reduce emergence reactions in pediatric patients given ketamine for emergency department procedures (65,66). Wathen et al. (66) reported an increased incidence of oxyhemoglobin desaturation in patients who received midazolam in addition to ketamine. Maldini (52) also observed respiratory depression when ketamine was combined with midazolam and recommended avoidance of this combination when using ketamine as an anesthetic for burn surgery. In our institution, benzodiazepines are administered for preoperative anxiolysis but large or intravenous doses are generally avoided in patients who will receive ketamine.

In our patient population emergence delirium is more common in patients who have not received ketamine (unpublished observation). When emergence agitation does occur regardless of what anesthetic drugs were used, we make sure that appropriate analgesic therapy has been administered then bring the parents into the recovery room to help reassure the patient. Benzodiazepines are administered if agitation continues. An α-2 adrenergic agonist, clonidine, has also proven effective in doses of $3–5 \mu g/kg$ body weight infused intravenously over 10 min (unpublished observation). Pretreatment with another α-2 agonist, dexmedetomidine has been reported to reduce emergence reactions after ketamine in adults (67).

Although techniques of fiberoptic intubation have been thoroughly reviewed (32,33), certain features of our experience with burn reconstruction patients are worthy of emphasis. If fiberoptic intubation is accomplished quickly after ketamine sedation, secretions are usually not a problem. When delays occur, however, secretions can obscure the view and impair the action of local anesthetics. Early administration of a drying agent such as glycopyrrolate or scopolamine will often facilitate fiberoptic intubation under ketamine sedation by reducing secretions. Nasal bleeding can also make pharyngoscopy difficult. Routine use of a decongestant should shrink nasal membranes making it easier to pass the endotracheal tube as well as the bronchoscope through the nose and decrease bleeding from nasopharyngeal membranes. Because significant morbidity and mortality have been reported with the intraoperative use of topical phenylephrine (68), we have adopted the use of an α-2 adrenergic nasal decongestant, oxymetazoline. Practitioners should be familiar with the principles guiding management of hypertensive crises associated with topical nasal decongestants (68). Especially avoiding interventions that will reduce myocardial contractility.

Since airway reflexes are preserved by ketamine it is important to anesthetize the glottic structures topically before contacting the larynx with the bronchoscope. This is most easily accomplished with a lidocaine solution applied through the working channel of the bronchoscope. An effective technique is to apply the lidocaine in two doses. First, to the epiglottis and vallecula (superior laryngeal nerve) and next to the glottis (inferior laryngeal nerve). The ultra-thin 2.2 mm fiberscope lacks a working channel and when this instrument is used for intubation a modification of technique utilizing a second fiberscope is helpful to anesthetize the glottis (34). Intubation with the ultra-thin fiberscope can be preceded by nasopharyngoscopy and lidocaine administration with a larger instrument with a working channel. Fiberoptic intubation with the ultra-thin fiberscope can then be more easily accomplished.

When fiberoptic intubation is attempted under sedation with ketamine, we prefer to pass the fiberscope through the larynx into the trachea before advancing the endotracheal tube into the nose. When nasal bleeding occurs in an awake patient the bronchoscope can be withdrawn, hemostasis achieved, and the patient can still protect the airway. In the sedated patient, bleeding not only makes visualization of structures difficult and impairs local anesthetic activity but can also cause laryngospasm.

A variety of techniques other than fiberoptic intubation have also been used for management of patients with difficult airways, including face and neck scars. One technique involves the surgical release of the neck scar contractures followed by direct laryngoscopy and intubation (44–46). Surgical release has been accomplished by these clinicians with local anesthesia with or without ketamine sedation. A problem with this technique is that direct laryngoscopy may still be difficult after surgical release (44).

The laryngeal mask airway (LMA) has gained popularity as a rescue device for the unanticipated difficult airway (69,70) and has also been described for management of patients with severe neck scars requiring frequent general anesthetics (46). The LMA has also been used as a conduit for intubation with a fiberoptic bronchoscope (69). The LMA is not appropriate for all surgical procedures, though, and when microstomia is present an LMA cannot be inserted.

A large number of devices have been developed for use in patients with difficult airways. These include lighted stylets, endotracheal tube guides, specialized laryngoscopes, the cuffed oropharyngeal airway, and esophageal tracheal combitube (71). Each of these devices has special advantages in certain situations. Each also has limitations. Use of any of these devices in patients with known or suspected difficult airway should be attempted only when the operator has gained experience with the device and is familiar with its limitations.

C. Regional Techniques

There are many advantages to the use of regional anesthesia techniques for patients undergoing reconstructive surgical procedures. Regional blocks may provide adequate anesthesia for certain procedures if it is acceptable to the patient. In this case certain risks of general anesthesia such as nausea and vomiting are avoided. In some patients with serious coexisting disease, significant risks of circulatory or pulmonary complications can be avoided by a regional anesthetic. Janezic (72) described performing full-thickness skin grafts solely under topical anesthesia with EMLA cream in two elderly and debilitated patients. Regional techniques may also be used to enhance postoperative care. Randalls (73) described successful management of 82-year-old burn patient with brachial pexus anesthesia via an indwelling catheter. The catheter position was confirmed radiologically. Bupivacaine was infused postoperatively for analgesia and to improve graft survival by immobilizing the affected extremity.

Even when a regional technique by itself is not acceptable (as with pediatric patients) a block may still be useful by providing postoperative analgesia. Munro et al. (74) found that postoperative pain control was better in their pediatric patients who had a regional anesthesia procedure in combination with their general anesthesia.

D. Pharmacologic Considerations in Patients Undergoing Burn Reconstruction

The physiologic and metabolic response to burn injury can markedly alter the response to drugs. Both pharmacokinetic and pharmacodynamic alterations occur. The altered drug response in burn patients may require adjustment of dosage in order to avoid toxicity or decreased efficacy (75). Interpatient variability, differences in the size and depth of burns among patients and differences in the time elapsed since the initial injury makes it difficult to provide specific dosing guidelines. However, trends in drug responsiveness have been observed that should be kept in mind during care of burn patients undergoing reconstructive procedures.

The hypermetabolic response to burn injury may persist for weeks to months after wounds have healed. Hepatic and renal metabolism may remain elevated during this time. Therefore, many drugs that are metabolized by the liver and kidneys are cleared more rapidly than in non burned individuals (76). Also, many drugs are highly protein bound (Table 7.2). Drug effects and elimination are related to the unbound fraction of drug. Free drug is more available to interact with receptors but is also more rapidly cleared by the liver or kidneys. The two major drug binding proteins, albumin and α-acid glycoprotein (AAG), have disparate responses to burn injury. Albumin levels tend to decrease after major burns resulting in increased free fractions of drugs that exhibit a high level of albumin binding (diazepam, thiopental). In general, acidic drugs ($pK_a < 7$, Table 7.3) bind to albumin most avidly (77). Basic drugs ($pK_a > 8$) also bind extensively to globulins, lipoproteins and glycoproteins. In addition, some drugs (lidocaine, propranolol) bind avidly to acute phase proteins such as AAG. AAG levels increase during the postburn period resulting in increased binding of drugs that have affinity for AAG. Since these drug-binding proteins respond in opposite ways, the effect of burn injury on drug metabolism and efficacy is dependent on the relative alterations in their plasma concentration. Based on this information, anesthetic drugs should be titrated carefully in burn patients.

Muscle relaxants exhibit the most clinically significant alterations in drug action following severe burns. The responses to both succinylcholine and nondepolarizing muscle relaxants are altered. During the postburn period

Table 7.2 Drug Binding to Plasma Proteins

Drug	Binding (%)	Drug	Binding (%)
Warfarin	99	Thiopental	80
Diazepam	98	Etomidate	75
Propofol	98	Lidocaine	65
Bupivacaine	95	Atracurium	51
Furosemide	95	Curare	45
Sufentanil	93	Morphine	40
Alfentanil	91	Vecuronium	30
Propranolol	90	Ketamine	12
Fentanyl	82		

Table 7.3 pK_a Values for Some Acidic and Basic Drugs

Drug	pK_a	Drug	pK_a
Diazepam	3.3	Morphine	7.9
Furosemide	3.9	Bupivacaine	8.1
Warfarin	5.0	Phenytoin	8.3
Alfentanil	6.5	Fentanyl	8.4
Chlorothiazide	6.8	Propranolol	9.4
Phenobarbitol	7.4	Atropine	9.7
Ketamine	7.5	Isoproteranol	10.1
Thiopental	7.6	Propofol	11.0

succinylcholine can produce exaggerated hyperkalemic responses severe enough to cause cardiac arrest (6). The enhanced potassium release after succinylcholine administration in burn patients is thought to be due to proliferation of extrajunctional acetylcholine receptors. Activation of these receptors allows more widespread depolarization of the muscle membrane that could result in amplified release of intracellular potassium. However, considerable individual variability in response exists. Most studies show that only a small percentage of burn patients exhibit dangerously high potassium levels after succinylcholine administration (6). The earliest reported exaggerated hyperkalemic response occurred 9 days after injury but normal responses were observed in the remaining patients for up to 20 days (78). The shortest postburn interval associated with succinylcholine-induced cardiac arrest was 21 days (79). Therefore, specific guidelines regarding the use of succinylcholine in severely burned patients are controversial. Various authors recommend avoiding succinylcholine use beginning from 24 h to 21 days after burn injury (80,81). As a result, most practitioners avoid the use of succinylcholine in all burn patients. However, there is no solid evidence to support this practice. The most current and comprehensive discussion of this issue is a pair of letters by Gronert (82) and Martyn (83) as responses to a review by MacLennon et al. (81). Martyn (83) reasoned that the best evidence indicates that succinylcholine is safe for up to 48 h after a large burn. After 48 h the risk is uncertain so it should probably be avoided. The time after healing before it is again safe to use succinylcholine is also uncertain with recommendations up to 1 year after healing.

Responses to nondepolarizing muscle relaxants are also altered after burn injury. Burn patients require three to fivefold greater doses of muscle relaxant to achieve adequate neuromuscular blockade (5). Resistance is apparent within 7 days of burn injury and persists to 40 days postinjury. Sensitivity returns to normal after ∼70 days after wound healing. Resistance to nondepolarizing muscle relaxants for up to a year after burn injury has been described (84). In most cases, increased amounts of nondepolarizing muscle relaxant are needed in burn patients. These agents should be administered in conjunction with neuromuscular monitoring to assure proper dosing.

E. Postoperative Nausea and Vomiting After Burn Reconstructive Surgery

The incidence of postoperative nausea and vomiting (PONV) in patients undergoing reconstructive surgery after burn injury is perceived to be high by many practitioners. However, few data exist on the incidence of PONV in this patient population. Stubbs and colleagues observed a 100% incidence of PONV after reconstructive procedures involving the scalp in burned children (85). PONV was reported in 45% of children undergoing surgical procedures that did not involve the scalp. In a follow-up study McCall et al. (86) noted a 69% overall incidence of PONV in burned children undergoing reconstructive procedures. This incidence was significantly decreased to 47% or 40%, respectively, in children treated prophylactically with ondansetron or dimenhydrate. Similarly, frank vomiting was observed in 61% of placebo-treated children compared to 29% and 40%, respectively, of children treated prophylactically with ondansetron or dimenhydrinate. Antiemetic agents were given within 30 min of the conclusion of surgery. This timing is based on studies that show antiemetic agents to be most effective if given at or near the conclusion of surgery (87). Studies assessing the incidence of PONV in adult patients undergoing reconstructive procedures after burn injury have not been published in the peer-reviewed literature.

Based on the current literature, it appears that the incidence of PONV in burned children undergoing reconstructive procedures is significant and would easily warrant classification as high risk. In addition, the incidence of PONV remains elevated in patients receiving prophylactic treatment with a single dose of ondansetron or dimenhydrinate. Studies of other high-risk patient populations show that a multimodal approach is needed for maximal efficacy in the treatment of PONV (88).

F. The Biology of Nausea and Vomiting

Emesis is a protective response that is designed to rid the host of toxic or harmful ingested substances (89). This response can be triggered by smell, taste, or sight. Postingestion emetic responses can be triggered both before and after a proemetic substance has been absorbed into the circulation. The presence of toxins or proemetic compounds in the gut lumen is detected by free nerve endings present in the gastric mucosa. Mechanoreceptors detect gastric distension and can also trigger an emetic response. Preabsorptive responses are transmitted by the vagus nerve to the dorsal motor nucleus of the vagus, nucleus tractus solitarius, and the area postrema. Emesis is then induced by activation of the "vomiting center," previously reported to be localized to the lateral reticular formation of the brain but likely to involve responses from several brainstem nuclei. Postabsorptive responses are mediated through activation of the chemoreceptor trigger zone (CTZ) in the area postrema. This highly vascular area possesses an incomplete blood–brain barrier that allows entry of substances from the blood or CSF and is likely to be the main center triggering PONV. Receptors for serotonin (5-HT3), histamine (H1), dopamine (DA-2), acetylcholine (muscarinic), and opiates are present in the CTZ. Activation of these receptors stimulates emesis. A variety of pharmacologic approaches for the treatment of PONV have been developed aimed at blocking specific receptors in the CTZ.

G. Antiemetic Agents

1. Antidopaminergic Agents

Several classes of antidopaminergic agents have efficacy in the treatment of PONV. These include phenothiazines, butyrophenones, and substituted benzamides (Table 7.4). The antiemetic effect of these agents is mediated by binding of the DA-2 receptor. Side effects include

Table 7.4 Classification of Antiemetic Agents

Drug class	Common side effect
Dopamine receptor antagonists (DA-2)	Sedation
Phenothiazines	Dissociation
Fluphenazine	Extrapyramidal effect
Chlorpromazine	
Prochlorperazine	
Butyrophenones	
Droperidol	
Haloperidol	
Substituted benzamide	
Metochlopromide	
Antihistamines (H1)	Sedation
Diphenhydramine	Dry mouth
Promethazine	
Anticholinergics	Sedation
Scopolamine	Dry mouth
Atropine	Tachycardia
Serotonin receptor antagonists	Headache
Ondansetron	
Dolasetron	
Corticosteroids	Glucose intolerance
Dexamethasone	Altered wound healing
Methylprednisolone	Immunosuppression
Hydrocortisone	Renal effects

dissociation and sedation. Extrapyramidal side effects have also been reported with use of these agents. In adults, the incidence of neurological side effects is low if droperidol is limited to a dose of 1.25 mg (90). However, children are perceived to exhibit prolonged drowsiness and a higher incidence of extrapyramidal effects compared to adults in some studies (91). Recent warnings by the FDA may limit future use of droperidol (92).

The use of metoclopramide as a prophylactic antiemetic in pediatric patients has also received mixed reviews. Some studies have shown efficacy for metoclopramide in PONV prophylaxis while others have not demonstrated benefit over placebo (93,94).

2. Antihistamines

Antihistamines such as diphenhydramine and promethazine are commonly used in the treatment of motion sickness and are also useful in PONV. Their antihistaminic and anticholinergic actions mediate the antiemetic effect of these agents. The most common side effects of these agents include sedation and dry mouth.

3. Anticholinergics

Scopolamine is commonly used in the treatment of motion sickness and also has efficacy for the treatment of PONV. The central potency of scopolamine is ~10-fold greater than atropine yet the visceral antimuscarinic effects, particularly tachycardia, are less. Therefore, scopolamine possesses the more desirable therapeutic index for the treatment of PONV. Common side effects include drowsiness and dissociation. Scopolamine patches have shown efficacy in the prophylaxis of PONV in pediatric patients undergoing strabismus or abdominal surgery (95,96). Glycopyrrolate is an anticholinergic agent with a quarternary ammonium structure that does not cross the blood brain barrier and is not effective in the treatment of PONV.

4. Serotonin Receptor Antagonists

The 5-HT3 receptor antagonists have emerged as a major class of drugs for the treatment of PONV. They possess efficacy for the treatment of PONV that is equal to that of other classes of antiemetics such as dopamine antagonists, but have a relatively benign side effect profile. The serotonin receptor antagonists are commonly used in the outpatient setting for prophylaxis and treatment of PONV. Their effectiveness as prophylactic and rescue agents for PONV has been shown in numerous studies (87). Because of their relatively high cost, some investigators have questioned the cost effectiveness of using these agents in PONV prophylaxis (97). However, many practitioners strongly recommend the use of serotonin receptor antagonists for PONV prophylaxis, particularly in the outpatient setting.

5. Corticosteroids

Corticosteroids such as dexamethasone are effective adjuncts for the treatment of PONV in high-risk patients. The mechanism of antiemetic action of these agents is unclear. However, their efficacy has been demonstrated in several studies (98). Overall, corticosteroids are not used as front-line agents for the treatment of PONV. However, many practitioners have recommended the use of these agents in association with other antiemetics in patients that are at high risk for PONV (88). Although chronic steroid use can have numerous and significant metabolic effects, a single dose of corticosteroids for treatment or prophylaxis of PONV is not likely to cause significant derangements.

H. Treatment of Patients at High Risk for PONV

PONV is one of the most common complications associated with surgical anesthesia. However, the optimal strategy for prevention or treatment of PONV remains controversial. Patients report the distress of PONV as being equal to that of postoperative pain. In addition, PONV can prolong the discharge of day surgery patients and result in unanticipated hospital admissions (99). Several factors have been identified that are predictive of increased risk for PONV. Risk factors can be divided into patient characteristics, surgical factors and anesthetic factors. Apfel et al. (100) reported that these risk factors are additive. Patient characteristics that are associated with PONV include a prior history of PONV or motion sickness, female gender, obesity, nonsmoking status, and pediatric age. Certain types of surgery are also associated with an increased incidence of PONV. These include intra-abdominal surgery, gynecologic procedures as well as surgery on the eye or middle ear. A surgical duration of >2 h is also associated with PONV. Based on the data presented earlier in this chapter, burn patients undergoing reconstructive procedures also have a high incidence of PONV. Anesthetic factors associated with PONV include the use of opioids, nitrous oxide, etomidate or anticholinesterases to reverse muscle relaxation. The use of propofol as an induction agent or maintenance anesthetic is associated with decreased PONV (101).

Many issues surround the use of antiemetics during the postoperative period. One major question is whether to use antiemetics prophylactically or as rescue therapy. Scuderi and colleagues (97) compared the use of ondansetron as antiemetic prophylaxis or rescue therapy in adult outpatient surgery. They reported no difference in discharge time from the hospital, readmission rate, or return to normal activity when comparing groups. They concluded that rescue therapy is more cost effective and is associated with similar patient satisfaction scores compared to prophylaxis in patients at low risk of PONV. However, patients at high risk of PONV reported greater satisfaction with the prophylactic regimen. Watcha and Smith (102) observed a decreased incidence of PONV in patients receiving prophylaxis with ondansetron or droperidol compared to patients receiving rescue treatment. They concluded that prophylaxis with ondansetron is justified if the incidence of PONV is $>30\%$ in a patient population and that prophylaxis with droperidol is indicated at a PONV incidence of $>13\%$. Similarly, Tang et al. (87) reported greater satisfaction in outpatient surgery patients receiving prophylaxis with ondansetron compared to patients treated for PONV in the postanesthesia recovery unit (PACU). In a later review of the literature, Watcha (88) proposed a decision tree for PONV treatment or prophylaxis based on patient risk factors (Fig. 7.10).

Overall, pediatric patients undergoing reconstructive surgery for burn wounds are at high risk of PONV. The incidence of PONV in a similar adult population has not been reported. Single agent prophylactic treatment of PONV with ondansetron or dimenhydrate has shown efficacy in pediatric patients. However, the incidence of PONV remained relatively high after single agent treatment. Based on studies in other patient populations at high risk of PONV, it is likely that multiagent prophylaxis will benefit pediatric burn patients undergoing reconstructive procedures. This multimodal approach should employ agents that interact with different receptors in the CTZ. For example, the combination of a serotonin receptor antagonist and dopamine receptor blocker would likely be more beneficial than the use of two different dopamine receptor antagonists. The use of propofol and avoidance of opioids, etomidate, and nitrous oxide may also decrease PONV in these patients. Furthermore, it is often useful to review the patient's medical records to determine the effectiveness of antiemetic agents given during previous anesthetics.

I. Postoperative Analgesia

Postoperative pain not only contributes to an unfavorable medical experience for the patient but as a significant source of physiological stress it can also contribute to postoperative morbidity in a variety of ways. Stress associated with postsurgical pain can be associated with increased nausea and vomiting, postoperative pulmonary complications, infections, and other complications (103). Patients who have survived large burn injuries may be experiencing chronic pain and may have reduced pain tolerance. Pain control is even more important in these patients who require many surgical procedures.

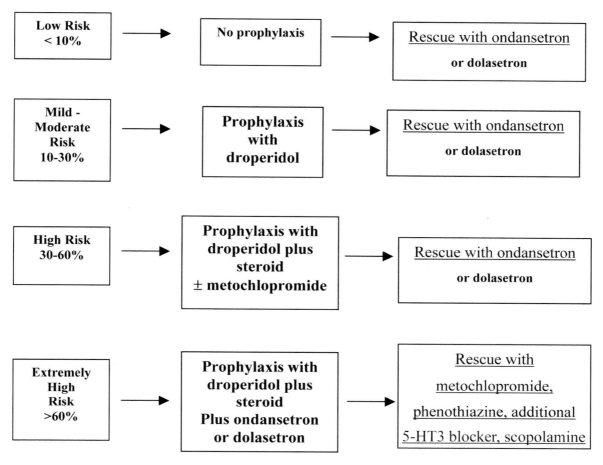

Figure 7.10 Possible approach to the treatment of PONV. [Adapted from Watcha (88).]

In the past, patients were often admitted to the hospital in the postoperative period to allow more effective pain control. With the increasing frequency of outpatient surgical procedures performed, it is important to know that postsurgical pain can be managed safely and effectively on an outpatient basis. Munro et al. (74) evaluated perioperative analgesia in 471 children from 10 months to 18 years of age who underwent a wide variety of outpatient surgical procedures that were expected to be associated with significant pain. Follow-up surveys documented 97% of patients had adequate to very good pain relief. In a subset of 185 of these patients who had genitourinary procedures, those who received regional anesthesia procedures reported better pain control.

Morphine is the first choice by many practitioners for postoperative pharmacological pain relief. Some patients may already be receiving opioids and require higher doses due to development of tolerance. This may not be apparent until after emergence in the postanesthesia care unit. Additional analgesia may be required to supplement opioids given intraoperatively.

Opiods used with patient-controlled analgesia (PCA) can be an especially effective technique of managing post surgical pain. PCA has also been found effective in select pediatric patients (104). Shin et al. (105) compared intravenous PCA with nalbuphine and ketorolac with intramuscular injection of meperidine in pediatric craniofacial patients. The PCA group had superior pain control and ambulated sooner than the patients treated with intramuscular meperidine. They found the PCA mode especially helpful for patients with moderate to severe pain associated with rib cartilage or iliac bone harvesting for grafts. PCA was also effective in providing postoperative analgesia for large flap surgeries.

Nonsteroidal anti-inflammatory drugs (NSAIDS) are also useful in treating postsurgical pain. Chauhan et al. (106) evaluated the safety of ketorolac in pediatric patients who underwent ureteroneocystostomy. They found no evidence of renal toxicity or increased bleeding. Ketorolac is used as part of a standard postoperative protocol after ureteroneocystostomy at their institution. A morphine-sparing effect of ketorolac was reported by Carney et al. (107) in pediatric general surgical patients. They also reported no increased bleeding or nephrotoxicity in this group of patients.

Local anesthetics are often effective in controlling certain types of postsurgical pain. Donor sites for split thickness skin-grafts are a significant source of pain for patients undergoing reconstructive procedures after burn injuries. Several strategies utilizing local anesthetics have been used to control pain from donor sites. Harvest of the skin for grafting is frequently preceded by local infiltration of solution to prepare the donor site. Addition of bupivacaine to the solution used for infiltration has been reported effective in reducing postoperative morphine requirements and pain scores up to 48 h after surgery (108,109). Plasma concentrations were well below toxicity levels when the total dose was limited to 3 mg/kg. Jellish et al. (110) compared effects of 2% lidocaine and 0.5% bupivacaine applied topically after harvest of split-thickness skin harvest sites. Pain scores and 24 h narcotic requirements were lower in patients treated this way with lidocaine. Alvi et al. (111) applied a bupivacaine gel (2.5 mg/mL) to denuded split-thickness skin donor sites up to 160 cm^2 and averaging 130 cm^2. Plasma bupivacaine concentration peaked at 0.07 μg/mL, well below toxic concentration of bupivacaine (4 μg/mL).

IV. SUMMARY

Advances in burn care have significantly improved the survival of severely burned patients. Subsequently, more patients will present to the operating room for surgical correction of burn-associated deformities. The sequelae of these injuries provide challenges in every phase of anesthetic management. The most notable challenges are related to airway management and securing vascular access. Altered drug responses, increased analgesic requirements, and a high incidence of PONV are also common problems encountered in this patient population. The requirement of multiple and staged procedures presents challenges but also allows tailoring of care to the individual patient's needs. The patients themselves and the medical record are invaluable sources of information regarding which drugs or techniques have been most effective during prior anesthetics. Management of severely burned patients for reconstructive surgery can be technically challenging. Development of an effective anesthetic plan and attention to detail is required to provide anesthesia in a safe and efficacious manner.

REFERENCES

1. Wolf SE, Rose JK, Desai MH, Mileski JP, Barrow RE, Herndon DN. Mortality determinants in massive pediatric burns: an analysis of 103 children with ≥80% TBSA burns (≥70% full-thickness). Ann Surg 1997; 225(5):554–569.

2. Ryan CM, Schoenfeld DA, Thorpe WP et al. Objective estimates of the probability of death from burn injuries. N Engl J Med 1998; 338:362–366.

3. Sheridan RL, Remensnyder JP, Schnitzer JJ, Schulz JT, Ryan CM, Tompkins RG. Current expectations for survival in pediatric burns. Arch Pediatr Adolesc 2000; 154:245–249.

4. Cote CJ, Petkan AJ. Thiopental requirements may be increased in children reanesthestized at least one year after recovery from extensive thermal injury. Anesth Analg 1985; 64(12):1156–1160.

5. Martyn J, Szyfelbein S, Ali H, Matteo R, Savares J. Increased D-tubocurarine requirement following major thermal injury. Anesthesiology 1980; 52:352–355.

6. Tolmie J, Joyce T, Mitchell G. Succinylcholine danger in the burned patient. Anesthesiology 1967; 18:467–470.

7. Thomas CR, Meyer WH, Blakeney PA. Psychiatric disorders associated with burn injury. In: Herndon DN, ed. Total Burn Care 2nd ed. London: W.B. Saunders, 2001:766–772.

8. American Society of Anesthesiologists Task Force on Preanesthesia Evaluation. Special article: practice advisory for preanesthesia evaluation. Anesthesiology 2002; 96(2):485–496.

9. Demling RH, Chen C. Pulmonary function in the burn patient. Semin Nephrol 1993; 13(4):371–381.

10. Colice GL. Long-term respiratory complications of inhalation injury. In: Haponik EF, Munster AM, eds. Respiratory Injury: Smoke Inhalation and Burns. New York: McGraw-Hill, 1990:329–345.

11. Perez-Guerra F, Walsh RE, Sagel SS. Bronchiolitis obliterans and tracheal stenosis. J Am Med Assoc 1971; 218:1568–1570.

12. Tasaka S, Kanazawa M, Mori M, Fujishima S, Ishizaka A, Yamasawa F, Kawashiro T. Long-term course of bronchiectasis and bronchiolitis obliterans as late complication of smoke inhalation. Respiration 1995; 62:40–42.

13. Slutzker D, Kinn R, Said SI. Bronchiectasis and progressive respiratory failure following smoke inhalation. Chest 1989; 95:1349–1350.

14. Cooper AB, Ferguson ND, Hanly PJ, Meade MO, Kachura JR, Grantson JT, Slutsky AS, Stewart TE. Long-term follow-up of survivors of acute lung injury: lack of effect of a ventilation strategy to prevent barotrauma. Crit Care Med 1999; 27(12):2616–2621.

15. Warner DO. Preventing postoperative pulmonary complications: the role of the anesthesiologist. Anesthesiology 2000; 92(5):1467–1472.

16. Tokics L, Hedenstierna G, Strandberg A, Brismar B, Lundquist H. Lung collapse and gas exchange during general anesthesia: effects of spontaneous breathing, muscle paralysis, and positive end-expiratory pressure. Anesthesiology 1987; 66(2):157–167.

17. Lawrence VA, Page CP, Harris GD. Preoperative spirometry before abdominal operations. Arch Intern Med 1989; 149:280–285.

18. Taal LA, Faber AW. Posttraumatic stress and maladjustment among adult burn survivors 1–2 years postburn. Burns 1998; 24:285–292.

19. Stoddard FJ, Nomzan DK, Murphy M, Beardslee WR. Psychiatric outcome of burned children and adolescents. J Am Acad Child Adolesc Psychiatry 1989; 28:589–595.

20. Kain ZN, Mayes LC, O'Connor TZ, Cicchetti DV. Preoperative anxiety in children: predictors and outcomes. Arch Pediatr Adolesc Med 1996; 150:1238–1345.

21. Egbert LD, Battit GE, Turndorf H, Beecher HK. The value of the preoperative visit by an anesthetist. J Am Med Assoc 1963; 185:553–555.

22. McCall JE, Fischer CG, Warden G, Kopcha R, Lloyd S, Young J, Schomaker B. Lorazepam given the night before surgery reduces preoperative anxiety in children undergoing reconstructive burn surgery. J Burn Care Rehabil 1999; 20(2):151–154.

23. McGraw TT, Striker TW, Liedhegner BG. Oral midazolam premedication and postoperative behavior in children. Anesth Analg 1993; 76:S255.

24. Gutstein HB, Johnson KL, Heard MB, Gregory GA. Oral ketamine preanesthetic medication in children. Anesthesiology 1992; 76(1):28–33.

25. White PF, Way WL, Trevor AJ. Ketamine: it's pharmacology and therapeutic uses. Anesthesiology 1982; 56(2):119–136.

26. Kamibayashi T, Harasawa K, Maze M. Alpha-2 adrenergic agonists. Can J Anaesth 1997; 44(5):R13–R18.

27. Tanaka M, Nichikawa T. Oral clonidine premedication attenuates the hypertensive response to ketamine. Br J Anaesth 1994; 73:758–762.

28. Bhana N, Goa KL, McClellan KJ. Dexmedetomidine. Drugs 2000; 59(2):263–268.

29. Smerling AL, Lieberman J, Rothstein P. Parents' presence during induction of anesthesia in children: parents' viewpoint, abstracted. Anesthesiology 1988; 69:A743.

30. Cauldwell CB. Induction, maintenance, and emergence. In: Gregory GA, ed. Pediatric Anesthesia. New York: Churchill Livingstone, 1994:227–229.

31. Hagberg CA. Handbook of Difficult Airway Management. Philadelphia: Churchill Livingstone, 2000.

32. Ovassapian A, Wheeler M. Flexible fiberoptic tracheal intubation. In: Hagberg CA, ed. Handbook of Difficult Airway Management. Philadelphia: Churchill Livingstone, 2000:83–111.

33. Ovassapian A. Fiberoptic Endoscopy and the Difficult Airway. Philadelphia: Lippincott-Raven, 1996.

34. Kleeman PP, Jantzen JP, Bonfils P. The ultra-thin bronchoscope in management of the difficult paediatric airway. Can J Anaesth 1987; 34(6):606–608.

35. Finfer SR, MacKenzie SI, Saddler JM, Watkins TG. Cardiovascular responses to tracheal intubation: a comparison of direct laryngoscopy and fiberoptic intubation. Anaesth Intensive Care 1989; 17(1):44–48.

36. Dombret MC, Juliard JM, Farinotti R. The risks of bronchoscopy in coronary patients. Rev Mal Respir 1990; 7:313–317.

37. Davies L, Mister R, Spence DPS, Calverley PMA, Earis JE, Pearson MG. Cardiovascular consequences of fiberoptic bronchoscopy. Eur Respir J 1997; 10:695–698.

38. Mathru M, Esch O, Lang J, Herbert ME, Chaljub G, Goodacre B, vanSonnenberg E. Magnetic resonance imaging of the upper airway: effects of propofol anesthesia and nasal continuous positive airway pressure in humans. Anesthesiology 1996; 84(2):273–279.

39. Wilson RD, Nichols RJ, McCoy NR. Dissociative anesthesia with CI-581 in burned children. Anesth Analg 1967; 46(6):719–724.

40. Demling RH, Ellerbe S, Jarrett F. Ketamine anesthesia for tangential excision of burn eschar: a burn unit procedure. J Trauma 1978; 18(4):269–270.

41. Wrigley SR, Black AE, Sidhu VS. A fiberoptic laryngoscope for pediatric anaesthesia. A study to evaluate the use if the 2.2 mm Olympus (LF-P) intubating fiberscope. Anaesthesia 1995; 50(8):709–712.

42. Tanzer RC. Burn reconstructive of the neck. Plast Reconstr Surg 1964; 33(3):207–212.

43. Defalque RJ. Ketamine for blind basal intubation. Anesth Analg 1971; 50(6):984–986.

44. Jíchová E, Königová R. Specific features of anaesthesia in the reconstruction period in severe burns. Acta Chirurgiae Plast 1980; 22(3):177–182.

45. Kreulen M, Mackie DP, Kreis RW, Groenevelt F. Surgical release for intubation purposes in postburn contractures of the neck. Burns 1996; 22(4):310–312.

46. Karam R, Ibrahim G, Tohme H, Moukarzel Z, Raphael N. Severe neck burns and laryngeal mask airway for frequent general anesthetics. Middle East J Anesth 1996; 13(5):527–535.

47. Jandová J, Königová R, Zapounková Z, Broz L. Combined technique of anesthesia in early and late neck reconstruction. Acta Chir Plast 1997; 39(2):56–59.

48. Lang J, Herbert M, Esch O, Chaljub G, Mathru M. Magnetic resonance of the upper airway: ketamine preserves airway patency compared to propofol. Anesthesiology 1996; 84:273.

49. Penrose BH. Aspiration pneumonitis following ketamine induction for general anesthesia. Anesth Analg 1972; 51(1):41–43.

50. Green SM, Rothrock SG, Lynch EL, Ho M, Harris T, Hestdalen R, Hopkins GA, Garrett W, Westcott K. Intramuscular ketamine for pediatric sedation in the emergency department: safety profile in 1,022 cases. Ann Emerg Med 1998; 31(6):688–697.

51. Corssen G, Oget S. Dissociative anesthesia for the severely burned child. Anesth Analg 1971; 50(1):95–102.

52. Maldini B. Ketamine anesthesia in children with acute burns and scalds. Acta Anaesthesiol Scand 1996; 40:1108–1111.

53. Barson PK, Scott ML, Lawson NW, Ochsner JL. Ketamine for bronchoscopy of children. South Med J 1974; 67(12):1403–1404.

54. Singh A, Girotra S, Mehta Y, Radhakrishnan S, Shrivastava S. Total intravenous anesthesia with ketamine for pediatric interventional cardiac procedures. J Cardiothorac Vasc Anesth 2000; 14(1):36–39.

55. Friedberg BL. Propofol-ketamine technique: dissociative anesthesia for office surgery (A 5-Year Review of 1264 Cases). Aesthetic Plast Surg 1999.

56. Reich DL, Silvay G. Ketamine: an update of the first twenty-five years of clinical experience. Can J Anaesth 1989; 36(2):186–197.

57. Haas DA, Harper DG. Ketamine: a review of its pharmacologic properties and use in ambulatory anesthesia. Anesth Prog 1992; 39:61–68.

58. Kohrs R, Durieux ME. Ketamine: teaching an old drug new tricks. Anesth Analg 1998; 87:1186–1193.

59. Soliman MG, Brindle F, Kuster G. Response to hypercapnia under ketamine anaesthesia. Canad Anaesth Soc J 1975; 22(4):486–494.

60. Bourke DL, Malit LA, Smith TC. Respiratory interactions of ketamine and morphine. Anesthesiology 1987; 66(2):153–156.

61. Fine J, Finestone SC. Sensory disturbances following ketamine anesthesia: recurrent hallucinations. Anesth Analg 1973; 52(3):428–430.

62. Moretti RJ, Hassan SZ, Goodman LI, Meltzer HY. Comparison of ketamine and thiopental in healthy volunteers: effects on mental status, mood, and personality. Anesth Analg 1984; 63:1087–1096.

63. Green SM, Johnson NE. Ketamine sedation for pediatric procedures: part 2, Review and implications. Ann Emerg Med 1990; 19(9):1033–1046.

64. Cartwright PD, Pingel SM. Midazolam and diazepam in ketamine anaesthesia. Anaesthesia 1984; 39:439–442.

65. Sherwin TS, Green SM, Khan A, Chapman DS, Dannenberg B. Does adjunctive midazolam reduce recovery agitation after ketamine sedation for pediatric procedures? A randomized, double-blind, placebo-controlled trial. Ann Emerg Med 2000; 35(3):229–238.

66. Wathen JE, Roback MG, Mackenzie T, Bothner JP. Does midazolam after the clinical effects of intravenous ketamine sedation in children? A double-blind, randomized, controlled, emergency department trial. Ann Emerg Med 2000; 36(6):579–588.

67. Levanen J, Makela ML, Scheinin H. Dexmedetomidine premedication attenuates ketamine-induced cardiostimulatory effects and postanesthetic delirium. Anesthesiology 1995; 82(5):1117–1125.

68. Groudine SB, Hollinger I, Jones J, DeBouno BA. Phenylephrine Advisory Committee. New York State guidelines on the topical use of phenylephrine in the operating room. Anesthesiology 2000; 92(3):859–864.

69. Brain AIJ. Three cases of difficult intubation overcome by use of the laryngeal mask. Anaesthesia 1985; 40:353–355.

70. Parmet JL, Colonna-Romano P, Horrow JC, Miller F, Gonzales J, Rosenberg H. The laryngeal mask airway reliably provides rescue ventilation in cases of unanticipated difficult tracheal intubation along with difficult mask ventilation. Anesth Analg 1998; 87:661–665.

71. Minkowitz HS. Airway gadgets. In: Hagberg CA, ed. Handbook of Difficult Airway Management. Philadelphia: Churchill Livingstone, 2000:49–167.

72. Janezic TF. Skin grafting of full thickness burns under local anesthesia with EMLA cream. Burns 1998; 24(3):259–263.

73. Randalls B. Continuous brachial plexus blockade. A technique that uses an axillary catheter to allow successful skin grafting. Anaesthesia 1990; 45(2):143–144.

74. Munro HM, Malviya S, Lauder GR, Voepel-Lewis T, Tait AR. Pain relief in children following outpatient surgery. J Clin Anesth 1999; 11(3):187–191.

75. Jaehde U, Sorgel F. Clinical pharmacokinetics in patients with burns. Clin Pharmacokinet 1995; 29:15–28.

76. Bonate PL. Pathophysiology and pharmacokinetics following burn injury. Clin Pharmacokinet 1990; 18(2):118–130.

77. Hull C. Principles of pharmacokinetics. In: Hemmings H, Hopkins P, eds. Foundations of anesthesiology. Basic and clinical sciences. London: Mosby, 2000:73–86.

78. Viby-Morgensen J, Hanel H, Hansen E, Graae J. Serum cholinesterase activity in burned patients II: anesthesia, suxamethonium and hyperkalemia. Acta Anesthesiol Scand 1975; 169–179.

79. McCaughey T. Hazards of anesthesia for the burned child. Can Anesth Soc J 1962; 9:220–233.

80. Yentis S. Suxamethonium and hyperkalemia. Anesth Intensive Care 1990; 18:92–101.

81. MacLennan N, Heimbach DM, Cullen BF. Anesthesia for major thermal injury. Anesthesiology 1998; 89:49–70.

82. Gronert GA. Succinylcholine hyperkalemia after burns. Anesthesiology 1999; 91:320.

83. Martyn JAJ. Succinylcholine hyperkalemia after burns. Anesthesiology 1999; 91:321–322.

84. Martyn JAJ, Matteo RS, Szyfelbein SK, Kaplan RF. Unprecedented resistance ti neuromuscular blocking effects of metocurine with persistence after complete recovery in a burned patient. Anesth Analg 1982; 61(7):614–617.

85. Stubbs T, Saylors S, Jenkins M, McCall J, Fischer C, Warden G. Pediatric patients experiencing postoperative nausea and vomiting after burn reconstruction surgery: an analysis. J Burn Care Rehabil 1999; 20:236–238.

86. McCall J, Stubbs K, Saylors S, Pohlman S, Ivers B, Smith S, Fischer C, Kopcha R, Warden G. The search for cost-effective prevention of post-operative nausea and vomiting in the child undergoing reconstructive burn surgery: ondansetron versus dimenhydrinate. J Burn Care Rehabil 1999; 20:309–315.

87. Tang J, Wang B, White P, Watcha M, Qi J, Wender R. The effect of timing of ondansetron administration on its efficacy, cost-effectiveness, and cost-benefit as a prophylactic antiemetic in the ambulatory setting. Anesth Analg 1998; 86:274–282.

88. Watcha MF. The cost-effective management of postoperative nausea and vomiting. Anesthesiology 2000; 92:931–935.

89. Simpson K, Lynch L. Physiology and pharmacology of nausea and vomiting. In: Hemmings H, Hopkins P, eds. Foundations of Anesthesia: Basic and Clinical Sciences. London: Mosby, 2000:623–630.

90. Hill R, Lubarsky D, Phillips-Bute B, Fortney J, Creed M, Glass P, Gan T. Cost-effectiveness of prophylactic antiemetic therapy with ondansetron droperidol, or placebo. Anesthesiology 2000; 92:958–967.

91. Baines D. Postoperative nausea and vomiting in children. Pediatr Anesth 1996; 6:7–14.

92. Food and Drug Administration Talk Paper: FDA strengthens warning for droperidol. Dec 5, 2001; T01–T62.

93. Broadman L, Ceruzzi W, Patane P, Hannallah R, Ruttimann U, Friendly D. Metocloprmide reduces the incidence of vomiting following strabismus surgery in children. Anesthesiology 1990; 72:245–248.

94. Pendeville P, Veyckemans F, van Boven M, Steinier J. Open placebo controlled comparison of the antiemetic effect of droperidol, metoclopramide or a combination of both in paediatric strabismus surgery. Acta Anesthesiol Belg 1993; 44:3–10.

95. Doyle E, Byers G, McNichol L, Morton N. Prevention of postoperative nausea and vomiting with transdermal hyoscine in children using patient controlled analgesia. Brit J Anesth 1994; 72:72–76.

96. Horimoto Y, Tomic H, Hanzawa K, Nishida Y. Scopolamine patch reduces postoperative emesis in paediatric patients following strabismus surgery. Can J Anesth 1991; 38:441–444.

97. Scuderi P, James R, Harris L, Grover M. Antiemetic prophylaxis does not improve outcomes after outpatient surgery when compared to symptomatic treatment. Anesthesiology 1999; 90:360–371.

98. Coloma M, Duffy LL, White PF, Kendall Tongier W, Huber PJ Jr. Dexamethasone facilitates discharge after outpatient anorectal surgery. Anesth Analg 2001; 92(1):85–88.

99. Gold B, Kitz D, Lecky J, Neuhaus J. Unanticipated admission to the hospital following ambulatory surgery. J Am Med Assoc 1989; 262:3008–3010.

100. Apfel C, Laara E, Koivuranta M, Greim C, Roewer N. A simplified risk score for predicting postoperative nausea and vomiting: conclusions from cross validations from two centers. Anesthesiology 1999; 91:693–700.

101. Visser K, Hassink EA, Bonsel GJ, Moen J, Kalkman CJ. Randomized controlled trial of total intravenous anesthesia with propofol versus inhalation anesthesia with isoflurane-nitrous oxide: postoperative nausea with vomiting and economic analysis. Anesthesiology 2001; 95(3):616–626.

102. Watcha MF, Smith I. Cost-effectiveness analysis of antiemetic therapy for ambulatory surgery. J Clin Anesth 1994; 6:370–377.

103. Lubenow TR, Ivankovich AD, McCarthy RJ. Management of acute postoperative pain. In: Barash PG, Cullen BF, Stoelting RK, eds. Clinical Anesthesia, 3rd ed. Philadelphia: Lippincott-Raven, 1997:305–1337.

104. Gaukroger P, Chapman M, Davey R. Pain control in pediatric burn the use of patient-controlled analgesia. Burns 1991; 17(5):396–399.

105. Shin D, Kim S, Kim CS, Kim HS. Postoperative pain management using intravenous patient-controlled analgesia for pediatric patients. J Craniofac Surg 2001; 12(2):129–133.

106. Chauhan RD, Idom CB, Noe HN. Safety of ketorolac in the pediatric population after ureteroneocystomy. J Urol 2001; 166(5):1873–1875.

107. Carney DE, Nicolette LA, Ratner MH, Minerd A, Baesl TJ. Ketorolac reduces postoperative narcotic requirements. J Pediatr Surg 2001; 36(1):76–79.

108. Edelman LS, Faucher L, Morris SE, Hill SM, Saffle JR. Subcutaneous clysis with bupivacaine reduces long-term pain following donor site harvest. J Burn Care Rehabil 2002; 23(2):S48.

109. McCall J, Fischer CG, Lloyd S, Kopsha R, Warden GD. Adding bupivacaine to subcutaneous infiltration solution reduces donor site pain in pediatric burn patients. J Burn Care Rehabil 2002; 23(2):S62.

110. Jellish WS, Gamelli RL, Furry PA, McGill VL, Fluder EM. Effect of topical local anesthetic application to skin harvest sites for pain management in burn patients undergoing skin-grafting procedures. Ann Surg 1999; 229(1):115–120.

111. Alvi R, Jones S, Burrows D, Collins W, McKiernan EP, Jones RP, Bunting P. The safety of topical anaesthetic and analgesic agents in a gel when used to provide pain relief at split skin donor sites. Burns 1998; 24(1):54–57.

8

Skin Grafts

PREMA DHANRAJ

Christian Medical College & Hospital, Vellore, Tamil Nadu, India

ROBERT L. McCAULEY

University of Texas Medical Branch and Shriners Hospital for Children—Galveston Unit, Galveston, Texas, USA

I. HISTORY

A. Autografts

Skin grafts appear to have originated in India with the Hindus 3000 years ago (1–7). However, it was not until 1570 that Fioravanti reported two successful tissue autografts. Subsequently, the concept of autografting was ignored until 1804, when Baronio published his success on free transplantation of skin on sheep. In 1817, Sir Astley Cooper reported the use of full-thickness skin grafts from an amputated thumb onto the stump for coverage. Later in 1921, Bunger reported the successful take of skin removed from the buttocks and transplanted to the nasal stump of a patient. In the mid 1800s, Warren and Pancoast published the use of full-thickness skin grafts from the arms to resurface defects of the nose and ear lobules. Thereafter, Reverdin stimulated worldwide interest in the use of skin grafts with his report on the successful

"take" pinch grafts. Over the next few years, numerous investigators stimulated interest in the use of skin grafts for coverage of soft tissue defects. In 1873, Thiersch reported the use of thin split-thickness grafts (0.005–0.010 in.) and 20 years later Krause popularized the use of full-thickness grafts, then known as Wolfe–Krause grafts. The role of skin grafts in the management of burn patients did not receive widespread attention until 1941, when Bown and McDowell reported their success with the use of thick split-thickness skin grafts (STSGs) for treatment of burns.

The next major advance in the use of skin grafts occurred in 1964, when Tanner, Vandeput, and Olley reported the use of expanded skin grafts. This technique allowed increased coverage of open defects when donor sites were limited. In 1975, Rheinwald and Green advanced the technology of autografting by employing epithelial skin culture techniques to grow epithelial cells, which were subsequently used for the resurfacing of burn patients. Essentially, this technique required full-thickness skin biopsies. The epidermal cells are separated from the dermis by using trypsin. After an *in vitro* culture period of 3–4 weeks for keratinocyte expansion, the autologous keratinocytes were available for wound coverage. The shortcomings of cultured epidermal cells are several. It takes time to culture the cells, the grafts are very fragile, and there is a low rate of graft "take." The patients require prolonged immobilization in order to facilitate graft "take." Later, blistering and the slough of epidermal grafts can occur, leading to less than optimal long-term results. Yet, under certain circumstances, this may be the only hope for patient survival.

Other advances in skin research occurred during these years. In 1960, Ponten reported that the sensory pattern of skin grafts was similar to that of the recipient site rather than that of the original donor site. In 1961, Mir y Mir reported the use of serial dermabrasion and chemical peels to reduce graft hyperpigmentation. Today, it is clear that skin grafts are the primary method of wound closure for patients who sustain major total body surface area burns (8). Yet, without the use of allografts and xenografts, advances in this field may not have been so rapid.

B.   Allografts and Xenografts

In 1877, Reverdin discussed the transplantation of pigskin to humans. In 1881, Girdner reported the first clinical use of allografts by harvesting skin from suicide victims to close burn wounds on another patient. Although significant portions of the graft survived, during the ensuing weeks "erysipelatous inflammation" developed, indicating allograft rejection. In 1910, Davis reported the clinical use of allografts and xenografts. However, the most significant advance was noted in 1938, when Bettman reported the successful use of allograft in two children with more than a 60% total body surface area burn.

In 1944, Webster reported the successful take of refrigerated skin grafts which were wrapped in vasaline gauze and stored at 4–7°C for 3 weeks. This success was followed by the report of Brown and Fryer when allografts were successfully used as biological dressings. In 1956, Sivetti also reported the use of bovine skin grafts as temporary biological dressings. The reason for the successful use of both xenografts and allografts as biological dressings was not clarified until 1958, when Eade reported a significant reduction in wound bacterial counts with the use of these techniques. By the mid-1960s, several investigators reported the beneficial effects of allografts and xenografts in the management of burn patients. In 1966, Zaroff reported his extensive experience with the use of allografts. The xenografts are also a physiologic and a biologic barrier.

Even today, the use of allografts has found its way in the management of nonburn wounds as well as in patients with major total body surface area burns.

C.   Skin Grafts

Skin grafts by definition are segments of tissue separated from the donor site and transplanted to the recipient site devoid of its blood supply. Grafts are classified according to species as autografts, isografts, allografts, and xenografts. An autograft is skin taken from one site of the body and transplanted to another site in the same person. Allografts (homografts) are skin taken from another individual of the same species. It is used in extensive burns where autograft donor sites are scarce. Allografts have important properties as temporary dressings (Table 8.1). They prevent protein and water loss, decrease bacterial count, and lessen pain. Allografts can also be used to test the readiness of a wound to accept an autograft. They perform well as a temporary biological dressing in patients too sick to undergo definitive autografting (9). Allografts, however, can revascularize before the rejection reaction is noted (10). Although O'Donoghue (11) noted the difference in the angiogenic properties of fresh skin allografts, he also noted that in spite of this difference, allografts were capable of neovascularization before being rejected.

Isograft refers to genetically identical donor and recipient individuals such as twins in humans. There are numerous reports of tissue transfers between identical twins that have been performed without incident. Xenograft is a graft taken from another species, used as a temporary biological dressing in cases of autograft and allograft shortage. The advantages are that it is relatively low cost, readily

Table 8.1   Properties of the Ideal Allograft

Prevents water loss
Barrier to bacteria
Inexpensive
Long shelf life
Does not become hypertrophic
Flexible
Conforms to irregular wound surfaces
Can be used "off the shelf"
Does not require refrigeration
Cannot transmit viral diseases
Does not incite inflammatory response
Durable
Easy to secure

Source: Modified with permission from Sheridan RL, Tompkins RG. Properties of allografts. IN: Herndon DN, ed. Total Burn Care. 2nd ed. St. Louis, MO: W.B. Saunders, 2002.

available, and can be easily stored. The most common temporary biological dressing is pig skin (12,13). Until allografts became more readily available, pigskin was widely used as a temporary dressing in burn wound management. The standardization of skin banking procedures in the United States has increased patient safety with respect to microbiological and serological tests to prevent transmission of bacterial and viral pathogens. With these guidelines in place, renewed interest in the use of amnion as a biological dressing has occurred.

Skin grafts consist of epidermis and dermis. Depending on the setting of the dermatome, the translucency of the graft, and the bleeding pattern of the donor site, one can refer to skin grafts as being thin, medium, or thick. STSGs involve the whole of the epidermis and a small part of the dermis. Depending on the depth of dermal involvement they can be further divided into thin STSGs or thick STSGs (14). A very thin STSG has great clinical application in the acute management of burn patients with large TBSA burns. The reconstruction of such patients is a challenge. Thin STSGs are those in which the thickness of the graft is between 5 and 12/1000 in. The advantage of STSG is that it revascularizes quickly (15). The disadvantages of using thin STSGs are that they contract and such grafts can produce unstable scars (16). Medium STSGs are very useful in reconstruction of various burn and new burn injuries. These grafts contain more dermal elements and contract less than the STSGs. The medium-depth STSGs that are used are between 0.012 and 0.018 in. Thick STSGs (>0.018 in.) are usually reserved for the reconstruction of burn patients. Revasculization is prolonged due to the thickness of the graft but secondary contraction is far less. The donor site for STSG can be anywhere in the body. Since it includes only a portion of the dermis, the epidermal appendages remain and are instrumental in the healing of donor sites. Moreover, skin can be harvested from the same site on multiple occasions many times. The grafted skin always maintains the epidermal characteristics of the donor area.

Full-thickness skin grafts (FTSGs) by definition include the epidermis and all of the dermis with varying portions of sweat glands, sebaceous glands, and hair follicles (17). Since the FTSG includes the entire thickness of the skin, it retains all the characteristics of the skin. Although secondary contraction occurs, it is far less than that of STSGs. In addition, the texture and pigment closely resemble the normal skin. A major disadvantage of using FTSG is that because of it's thickness, revascularization is prolonged and the graft is more sensitive to loss due to hematoma or seroma formation. In cases where large FTSGs are utilized, a two-stage approach may be more valuable in assuring 100% graft take. An incisional release may be carried out and the defect covered with allograft. Several days later an FTSG is used to resurface the defect.

Composite grafts are grafts that include two different tissue types. Composite cartilage grafts, for instance, include both skin and cartilage. A common use of such a graft is for the reconstruction of nasal ala defects (18). However, the risk of nonvascularization of this type of graft limits its size.

Selection of the site and type of graft is an important decision (19). During the acute phase of care, obviously the most important decision is to save lives. Hence, STSGs are the choice of treatment for wound coverage. However, during the reconstructive phase of burn care, the decision to use the skin grafts and the donor site from which they are used become important as we evaluate aesthesis, color match, and the prevention of further contractures. STSGs are often the first choice of treatment for the correction of scar contractures. Despite many disadvantages, such as contraction, abnormal pigmentation, and lack of growth in children, the ease and accessibility of this tissue often pushes it into to the forefront of burn reconstruction. It can be taken from anywhere in the body including the scalp and extremities. When possible, it should be taken from areas where concealment of the donor site is possible. When utilized in the face, STSGs produce optimal results when taken from the scalp, upper inner arms, or the supraclavicular areas. The use of lower-extremity and buttock grafts, especially, should be discouraged in the face.

FTSG are often used for the face and neck. The donor site for the face is usually from the postauricular or supraclavicular region. The donor site is usually closed primarily. McCauley et al. have successfully used FTSGs of large dimensions, measuring 30 cm × 20 cm, from the abdomen and flank to resurface extensive defects following release of burn scar contractures of the neck (20). Although they uniformly had 100% take of these FTSGs, all operations were performed in two stages. The donor sites are often closed primarily with STSGs. The other useful donor site includes skin from the upper medial aspect of the thigh in reconstructing the areola.

II. HARVESTING

A. Free-Hand Harvesting

The Humby knife is a common free-hand dermatome for harvesting grafts. The basic maneuver is a gradual back and forth movement. A roller is attached to the knife and the distance between the blade and the roller is calibrated to permit varying thickness of graft. Large skin grafts can be harvested in the best of hands. However, the edges of the graft are always irregular. The Goulian knife is a smaller knife and very useful for taking grafts in the outpatient setting. The technique of graft harvesting is similar to that of the Humby knife. The scalpel is a very useful tool for harvesting FTSGs. These grafts may require postharvest defatting prior to placement in the intended defect (Fig. 8.1).

B. Power Dermatome

The Padgett® dermatome is an electricity-driven dermatome. It is light and easy to use. It has a rapidly vibrating movement and the width of the graft depends on the width setting of the dermatome. The thickness of the graft can be adjusted by using this instrument. The Castroviejo® is a small electric dermatome. It is very useful in the harvesting of mucous membrane grafts. Briggman and Wheeler (21) have used this instrument to remove mucosal grafts. The Zimmer® dermatome is a compressed air-driven device. The advantage over electric dermatome is that it allows control of the blade speed and depth of graft harvesting (Figs. 8.2 and 8.3).

C. Hand-Driven Dermatomes

The Reese dermatome is precise when compared to other drum dermatomes. It comes with a set of shims and can be difficult to change thickness in midstream. The movement is by gradual rotation of the drum over the rotating blade. The Padgett® dermatome is less precise than the Reese type, but it is lighter and easier to use and allows recalibration of the depth while cutting.

Skin grafts can be expanded to increase the amount of surface area covered when skin donor site areas are insufficient. Expansion can be increased from 6 to 12 times the original size through a process known as meshing (22). The meshing of grafts is also useful when a copious amount of drainage is expected. A number of instruments are available for meshing, including the simple hand mesh using scalpel blade, the Zimmer skin graft mesher, or the Brennen mesher (23–25).

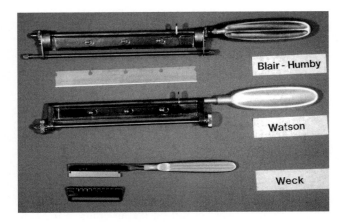

Figure 8.1 Various types of free-hand knives for harvesting of skin grafts.

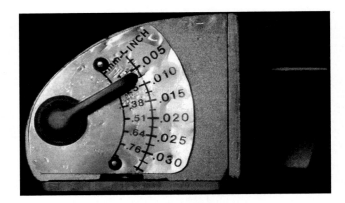

Figure 8.2 Calibration of Padgett® dermatome.

III. GRAFT SURVIVAL

For a graft to "take" it must have a vascular bed. In chronic wounds, proper preparation of the wound bed to receive an STSG may be required. If the wound is infected (bacterial counts are $>10^5$ organisms per gram of tissue), either excision of the wound or jet lavage helps to reduce the bacterial count. To test the adequacy of a vascular bed, allografts have been used prior to the application of an autograft. Skin grafts will not take on bare bone, cartilage, or tendons. However, the bridging phenomenon allows revascularization of these areas if they are <1 cm. For grafts to survive, contact of the graft with the recipient is crucial. Although there are a number of methods utilized to assist with grafts–recipient site contact, the tie over bolster or other compressive wraps ensures this contact (26,27). Splinting may also be necessary depending on the location of the graft.

A. Revascularization

There are three steps to the revascularization of the grafts: plasmatic inhibition, inosculation, and neovascularization.

Plasmatic imbibition occurs immediately after the skin graft comes into contact with the recipient bed. It begins to absorb a plasma-like fluid by osmotic diffusion (28). At the same time, a fibrin network is formed between the graft and the recipient bed (29). The entire process lasts ~48 h, during which time fibrin bonds cause grafts to adhere to the recipient bed. Several investigators believe that serum also helps to keep the graft moist during this stage (30–32). Inosculation is budding of new capillaries, which probably occurs from both the graft site and the recipient site. This development of new vascular anastomoses allows the flow of blood in establishing this new circulating pattern (33,34). Once the circulation is established, new blood vessels start forming between the graft and the recipient bed (35). According

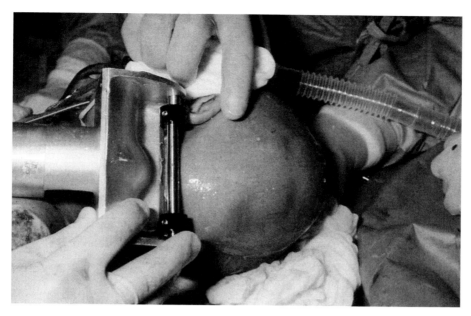

Figure 8.3 Use of power-driven dermatome for harvesting of a scalp STSG.

to Mir, graft survival initially is by vascular connection followed later by vascular ingrowth (36). Medawar noted the ingrowth of capillaries from the host bed on the fourth postgraft day (37).

IV. GRAFT FAILURE

The failure of grafts can occur for multiple reasons. In assessing the process, one must evaluate preoperative factors, intraoperative conditions, and postoperative care. Preoperative factors encompass the evaluation of the patient's overall health, including the assessment of nutritional factors. In addition, the status of the wound bed and associated comorbid conditions, that is, diabetus mellitus, are assessed. If the wound is chronically open and infected (bacterial count $>10^5$ organisms per gram of tissue), graft survival is markedly reduced. It should be noted that fibrotic open wounds have less of a vascular bed and may compromise a graft take. Introperative considerations are in part dictated by our preoperative evaluation. The tangential excision of burn wounds removes necrotic debris and provides a fresh vascular bed for graft "take". The excision of chronically open wounds also removes nonvascularized tissue and provides a fresh bed. As noted, the use of jet lavage can further reduce bacterial count by two logs to ensure graft take. Hemostasis is crucial prior to graft placement to decrease the possibility of hematoma formation. In addition, assuring contact of the graft with the underlying surface is crucial. Postoperatively, the crucial issue is the prevention of shearing.

Shearing forces disrupt the delicate relationship between the graft and the recipient site (38). This interrupts the process of graft revascularization and may contribute to graft failure.

Skin grafts undergo two types of contraction: primary contraction and secondary contraction. Primary contraction is the immediate recoil of the harvested graft and is a function of the amount of elastic fibers present in the dermis. The thicker the graft, the more elastin is present in the dermis and, consequently, the greater the degree of primary contraction (39). Davis and Kitlowski (40) found that STSGs had 9% primary contraction rate and full thickness grafts had 41% contraction rate. Regnell (41) also noted that the tendency of full-thickness free-skin graft to contract may be more due to elastic recoil. Secondary contraction of skin grafts is dependent on the recipient bed and the graft itself. The thinner the graft, the greater the secondary contraction. Thicker grafts have less of a tendency to contract. To some extent, secondary contraction can be prevented by using splints. Various authors feel that at least 75% of the dermis should be incorporated in an STSG to maximally inhibit wound contraction (42–45). Rudolph (44) noted the inhibition of myofibroblast function in the wound bed upon application of skin grafts when compared to nongrafted sites.

Skin grafts can develop major pigment mismatch problems (46). The stimulation of melanocytes is a common occurrence. To date, control of melanocytic activity has eluded investigators. Until this problem is solved, pigmentation changes after placement of skin grafts will continue to be a problem. STSGs tend to hyperpigment. There are various treatment options utilized to lessen hyperpigmentation, such as avoiding UV light exposure and using sun-blocking agents. Detailed treatment of hyperpigmentation is later addressed in this book.

Skin grafts slowly regain normal sensation. Nerve growth occurs from the wound margins. Sensation usually returns between 1 and 6 months' duration (47). Ponten (48) found that grafts assumed the pattern of innervation similar to the recipient tissue, whereas Fitzgerald et al. (49) believed that the pattern of innovation reflects that of the donor site.

The STSG donor site heals secondarily by epithelialization from the epidermal elements. Immediately after harvesting, there is a brisk blood loss. Robinson (50) measured blood loss as 46 cm^3 from a 4 in. $\times$ 8 in. area. Coverage of wound donor sites is variable. The various types of dressing are Scarlet Red® and Xeroform® gauze, which is covered with a bulky dressing. In general, the dressing is removed the next day and the graft is allowed to air dry. Opsite®, an artificial semipermeable membrane, can also be used when donor sites are small. This results in improved reduction of pain (51–54). Various authors have compared Biobrane®, Duoderm®, and Xeroform® as covers for skin graft donor sites (55,56). Shepard (57) even reported successful storage of skin grafts on donor sites. However, all of these products have their advantages and disadvantages. Various skin substitutes have also been used for donor site dressings to reduce the pain they range, all in the hope of accelerating epithelialization and reducing pain (58–65).

REFERENCES

1. Davis JS. Story of plastic surgery. Ann Surg 1941; 113:651.
2. Hauben DJ, Baruchin A, Mahler D. On the history of the free skin graft. Ann Plast Surg 1982; 9:242–245.
3. Gibson T. Early free grafting. The restitution of parts completely separated from the body. Br J Plast Surg 1965; 18:1–11.
4. Borges AF. Improvement of antitension lines scar by the "W-plasty" operation. Br J Plast Surg 1959; 12:29.
5. Borges AF. The W-plastic versus the Z-plastic scar revision. Plast Reconstr Surg 1969; 44: 58–62.
6. Hoffacker W. Case history of a severed portion of the nose. Med Ann 1836; 2:149.
7. Rogers. Historical development of free skin grafts. Surg Clin North Am 1959; 39:289.
8. Vistnes LM. Grafting of skin. Surg Clin North Am 1977; 57:939–960.
9. Brown JB, Fryer MP, Randall P, Lu M. Postmortem homografts as "biological dressings" for extensive burns and denuded areas. Immediate and preserved homografts as life-saving procedures. Ann Surg 1953; 138:618–630.
10. McGregor IA. The vascularization of human skin. Br J Plast Surg 1955; 7:331–337.
11. O'Donoghue MN, Zarem HA. Stimulation of neovascularization—comparative efficacy of fresh and preserve skin grafts. Plast Reconstr Surg 1971; 48:474–478.
12. Bromberg BD, Chul SI, Mohn MP. The use of pig skin as a temporary biologic dressing. Plast Reconstr Surg 1965; 36:80–90.
13. Raven TF. Skin grafting from the pig. Br Med J 1887; 2:623.
14. Blair VP, Brown JB. The use and uses of large split skin grafts of intermediate thickness. Surg Gynecol Obstet 1929; 49:82.
15. Smahel J. The healing of skin grafts. Clin Plast Surg 1977; 4:409–424.
16. Rudolph R, Klein L. Healing process in skin grafts. Surg Gynecol Obstet 1973; 136:641–654.
17. Grabb WC. Basic techniques of plastic surgery. In: Grabb WC, Smith JW, eds. Plastic Surgery. 3rd ed. Boston: Little, Brown, 1979:1–30.
18. Dingman RO, Walter C. Use of composite ear grafts in correction of short nose. Plast Reconstr Surg 1969; 43:117–124.
19. O'Connor NE et al. Grafting of burns with cultured epithelium prepared from autologous epidermal cells. Lancet 1981; 1:75.
20. McCauley RL, Owesy F, Dhanraj P. Management of grade IV burn scar contracture of the neck in children. Proc Amer Burn Assoc 2001; 22(2):90.
21. Briggaman RA, Wheeler CE Jr. Epidermal–dermal interactions in adult human: role of dermis in epidermal maintenance. J Invest Dermatol 1968; 51:454–465.
22. Tanner JC Jr, Vandeput J, Olley JF. The mesh skin graft. Plast Reconstr Surg 1964; 34:287–292.
23. Davison PM, Batchelor AG, Lewis-Smith PA. The properties and uses of non expanded machine-meshed skin grafts. Br J Plast Surg 1986; 39(4):462–468.
24. Richard R, Miller SF, Steinlage R, Finley RK Jr. A comparison of the Tanner and bioplasty skin mesher system for maximal skin graft expansion. J Burn Care Rehabil 1993; 14:690–695.
25. Dziewulski P, Phipps AR. Modification of the dermacarrier to obtain meshed split skin grafts of different expansion ratios. Br J Plast Surg 1991; 44:315–317.
26. Watson SB, Miller JG. Optimizing skin graft take in children's hand burns-the use of Silastic foam dressings. Burns 1993; 19:519–521.
27. Balakrishnan C. Simple method of applying pressure to skin grafts of neck with foam dressing and staples. J Burn Care Rehabil 1994; 15:432–433.
28. Hinshaw JR, Miller ER. Histology of healing split thickness, full-thickness autogenous skin grafts and donor sites. Arch Surg 1965; 91:658–676.
29. Travis MJ et al. Graft adherence to de-epithelialized surfaces: a comparative study. Ann Surg 1976; 184:594.
30. Clemmesen T. The early circulation in split skin grafts. Acta Chir Scand 1962; 124:11–18.
31. Converse JM, Smahel J, Ballantyne D, Harper D. Inosculation of vessels of skin graft and host bed: a fortuitous encounter. Br J Plast Surg 1975; 28:274–282.
32. Peer LA, Walker JC. The behavior of autogenous human tissue grafts, I. Plast Reconstr Surg 1951; 7:623.

33. Haller JA, Billingham RE. Studies of the origin of the vasculature in free skin grafts. Ann Surg 1967; 166:896–901.

34. Birch J, Branemark PI. The vascularization of a free full thickness skin graft. 1. A vital microscopic study. Scand J Plast Reconstr Surg 1969; 3:1–10.

35. Converse JM, Rapaport FT. The vascularization of skin autografts and homografts; an experimental study in man. Ann Surg 1956; 143:306–315.

36. Mir y Mir L. Biology of the skin graft. New aspects to consider in its revascularization. Plast Reconstr Surg 1951; 8:378–389.

37. Medawar PB. The storage of living skin. Proc R Soc Med 1954; 47:62–64.

38. Tsukada S. Transfer of free skin grafts with a preserved subcutaneous vascular network. Ann Plast Surg 1980; 4:500–506.

39. Brown, McDowell. Skin Grafting. 3rd ed. Philadelphia: JB Lippincott Company, 1958.

40. Davis JS, Kitlowski EA. The immediate contraction of cutaneous grafts and its cause. Arch Surg 1931; 23:954.

41. Regnell A. The secondary contracting tendency of free skin grafts. Br J Plast Surg 1953; 5–6.

42. Padgett EC. Calibrated intermediate skin graft. Plast Reconstr Surg 1967; 39:195.

43. Corps BV. The effect of graft thickness, donor site and graft bed on graft shrinkage in the hooded rat. Br J Plast Surg 1969; 22:125–133.

44. Rudolph R. The effect of skin graft preparation on wound contraction. Surg Gynecol Obstet 1976; 142:49–56.

45. Rudolph R. Inhibition of myofibroblasts by skin graft. Plast Reconstr Surg 1979; 63:473–480.

46. Mir y Mir L. The problem of pigmentation in the cutaneous graft. Br J Plast Surg 1961; 14:303–307.

47. Hutchison J, Tough JS, Wyburn GM. Regeneration in grafted skin. Br J Plast Surg 1949; 2:82.

48. Ponten B. Grafted skin. Acta Chir Scand 1960; 257(suppl): 1–78.

49. Fitzgerald MJ, Martin F, Paletta FX. Innervation of skin grafts. Surg Gynecol Obstet 1967; 124:808–812.

50. Robinson. Blood loss from donor sites in skin grafting procedures. Surg 1949; 25:105.

51. Feldman DL. Which dressing for split thickness skin graft donor sites. Ann Plast Surg 1991; 27:288–291.

52. Feldman DL, Karpinski RH. A prospective trial comparing Biobrane, Duoderm, and xeroform for skin graft donor sites. Surg Gynecol Obstet 1991; 173:1–5.

53. Morris WT, Lamb AM. Painless split skin donor sites: a controlled double-blind trial of Op-Site, scarlet red, and bupivacaine. Aust N Z J Surg 1990; 60:617–620.

54. Barnett A, Berkowitz RL, Mills R, Vistnes LM. Comparison of synthetic adhesive moisture vapor permeable and fine mesh gauze dressing for split-thickness skin graft donor sites. Am J Surg 1983; 145:379–381.

55. Zapata-Sirvent R, Hansbrough JF, Carroll W, Johnson R, Wakimoto, A. Comparison of Biobrane and Scarlet Red dressings for treatment of donor sites wounds. Arch Surg 1985; 120:743–745.

56. James JH, Watson AC. The use of Opsite, a vapour permeable dressing, on skin graft donor sites. Br J Plast Surg 1975; 28:107–110.

57. Shepard GH. The Storage of split-skin grafts on their donor sites. Plast Reconstr Surg 1972; 49:115–122.

58. Gallico GG III. Biologic Skin substitutes. Clin Plast Surg 1990; 17:519–526.

59. Hoekstra MJ, Kreis RW, du Pont JS. History of the Euro Skin Bank: the innovation of preservation technologies. Burns 1994; 20:S43–S47.

60. de Backere AC. Euro Skin Bank: large scale skin banking in Europe based on glycerol-preservation of donor skin. Burns 1994; (suppl 1):S4–S9.

61. Robson MC, Krizek TJ. The effect of human amniotic membranes on the bacterial population of the infected rat burns. Ann Surg 1973; 177:144–149.

62. Pruitt BA, Levine NS. Characteristics and uses of biologic dressings and skin substitutes. Arch Surg 1984; 119:312–322.

63. Burke JF, Yannas IV, Quinby MC Jr, Bonoloc CC, Jung WK. Successful use of a physiologically acceptable artificial skin in the treatment of extensive burn injury. Ann Surg 1981; 194:413–428.

64. Georgiade N, Perschel E, Brown I. A clinical and experimental investigation of the preservation of skin. Plast Reconstr Surg 1956; 17:267–275.

65. Brady SC, Snelling CFT, Chow G. Comparison of donor site dressings. Ann Plast Surg 1980; 5:238–243.

9

Skin Substitutes: Theoretical and Developmental Considerations

STEVEN T. BOYCE, DOROTHY M. SUPP

University of Cincinnati and Shriners Burn Hospital, Cincinnati, Ohio, USA

I. OBJECTIVES OF SKIN SUBSTITUTES

Burn injury remains an important medical problem in the United States. Recent estimates indicate that over 1 million burn injuries occur annually, resulting in over 50,000 acute hospital admissions and more than 5000 deaths (1). These medical needs have stimulated new developments in burn care that have resulted in reduced mortality and morbidity. Advances in fluid resuscitation, infection control, nutritional support, and burn wound excision have contributed to improved survival, even in patients with catastrophic burn injuries (2,3). Because most patients survive the initial resuscitation phase, timely wound closure is critical for recovery. In patients with large wounds, permanent wound closure is problematic because of the lack of donor sites for skin autografting. Delayed wound coverage increases the likelihood of infection, which is a major cause of mortality (4).

The need for timely wound closure has led to the development of a number of skin substitutes as alternatives to split-thickness autograft (Table 9.1). These include biological dressings, which provide temporary wound

Table 9.1　Examples of Engineered Skin Substitutes

Skin substitute	Source	Description
Acellular		
Integra®	Integra Life Science Corporation	Artificial dermis, consists of porous bovine collagen–glycosaminoglycan membrane with silastic coating; once vascularized, silastic layer removed, thin split-thickness autograft applied (5–8)
Biobrane™	Dow Hickam/Bertek Pharmaceuticals	Temporary wound cover; bilaminate membrane consisting of collagen-coated nylon mesh fabric bonded to thin layer of silicone (9,10)
Alloderm®	LifeCell Corporation	Allogeneic acellular human dermis; matrix preserved by freeze-drying; can be used as a template for dermal regeneration in conjunction with thin split-thickness autograft (11)
Cellular		
Transcyte® (formerly Dermagraft-TC)	Smith & Nephew	Temporary dermal replacement; Biobrane™ seeded with human allogeneic neonatal fibroblasts, then frozen; fibroblasts not viable at time of grafting (12–14)
Dermagraft®	Smith & Nephew	Cryopreserved living dermal replacement; allogeneic human neonatal fibroblasts seeded on polymer mesh scaffold; fibroblasts viable at time of grafting (15,16)
Epicel™	Genzyme Biosurgery	Cultured autologous keratinocyte sheets prepared from cells isolated from patient skin biopsy (17)
Laserskin™	Fidia Advanced Biopolymers	Laser-perforated hyaluronic acid-derived membrane populated with autologous cultured keratinocytes (18)
Orcel™	Ortec International, Inc.	Bovine collagen sponge containing human allogeneic cultured keratinocytes and fibroblasts (19)
Apligraf®	Organogenesis, Inc.	Bovine collagen gel containing human allogeneic fibroblasts and keratinocytes (20–22)
Cultured Skin Substitutes (CSS)	Shriners Hospitals (Investigative)	Collagen–glycosaminoglycan sponge containing autologous human fibroblasts and keratinocytes (23–25)

Note: This list includes examples of both acellular and cellular skin substitutes used clinically for wound healing purposes, but is not intended to be all-inclusive.

coverage to facilitate wound closure, but do not persist after healing, as well as permanent skin replacements. An example of a synthetic dressing is Biobrane™, an acellular peptide-coated nylon mesh material bonded to a layer of silicone (9). This has been used on excised full-thickness burn wounds as a temporary coverage before autografting, and has been shown to be as effective as frozen cadaver allograft for this purpose (10). Other examples of temporary wound covers, such as Transcyte and Apligraf, contain allogeneic human cells isolated from neonatal foreskin. Transcyte is composed of Biobrane seeded with allogeneic fibroblasts (12,13), and Apligraf consists of a bovine type I collagen gel populated with both allogeneic fibroblasts and keratinocytes (20,21). Because these products contain allogeneic cells, they can provide wound coverage and supply cytokines that facilitate wound repair, but they do not persist on the patient after healing is complete. In general, allogeneic cells are replaced within 1–6 weeks after grafting by the patient's own cells (26–29). Skin substitutes that are populated with patient-derived cells can provide permanent wound closure for the healing of large burns and other wounds. Integra™ is an example of a synthetic

dermal substitute that is used to facilitate wound closure which does not contain cells at the time of grafting. It consists of a cross-linked collagen–glycosaminoglycan membrane as a dermal matrix, and a silastic coating which provides a synthetic epidermal structure for barrier replacement (5,6). The artificial dermis becomes populated with cells from the wound bed and is vascularized within a few weeks; the silastic coating can then be removed and replaced with a thin sheet of split-thickness skin (7,8). Other skin substitutes can be populated *in vitro* with autologous keratinocytes and fibroblasts, which are derived from biopsies of the patient's uninjured skin and expanded in culture. Grafted as epithelial sheets (17) or as composites of biopolymers and cells (23–25), these are theoretically permanent skin substitutes once engraftment is achieved.

Skin replacements can be used as adjunctive therapies in patients who are also receiving conventional skin grafts to facilitate wound closure (23–25,30,31). By increasing availability of skin grafts, skin substitutes can provide several advantages over conventional therapy, including reduction of donor site area required to close wounds permanently, reduction in number of surgical procedures and hospitalization time, and reduction of mortality and morbidity from scarring (14,32).

The primary goal of skin substitutes is restoration of epidermal barrier, to minimize protein and fluid loss, and prevent infection (33). To be useful in a clinical setting, the ideal skin replacement should be ready to be used when needed, promote complete engraftment without contraction or the need for regrafting, allow rapid healing to form both dermal and epidermal layers, achieve favorable functional and cosmetic outcome, be free from risk of disease transmission, and have minimal immunological reaction (4). The ultimate objective for skin substitutes is restoration of the anatomy and physiology of uninjured skin after healing of the wound. There are currently no skin substitutes available which fully replace all of the structures or functions of uninjured skin. Skin substitutes that contain cultured cells can provide large quantities of grafts for wound treatment, but restore only a subset of anatomic structures and physiologic functions of skin (Table 9.2). Therefore, the full potential for engineering of skin substitutes has not yet been realized.

II. REQUIREMENTS

A. Anatomic and Physiologic

Normal human skin performs a wide variety of protective (barrier, UV light absorption, immune surveillance, mechanical), perceptive (touch, temperature, pain), and regulatory (thermal, hydration, excretory) functions that help the body maintain homeostasis. Skin performs these functions by integration of epidermis and dermis, transducing energy through cellular and extracellular mechanisms to provide information to the brain for appropriate responses. The predominant cell type found in the epidermis is the keratinocyte. Other epidermal cells include adnexal cells

(glands, hair, nails), melanocytes, dendritic cells of the immune system (i.e., Langerhans cells), and sensory structures of nerves (i.e., Merkel cells). Dermal cells include fibroblasts, vascular components (endothelial cells, smooth muscle cells), nerve cells (temperature, pain), immune-response cells (mast cells), and pilo-erector muscles. The bulk of dermal tissue consists of extracellular matrix (collagens, elastin, reticulin, polysaccharides) that gives mechanical strength to the skin. Epidermis contains only very small amounts of extracellular matrix, predominantly carbohydrate polymers (34) and stratum corneum lipids (35,36) that organize as a liquid crystal to form a barrier to permeability of aqueous fluids. The extracellular matrix of the skin is synthesized by cells of the dermis and epidermis, and is organized into a correct anatomy. The composition and structure of extracellular matrix are essential to skin function. Because morbidity is defined and characterized by loss of tissue structure and function, full recovery after skin injury may not be expected without full restoration of all cell types. Although cells from the wound bed are a source of fibrovascular tissue, closure of full-thickness wounds requires transplantation of epithelial skin cells. However, epithelial closure alone does not restore full skin function. Therefore, complete re-establishment of skin function and medical recovery require restoration of all types of skin cells from the graft and/or the wound in an anatomically correct structure. This is currently a major limitation of engineered skin substitutes. For example, no skin substitute contains a functional vascular plexus, although experimental models have been described (37,38). Consequently, both the mechanism and the time for vascularization of engineered skin substitutes may be distinguished from grafts of native skin. This anatomic deficiency in skin substitutes may cause them to become ischemic and nutrient deprived after grafting, contributing to secondary wound infection and graft failure.

Table 9.2 Comparison of Native Skin Structures in Split-Thickness Autograft, Clinical Models of Engineered Skin, and Healed Skin After Grafting

Cell type/ structure	Tissue	Split-thickness autograft	Engineered skin substitute	Healed skin after grafting
Keratinocytes	Epidermis	+	+	+
Melanocytes	Epidermis	+/−	+/−	+/−
Hair follicle	Epidermis	−	−	−
Sebaceous gland	Epidermis	−	−	−
Sweat gland	Epidermis	−	−	−
Immune cells	Epidermis/Dermis	+	−	+
Nerve cells	Epidermis/Dermis	+	−	+/−
Fibroblasts	Dermis	+	+/−	+
Endothelial cells	Dermis	+	−	+
Smooth muscle	Dermis	+	−	+/−

B. Surgical

The standard of care for rapid closure of full-thickness excised burns is split-thickness autologous skin. Autograft can be applied either as a sheet (39), or it can be expanded by meshing (40). Functional and cosmetic recovery after grafting is generally acceptable, allowing the return of patients to productive roles in society (41). Successful outcome for conventional skin grafts depends on several factors, including adherence of grafts to wounds, histocompatibility, control of fluid loss and infection, absence of toxicity, mechanical stability and patient compliance, cost-effectiveness, and availability (42,43). These requirements must also be satisfied by skin substitutes prepared through tissue engineering. However, anatomic deficiencies in engineered skin substitutes decreases the probability that these requirements can be satisfied. Limitations of skin substitutes prepared by laboratory fabrication, compared with split-thickness skin grafts, include reduced rates of engraftment (44), increased microbial contamination (45), mechanical fragility (46), increased time to healing (47), increased regrafting, and very high cost (48). These complications of skin substitutes may increase, rather than decrease, the risks to patient recovery. Therefore, the use of engineered skin substitutes may be advisable as an adjunctive therapy in cases without other alternatives, such as very large burns, until efficacy comparable to split-thickness skin is demonstrated. Nevertheless, complications with early models of skin substitutes do not preclude their long-term potential for medical advantages in burn wound care.

III. PRINCIPLES OF TISSUE ENGINEERING OF HUMAN SKIN

The engineering of skin substitutes removes constraints for the structure and function of skin for transplantation. Hypothetically, skin pigment, texture, pliability, tensile strength, barrier, matrix, and cytokine expression may be altered by regulation of the composition of engineered skin (49,50). For the purpose of this discussion, it is assumed that the ultimate goal for engineered skin is complete restoration of the anatomy and physiology of uninjured human skin. After this milestone has been reached, modifications of the native structures and functions can be evaluated to determine whether any advantage is conferred to the recipient.

A. Components

Human skin is comprised of various cells, biopolymers, and soluble factors. Ultimately, wound closure is defined by restoration of epidermal barrier, which provides protection from fluid loss and infection. Barrier components are synthesized by the parenchymal cells of the epidermis, the keratinocytes (51). Many investigators have evaluated the use of cultured keratinocytes for treatment of excised, full-thickness burns (52–56). A consensus has developed that replacement of connective tissue was also required for satisfactory outcome (46,57). Fibro-vascular connective tissue provides the mechanical strength and blood supply to skin, to facilitate attachment and nourishment for the epidermis. Therefore, repopulation with fibroblasts, endothelial cells, and smooth muscle is required to form stable skin. These components may populate grafts from the wound bed. Recently, several models of engineered skin have been developed which include cultured dermal fibroblasts, in addition to epidermal keratinocytes, to facilitate predictable repair of connective tissue in treated wounds (24,58-61). Pigment cells, the melanocytes, can be cultured and transplanted (62) for treatment of vitiligo and burn scars, and have been added into cell–polymer constructs (63–65). Nerve cells may extend dendrites into healing grafts, but full restoration of skin sensation has not been demonstrated to date with either split-thickness skin grafts or transplanted engineered skin (66,67). Glands (sweat, sebaceous) and hair follicles have been transplanted in preclinical studies (68,69), but currently neither engineered skin nor skin autografts can restore these structures. Because of this limitation, thermal regulation in healed wounds treated with engineered skin is inadequate. However, these deficiencies do not reduce the importance of engineered skin for definitive closure of wounds, and therapeutic benefits to patients.

Table 9.3 summarizes some of the current materials used for engineered skin substitutes (70). These materials range from cultured dermal and epidermal cells (autologous or allogeneic) to tissue derivatives and synthetic polymers. Combinations of dermal and epidermal substitutes have also been reported to effectively close

Table 9.3 Components of Engineered Skin Substitutes

Dermal substitutes	Epidermal substitutes
Collagen gel	Silastic sheet
Collagen–glycosaminoglycan matrix	Thin epidermal autograft
Acellular cadaveric human skin matrix	Epidermal suction blisters
Polylactic acid/ polyglycolic acid	Keratinocyte/fibrin glue suspensions
Allogeneic cultured fibroblasts	Allogeneic cultured keratinocytes
Autologous cultured fibroblasts	Autologous cultured keratinocytes

excised, full-thickness burns and experimental wounds (30,71–75). Commercial products and experimental models for dermal and/or epidermal repair have been configured from individual and combined materials, as shown in Table 9.1.

B. Process

Skin substitutes can be engineered to meet specific functional objectives. Their fabrication requires a deliberate process that will result in a composition meeting the design specifications. For engineering of tissues such as skin, recapitulation of the organ's developmental process would result in correct structures and functions. Skin develops through sequential cytogenesis, morphogenesis, histogenesis, and organogenesis. Although wound healing involves the processes of cytogenesis, morphogenesis, and histogenesis, organogenesis in wounded skin does not occur. Current technologies promote wound healing phenotypes in skin cells, and consequently many of the structures that result from developmental processes, such as glands, follicles, and nerves, are not formed in skin substitutes (76).

1. Cytogenesis

Increased numbers of epidermal and dermal cells are required to repopulate wounds and restore skin structure. Selective *in vitro* culture of skin cells, including keratinocytes, melanocytes, fibroblasts, and endothelial cells, stimulates exponential increases in cell populations. This increase can be expressed using the equation $(P_I)(2^n) = (P_F)$, where P_I is the initial population, n is the number of population doublings, and P_F is the final population (77). By this exponential function, a population of cells can increase in number $\sim$1 million-fold in 20 generations. With an approximate doubling time of 1 day or less for keratinocytes and fibroblasts, very large populations of skin cells can be prepared in only 2–3 weeks of culture. The technological advances that allowed for the rapid growth of cells in culture have provided the fundamental basis for generation of tissue substitutes for skin repair. For keratinocytes, these advances have included culture in serum-containing (78) or serum-free media (79), both of which are now commonly practiced.

2. Morphogenesis

After preparation of large populations of skin cells in culture, organization into skin substitutes increases homology to native skin. Cultured human keratinocytes may be combined with dermal substitutes *in vitro* (80–82), and exposed to the air to stimulate epithelial stratification and cornification (83–85). Culture at the air–liquid interface provides a polarized environment with nutrient

medium contacting the dermal substitute, and air contacting the epidermal substitute. Keratinocytes in skin substitutes respond to this gradient of hydration by orienting proliferating cells toward the medium and cornified cells toward the air. This results in establishment of a stratified, squamous epithelium in culture. Fibroblasts fill the biopolymer substrate, begin to degrade it, and generate new extracellular matrix (Fig. 9.1).

Two biologic changes occur in skin substitutes prepared with keratinocytes and fibroblasts inoculated at very high cell densities. First, the proliferation rates of the cells decrease, resulting in a decrease in the nutritional requirements per cell. However, the nutritional requirements of the entire population may increase because skin substitutes generally contain significantly more cells per unit volume than monolayer cell cultures. Second, the increase in cell density causes an increase in concentration of growth factors secreted by cells in the tissue substitute. Higher concentrations of secreted factors can confer independence from exogenous growth factors supplied by the culture medium (86,87). Addition of certain mitogens under conditions of high cell densities may result in cytotoxicity. Keratinocytes and fibroblasts are known to secrete a wide variety of cytokines, including inflammatory mediators, growth factors, extracellular matrix components, and catabolic enzymes (49). Combining epithelial and mesenchymal cells in cultured skin substitutes may facilitate operation of paracrine mechanisms

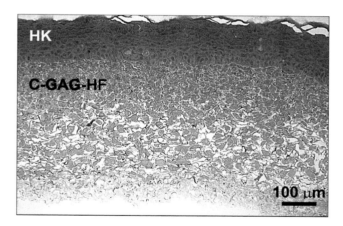

Figure 9.1 Histology of a clinical cultured skin substitute. Shown is a toluidine blue-stained section of a skin substitute cultured for 1 week at the air–liquid interface. To prepare this graft, a collagen-based membrane was inoculated with 5×10^5 cultured human fibroblasts per square cm; 1×10^6 cultured human keratinocytes per square cm were inoculated on top of the dermal substitute 1 day later. After a total of 10 culture days, this skin substitute was used to heal an excised burn wound on a pediatric patient. Abbreviations: HK = human keratinocytes; C-GAG-HF = collagen-glycosaminoglycan substrate populated with human fibroblasts. Scale bar = 100 μm.

between cell types. For example, the mesenchymal-cell mitogen platelet-derived growth factor (PDGF) is synthesized by keratinocytes in normal epidermis, and its receptors are expressed in cells of the dermis (88,89). PDGF and other factors, including fibroblast growth factors 7 and 10, transforming growth factors alpha and beta, and epidermal growth factor, are believed to stimulate the mechanisms of action for healing of skin wounds (90). The same mechanisms have been demonstrated by topical applications of recombinant growth factors (91–94). Unlike topical application of exogenous cytokines to facilitate wound healing, synthesis and delivery of these factors by engineered skin provides a continuous supply, and may regulate delivery of factors according to mechanisms endogenous to the wound.

3. Histogenesis

There are currently no models of engineered skin substitutes that reproduce the anatomy, physiology or biologic stability of uninjured skin. Stable recovery of skin function occurs only after transplantation, vascularization and healing of engineered grafts according to *in vivo* mechanisms. This step in the process of tissue engineering requires survival of cells after transplantation and incorporation into the healing wound. Therefore, skin substitutes must respond to the regulatory mechanisms of the wound environment to restore function. In acute wounds, such as excised burns, skin substitutes must respond to inflammatory processes and integrate with the underlying fibro-vascular tissue to support grafted epithelium. If skin substitutes engraft, a healed epithelium should develop within 2 weeks after application. Clinical characteristics of healed epithelium include repelling of water, suppression of granulation tissue, and capillary blanching and refill after punctate depression.

4. Organogenesis

Recovery of all functions of uninjured skin is a current goal of tissue repair, and the ultimate goal of engineered skin substitutes. Even split-thickness skin grafts do not accomplish this goal at the present time. Only transplantation of full-thickness skin can restore organotypic functions such as perspiration, hair growth, and normal pigmentation (95,96). Because development of epidermal appendages occurs *in utero*, but not in wound healing, these structures may be transplanted, but cannot yet be prepared from postnatal cells after selective culture.

IV. CLINICAL CONSIDERATIONS

Multiple factors of clinical care can determine whether treatment of wounds with engineered skin substitutes results in skin repair. Modifications of care protocols for debrided, full-thickness wounds must be used to compensate for the anatomic and physiologic deficiencies in engineered skin. Currently available skin substitutes are avascular, tend to heal more slowly than skin autograft, and may be mechanically fragile. Factors which affect the outcome with engineered skin grafts include wound bed preparation, control of microbial contamination, dressings and nursing care, and survival of transplanted cells during vascularization of grafts.

A. Surgical Considerations

Clinical complications with engineered skin generally result from anatomic and physiologic deficiencies that compromise responses of the graft to the wound healing process. Split-thickness skin contains a vascular plexus and adheres to debrided wounds by coagulum. This is followed by inosculation of vessels in the graft to vessels in the wound within 2–5 days. Although healing is not complete at this time point, native skin is engrafted and reperfused within 1 week after grafting. In contrast, current clinical models of engineered skin substitutes are avascular, requiring reperfusion from *de novo* angiogenesis. If the rate of vascularization is considered constant, then the time required for perfusion is directly proportional to the thickness of the dermal component of the skin substitute, and is longer than perfusion of split-thickness skin. Vascularization can be accelerated by secretion of angiogenic factors from engineered skin containing keratinocytes and/or fibroblasts (97,98), but growth factors alone cannot compensate for the lack of a vascular plexus prior to grafting. The additional time required for vascularization may contribute to epithelial loss from microbial destruction and/or nutrient deprivation.

Attachment of cultured epithelium to a dermal substitute *in vitro* is advantageous because both epidermal and dermal components are applied in a single surgical procedure, similar to skin autograft. Biopolymers in composite skin substitutes are adsorbed and replaced as cells secrete enzymes and extracellular matrix components, contributing to formation of functional skin tissue. Culture conditions can be optimized to promote deposition of basement membrane proteins at the dermal–epidermal junction prior to grafting (99), thereby eliminating the problem of blistering that is frequently observed after grafting of epithelial sheets (17). Alternatively, dermal and epidermal components of skin substitutes may be applied in two stages: first, application of a dermal substitute followed by vascularization and second, grafting of an autologous epidermal substitute (7,57,100). This two-step approach increases the density of blood vessels and extracellular matrix in the graft bed, and has been reported to improve efficacy of cultured keratinocyte sheets.

However, it requires two surgical procedures to accomplish permanent wound closure.

Topical antimicrobial agents are more effective for control of wound contamination than parenteral antimicrobials (101). Topical antimicrobial treatments must provide effective coverage of a broad spectrum of gram-negative and gram-positive bacteria as well as common fungal contaminants. In burns, common wound contaminants include *Pseudomonas aeruginosa*, *Staphylococcus aureus*, and *Candida albicans*. For use with engineered skin substitutes, topical antimicrobials must have low cytotoxicity to allow healing to proceed. It is also important to avoid overlap of topical agents with parenteral drugs used for treatment of sepsis. This can lead to development of organisms resistant to the topical agents, and subsequent sepsis from a resistant organism may be untreatable. For example, if aminoglycosides are routinely used for parenteral treatment of sepsis, then they should not be used topically. Silver compounds, such as silver sulfadiazine and silver nitrate, can be toxic to cells in cultured skin substitutes because they act by precipitation of chloride from biological material, although very low concentrations have been reported to be noncytotoxic (102). Parallel assays of cellular toxicity and antimicrobial activity have been used to determine effective concentrations of agents that preserve cell viability (103). Several studies have identified individual agents, and formulations of multiple agents, that are not inhibitory to proliferation of keratinocytes and fibroblasts and that remain effective against common wound organisms (104–108). Investigative formulations for management of microbial contamination of skin substitutes include neomycin and polymyxin B for gram-negative organisms; mupirocin for gram-positive bacteria; and nystatin or amphotericin B for fungi (108). Quinolone drugs (i.e., norfloxacin, ciprofloxacin) may be added to broaden coverage of bacteria (107), if they are not part of the routine parenteral therapy for bacteremia, septicemia, or sepsis.

B. Nursing Considerations

A major limitation of engineered skin substitutes is mechanical fragility. This contributes to graft failure due to shear and maceration. For delicate grafts, a backing material that allows convenient handling and stapling to the wound may be added for mechanical reinforcement. For example, cultured epithelial autografts are routinely attached to petrolatum-impregnated gauze for surgical application (109). However, this material is not compatible with wet dressings that are frequently used to combat infection. Alternatively, composite skin substitutes may be handled and stapled to wounds with a backing of N-Terface™ (Winfield Laboratories, Richardson, TX), a relatively strong, nonadherent, highly porous material

(23,24). Similarly, Surfasoft™ (Mediprof, Amsterdam, Holland) has been used in Europe as a porous, nonadherent backing for cultured epithelial autografts (110). Porous dressings do not interfere with the delivery of topical solutions, and permit drainage of wound exudate from grafts until engraftment is achieved. To avoid mechanical disturbance, frequency of dressing changes is kept to a minimum during the first week after grafting. As the mechanical strength of grafted skin substitutes improves, due to development of fibro-vascular tissue and epidermal barrier, the frequency of dressing changes can increase. With close attention to these surgical and nursing factors, closure of excised, full-thickness burns can be accomplished with reduction of requirements for donor skin autograft.

C. Assessment

The outcome after treatment of wounds with engineered skin substitutes must be measured to determine whether the benefits justify any risks associated with the therapy. Qualitative outcome is assessed through clinical evaluation and relies most heavily on the trained eye of the clinician. Clinical examination integrates multiple properties in the wounds according to the perceptions of the physician. For example, the Vancouver Scale is used for assessment of burn scar by trained clinicians, and provides an ordinal score for properties of skin including pigmentation, vascularity, pliability, and scar height (111). Similar comparative scales developed for engineered skin substitutes have shown no statistical difference from skin autograft at 1 year after grafting (25). These scales are used to assign quantitative values to qualitative measurements, and as such provide a relative comparison for evaluation. However, they are inherently subjective and dependent on the examiner.

Objectivity may be increased by assessment of wounds with noninvasive instruments that measure biophysical properties in skin, including vascular perfusion, epidermal barrier, pliability, color, and surface pH (Table 9.4). These instruments may be used to measure the normal, healthy condition of skin, as a standard of comparison for dermatological pathology. In extreme conditions, such as full-thickness skin wounds, virtually all of the biophysical properties of skin are outside of the normal range, and can easily be distinguished statistically from uninjured skin. Quantitative assessment of parameters of engineered skin substitutes can highlight deficiencies compared to normal skin or split-thickness autograft. Instrumentation can provide a means to assess the benefit of skin substitutes to the patient, without interfering with recovery. Although no single property is definitive, multiple measurements can provide a general assessment for evaluation of outcome. For example, measurements of surface electrical

Table 9.4 Noninvasive Biophysical Instruments for Assessment of Skin

Assessment	Property measured	Instrument
Percent engraftment	Percent original wound area	Planimetry
Vascular perfusion	Blood flow	Laser Doppler
Epidermal barrier	Surface electrical capacitance	Dermal phase meter
Surface hydration	Transepidermal water loss	Evaporimeter
Elasticity	Pliability	Dermal torque meter
Pigmentation	Color	Chromameter
Acid mantle of skin surface	pH	Surface pH meter
Heat	Temperature	Infrared camera

capacitance can be used to define the degree of skin barrier development. Skin capacitance is measured using a dermal phase meter, an instrument that is easily used in a clinical setting, with minimal pain or discomfort for the patient (112). However, this value alone does not predict functional recovery. Similarly, pigmentation of wounds treated with engineered skin substitutes can be measured quantitatively and kinetically with the chromameter, but it does not assess scar formation. Therefore, multiple parameters of skin function must be measured to quantify overall benefit from treatment with skin substitutes.

D. Cost

An important practical obstacle to the routine clinical use of skin substitutes remains the high cost of their preparation and care. Estimates for the cost of keratinocyte sheets range from $1000 to $13,000 for each percentage of body surface area covered (48,113). If a dermal substitute is also included, the cost can approximately double (7,11). Therefore, expense can become a limiting factor for treatment of very severely burned patients with cultured skin substitutes. Unfortunately, patients with burns covering a very large percentage of their body, who have limited donor sites for autografting, are the patients most in need of skin substitutes. Although the use of skin substitutes can theoretically reduce the number of surgeries required to heal large burns, which should decrease the total time of hospitalization, there are presently no studies that clearly demonstrate a decrease in hospitalization costs by use of skin substitutes of any kind. The use of engineered skin grafts remains an important adjunct to conventional skin grafting in the treatment of burns (46), but cannot be used as a primary modality of wound closure except in the most extreme cases.

V. REGULATORY ISSUES

It is the responsibility of the U.S. Food and Drug Administration (FDA) to protect the public from health risks associated with new therapies. As such, FDA approval requires that new therapies be safe and effective, and that the probable benefits to health outweigh the probable risks of the therapy, or of the untreated disease or condition (114). Safety considerations for engineered skin substitutes must take several factors into account, including media composition, tissue acquisition, implant fabrication and storage, and testing of the final product for sterility (114). For example, cell culture media must be of the greatest possible purity and free from toxic chemical contaminants. Cells derived from allogeneic donors must be determined to be free of transmissible pathogens, according to tissue-banking standards. Autologous cells must be carefully handled as well. Because autologous tissues are not routinely screened for bloodborne pathogens, laboratory personnel must take precautions to protect themselves, and to prevent infection during processing of cells for transplantation. Xenogeneic components, such as bovine collagen, must not only be free from pathogens that can cross species boundaries, but must also be nonimmunogenic. The final product must be tested to assure that contamination of materials has not resulted from improper handling during laboratory preparation.

Engineered skin substitutes may be regulated primarily as devices or biologics, depending on their specific composition. In most cases, cells combined with biopolymers are considered class III (significant risk) devices that require demonstration of effectiveness in addition to safety (114). Preclinical testing generally includes *in vitro* characterization of anatomy and physiology, as well as animal studies to determine host response, changes over time, and restoration of function. Skin substitutes consisting of autologous cells only, or an acellular human tissue matrix, are considered low-risk and may not require collection of effectiveness data. Living autologous cell populations intended for structural repair are considered to be inherently efficacious (115). However, if no effectiveness data are collected, no claims of effectiveness can be advertised. The clinician must use caution, realizing that the commercial availability of an engineered skin substitute does not assure that it is efficacious.

VI. CLINICAL EXPERIENCE: BURNS

Favorable qualitative results have been obtained by a combination of cultured autologous keratinocytes and fibroblasts with collagen-based dermal substitutes (24). Termed cultured skin substitutes (CSS), these engineered skin grafts have been transplanted for treatment of burns, chronic wounds, and reconstructive surgery of the skin. Each of these medical indications requires specific considerations to optimize the outcome after surgery. For the purpose of this review, discussion of clinical experience with CSS will be limited to the treatment of burn wounds.

The most extensive experience with autologous CSS has been in the treatment of patients with burns affecting >50% total body surface area (TBSA). Progressive improvement of the anatomy and physiology of CSS has correlated well with increased efficacy of burn wound closure. For preparation of CSS, primary cultures of keratinocytes and fibroblasts are isolated using standard techniques (77,79,116) from small split-thickness skin biopsy samples that are usually taken during a patient's first autografting procedure (24,25,117). Grafting to patients can generally be performed within 2 weeks of inoculation of CSS, which corresponds to 4–5 weeks after the initial patient biopsy. Future technical improvements which accelerate cell growth in culture, reduce the density of cells inoculated, or enhance maturation of the CSS can be expected to decrease the time from initial patient biopsy to treatment with CSS.

Improved engraftment has resulted from development of an irrigation solution consisting of nutrients and non-cytotoxic antimicrobial agents (25). Enhanced epidermal barrier and basement membrane formation, by addition of ascorbic acid to the incubation medium, have further increased engraftment (99). Another important advance was realized by the successful combination of autologous CSS with the dermal substitute Integra Artificial Skin® (30). It was observed that CSS attach rapidly by connections between the neo-dermis formed by grafted Integra® and the dermal component of the CSS, resulting in >90% engraftment.

Figure 9.2 shows a pediatric patient with 94% burns who was covered over more than 60% of his TBSA with autologous CSS grafts. The healed skin is smooth, pliable, and strong. The anterior trunk was treated with cadaveric allograft and Integra as temporary covers. The very smooth surface is attributed to the use of Integra as a graft base. Because CSS is composed of both keratinocytes and fibroblasts, basement membrane develops in the laboratory, thus no epidermal blistering occurs after grafting. Protective skin barrier develops within 1 week after grafting due to the development of stratum corneum in CSS *in vitro*. Because the cultured skin cells

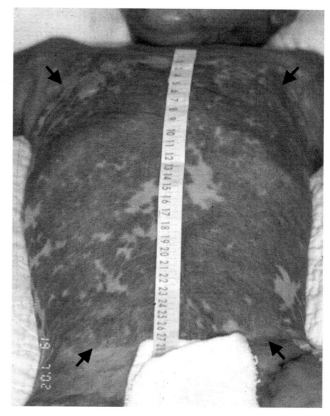

Figure 9.2 Clinical outcome at 14 months after grafting of cultured skin substitutes to excised, full-thickness burns. The arrows indicate the region of the anterior trunk grafted with cultured skin. Healed skin is soft, smooth, and strong. Pigmentation has irregular distribution, but uniform intensity. No reconstruction has been required, and the skin remains fully pliable suggesting that it is growing with the patient. Scale is in centimeters.

can be cryopreserved for several years in liquid nitrogen, additional CSS can be prepared at a later date with no additional donor site harvesting. Serial tracings of grafted areas over extended periods of time have demonstrated that skin healed with autologous CSS continues to grow as pediatric patients grow. This finding illustrates that connective tissue which develops after grafting of CSS may be distinguished from contracted bands of collagenous scar.

VII. FUTURE DIRECTIONS

Despite encouraging clinical results with CSS for the adjunctive treatment of excised burns, skin substitutes containing just two cell types are limited by anatomic and physiologic deficiencies compared to split-thickness skin autograft. Several areas of preclinical investigation suggest that skin substitutes can be further engineered to increase homology to native human skin. These include the incorporation of additional cell types to improve functional and cosmetic outcome, and the use of genetically modified skin cells to enhance performance after grafting.

A. Regulation of Pigmentation

Normal skin pigmentation results from the appropriate distribution and function of epidermal melanocytes. These cells serve important physiological functions, most notably protection from UV irradiation (118,119). Melanocyte function is also important psychologically, as a patient's body image and personal identity can impact recovery from massive burn injury (120).

Pigmentation of cultured skin grafted clinically for treatment of burn injury results from transplantation of "passenger" melanocytes (30,117). The term "passenger" refers to the persistence of melanocytes in selective cultures of epidermal keratinocytes. Melanocytes can survive under conditions used for keratinocyte culture, though they proliferate at slow rates and tend to be depleted upon serial passage or cryopreservation of cultures (53,121,122). Pigmented areas resulting from passenger melanocytes in grafted CSS develop as individual foci within 2 months after transplantation (117). By 1–2 years after healing, the foci increase in area and occasionally fuse together to form regions of uniform pigmentation (Fig. 9.2). The enlargement of the pigmented areas was shown to correspond to transfer of melanosomes to adjacent keratinocytes (117). Hypothetically, increasing the number of melanocytes transplanted in engineered skin should result in regular distribution of pigmentation after healing.

Uniform pigmentation has been demonstrated in preclinical studies with cultured composite skin grafts deliberately populated with selectively cultured human melanocytes (64,65). CSS inoculated with a mix of keratinocytes with 3% melanocytes resulted in uniform dark pigmentation after grafting to athymic mice (65). Cytometric cell sorting was used to selectively deplete melanocytes from keratinocyte cultures, resulting in lack of pigmentation after grafting (65). Future studies will be needed to address regulation of the level of pigmentation in uniformly pigmented cultured skin.

B. *In Vitro* Angiogenesis

As previously described, a major limitation of CSS is lack of a vascular plexus. This necessitates vascularization to occur *de novo* rather than through inosculation of the graft with the wound, increasing the time of nutrient deprivation and susceptibility to microbial contamination for grafted wound. This limitation has been addressed clinically by irrigating the grafted CSS with a solution of nutrients and antimicrobial agents for several days after transplantation (25,30,123). The use of topical nutrients and antimicrobials addresses the vascular deficiency in CSS indirectly. A direct approach would be to initiate angiogenesis in the skin substitutes *in vitro*, prior to grafting, hypothetically permitting vascularization of the CSS to occur through both inosculation of existing vessels in the grafts with vessels from the wound bed and neovascularization, as occurs for grafted split-thickness skin (124).

Initiation of angiogenesis *in vitro* requires the addition of endothelial cells to the dermal compartment of the engineered skin substitute. Cultured endothelial cells have been demonstrated to organize into vascular structures under certain culture conditions through the use of biomaterial supports and/or coculture with other cell types. For example, engineered human blood vessels have been constructed *in vitro* using mixtures of vascular smooth muscle cells, dermal fibroblasts, and human umbilical vein endothelial cells (HUVEC) in a collagen matrix (125), or using isolated cells grown along a tubular support to facilitate lumen formation (126). A preclinical study involving transplantation of engineered blood vessels constructed by culture of HUVEC in three-dimensional collagen/fibronectin gels has been reported (127). These engineered tissues organized into multilayered structures after implantation in mice, illustrating the feasibility of grafting synthetic vessels, but overexpression of Bcl-2 through retroviral modification was required to promote survival of the transplanted endothelial cells (127). In a similar study, human dermal microvascular endothelial cells (HDMEC) in a porous poly-L-lactic acid sponge were implanted under the skin of recipient mice to form functional microvessels (128).

Similar approaches have been applied to the problem of vascular deficiency of cultured skin grafts in preclinical studies. For example, preparation of a skin equivalent containing dermal fibroblasts, epidermal keratinocytes, and HUVEC was reported, but transplantation to wounds was not performed (37).

A potential limitation of this and other studies that may impede their clinical application in cultured skin grafting is the reliance on nondermal (e.g., HUVEC) or nonautologous endothelial cells. Preparation of endothelialized skin substitutes for grafting to a patient with a competent immune system should ideally be performed using multiple cell types (keratinocytes, fibroblasts, and HDMEC) derived from a single autologous skin sample. Recently, transplantation of HDMEC in a composite skin substitute containing isogenic keratinocytes and fibroblasts was demonstrated in an athymic mouse model (38). HDMEC persisted in the dermal compartments of the skin substitutes and formed multicellular aggregates *in vitro* and *in vivo*. By 4 weeks after grafting to athymic mice, HDMEC were found in linear and circular organizations resembling vascular analogs associated with basement membrane deposition and mouse smooth muscle cells. The transplantation of HDMEC in a clinically relevant cultured skin model showed the feasibility of preparing CSS containing autologous HDMEC for grafting to patients. Initiation of angiogenesis *in vitro* may result in engineered skin with greater homology to split-thickness autograft. Future studies must demonstrate inosculation of vascular analogs from the engineered skin with severed vessels in the wound bed to yield improved performance after grafting.

C. Cutaneous Gene Therapy

Cultured human keratinocytes and fibroblasts are amenable to genetic modification by a variety of methods. Genetically modified cells can be used to populate engineered skin substitutes, resulting in skin grafts that act as vehicles for cutaneous gene therapy. This type of gene therapy is termed "*ex vivo*" because cells are removed from the body and genetically modified in culture before being transplanted back to the recipient. There has been substantial interest recently in the use of genetically modified skin substitutes for the treatment of cutaneous diseases. For example, preclinical studies suggest that *ex vivo* gene therapy can be useful for treatment of lamellar ichthyosis, characterized by a defective epidermal barrier (129,130), and the blistering skin disease junctional epidermolysis bullosa (JEB) (131,132). Cultured keratinocytes can theoretically be genetically modified and transplanted for secretion of circulating factors to treat disease. Keratinocytes have been genetically modified to secrete human growth hormone (133,134) and clotting factor IX (135–137), but therapeutic circulating levels after experimental transplantation of cells have been difficult to obtain.

Another application of cutaneous gene therapy is the regulation of wound healing with engineered skin substitutes. Genetic modification can hypothetically be used to overcome limitations inherent to cultured skin grafts, or to enhance their biological activity. For example, retroviral transduction was used to overexpress the gene encoding PDGF-A, a mesenchymal cell mitogen, in human keratinocytes (138,139). PDGF-A modified keratinocytes seeded on an acellular dermal matrix showed improved performance after grafting to full-thickness wounds on athymic mice (139). The PDGF-A-modified grafts showed increased cellularity, vascularization, and collagen deposition compared to control grafts (139), suggesting improved function due to PDGF-A overexpression. Interestingly, no effect was seen in similar studies performed with composite grafts containing both keratinocytes and fibroblasts (140), suggesting that genetic modification with PDGF-A could be used to compensate for the absence of fibroblasts in engineered skin models

containing only keratinocytes. In other studies, keratinocytes were genetically modified by retroviral transduction to overexpress the angiogenic cytokine vascular endothelial growth factor (VEGF) (97,98). After transplantation to athymic mice, skin substitutes containing fibroblasts and VEGF-modified keratinocytes showed enhanced and accelerated vascularization, decreased contraction, and increased engraftment compared to control grafts containing unmodified cells (97,98). Thus, genetic modification of keratinocytes can hypothetically be used to overcome the lack of a vascular plexus in engineered skin grafts.

Many of the genes involved in the processes of normal skin development and wound healing have been identified and cloned. Thus, genetic modification of keratinocytes, fibroblasts, or other cells in skin substitutes can be used to regulate the process of wound healing for specific applications, or to compensate for anatomic or physiologic deficiencies of engineered skin. Additionally, genetically modified cultured skin grafts can theoretically be used to secrete cytokines or other factors into the circulation for systemic treatment of genetic disease or acute injuries such as burns. Future studies must be guided toward the identification of relevant target genes, appropriate physiological regulation of gene expression, and safety of transplantation of modified cells.

VIII. CONCLUSIONS

Technological advances in the culture of skin cells have permitted the production of engineered skin substitutes. Continued research will be needed to identify more efficient methods to utilize precious autologous tissue, provide greater amounts of skin substitutes for grafting, and shorten the time required for their preparation. Additional research is aimed at improving the anatomy and physiology of skin substitutes, working toward better homology to native skin autograft. These efforts will lead to enhanced performance of engineered skin grafts, greater clinical efficacy, and reduction of morbidity and mortality for patients with burn injuries.

ACKNOWLEDGMENTS

The authors' studies are supported by grants from The National Institutes of Health (GM50509), The Food and Drug Administration (FD-R000672), and The Shriners Hospitals for Children (#8670, #8450, and #8680).

REFERENCES

1. Brigham P, McLoughlin E. Burn incidence and medical care use in the United States: estimates, trends, and data sources. J Burn Care Rehabil 1996; 17:95–107.

2. Rose JK, Herndon DN. Advances in the treatment of burn patients. Burns 1997; 23:S19–S26.

3. Fratianne RB, Brandt CP. Improved survival of adults with extensive burns. J Burn Care Rehabil 1997; 18:347–351.

4. Berthod F, Damour O. In vitro reconstructed skin models for wound coverage in deep burns. Br J Dermatol 1997; 136(6):809–816.

5. Yannas IV, Burke JF. Design of an artificial skin. I. Basic design principles. J Biomed Mater Res 1980; 14:65–81.

6. Yannas IV, Burke JF, Gordon PL, Huang C, Rubenstein RH. Design of an artificial skin II. Control of chemical composition. J Biomed Mater Res 1980; 14:107–131.

7. Heimbach D, Luterman A, Burke JF, Cram A, Herndon D, Hunt J, Jordon M, McManus W, Solem L, Warden G, Zawacki B. Artificial dermis for major burns; a multicenter randomized clinical trial. Ann Surg 1988; 208:313–320.

8. Sheridan RL, Hegarty M, Tompkins RG, Burke JF. Artificial skin in massive burns—results to ten years. Eur J Plast Surg 1994; 17:91–93.

9. Tavis MN, Thornton NW, Bartlett RH, Roth JC, Woodroof EA. A new composite skin prosthesis. Burns 1980; 7:123–130.

10. Purdue GF, Hunt JL, Gillespie RW, Hansbrough JF, Dominic WJ, Robson MC, Smith DJ, MacMillan BG, Waymack JP, Herndon DN. Biosynthetic skin substitute versus frozen human cadaver allograft for temporary coverage of excised burn wounds. J Trauma 1987; 27(2):155–157.

11. Wainwright D, Madden M, Luterman A, Hunt J, Monafo W, Heimbach D, Kagan R, Sittig K, Dimick A, Herndon D. Clinical evaluation of an acellular allograft dermal matrix in full-thickness burns. J Burn Care Rehabil 1996; 17:124–136.

12. Hansbrough JF, Mozingo DW, Kealey GP, Davis M, Gidner A, Gentzkow GD. Clinical trials of a biosynthetic temporary skin replacement, Dermagraft-transitional covering, compared with cryopreserved human cadaver skin for temporary coverage of excised burn wounds. J Burn Care Rehab 1997; 18:43–51.

13. Purdue GF, Hunt JL, Still JM Jr, Law EJ, Herndon DN, Goldfarb IW, Schiller WR, Hansbrough JF, Hickerson WL, Himel HN, Kealey GP, Twomey J, Missavage AE, Solem LD, Davis M, Totoritis M, Gentzkow GD. A multicenter clinical trial of a biosynthetic skin replacement, Dermagraft-TC, compared with cryopreserved human cadaver skin for temporary coverage of excised burn wounds. J Burn Care Rehab 1997; 18:52–57.

14. Lukish JR, Eichelberger MR, Newman KD, Pao M, Nobuhara K, Keating M, Golonka N, Pratsch G, Misra V, Valladares E, Johnson P, Gilbert JC, Powell DM, Hartman GE. The use of a bioactive skin substitute decreases length of stay for pediatric burn patients. J Pediatr Surg 2001; 36(8):1118–1121.

15. Cooper ML, Hansbrough JF, Spielvogel RL, Cohen R, Bartel RL, Naughton G. In vivo optimization of a living dermal substitute employing cultured human fibroblasts on a biodegradable polyglycolic or polygalactin mesh. Biomaterials 1991; 12:243–248.

16. Hansbrough JF, Cooper ML, Cohen R, Spielvogel RL, Greenleaf G, Bartel RL, Naughton G. Evaluation of a biodegradable matrix containing cultured human fibroblasts as a dermal replacement beneath meshed skin grafts on athymic mice. Surgery 1992; 111(4):438–446.

17. Carsin H, Ainaud P, Le Bever H, Rives J, Lakhel A, Stephanazzi J, Lambert F, Perrot J. Cultured epithelial autografts in extensive burn coverage of severly traumatized patients: a five year single-center experience with 30 patients. Burns 2000; 26:379–387.

18. Lam PK, Chan ES, To EW, Lau CH, Yen SC, King WW. Development and evaluation of a new composite Laser-skin graft. J Trauma 1999; 47(5):918–922.

19. Stephens R, Wilson K, Silverstein P. A premature infant with skin injury successfully treated with bilayered cell matrix. Ostomy Wound Manag 2002; 48(4):34–38.

20. Falanga V, Margolis DJ, Alvarez O, Auletta M, Maggiacomo F, Altman M, Jensen J, Sabolinski M, Hardin-Young J. Rapid healing of venous ulcers and lack of clinical rejection with an allogeneic cultured human skin equivalent. Arch Dermatol 1998; 134(3):293–300.

21. Eaglstein WH, Iriondo M, Laszlo K. A composite skin substitute (Graftskin) for surgical wounds: a clinical experience. Dermatol Surg 1995; 21:839–843.

22. De SK, Reis ED, Kerstein MD. Wound treatment with human skin equivalent. J Am Pediatr Med Assoc 2002; 92(1):19–23.

23. Hansbrough JF, Boyce ST, Cooper ML, Foreman TJ. Burn wound closure with cultured autologous keratinocytes and fibroblasts attached to a collagen-glycosaminoglycan substrate. J Am Med Assoc 1989; 262:2125–2130.

24. Boyce ST, Greenhalgh DG, Kagan RJ, Housinger T, Sorrell JM, Childress CP, Rieman M, Warden GD. Skin anatomy and antigen expression after burn wound closure with composite grafts of cultured skin cells and biopolymers. Plast Reconstr Surg 1993; 91(4):632–641.

25. Boyce ST, Goretsky MJ, Greenhalgh DG, Kagan RJ, Rieman MT, Warden GD. Comparative assessment of cultured skin substitutes and native skin autograft for treatment of full-thickness burns. Ann Surg 1995; 222(6):743–752.

26. Brain A, Purkis P, Coates P, Hackett M, Navsaria H, Leigh I. Survival of cultured allogeneic keratinocytes transplanted to deep dermal bed assessed with probe specific for Y chromosome. Brit Med J 1989; 298:917–919.

27. Phillips TJ, Bhawan J, Leigh IM, Baum HJ, Gilchrest BA. Cultured epidermal autografts and allografts: a study of differentiation and allograft survival. J Am Acad Dermatol 1990; 23:189–195.

28. Thivolet J, Faure M, Demidem A, Mauduit G. Long-term survival and immunological tolerance of human epidermal allografts produced in culture. Transplantation 1986; 42(3):274–280.

29. Zhao YB, Zhao XF, Li A, Lu SZ, Wang X, Huang SZ, Zhuo XT. Clinical observations and methods for identifying the existence of cultured epidermal allografts. Burns 1992; 18(1):4–8.

30. Boyce ST, Kagan RJ, Meyer NA, Yakuboff KP, Warden GD. The 1999 Clinical Research Award. Cultured skin substitutes combined with Integra to replace native

skin autograft and allograft for closure of full-thickness burns. J Burn Care Rehabil 1999; 20(6):453–461.

31. Boyce ST, Kagan RJ, Yakuboff KP, Meyer NA, Rieman MT, Greenhalgh DG, Warden GD. Cultured skin substitutes reduce donor skin harvesting for closure of excised, full-thickness burns. Ann Surg 2002; 235(2):269–279.

32. Boyce ST, Warden GD. Principles and practices for treatment of cutaneous wounds with cultured skin substitutes. Am J Surg 2002; 183:445–456.

33. Gallico GG III. Biologic skin substitutes. Clin Plast Surg 1990; 17(3):519–526.

34. Sorrell JM, Caterson B, Caplan AI, Davis B, Schafer IA. Human keratinocytes contain carbohydrates that are recognized by keratan sulfate-specific monoclonal antibodies. J Invest Dermatol 1990; 95(3):347–352.

35. Schurer NY, Elias PM. The biochemistry and role of epidermal lipid synthesis. Adv Lipid Res 1991; 24:27–56.

36. Elias PM. Stratum corneum architecture, metabolic activity and interactivity with subjacent cell layers. Exp Dermatol 1996; 5(4):191–201.

37. Black AF, Berthod F, L'Heureux N, Germain L, Auger FA. In vitro reconstruction of a human capillary-like network in a tissue-engineered skin equivalent. FASEB J 1998; 12:1331–1340.

38. Supp DM, Wilson-Landy K, Boyce ST. Human dermal microvascular endothelial cells form vascular analogs in cultured skin substitutes after grafting to athymic mice. FASEB J 2002; 16:797–804.

39. Housinger TA, Hills J, Warden GD. Management of pediatric facial burns. J Burn Care Rehabil 1994; 15(5):408–411.

40. Tanner JC, Vandeput J, Olley JF. The mesh skin autograft. Plast Reconstr Surg 1964; 34:287–292.

41. Staley M, Richard R, Warden GD, Miller SF, Shuster DB. Functional outcomes for the patient with burn injuries. J Burn Care Rehabil 1996; 17(4):362–368.

42. Pruitt BA Jr, Levine S. Characteristics and uses of biologic dressings and skin substitutes. Arch Surg 1984; 199:312–322.

43. Hansbrough JF. Wound Coverage with Biologic Dressings and Cultured Skin Substitutes. 1st ed. Austin, TX: R.G. Landes, 1992.

44. Odessey R. Addendum: multicenter experience with cultured epithelial autografts for treatment of burns. J Burn Care Rehabil 1992; 13:174–180.

45. Pittelkow MR, Scott RE. New techniques for the in vitro culture of human skin keratinocytes and perspectives on their use for grafting of patients with extensive burns. Mayo Clin Proc 1986; 61:771–777.

46. Desai MH, Mlakar JM, McCauley RL, Abdullah KM, Rutan RL, Waymack JP, Robson MC, Herndon DN. Lack of long term durability of cultured keratinocyte burn wound coverage: a case report. J Burn Care Rehabil 1991; 12:540–545.

47. Williamson J, Snelling C, Clugston P, Mac Donald I, Germann E. Cultured epithelial autograft: five years of clinical experience with twenty-eight patients. J Trauma 1995; 39:309–319.

48. Rue LW, Cioffi WG, McManus WF, Pruitt BA. Wound closure and outcome in extensively burned patients treated with cultured autologous keratinocytes. J Trauma 1993; 34(5):662–667.

49. Boyce ST. Skin repair with the cultured cells and biopolymers. In: Wise D, ed. Biomedical Applications. Totowa, NJ: Humana Press, Inc., 1996:347–377.

50. Boyce ST. Cultured skin substitutes: a review. Tiss Eng 1996; 2(4):255–266.

51. Elias PM. Epidermal lipids, barrier function, and desquamation. J Invest Dermatol 1983; 80:44s–49s.

52. Gallico III GG, O'Connor NE, Compton CC, Kehinde O, Green H. Permanent coverage of large burn wounds with autologous cultured human epithelium. N Engl J Med 1984; 311:448–451.

53. Compton CC, Gill JM, Bradford DA, Regauer S, Gallico GG, O'Connor NE. Skin regenerated from cultured epithelial autografts on full-thickness burn wounds from 6 days to 5 years after grafting. Lab Invest 1989; 60(5):600–612.

54. Clugston PA, Snelling CFT, Macdonald IB, Maledy HL, Boyle JC, Germann E, Courtemanche AD, Wirtz P, Fitzpatrick DJ, Kester DA, Foley B, Warren RJ, Carr NJ. Cultured epithelial autografts: three years of clinical experience with eighteen patients. J Burn Care Rehabil 1991; 12:533–539.

55. Herndon DN, Rutan RL. Comparison of cultured epidermal autograft and massive excision with serial autografting plus homograft overlay. J Burn Care Rehabil 1992; 13:154–157.

56. Coleman JJ, Siwy BK. Cultured epidermal autografts: a life-saving and skin-saving technique in children. J Pediatr Surg 1992; 27(8):1029–1032.

57. Cuono C, Langdon R, Birchall N, Barttelbort S, McGuire J. Composite autologous-allogeneic skin replacement: development and clinical application. Plast Reconstr Surg 1987; 80:626–635.

58. Hansbrough JF, Dore C, Hansbrough WB. Clinical trials of a living dermal tissue replacement placed beneath meshed, split-thickness skin grafts on excised wounds. J Burn Care Rehabil 1992; 13:519–529.

59. Parenteau NL, Bilbo P, Nolte CJ, Mason VS, Rosenberg M. The organotypic culture of human skin keratinocytes and fibroblasts to achieve form and function. Cytotechnology 1992; 9(1–3):163–171.

60. Kuroyanagi Y, Kenmochi M, Ishihara S, Takeda A, Shiraishi A, Ootake N, Uchinuma E, Torikai K, Shioya N. A cultured skin substitute composed of fibroblasts and keratinocytes with a collagen matrix: preliminary results of clinical trials. Ann Plast Surg 1993; 31(4):340–349.

61. Coulomb B, Friteau L, Baruch J, Guilbaud J, Chretien-Marquet B, Glicenstein J, Lebreton-Decoster C, Bell E, Dubertret L. Advantage of the presence of living dermal fibroblasts within in vitro reconstructed skin for grafting in humans. Plast Reconstr Surg 1998; 101:1891–1903.

62. Lerner AB, Halaban R, Klaus SN, Moellmann GE. Transplantation of human melanocytes. J Invest Dermatol 1987; 89(3):219–224.

63. Stoner ML, Wood FM. The treatment of hypopigmented lesions with cultured epithelial autograft. J Burn Care Rehabil 2000; 21(1):50–54.

64. Boyce ST, Medrano EE, Abdel-Malek ZA, Supp AP, Dodick JM, Nordlund JJ, Warden GD. Pigmentation and inhibition of wound contraction by cultured skin substitutes with adult melanocytes after transplantation to athymic mice. J Invest Dermatol 1993; 100(4):360–365.

65. Swope VB, Supp AP, Cornelius JR, Babcock GF, Boyce ST. Regulation of pigmentation in cultured skin substitutes by cytometric sorting of melanocytes and keratinocytes. J Invest Dermatol 1997; 109(3):289–295.

66. Ward RS, Tuckett RP. Quantitative threshold changes in cutaneous sensation of patients with burns. J Burn Care Rehabil 1991; 12(6):569–575.

67. Ward RS, Saffle JR, Schnebly WA, Hayes-Lundy C, Reddy R. Sensory loss over grafted areas in patients with burns. J Burn Care Rehabil 1989; 10(6):536–538.

68. Jahoda CA, Oliver RF, Reynolds AJ, Forrester JC, Horne KA. Human hair follicle regeneration following amputation and grafting into the nude mouse. J Invest Dermatol 1996; 107(6):804–807.

69. Michel M, L'Heureux N, Pouliot R, Xu W, Auger F, Germain L. Characterization of a new tissue-engineered human skin equivalent with hair. In Vitro Cell Dev Biol 1999; 35:318–326.

70. Boyce ST. Cultured skin for wound closure. In: Rouahbia M, ed. Skin Substitute Production by Tissue Engineering: Clinical and Fundamental Applications. Austin, TX: R.G. Landes, 1997:75–102.

71. Compton CC, Hickerson W, Nadire K, Press W. Acceleration of skin regeneration from cultured epithelial autografts by transplantation to homograft dermis. J Burn Care Rehabil 1993; 14(6):653–662.

72. Pandya AN, Woodward B, Parkhouse DM. The use of cultured autologous keratinocytes with integra in the resurfacing of acute burns. Plast Reconstr Surg 1998; 102(3):825–830.

73. Medalie DA, Eming SA, Tompkins RG, Yarmush ML, Krueger GG. Evaluation of human skin reconstituted from composite grafts of cultured keratinocytes and human acellular dermis transplanted to athymic mice. J Invest Dermatol 1996; 107(1):121–127.

74. Compton CC, Butler CE, Yannas IV, Warland G, Orgill DP. Organized skin structure is regenerated in vivo from collagen-GAG matrices seeded with autologous keratinocytes. J Invest Dermatol 1998; 110:908–916.

75. Horch RE, Bannasch H, Stark GB. Cultured human keratinocytes as a single cell suspension in fibrin glue combined with preserved dermal grafts enhance skin reconstitution in athymic mice full-thickness wounds. Eur J Plast Surg 1999; 22:237–243.

76. Clark RAF. Cutaneous wound repair. In: Goldsmith LA, ed. Physiology, Biochemistry, and Molecular Biology of the Skin. New York: Oxford University Press, 1991:576–601.

77. Boyce ST, Ham RG. Calcium-regulated differentiation of normal human epidermal keratinocytes in chemically defined clonal culture and serum-free serial culture. J Invest Dermatol 1983; 81(suppl 1):33s–40s.

78. Rheinwald JG, Green H. Serial cultivation of strains of human epidermal keratinocytes: the formation of keratinizing colonies from single cells. Cell 1975; 6:331–343.

79. Boyce ST, Ham RG. Cultivation, frozen storage, and clonal growth of normal human epidermal keratinocytes in serum-free media. J Tiss Cult Methods 1985; 9:83–93.

80. Boyce ST, Hansbrough JF. Biologic attachment, growth, and differentiation of cultured human epidermal keratinocytes on a graftable collagen and chondroitin-6-sulfate substrate. Surgery 1988; 103:421–431.

81. Slivka SR, Landeen L, Zeigler F, Zimber MP, Bartel RL. Characterization, barrier function and drug metabolism of an in vitro skin model. J Invest Dermatol 1993; 100(1):40–46.

82. Parenteau NL, Nolte CM, Bilbo P, Rosenberg M, Wilkins LM, Johnson EW, Watson S, Mason VS, Bell E. Epidermis generated in vitro: practical consideration and applications. J Cell Biochem 1991; 45(3):245–251.

83. Boyce ST, Williams ML. Lipid supplemented medium induces lamellar bodies and precursors of barrier lipids in cultured analogues of human skin. J Invest Dermatol 1993; 101:180–184.

84. Prunieras M, Regnier M, Woodley DT. Methods for cultivation of keratinocytes at the air-liquid interface. J Invest Dermatol 1983; 81(1):28s–33s.

85. Ponec M, Kempenaar J, Weerheim A, de Lannoy L, Kalkman I, Jansen H. Triglyceride metabolism in human keratinocytes cultured at the air-liquid interface. Arch Dermatol Res 1995; 287(8):723–730.

86. Boyce ST, Hoath SB, Wickett RR, Harriger MD, Williams ML. Loss of EGF requirement by cultured analog of human skin: biochemical and physiologic analyses. J Invest Dermatol 1993; 100(4):579.

87. Chen C-SJ, Lavker RM, Rodeck U, Risse B, Jensen PJ. Use of a serum-free epidermal culture model to show deleterious effects of epidermal growth factor on morphogenesis and differentiation. J Invest Dermatol 1995; 104(1):107–112.

88. Ansel JC, Tiesman JP, Olerud JE, Krueger JG, Krane JF, Tara DC, Shipley GD, Gilbertson D, Usui ML, Hart CE. Human keratinocytes are a major source of cutaneous platelet-derived growth factor. J Clin Invest 1993; 92:671–678.

89. Beer H-D, Longaker MT, Werner S. Reduced expression of PDGF and PDGF receptors during impaired wound healing. J Invest Dermatol 1997; 109:132–138.

90. Greenhalgh DG, Sprugel KH, Murray MJ, Ross R. PDGF and FGF stimulate wound healing in the genetically diabetic mouse. Am J Pathol 1990; 136(6):1235–1246.

91. Lynch SE, Colvin RB, Antonaides HN. Growth factors in wound healing: single and syneristic effects on partial thickness porcine skin wounds. J Clin Invest 1989; 84:640–646.

92. Robson MC, Phillips LG, Lawrence WT, Bishop JB, Youngerman JS, Hayward PG, Broemeling LD, Heggers JP. The safety and efficacy of topically applied recombinant basic fibroblast growth factor on the healing of chronic pressure sores. Ann Surg 1992; 216:401–408.

93. Brown GL, Nanney LB, Griffen J, Cramer AB, Yancey JM, Curtsinger LJ, Holtzin L, Schultz G, Jurkiewicz S, Lynch JB. Enhancement of wound healing by topical treatment with epidermal growth factor. N Engl J Med 1989; 321:76–79.

94. Brown RL, Breeden MP, Greenhalgh DG. PDGF and TGF-alpha act synergistically to improve wound healing in the genetically diabetic mouse. J Surg Res 1994; 56:562–570.

95. Mast BA, Newton ED. Aggressive use of free flaps in children for burn scar contractures and other soft-tissue deficits. Ann Plast Surg 1996; 36(6):569–575.

96. Isenberg JS, Price G. Longitudinal trapezius fasciocutaneous flap for the treatment of mentosternal burn scar contractures. Burns 1996; 22(1):76–79.

97. Supp DM, Supp AP, Bell SM, Boyce ST. Enhanced vascularization of cultured skin substitutes genetically modified to overexpress vascular endothelial growth factor. J Invest Dermatol 2000; 114(1):5–13.

98. Supp DM, Boyce ST. Overexpression of vascular endothelial growth factor accelerates early vascularization and improves healing of genetically modified cultured skin substitutes. J Burn Care Rehabil 2002; 23:10–20.

99. Boyce ST, Supp AP, Swope VB, Warden GD. Vitamin C regulates keratinocyte viability, epidermal barrier, and basement membrane formation in vitro, and reduces wound contraction after grafting of cultured skin substitutes. J Invest Dermatol 2002; 118:565–572.

100. Burke JF, Yannas IV, Quinby WC, Bondoc CC, Jung WK. Successful use of a physiologically acceptable skin in the treatment of extensive burn injury. Ann Surg 1981; 194:413–428.

101. Monafo WW, West MA. Current treatment recommendations for topical burn therapy. Drugs 1990; 40:364–373.

102. McCauley RL, Linares RL, Pelligrini V, Herndon DN, Robson MC, Heggers JP. In vitro toxicity of topical antimicrobial agents to human fibroblasts. J Surg Res 1989; 46:267–274.

103. Lineaweaver W, McMorris S, Soucy D, Howard R. Cellular amd bacterial toxicities of topical antimicrobials. Plast Reconstr Surg 1985; 75:394–396.

104. Holder IA. The wet disc antimicrobial solution assay: an in vitro method to test efficacy of antimicrbial solutions for topical use. J Burn Care Rehabil 1989; 10:203–208.

105. Kuroyanagi Y, Kim E, Shioya N. Evaluation of synthetic wound dressing capable of releasing silver sulfadiazine. J Burn Care Rehabil 1991; 12:106–115.

106. Boyce ST, Holder IA. Selection of topical antimicrobial agents for cultured skin for burns by combined assessment of cellular cytotoxicity and antimicrobial activity. Plast Reconstr Surg 1993; 92(4):493–500.

107. Boyce ST, Warden GD, Holder IA. Cytotoxicity testing of topical antimicrobial agents on human keratinocytes and fibroblasts for cultured skin grafts. J Burn Care Rehabil 1995; 16(2):97–103.

108. Boyce ST, Warden GD, Holder IA. Non-cytotoxic combinations of topical antimicrobial agents for use with cultured skin. Antimicrob Agents Chemother 1995; 39(6):1324–1328.

109. Compton CC. Wound healing potential of cultured epithelium. Wounds 1993; 5(2):97–111.

110. Teepe RGC, Kreis RW, Koebrugge EJ, Kempenaar JA, Vloemans AF, Hermans RP, Boxa H, Dokter J, Hermans J, Ponec M, Vermeer BJ. The use of cultured autologous epidermis in the treatment of extensive burn wounds. J Trauma 1990; 30:269–275.

111. Sullivan T, Smith H, Kermode J, McIver E, Courtemanche DJ. Rating the burn scar. J Burn Care Rehabil 1990; 11(3):256–260.

112. Goretsky MJ, Supp AP, Greenhalgh DG, Warden GD, Boyce ST. The 1995 Young Investigator Award: Surface electrical capacitance as an index of epidermal barrier properties of composite skin substitutes and skin autografts. Wound Repair Reg 1995; 3(4):419–425.

113. Munster AM, Weiner SH, Spence RJ. Cultured epidermis for coverage of burn wounds: a single center experience. Ann Surg 1990; 211:676–680.

114. Boyce ST. Regulatory issue and standardization. In: Atala A, Lanza R, eds. Methods of Tissue Engineering. San Diego, CA: Academic Press, 2001:3–17.

115. US Food and Drug Administration. Guidance on applications for products comprised of living autologous cells manipulated ex vivo and intended for structural repair or reconstruction. Fed Regist 1996; 61(103):26523–26524.

116. Boyce ST. Methods for serum-free culture of keratinocytes and transplantation of collagen-GAG based composite grafts. In: Morgan JR, Yarmush M, eds. Methods in Tissue Engineering. Totowa, NJ: Humana Press, Inc., 1998:365–389.

117. Harriger MD, Warden GD, Greenhalgh DG, Kagan RJ, Boyce ST. Pigmentation and microanatomy of skin regenerated from composite grafts of cultured cells and biopolymers applied to full-thickness burn wounds. Transplantation 1995; 59(5):702–707.

118. Abdel-Malek ZA. Endocrine factors as effectors of integumental pigmentation. Dermatol Clin 1988; 6(2):175–183.

119. Nordlund JJ, Abdel-Malek ZA, Boissy RE, Rheins LA. Pigment cell biology: an historical review. J Invest Dermatol 1989; 92:53S–60S.

120. Fauerbach JA, Heinberg LJ, Lawrence JW, Munster AM, Palombo DA, Richter D, Spence RJ, Stevens SS, Ware L, Muehlberger T. Effect of early body image dissatisfaction on subsequent psychological and physical adjustment after disfiguring injury. Psychosom Med 2000; 62(4):576–582.

121. DeLuca M, Franzi A, D'Anna F, Zicca A, Albanese E, Bondanza S, Cancedda R. Co-culture of human keratinocytes and melanocytes: differentiated melanocytes are physiologically organized in the basal layer of the cultured epithelium. Eur J Cell Biol 1988; 46:176–180.

122. Compton CC, Warland G, Kratz G. Melanocytes in cultured epithelial autografts are depleted with serial subcultivation and cryopreservation: implications for clinical outcome. J Burn Care Rehabil 1998; 19(4):330–336.

123. Boyce ST, Supp AP, Harriger MD, Greenhalgh DG, Warden GD. Topical nutrients promote engraftment and inhibit wound contraction of cultured skin substitutes in athymic mice. J Invest Dermatol 1995; 104(3):345–349.

124. Young DM, Greulich KM, Weier HG. Species-specific in situ hybridization with fluorochrome-labeled DNA probes to study vascularization of human skin grafts on athymic mice. J Burn Care Rehabil 1996; 17:305–310.

125. Lin SD, Chai C-Y, Lai C-S, Chou C-K. A mixture of allogeneic and autologous microskin grafting of rabbit skin wounds with Biobrane overlay. Burns 1994; 20(1):30–35.

126. L'Heureux N, Paquet S, Labbe R, Germain L, Auger F. A completely biological tissue-engineered human blood vessel. FASEB J 1998; 12:47–56.

127. Schechner JS, Nath AK, Zheng L, Kluger MS, Hughes CCW, Sierra-Honigmann MR, Lorber MI, Tellides G, Kashgarian M, Bothwell ALM, Pober JS. In vivo formation of complex microvessels lined by human endothelial cells in an immunodeficient mouse. Proc Natl Acad Sci USA 2000; 97:9191–9196.

128. Nor JE, Peters MC, Christensen JB, Sutorik MM, Linn S, Kahn MK, Addison CL, Mooney DJ, Polverini PJ. Engineering and characterization of functional microvessels in immunodeficient mice. Lab Invest 2001; 81:453–463.

129. Bale SJ, Doyle SZ. The genetics of ichthyosis: a primer for epidemiologists. J Invest Dermatol 1994; 102:49S–50S.

130. Choate KA, Medalie DA, Morgan JR, Khavari PA. Corrective gene transfer in the human skin disorder lamellar ichthyosis. Nature Med 1996; 2(11):1263–1267.

131. Vailly J, Gagnouz-Palacios L, Dell'Ambra E, Romero C, Pinola M, Zambruno G, De Luca M, Ortonne JP, Meneguzzi G. Corrective gene transfer of keratinoyctes from patients with junctional epidermolysis bullosa restores assembly of hemidesmosomes in reconstructed epithelia. Gene Ther 1998; 5(10):1322–1332.

132. Dellambra E, Vailly J, Pellegrini G, Bondanza S, Golisano O, Macchia C, Zambruno G, Meneguzzi G, De Luca M. Corrective transduction of human epidermal stem cells in laminin-5-dependent junctional epidermolysis bullosa. Hum Gene Ther 1998; 9(9):1359–1370.

133. Vogt PM, Thompson S, Andree C, Liu P, Breuing K, Hatzis D, Brown H, Mulligan RC, Ericksson E. Genetically modified keratinocytes transplanted to wounds reconstitute the epidermis. Proc Natl Acad Sci USA 1994; 91(20):9307–9311.

134. Morgan JR, Barrandon Y, Green H, Mulligan RC. Expression of an exogenous growth hormone gene in transplantable human epidermal cells. Science 1987; 237:1476–1479.

135. Gerrard AJ, Hudson DL, Brownlee GG, Watt FM. Towards gene therapy for haemophilia B using primary human keratinocytes. Nat Genet 1993; 3:180–183.

136. Page SM, Brownlee GG. An ex vivo keratinocyte model for gene therapy of hemophilia. Br J Invest Dermatol 1997; 108:139–145.

137. White SJ, Page SM, Margaritis P, Brownlee GG. Long-term expression of human clotting factor IX from retrovirally transduced primary human keratinocytes in vivo. Hum Gene Ther 2002; 9:1187–1195.

138. Eming SA, Lee J, Snow RG, Tompkins RG, Yarmush ML, Morgan JR. Genetically modified human epidermis overexpressing PDGF-A directs the development of a cellular and vascular connective tissue stroma when transplanted to athymic mice—implications for the use of genetically modified keratinocytes to modulate dermal regeneration. J Invest Dermatol 1995; 105:756–763.

139. Eming SA, Medalie DA, Tompkins RG, Yarmush ML, Morgan JR. Genetically modified human keratinocytes overexpressing PDGF-A enhance the performance of a composite skin graft. Hum Gene Ther 1998; 9(4):529–539.

140. Supp DM, Bell SM, Morgan JR, Boyce ST. Genetic modification of cultured skin substitutes by transduction of keratinocytes and fibroblasts with platelet derived growth factor A. Wound Repair Reg 2000; 8:26–35.

10

Microsurgical Free Tissue Transfer in Burn Reconstruction: Overview

FU-CHAN WEI, TEWODROS M. GEDEBOU
Chang Gung University and Medical College, Taipei, Taiwan

I. INTRODUCTION

Burn injury to the external surface of the human body (integument or mucosa) may be caused by a variety of methods (thermal, chemical, cold, radiation, abrasion, or electricity) with variable depths of injury. The significant improvement of mortality rates during the past few decades has shifted the focus of management from merely survival to the restoration of quality of life to the patient as well. Since Janzekovich's (1) report, current management of deep burns dictates early excision and resurfacing to minimize both local and potential systemic complications.

Resurfacing is traditionally accomplished with split-thickness skin grafts (STSG), which is followed by physical therapy, wound care, and compression garments in the hope of reducing hypertrophic scarring. Despite the multiple reports focusing on the management of the burn cicatrix, a distressingly large number of postburn patients eventually develop extensive scar hypertrophy. Depending on the extent as well as location, the burn cicatrix often causes tremendous functional and aesthetic "disability." Reconstruction in such patients has to, therefore, incorporate restoration of both function and form while avoiding significant morbidity. To this end, skin grafts, skin expansion, local flaps, Z-plasties, and pedicled flaps have all been utilized with varying degrees of success but also with major drawbacks. The recent advent of microsurgical tissue transfer, however, has allowed a veritable explosion in the number of methods available to accomplish the ultimate goals of restoration to these otherwise "terminal" patients.

II. PATHOLOGY OF BURN WOUNDS

Burns to the external surface of the body are classified according to the depth of injury, which ranges from superficial (epidermis or mucosa) to underlying structures. The zone of injury may be extended beyond the initial area due to secondary effects of ischemia, infection, or overzealous debridement. Additionally, after debridement of full-thickness burns, vital underlying structures such as cornea, viscera, tendons, bone, cartilage, nerves, or vessels, which are unable to stand the rigors of the external environment, may be exposed.

The topic of wound healing as well as its manipulation has been and continues to be of significant interest to the surgical community. All wounds proceed through the inflammatory, proliferative, and maturation phases and those associated with burn injury usually result in hypertrophy. Despite the plethora of reports in the literature,

sufficient control of the wound healing process has remained elusive (2). Despite "appropriate" management, the combination of contraction and hypertrophy leads to distortional healing, especially in deep burns, which are associated with prolonged inflammatory or proliferative stages as well as wounds resurfaced with inadequate tissue such as STSG (3–5).

The process of burn scar contraction and hypertrophy develops into a contracture when overlying an area of mobility such as the face or the various joints of the body. The immobilizing effects of extrinsic contractures over time lead to intrinsic ones as underlying tissue (muscle, ligaments, joint capsules, and tendons) undergoes fibrotic shortening. The powerful nature of the burn contracture may over time lead to significant baseline deformity beyond the mere prevention of motion as demonstrated in Case 1 [Fig. 10.1(A–D)]. In young children, subluxation and dislocation of the small joints may even result

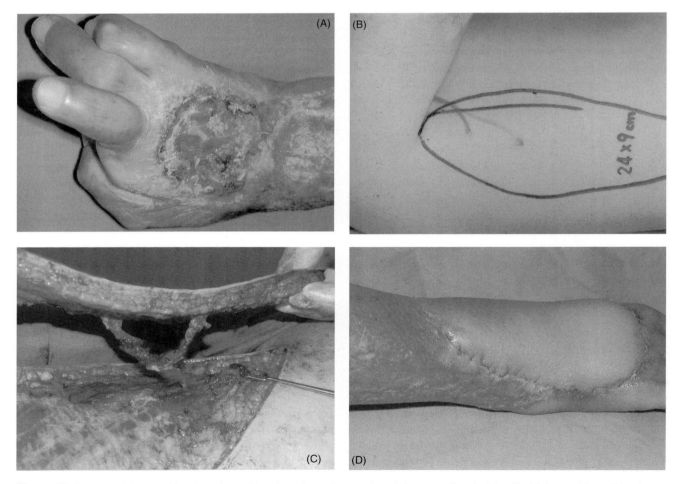

Figure 10.1   (A) A 34-year-old male patient with a deep thermal grease burn injury resurfaced with split-thickness skin grafting 2 years previously presenting with a chronic recalcitrant ulcer and disabling dorsal contracture of the wrist. (B) A thin thoracodorsal perforator flap is designed. (C) Harvest of the thoracodorsal perforator flap demonstrated two sizable perforator vessels dissected to the thoracodorsal vessels. (D) Improved range of motion of the wrist and fingers was observed at early postoperative follow-up.

(6,7). Similarly, scoliosis, leg length discrepancies, scapular protraction, and thoracic kyphosis have all been described (3,8). Furthermore, if involving the loose structures of the face as in Case 2 [Fig. 10.2(A–C)], secondary problems such as exposure keratitis or inadequate oral aperture may arise in addition to the obvious aesthetic distortion. Corrosive esophageal burns likewise, may over time develop several strictures that disallow normal passage of food, and even air, as the laryngeal obliteration continues unabated long after the initial injury. Besides such functional disability, the "burned" esophagus over time may undergo malignant transformation. Similarly, the neglected or inadequately managed chronic burn ulcer over a period of years could also develop into a Marjolin's ulcer. It therefore, behooves the clinician to wlook beyond merely the external pathology of the burn cicatrix and anticipate additional problems that could develop secondarily and with even greater implications to the patient.

III. PREOPERATIVE EVALUATION

Evaluation of the patient begins with an overall detailed history and examination. The patient's basic metabolic, nutritional, cardiopulmonary, immunological, hematological, and psychological status needs to be systematically evaluated and documented. Regardless of surgical proficiency, biology is king in dictating the final outcome; therefore, optimization of the patient on all fronts needs to be undertaken aggressively prior to embarking on microsurgical reconstruction.

During the acute stage, the main focus is prevention of extension of the zone of injury. The extent of injury both in depth and in surface area is documented, and exposure of underlying vulnerable structures sought for. Compartment syndrome, infection, edema, or injury to neurovascular structures affecting uninjured areas need to be diagnosed early. Re-evaluation of the wound should be vigilant during the entire acute phase period, which may last a few weeks, as proper management is dependent not only on the original extent of the burn, but also on variability of the clinical progress of the patient.

The "late" evaluation of the burn patient requires a different approach than during the acute period. At this point, severe systemic disturbances have abated, and the focus has become the local effect of the burn cicatrix. Cicatricial maturity and involvement of adjacent or underlying structures need to be documented. Depending on the time from original injury or the stage of growth of the patient, the dynamic nature of the burn cicatrix must be realized and expectations made on possible secondary

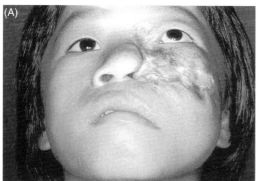
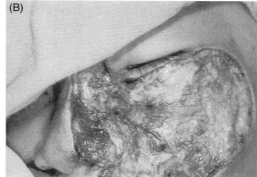
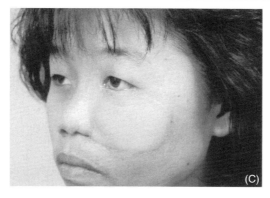

Figure 10.2 (A) A 4-year-old girl sustained a deep thermal burn to the left upper face distorting her nose and causing worsening ectropion of the left lower eyelid. (B) Intraoperative appearance after excision of all healed burn tissue. (C) Follow-up appearance 8 years after radial forearm free-flap reconstruction.

effects in the future. For example, the presence of a finger flexion contracture during a patient's growth period may lead to shortening of the entire structure, or of the neurovascular structures relative to the finger, thereby imposing restrictions on straightening the finger despite adequate contracture release (8). Furthermore, since the burn cicatrix involves a tissue deficient state, an estimation of the total surface area needed to resurface its excision and contracture release must be made. Vascular examination of both donor and recipient areas is undertaken by both palpation and Doppler ultrasound in most instances; however, it may require angiography if the burn cicatrix does not permit adequate examination.

The functional and aesthetic disability faced by the patient must therefore be understood prior to any therapeutic effort. More important, however, is the evaluation of the patient as a candidate for reconstructive surgery in relation not only to his/her medical condition, but also to age, lifestyle, compliance, motivation, education, and expectation.

IV. LIMITATIONS OF TRADITIONAL MANAGEMENT

Skin grafts either as partial or full-thickness, are most commonly used for resurfacing due to simplicity and high rates of initial "success." The prolonged period of immobilization as well as intensive wound management with compression garments and the physical therapy that follows tax the resources of both the patient and the care providers. Even so, "late" failure is characteristic due to frequent recurrence of contracture as the contractile forces of the wounds overcome the weak resistance of skin graft coverage. Z-plasty in all its variations (butterfly-plasty, double to seven flap-plasty) is a valuable technique, and is used to improve the range of the smaller joints of the extremities (9,10). Restrictions are imposed, however, by availability of uninjured local tissue as well as limited lengthening potential. Local axial or random expanded flaps are useful techniques to utilize as long as the local tissue is spared and the arc of rotation allows for proper inset. Unfortunately, such flaps, like skin grafts, behave like parasites in the new wound bed, and require it to be healthy and well vascularized (2). Finally, although invaluable in the management of burns of the head and neck area, tissue expansion procedures are associated with multiple operations, several painful expansion events, and potential complications such as extrusion or infection. Furthermore, areas such as the distal extremities are not amenable to tissue expansion.

Microvascular transfer of tissue, however, avoids the majority of restrictions imposed by all previous methods of reconstruction, allowing significant versatility in tissue type, donor area, amount of tissue, and could incorporate other methods such as pre-expansion or prefabrication (11). Free-tissue survival rates are at a minimum equivalent to those of skin grafts; however, they do not undergo significant contraction (except muscle flaps) and the prolonged, postoperative immobilization period is avoided. Given the "surgical reticence" of patients with significant postburn deformities, it is important to "get it right the first time," therefore free-tissue transfer should be considered as first-line therapy when indicated.

V. INDICATIONS FOR MICROSURGICAL RECONSTRUCTION

Microsurgical reconstruction following burn injury is applicable at the different phases of the healing process, although on different grounds. Functional considerations are pre-eminent at all stages of healing: acute, dynamic, and chronic. Although aesthetic motivations behind the application of microsurgical procedures usually predominate at the late stages, "pre-emptive" applications may be undertaken in anticipation of future problems.

A. Functional Considerations

1. Acute Stage

Truly "emergent" free flaps are indicated in extremely rare circumstances. One absolute indication for immediate microsurgical reconstruction is when revascularization is required (12). A burn injury leading to segmental loss of vascular structures of an extremity will require bridging vascular grafts for salvage of the distal part. Vein grafts suffice in this instance; however, if coverage is also needed to protect the vascular repair then flow-through free flaps may accomplish both requirements singularly (13,14). Aside from this rare clinical situation, all other deep burns including those that lead to exposure of vital structures can be managed "urgently" and not rushed to the operating room. Wounds can be cared for meticulously while the patient's overall condition is stabilized. If a full-thickness burn is overlying a critical joint whereby contracture development is expected to have significant disability, consideration should be made to undertake primary resurfacing with free-tissue transfer. An example would be a full-thickness burn of the dorsum of the wrist and hand exposing extensor tendons. Skin grafting will assuredly lead to contracture formation as in Case 1 [Fig. 10.1(A–D)], and use of the reversed radial forearm pedicled flap further reduces the vascularity of the hand (15). Free-tissue transfer can accomplish the desired effect of an aesthetic, sturdy, and well-vascularized coverage. Although there is difficulty in assessment of adequacy of debridement as well as recipient vessels for microsurgical reconstruction during the acute stage, adherence to basic principles allows for safety (16,17). The general condition of burn patients limits the universal application of microsurgery during the acute stage, and the reconstructive surgeon is most often consulted after functional and aesthetic complications have developed in the postburn period.

2. Maturation Stage

Inadequate initial resurfacing methods overlying areas of frequent motion, such as the joints of the hand, may be plagued by epidermal breakdown, frequent ulceration, and pain, which further limit the use of the involved structure. Such chronic burn ulcers are recalcitrant to skin grafting. In these instances, a more sturdy soft tissue cover is essential after radical debridement. When local flaps are not available, then distant tissue transfer will achieve stable coverage.

Albeit the variability of clinical disability caused by burns, the underlying mechanism remains that of contraction and immobility. Therefore, with regard to the burn wound hypertrophy, time is the enemy, and early restoration must be undertaken aggressively. Optimal management of such patients requires the early release of the cicatrix and resurfacing with tissue that best resists the contraction and hypertrophy process (18). To this end, either local tissue rearrangement (local flaps, Z-plasty), if available, or distant tissue transplantation offers the best solution. Case 3 [Fig. 10.3(A–D)] demonstrates application of free-tissue transfer for a palmar flexion contracture disabling the hand during this dynamic stage.

3. Late Stage

Unfortunately, most patients present after secondary problems have matured, further complicating the reconstructive effort. Release of all contractures restricting motion

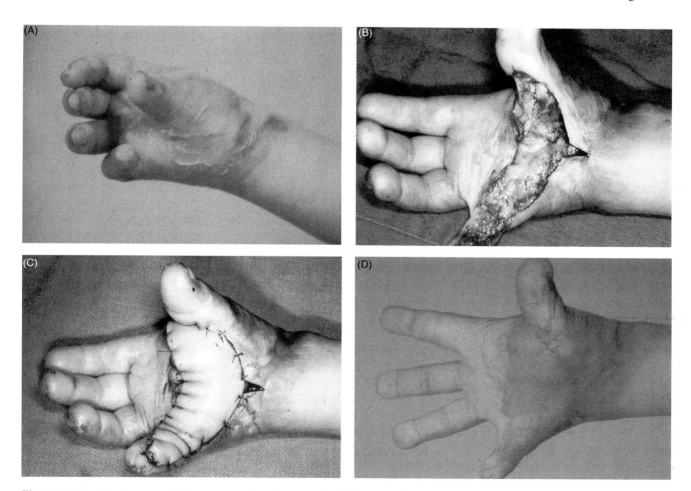

Figure 10.3 (A) A 4-year-old boy presented with progressive bilateral palmar contracture injury 5 months following burn injury. (B) Intraoperative appearance after excision of the palmar scar. (C) Appearance immediately after resurfacing with a thin lateral arm free-flap. (D) Final result more than 2 years postoperatively demonstrating almost normal range of motion and function.

entails removal of the external cicatrix, as well as the underlying muscular or ligamentous structures that have thickened and shortened. For example, oropharyngeal burns from corrosive fluid ingestion may lead to problems with speech, respiration, and swallowing due to progressive, obliterative fibrosis of the oropharynx and upper gastrointestinal tract. Restoration of upper esophageal continuity and voice are currently possible only through the microsurgical transfer of intra-abdominal segments of the intestinal tract. Similarly, cervicomental burns may lead to a flexion contracture of the head and, if severe enough, prevent mouth closure. Excision of the burn cicatrix and release of fibrosed underlying platysma and strap muscles often result in extensive defects, which require large soft tissue free flaps adhering to aesthetic unit principles (19,20) [see Case 4, Fig. 10.4(A–C)]. Upper-extremity burn contractures involving the axilla, elbow, wrist, and fingers also frequently require free-tissue transfer for stable resurfacing. When structures such as tendons have shortened and require tenotomy for lengthening, accurate reconstruction is best achieved with a composite tendon-cutaneous free flap. Reconstruction after loss of the digits of the hand, especially the thumb, is best achieved from toe transfers. Depending on the missing parts of the digit(s), toe pulp, great or lesser toe wrap around, vascularized joint, total great toe, trimmed great toe, total lesser toe, or combined lesser toes can be transferred to the hand (21–25). Severe burn injury to the penis also requires reconstructive efforts to focus on urinary and sexual function as well as appearance. Free flap phalloplasty is best able to address such requirements, with the radial forearm flap as the current gold standard, although the prefabricated free fibula osteocutaneous flap may rise to prominence in this arena (26–30). Electric burns may cause injury to multiple structures with resultant complex, multifaceted injury such as Volkmann's contracture. Functioning muscle transfer, such as the gracilis or rectus femoris free flaps, offers the only hope for restoration of some degree of function to the injured extremity. As the primary structure with which we interact with the external world, the foot is similarly exposed to burn injury with significant disability if affecting weight-bearing areas or the toes [Case 5, Fig. 10.5(A–D)].

B. Aesthetic Considerations

Body image is a basic part of personal identity, and its significance to the patient should not be underestimated. In contrast to the patient desiring cosmetic surgery, who is looking to enhance the positive attention received from other individuals, the postburn patient is seeking for ways to reduce the negative attention endured. Therefore, aesthetic reconstruction of any burn wound entails the accurate restoration of what is missing as well as the "hiding" of incision lines along the borders of the aesthetic unit or subunit. Replacement of tissue matched by color, texture, contour architecture, appendages, and thickness is paramount. Besides blending in with the surrounding normal tissue, the wound also needs to be judged on how it affects the surrounding structures. This is especially true around the loose structures of the face, such as the eyelids, nasal alae, and mouth (31). Finally, the location of the wound will also dictate whether the aesthetic deficit is worth correcting. It is more likely that wounds affecting exposed areas such as the face and hands are corrected instead of those "hidden," such as the torso. The decision to undertake reconstruction of a burn wound for aesthetic purposes should be individualized in such a manner as to allow the priorities as well as expectations of the patient and physician to coincide. Free-tissue transfer best allows for aesthetic unit reconstruction, although color match may be inferior compared to local flaps or tissue expansion especially important in the head and neck.

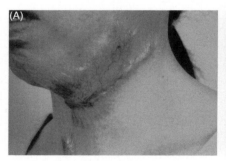 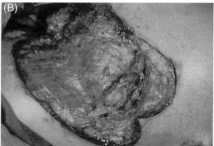 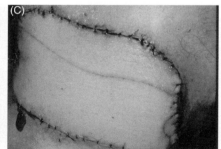

Figure 10.4 (A) A 20-year-old woman presented with a left neck contraction after a healed deep thermal burn several years ago. (B) Intraoperative appearance after excision of the burn wound and release of any underlying contractures. (C) Appearance immediately after reconstruction with a thinned anterolateral thigh flap. There was no contracture recurrence 2 years postoperatively, and the appearance was satisfactory.

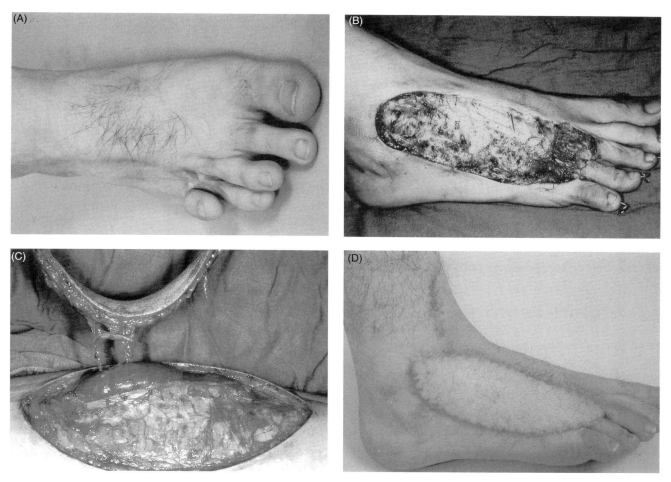

Figure 10.5 (A) A young man presented with a healed burn of the dorsolateral aspect of the right foot with significant disability with ambulation. (B) Intraoperative appearance after excision and release of all contractures and k-pinning of the lateral three toes in extension. (C) Harvest of a thinned anterolateral thigh flap demonstrating two hearty perforator vessels prior to vascular disconnection. (D) Appearance 5 months postoperatively with restoration of normal ambulation and satisfactory appearance.

VI. CONTRAINDICATIONS TO MICROSURGICAL RECONSTRUCTION

Because microsurgical free flap reconstruction is lengthy, the surgeon must select patients carefully. Although systemic complications are rare following free-flap reconstruction, the decision regarding patient suitability should be individualized based on clinical evaluation of the patient. Factors that play a role in this decision include current tobacco use, cardiovascular, pulmonary, nutritional, metabolic, psychological, and immune status. Age by itself is not a contraindication as free flaps have been undertaken successfully at both extremes of age. More important than chronological age, however, is the physiologic age of the patient. Coagulation disorders or various vessel inflammatory disorders also pose significant challenges for the safe microvascular transfer of tissue. In

general, however, the superficial level of dissection, lack of significant blood loss, and elective status of free-flap reconstruction make it a relatively safe procedure.

VII. TIMING OF MICROSURGICAL RECONSTRUCTION

Technically, microsurgical free-tissue transfer can be undertaken at any stage after severe burn injury. Although reports of "emergent free flaps" have surfaced in the literature, there are truly very few cases where they are required (16,17). The only indication is to revascularize acutely devascularized tissue, which can be reconstituted with a flow-through free flap (13,14,32). Difficulty in performing microvascular anastomosis during the acute stage is often due to inability in assessment of suitable vessels as well as viable tissue margins. Furthermore, unlike the simple amputation of a digit, major burns are plagued by systemic complications prohibitive of lengthy operations.

"Urgent" free flaps may be indicated, however, when vital structures are exposed after debridement, and are undertaken when the patient's medical status permits. In situations when secondary complications may result from a contracture, such as lid ectropion or immobilization of an important joint, intervention is more elective, although it should be timely. In the vast majority of patients, however, microsurgical reconstruction is performed after disabling scar contractures have been established. With the accumulation of experience, it seems reasonable to choose free-tissue transfer in earlier stages for patients with suitable indications. The reconstructive ladder, as originally defined, should be reconfigured to correlate with the therapeutic methods available today.

VIII. SELECTION OF FREE FLAPS

There are numerous tissues available for transfer depending on the need (Table 10.1). Although the advent of perforator flaps has introduced several new flaps, the reconstructive microsurgeon needs to familiarize himself/herself with only a few versatile flaps with minimal donor morbidity. As such, one of the most ideal single soft tissue flaps in our experience has been the anterolateral thigh (ALT) flap. Based on dissection of direct cutaneous vessels from the lateral descending branch of the deep femoral vessels regardless of the pedicle course (i.e., septocutaneous vs. musculocutaneous), the ALT flap can be harvested to be thin cutaneous, adipofascial, fasciocutaneous, musculocutaneous (vastus lateralis), chimeric (including the tensor fascia lata, rectus femoris, or ALT), or be designed to be sensate.

IX. COMPLICATIONS AND LIMITATIONS

Systemic complications following free-tissue transfer (except visceral) are rare. Improper patient selection or negligence of the general care of the patient will result in a poor outcome. Survival of free-tissue transfer is generally accepted to be >95% at most centers. Inadequate wound debridement, use of vein grafts, hematologic disorders, surgical technique, infection, all contribute to flap failure among burn patients, but overall success rates remain similar to other clinical conditions (15,19,33–37). Although patients of a wide range of ages tolerate free tissue transfer well, it has been suggested that medical complications are higher for those older than 70 years (38). More important than age by itself, however, is the health of the patient, therefore individualization remains

Table 10.1   Selection of Free Flaps

Tissue requirement	Available flaps
Thin surface coverage	RF, lateral arm, dorsalis pedis, medialis pedis, temporoparietal fascia thenar, thinned ALT
Thick surface coverage	Scapular, parascapular, TRAM, ALT, groin, thoracodorsal perforator, tensor fascia lata
Conforming to irregular areas	Omentum, rectus abdominis, ALT with vastus lateralis, latissimus dorsi, serratus anterior
Bone	Fibula, iliac crest, scapula
Specialized: hair bearing	Temporoparietal scalp
Composite: tendon	Dorsalis pedis-toe extensors, RF palmaris longus. ALT-tensor fascia lata
Flow-through	RF, ALT, lateral arm
Structural: esophageal	Colon, jejunum, ileocolic complex, RF, ALT
Structural: digits	Great toe, trimmed great toe, great toe wrap-around, lesser toe, combined lesser toes, pulp
Structural: breast	DIEP, TRAM, SGAP, ALT
Structural: penis	RF, fibula
Functional: muscle/tendon	Gracilis, latissimus dorsi, serratus anterior
Custom-fit unit	Pre-expansion, pre-lamination, pre-fabrication

Note: Abbreviations: ALT, anterolateral thigh; TRAM, transverse rectus abdominis muscle; RF, radial forearm; SGAP, superior gluteal arterial perforator; DIEP, deep inferior epigastric perforator flaps.

the basis for proper patient selection in the hope of minimizing morbidity.

X. INTRAOPERATIVE CONSIDERATIONS IN FREE-FLAP RECONSTRUCTION

Reconstructive microsurgery requires knowledge of the normal function of the affected structure, ability to raise a variety of flaps and capability of anastomosing vessels of 1–2 mm diameter, and general management of the patient. Basic strategy in microsurgical transfer of tissue is preparation of the recipient site, harvest of the flap, its inset, and microscopic anastomosis. Ideal operative strategy employs a team approach to reduce ischemia time as well as the overall operative period. The operating microscope should be of high quality, with good optics and a strong light source. Microinstruments include forceps, needle holder, vessel clamps (double or single), scissors, and a vessel dilator as a minimum. Non-absorbable suture (9-0 to 11-0) with a curved, round-bodied sharp microneedle is needed for vessel anastomosis. Surgical loupes allow for an expeditious and safe dissection of most free flaps, and also may be safely used for anastomosis of the larger vessels. The donor vessels are anastomosed end-to-end or end-to-side to recipient vessels. Basic principles of handling vessels should be followed religiously limiting trauma to the intima and spatulating the ends prior to anastomosis, which may be achieved by either interrupted or simple running techniques depending on surgeon preference. Heparinized saline should be used to flush out any thrombus formation and topical papaverine (30 mg/cm^3) or lidocaine (200 mg/cm^3) solution used liberally to prevent or treat vascular spasm. Arterial adventitiectomy is undertaken to achieve a local sympathectomy and reduce spasm events, especially when digital vessels are involved (39). Ischemia time is minimized in general, with special attention given to more sensitive tissues such as jejunum. Preparation is the key to expedition of free-tissue transfer: isolating adequate recipient vessels, providing adequate length of donor vessels, proper design of donor tissue for accurate inset, and proper positioning of the patient and surgeon. If necessary, bridging vein grafts from the saphenous system are easy to harvest and reliable, although a higher rate of failure may result (34,37). Perfusion is assessed on the table by testing the patency of each anastomosis, assessing venous return (if arterial anastomosis is done first), and checking flap dermal bleeding, surface color, or capillary refill. The donor site is closed primarily if possible, and if not, skin grafts are applied. In amenable areas, secondary procedures may be undertaken to improve the appearance of the donor scar, possibly even using tissue expansion.

XI. POSTOPERATIVE CARE AND REHABILITATION

Special attention needs to be made to ensure flap survival during the early postoperative period. Maintaining adequate fluid balance and body temperature, occasionally providing anticoagulation, and intensive flap monitoring are essential. Monitoring may be via the frequent clinical examination of the flap (color, temperature, turgor, capillary refill, and pin prick bleeding) or the use of a variety of methods (laser Doppler, Doppler arterial probes, thermocouple probe, photoplethysmography, color-flow ultrasound, surface temperature, dermofluorometry, fluorescein photography, flourescein, PO$_2$ tension monitoring, bone scintigraphy, etc.) depending on preference or availability (40). A microsurgical intensive care unit in our experience provides an ideal setting for acute patient care and flap monitoring. Close and frequent examination is necessary for a minimum of 5 days in that salvage is possible in the vast majority of compromised flaps (15,40). Although

free-tissue transfer in general does not add significant stress to the overall physiology of the patient, systemic issues should not be neglected during the postoperative period to prevent medical complications (41). For the ensuing few weeks, the patient has to be instructed to avoid posture or dressings that may compromise the pedicle supplying the flap. Upon adequate wound healing, physical therapy may be instituted for any residual motor or sensory impairment, without the need for intensive scar management. Whereas resurfacing free flaps allow early mobility (within 2 weeks), composite tissue transfers such as the toes require specific routines and timelines to allow for adequate healing of specific tissues.

XII. ADVANTAGES AND DISADVANTAGES OF MICROSURGICAL TISSUE TRANSFER

The significance of the various pros and cons of microsurgical tissue transfer is dependent on a wide variety of factors regarding the patient, physician, and clinical setting. Overall, however, for the majority of patients in a modern clinical setting with availability of well-trained microsurgeons, free flaps provide an invaluable service in the reconstruction of burn patients (Table 10.2).

XIII. CONCLUSION

Although affecting a relatively superficial organ, major burns impart significant impact on human life in a multi-dimensional way. During the acute stage, systemic disturbance may cause immediate loss of life itself, whereas local

Table 10.2 Advantage and Disadvantages of Free-Tissue Transfer Reconstruction

Advantages	Disadvantages
Versatility in design	Long operative time
Composite tissue transfer	Equipment intensive
Reliable	Possible long hospitalization
Effective prevention of contracure	Donor site expended permanently
Multiple possible donor sites	1–5% Failure rate
Postoperative garment unnecessary	Specialized training and facility necessary
Custom-fit preparation prior to transfer possible (prefabrication, pre-expansion)	
Improves local vascular supply	
Large surface area coverage possible	

complications may lead to loss of the underlying structure or organ. After abatement of the initial inflammatory phase, however, the "healing" burn may further inflict heavy damage to quality of life. Hypertrophy of the burn wound over critical areas leads to disabling a given structure in addition to resulting in significant aesthetic disturbance. Unfortunately, this process of hypertrophy does not spontaneously resolve and the resultant burn cicatrix permanently influences the patient's ensuing life.

Restoration of normal quality of life to these patients is as important as the preservation of life itself, and they may become surgical nomads searching for the holy grail of reconstructive surgery. Eventually, after failure of traditional methods of reconstruction, such patients develop medical reticence and distrust as both patient and doctor develop "fatalistic" attitudes. Therefore, the surgeon should undertake the restorative effort most likely able to address the compromise of both function and form primarily. Free-tissue transfer represents one of the most versatile reconstructive methods yielding results generally superior to other techniques due to its ability to be "custom-fitted." High demands on microsurgical skills, intraoperative time, and availability of donor tissue, however, behooves the reconstructive surgical community to continue the search for new methods that maximize restoration of form and function while minimizing morbidity. At the start of this new millennium, however, microsurgery provides the gold standard method for reconstruction and rehabilitation of the severely burned patient restore to the normal quality of life.

REFERENCES

1. Janzekovic Z. A new concept in the early excision and immediate grafting of burns. J Trauma 1970; 19:1103–1108.
2. Gibran NS, Heimbach DM. Current status of burn wound pathophysiology. Clin Plast Surg 2000; 27(1):11–22.
3. Deitch EA, Wheelahan TM, Rose MP, Clothier J, Cotter J. Hypertrophic burn scar. J Trauma 1983; 23(10):895–898.
4. Rudolph R. Inhibition of myofibroblasts by skin grafts. Plast Reconstr Surg 1970; 63:473–480.
5. Rudolph R, Guber S, Suzuki M, Woodward M. The life-cycle of the myofibro-blast. Surg Gynecol Obstet 1977; 145:389–394.
6. Woo SH, Seul J-H. Optimizing the correction of severe postburn hand deformities by using aggressive contracture releases and fasciocutaneous free-tissue transfers. Plast Reconstr Surg 2001; 107(1):1–8.
7. Salisbury RE. Reconstruction of the burned hand. Clin Plast Surg 2000; 27(1):65–69.
8. Germann G, Cedidi C, Hartmann B. Post-burn reconstruction during growth and development. Ped Surg Int 1977; 12:321–326.
9. Wang S-W et al. Early vascular grafting to prevent upper extremity necrosis after electrical burns. Chin Med J 1984; 97:53.
10. Brandt K, Khouri RK, Upton J. Free flaps as flow-through vascular conduits for simultaneous coverage and revascularization of the hand or digit. Plast Reconstr Surg 1990; 98(2):321–327.
11. Koshima I, Inagawa K, Sahara K, Tsuda K, Moriguchi T. Flow-through vascularized toe-joint transfer for reconstruction of segmental loss of an amputated finger. J Reconstr Microsurg 1998; 14(7):453–457.
12. Asko-Seljavaara S, Pitkänen J, Sundell B. Microvascular free flaps in early reconstruction of burns in the hand and forearm. Scand J Plast Reconstr Surg 1984; 18:139–144.
13. Chick LR, Lister L, Sowder L. Early free flap coverage of electrical and thermal burns. Plast Reconstr Surg 1992; 89:1013–1019.
14. Grotting J, Walkinshaw M. The early use of free flaps in burns. Ann Plast Surg 1985; 15:127–131.
15. Nappi J, Lubbers L, Carl B. Composite tissue transfer in burn patients. Clin Plast Surg 1986; 13(1):137–144.
16. Angrigiani C. Aesthetic microsurgical reconstruction of anterior neck burn deformities. Plast Reconstr Surg 1994; 93(3):507–518.
17. Koshima I, Soeda S. Repair of a wide defect of the lower leg with combined scapular and parascapular flap. Br J Plast Surg 1985; 38:518–521.
18. Wei F-C et al. Microsurgical thumb reconstruction with toe transfer. Plast Reconstr Surg 1992; 93:345–351.
19. Wei F-C, Colony L. Microsurgical reconstruction of opposable digits in mutilating hand injuries. Clin Plast Surg 1989; 16:491–504.
20. Wei F-C et al. Simultaneous multiple toe transfer in hand reconstruction. Plast Reconstr Surg 1988; 81:366–377.
21. Morrison W, O'Brien McC, Macleod M. Thumb reconstruction with a free neurovascular wrap-around flap from the big toe. J Hand Surg 1980; 5:575–583.
22. Logan A, Elliot D, Foucher G. Free toe pulp transfer to restore traumatic digital pulp loss. Br J Plast Surg 1985; 38:497–500.
23. Chang TS, Hwang WY. Forearm flap in one stage reconstruction of the penis. Plast Reconstr Surg 1984; 74:251–258.
24. Hage JJ, Winters HA, Van Lieshout J. Fibula free flap phalloplasty. Microsurgery 1996; 17:358–365.
25. Gilbert DA et al. New concepts in phallic reconstruction. Ann Plast Surg 1987; 18:128–365.
26. Santanelli F, Scuderi N. Neophalloplasty in female-to-male transsexuals with the island tensor fascia lata flap. Plast Reconstr Surg 2000; 6:1990–1996.
27. Hage JJ, DeGraafi FH. Addressing the ideal requirements by free flap phalloplasty. Microsurgery 1993; 14:592–598.
28. Angrigiani C, Grilli D. Total face reconstruction with one free flap. Plast Reconstr Surg 1997; 99(6):1566–1575.
29. Krizek TJ, Robson MC, Headley BJ. Management of burn syndactyly. J Trauma 1974; 14:587–593.
30. Beasley RW. Secondary repair of burned hands. Hand Clin 1990; 6:319–341.

31. Pribaz JJ. Prelaminated free flap reconstruction of complex central facial defects. Plast Reconstr Surg 1999; 104(2):357–365.

32. Flatt AE. Digital artery sympathectomy. J Hand Surg 1990; 5:550–556.

33. Khouri RK, Cooley BC, Kunselman AR, Landis JR, Yeramian P, Ingram D, Natarajan N, Benes CO, Wallemark C. A prospective study of microvascular free-flap surgery and outcome. Plast Reconstr Surg 1998; 102(3):711–721.

34. Kroll SS et al. Choice of flap and incidence of free flap success. Plast Reconstr Surg 1996; 98(3):459–463.

35. Moelleken BR et al. Flap monitoring. Perspect Plast Surg 1990; 4(1):94.

36. Kuo YR, Jeng SF. Acute pulmonary edema after microsurgery. J Reconstr Microsurg 1998; 14(2):97–99.

37. Tseng W-S et al. "Flow-through" type free flap for revascularization and simultaneous coverage of a nearly complete amputation of the foot. J Trauma 2000; 48(4):773–776.

38. Berger A, Tizian C, Schneider W. Microsurgery as an integrated part of the rehabilitation of severly burned patients. Scand J Plast Reconstr Surg 1987; 21:261–264.

39. Sharzer LA et al. Clinical application of free-flap transfer in the burn patient. J Trauma 1975; 15:766–771.

40. Grotting JC. Prevention of complications and correction of postoperative problems in microsurgery of the lower extremity. Clin Plast Surg 1991; 18(3):485–489.

41. Silverberg B, Banis JC Jr, Verdi GD, Acland RD. Microvascular reconstruction after electrical and deep thermal injury. J Trauma 1986; 26(2):128–134.

42. Shen T, Shen TY, Sun YH, Cao DX, Wang NZ. The use of free flaps in burn patients. Plast Reconstr Surg 1988; 81(3):352–357.

43. Shaari CM, Shaari CM, Buchbinder D, Costantino PD, Lawson W, Biller HF, Urken ML. Complications of microvascular head and neck surgery in the elderly. Arch Otolaryngol Head Neck Surg 1998; 124(4):407–411.

11

Principles of Tissue Expansion

ROBERT L. McCAULEY

University of Texas Medical Branch and Shriners Hospital for Children—Galveston Unit, Galveston, Texas, USA

MICHAEL K. OBENG

University of Texas Medical Branch, Galveston, Texas, USA

I. INTRODUCTION

The human skin does not heal through tissue regeneration. Scarring is the normal end result of any traumatic injury to the skin. Burn injury only represents a segment of traumatic injuries in which scarring may become problematic. Yet, with patients continuing to survive large total body surface area burns, scarring can not only limit mobility, but can also become aesthetically disfiguring. Without question, one of the most challenging tasks we face today is the aesthetic and functional reconstruction of the burn patient. The extensive use of skin grafts, local skin flaps, distant flaps, and microvascular free-tissue transfer has given reconstructive surgeons significant tools in approaching this daunting task. However, inherent in each of these techniques are problems with color match and texture. In addition, donor site disfigurement may also play a role both psychologically and physically. Skin expansion is based on the dynamic nature by which living tissue responds to mechanical stress. The growth of the uterus during pregnancy or massive changes in weight demonstrate the ability of the skin to accommodate changes in body habitus. Controlled soft tissue expansion offers many advantages over other modalities in the reconstruction of burn patients. The color and texture of expanded skin is a better match to the surrounding tissues than skin grafts or even distant flaps. Donor site morbidity is minimized or eliminated. Lastly, expanded skin can maintain sensibility. Although tissue expansion has numerous advantages, it is not recommended in all situations. Yet, it is such a valuable technique that it has become an integral part of the armamentarium in the reconstruction of burn patients.

II. HISTOMORPHOLOGY OF TISSUE EXPANSION

As noted, the concept of tissue expansion has occurred both under natural conditions (i.e., pregnancy and breast development) and in abnormal circumstances (i.e., tumor growth). As part of the exotic aesthetics of various cultures, tissue expansion has long been noted as a method to document the positions of social hierarchy. The Chadian women of Africa, the Paduang women of Burma, and the Brazilian Indians are noted for insertion of disks into the lower lip, ear lobules, and neck as a symbol of beauty and their position within the tribal society (1,2). However, the use of tissue expansion medically dates back to the early 1900s. In 1905 Codivilla (3) reported the use of a bone traction device to lengthen the lower limbs. This concept was further popularized by Putti (4) in 1921. The first clinical case of pure soft tissue expansion was reported by Neumann when he reconstructed the upper two-thirds of the right ear in a 52-year-old man by inserting a rubber balloon above the ear with a polyethylene tubing exiting through the stab wound in the neck (5). The balloon was gradually inflated over a 6-week period with a ~50% increase in postauricular skin. This expanded flap was then advanced to cover the cartilaginous framework. However, the concept of soft tissue expansion to correct traumatic defects did not become popular for another 20 years.

In 1975, both Radovan (6) and Austad (7) began pioneering work on soft tissue expansion. Experimental data on the biology of tissue expansion have largely come from animal data. Although it is clear that Radovan became the first surgeon to gain extensive experience with tissue expanders, Austad et al. (7,8) first reported the laboratory experience with expanders prior to clinical use.

A number of histological studies have been performed to delineate some of the histological changes that occur in expanded skin.

A. Epidermis

Initial studies of the epidermis revealed several interesting findings. Examination of tissues in both guinea pigs and humans revealed epidermal thickening (7,8,10). Further studies by Paysk et al. (9) showed that epidermal thickening persisted for 2 years after expansion. Interestingly enough, there was no correlation of epidermal thickening with expansion time, volume, location, or patient age. Paysk et al. (10) also showed that the epidermal thickening appeared to occur in the stratum spongiosum. Light microscopy revealed several interesting findings. The basal lamina appeared undulated. The tonofilaments in the basal and prickle cells revealed increased bundles of tonofibrils. These findings, along with the decrease in the intracellular spaces noted in all epidermal layers suggested increased mitotic activity. Later, Austad et al. (8) quantitatively documented epidermal mitotic activity using tritiated thymidine. He noted that epidermal mitosis increased threefold during inflation, but returned to baseline over the next 2–5 days.

B. Dermis

The expansile and recoil properties of the skin are related to the amount of collagen and elastic fibers in the dermis (11,12). Unlike the epidermis, the dermis undergoes significant changes during the expansion process. The thickness of the dermis is reduced dramatically. Again, this is not related to expander volume or anatomic location (9). Most of the dermal thinning occurs in the reticular dermis. Although thinning of the papillary dermis is noted, this is less dramatic. During the first few weeks of expansion, the dermis thins significantly, but less so toward the end of the expansion process. After expansion, the reticular dermis is noted to have increased amounts of thick bundles of collagen fibers parallel to the skin. In addition, the elastic fibers in the expanded dermis were thicker and longer. It is believed that the presence of increased numbers of active fibroblasts in the dermis is responsible for the immature collagen fibers. Collagen bundles populate both the reticular and the papillary dermis from the multiplication of fibroblasts (11,12).

Skin has the ability to stretch and recoil. Elastic fibers, linked to each other by end-to-side junctions are each interspersed among collagen fibers, which are often larger and unlinked to another. Elastin fibers, unlike collagen, have the ability to stretch and retract. Collagen fibers in their relaxed state are disoriented and unparalleled. These fibers, in the presence of applied stress, align in a parallel fashion (9). This response is linearly proportional to the magnitude of the applied stress. In the presence of excess stress, striae formation is inevitable. In addition, too much stress during expansion of skin can cause constriction in the tiny blood vessels inducing ischemia. Our goal is to take advantage of this regeneration process without causing flap loss secondary to necrosis. It should be noted that hair follicles, sebaceous and sweat glands, and sensory nerves might undergo subtle changes, if any at all. Hair follicles and glandular tissues remain unchanged qualitatively, but remain active. The lumens of various glands remain open even though adjacent structures have been compressed (11,12). In addition, sensory fibers do not undergo any appreciable structural changes (9).

C. Skeletal Muscle

Skeletal muscles under expansion undergo some atrophy. Although, muscle is more tolerant than other tissues to expansion, there is a significant decrease in muscle mass and thickness (12). Even with these drastic changes during expansion, no significant functional loss has been noted. Striated muscles tolerate expansion better then facial muscles, and there is no decline in power, excursion, or repetitive activity. However, some ultrastructural changes do occur. There is enlargement of the sarcoplasmic reticulum, as well as an increase in the size and number of mitochondria within skeletal muscles (9,11).

D. Adipose Tissue

Fat appears to be the most intolerant of tissues to expansion. There is a marked decrease in the thickness of the adipose layer (9,11). The adipocytes become flattened and smaller. Experimental data noted replacement of adipocytes with fibrous tissue. Although frank fat necrosis has not been observed experimentally, the loss of fatty tissue appears to be permanent.

E. Blood Vessels

Numerous investigators have noted a significant proliferation of blood vessels associated with tissue expansion. This proliferation occurs primarily at the junction of the capsule and host tissues. Within days of expansion, small capillaries become distended, and the number of arterioles and venules increases. Cherry et al. (13) noted an increase in the surviving length of expanded random-patterned skin flaps when compared to delayed skin flaps. Sasaki et al. (14) later confirmed previous studies by documenting increased blood flow in expanded flaps. Lantieri et al. (15) later suggested that vascular endothelial growth factor (VEGF) might play a part in the development of the increased vascularity of expanded flaps since VEGF was only expressed in expanded flap.

F. Molecular Basis for Tissue Expansion

Initial studies by several investigations documented an increased mitotic index in the epidermal layer of the skin with expansion (7,16). Takei et al. (17) felt that a number of growth factors were involved in this strain induced cellular activity. The process of expansion is believed to affect not only the adjacent tissue, but also a number of cell types. This group postulated that platelet derived group factors (PDGF) as well as other growth factors could stimulate cutaneous cells. While it is well known that transforming growth factor-beta (TGF-B) can influence extracellular matrix production, this growth factor can also enhance fibroblast proliferation. Last, membrane bound molecules may also play a role in the regulation of intercellular signal transduction pathways (Fig. 11.1). However, the exact mechanism by which strain influences skin biology is still unclear. Whether or not we can modulate this response chemically remains to be seen.

III. PRINCIPLES OF TISSUE EXPANSION

Correction of burn deformities using tissue expansion is a multistage process. Not only is patient selection crucial, so is individualized preoperative planning. The expectations of the patient and those of the surgeon should match. Patient acceptance of the weekly or biweekly injection processes and the progressive deformity caused by the expander is essential. A number of parameters must be considered prior to expansion. Issues related to the insertion process are less controversial when compared to the details as to how this should be done. Most surgeons feel that the use of perioperative antibiotics is crucial. However, other issues are controversial. The type of incision used is still under scrutiny: paralesional or remote. The orientation and the number of expanders used have also been scrutinized. What size expander should one use, and how much flap advancement can be expected? These are still debated issues. Internal vs. external port placement may be individualized based on circumstances. How this affects the success of expansion is not always clear. Since all of these concerns are key to the successful use of expanders and influence preoperative planning, they should be addressed.

A. Incisions: Paralesional or Remote

The type of incision used to insert a tissue expander is still an issue. Clearly, healing of the incision is crucial to the initiation of the expansion process. One issue which does not appear to be controversial is that, regardless of the type of incision used, it should be as small as possible. Proponents of paralesional incisions, that is, incisions at the junction of normal tissue and the scarred area, believe that minimal undermining of tissues is required for insertion of expanders. In addition, no statistically sound data have proven that infection rates, wound dehiscence rates, and implant exposure rates are significantly different. Proponents of the remote incision believe that healthy tissue approximated to healthy tissue affords better healing. In addition, the migration of expanders during

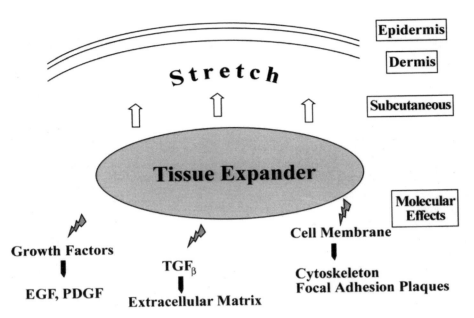

Figure 11.1   Influence of tissue expansion on the expression of growth factors and the production of extracellular matrix. [Reproduced with permission from Takei et al. (17).]

the expansion process will not interfere with the weakness point in the skin, the incision. Complication rates have been cited to be less. However, a number of factors may influence these data. Currently, no controlled, randomized studies exist on site-specific expansion to settle this controversy. Complications may simply be related to the quality and quantity of tissues undergoing expansion and the donor site location.

B.   Implant Type and Size

Tissue expanders come in all shapes and sizes. They can be bought "off the rack" or custom made. The choices of remote vs. *in situ* ports are also available. In addition, differential expanders are also currently utilized. In 1984, Gibney recommended the use of expanders with a base width that is $2\frac{1}{2}$–3 times the width of the defect to be covered (18). Later, Manders et al. (19) recommended the use of as large an expander as possible. Brobmann and Huber (20) in an experimental study on pigs addressed the issue of expander size and shape relative to the amount of expansion obtained. It was determined that less time, pressure, and volume are needed in a larger expander to achieve gain in the same surface area when compared to smaller implants (20). Several investigators have proposed the use of a mathematical model for determining the size, amount of inflation required, and expected advancement (21,22). Although this sophisticated model is mathematically sound, its complexity has not led to widespread use. When expanders are placed over rigid flat surfaces, predicting the amount of flap advancement is straightforward. It is only when expanders are placed over soft

tissues with the capacity for inward compression, that is, the abdomen, or in areas of concavity, that is, the neck, that the prediction of advancement is less reliable. Nevertheless, the use of as large an expander as the donor site will accept is reasonable. In the scalp, prediction of flap advancement is reliable. In the author's experience, measuring the dome of the expander and subtracting the width of the expander is fairly accurate in determining the amount of flap advancement (Fig. 11.2).

C.   Internal vs. External Ports

Several investigators have documented safety in the use of external ports (23–25). Although, individual circumstances and location are the best determinants as to how the port is placed, issues of safety and efficiency are not abandoned by either technique. In the pediatric population, the use of external ports can alleviate pain and anxiety associated with weekly injections (26).

D.   Rate of Expansion

Intraoperative expansion, as described by Sasaki, is a valuable technique for resurfacing small defects. Its efficacy has been shown experimentally and clinically. However, the technique and indications may be limited in large burn defects.

The rate at which expansion occurs postoperatively varies by site and by surgeon. Depending on the area of the body, expansion has been recommended anywhere from 1 week to $2\frac{1}{2}$ weeks after placement. Injection

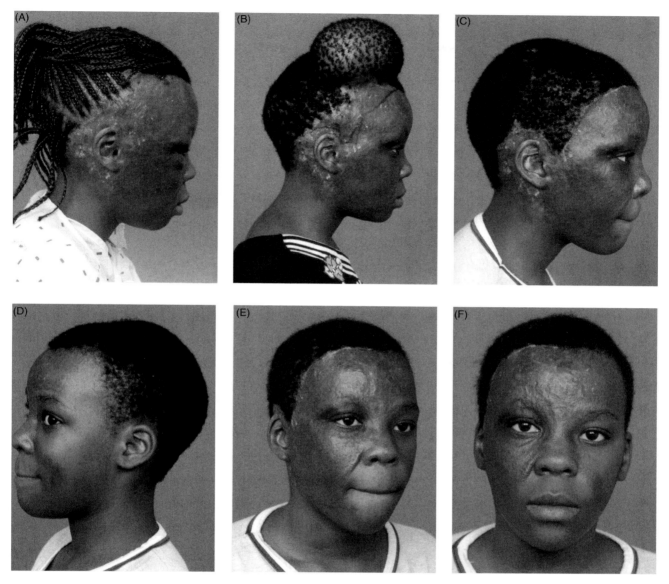

Figure 11.2   (A) Ten-year-old black female with scalp alopecia (Type 1B). (B) Placement of a 340 cm^3 expander inflated to 500 cm.^{3} (C) Complete coverage after estimating flap length by measuring the dome of the expander and subtracting the width of the expander. (D) Comparison with contralateral side. (E, F) Frontal views.

fractions vary, but 10% of the volume per week is required to complete expansion within a 3-month period. However, individual variations exist and one must be aware of pressure changes which occur with expansion so that flap ischemia and subsequent exposure of the expander does not become a problem. Pietila et al. (27) addressed the issue of accelerated expansion with the "overfilling" technique. This group defined overexpansion as expansion to the point where dermal capillary flow is zero by laser doppler flow meter and patient discomfort is high. Reportedly, fluid was then removed until capillary refill returned and the patient no longer experienced discomfort. In a series of 14 patients, they confirmed an average increase

of 59% using this technique. However, complications in these patients were not addressed.

E.   Techniques in Tissue Expansion

1.   Patient Selection

Because of the extent of skin damage in burns as well as its poor expansive nature, patient selection in deciding the best donor area to be expanded is of paramount importance. Tissue expansion is a dynamic process and it requires a favorable donor site for insertion and subsequent filling. Most burn patients present with extensive skin grafts. Patients in the acute phase of healing their wounds or patients with open wounds or infections should be avoided. In addition, poorly vascularized skin as well as scars do not favor placement of tissue expanders. Normally, donor sites are chosen based on clinical availability. In patients with large TBSA burns, ideal donor sites may not exist. Donor sites uninvolved with burn injury can provide an excellent aesthetic and functional outcome. In the head and neck region, respecting the boundaries of the aesthetic units is essential for optimal outcomes.

2. Intraoperative Considerations

In most cases, expanders are placed either below the galea or at the fascial layer, depending on location. Meticulous hemostasis is crucial. Irrigation of the expander packet with antibiotic solution is also a common practice. Checking the expander for leakage is an important part of the procedure. The injection of air with the submersion of the expander in saline is reliable for detecting leaks. Alternatively, the use of methylene blue helps to identify expander leaks prior to insertion (28).

3. Operative Techniques

Once the expander has been successfully inflated and is ready for removal, advancement or rotation of the flap has usually been decided. Hudson (29) feels that the best method for maximizing the use of expanded tissue in both a vertical and a horizontal direction is to add back cuts to the sides as well as the base of the flap. Scoring the capsule to increase flap advancement has been touted by several authors. However, limitations exist. The absolute increase in flap advancement gained with scoring is not clear. In addition, increased bleeding and potential damage to the overlying blood vessels may cause vascular compromise.

4. Postoperative Issues

The timing of postoperative expansion has also been debated. Most surgeons believe the timing for the first injection is site specific if no problems occur with the healing of the incision line. The expansion process is best started before the development of firm capsule formation. This process can be safely done in the office under sterile conditions and does not require anesthesia. Patient discomfort and tightness of the expanded tissue should serve as guidelines for determining the amount of fluid placed. After every injection, the skin is checked for blanching.

IV. BURN RECONSTRUCTION: THE ROLE OF TISSUE EXPANSION

Historically, the surgical treatment for burn scars and burn scar contractures has been excision of the scars and resurfacing of the defect with a number of previously described techniques. However, Radovan (6) ushered in a new era of reconstruction in 1976, when he first placed a tissue expander in the arm of a patient to resurface a 77 cm² defect. His initial experience of 130 patients was reported in 1984. Expansion was described as a two-stage process which yielded impressive results in the resurfacing of both burn and nonburn deformities. During this time, independent work by Austad (30) was carried out using the self-inflating tissue expander. In 1984, Manders et al. (19) reported their success with scalp expansion resurfacing areas of burn alopecia children. Later, Manders et al. (31) reported a larger series of 35 patients undergoing 41 expansions for a wide spectrum of problems. Here, complications associated with expansion were addressed and separated into minor and major complications. Major complications were defined as those which interrupted the expansion process and prevented achievement of the desired results. Marks et al. (32) reported one of the earlier series of patients with burns only, who were treated with tissue expansion. In his series of 45 patients with burns, expanders were used to reconstruct areas of the head and neck, trunk, and extremities. This group concluded that tissue expansion was a valuable technique for correction of small- and moderate-sized burn scars, if surrounded by normal tissue. It was also felt that in the head and neck region, larger defects could be addressed. MacLennon et al. (33) later reviewed their experience with expansion in the head and neck region in burn patients. Although results were uniformly encouraging, caution was expressed in the use of expanders to resurface the lower face and cheeks because of the risk for the development of ectropions of the eyelids and lips. Most recently, Pitanguy et al. (2) addressed the issue of repeated expansion in burn patients. Between 1985 and 2000, 346 expanders were used in 132 patients. In 42 of these patients repeated expansions were performed. Although complication rates were low, two points were brought to light. First, repeated expansions required an interval of 6 months to 1 year. Second, the area of re-expansion should be prepared with dermotomy, a mechanical massage method which consists of positive pressure rolling in conjunction with applied suction to the skin and subcutaneous tissues. Although this technique has not gained widespread use, Pitanguy et al. (2) believe that it increases vascularization and elasticity of the skin targeted for re-expansion.

A. Burn Alopecia

Prior to expansion, burn alopecia was managed with serial excision and local flaps. Huang et al. (34) showed that burn alopecia up to 15% of the hair-bearing scalp could be managed with serial excision of the alopecia segment.

Areas >15% required extensive use of scalp flaps to camouflage defects. The next stage of evolution for closure of scalp defects came from Orticochea (35,36). The three- and four-limb Orticochea flaps were successfully used to close scalp defects >15% of the hair-bearing scalp. The Juri flap, the lateral pedicled scalp flap, was described to reconstruct the anterior hairline in bald patients (37,38). Its use in combination with tissue expansion has been described (39). However, tissue expansion has added an entirely new dimension to the treatment of burn alopecia. Presently, it is the gold standard by which other techniques must be measured.

Many investigators have demonstrated the safety and efficiency of tissue expansion in the correction of burn alopecia (19,40,41). McCauley et al. (40) classified both the

pattern of alopecia and the extent of alopecia. This classification system was designed as a template by which reconstruction efforts could be designed to address specific problems with burn alopecia (Table 11.1). It is important to note that scalp expansion only allows redistribution of a healthy scalp tissue without creating new hair follicles. It has been noted that the interfollicular distance can increase twofold without noticeable thinning of the hair (31). Several investigators have been reluctant to address burn alopecia, which is >50% of the hair-bearing scalp, citing poor results. However, alternatives to resurfacing of the scalp are limited and some patients feel that some hair is better than no hair (Fig. 11.3).

Table 11.1 Classification of Burn Alopecia

Type I	Single alopecia segment
	A <25% of the hair-bearing scalp
	B 25–50% of the hair-bearing scalp
	C 50–75% of the hair-bearing scalp
	D >75% of the hair-bearing scalp
Type II	Multiple alopecia segments amenable to tissue expansion placement
Type III	Patchy burn alopecia not amenable to tissue expansion
Type IV	Total alopecia

Source: Reproduced with permission from McCauley et al. (40).

B. Face and Neck

When burn scar contractures of the face and neck are present, it is usually difficult to gauge the amount of soft tissue expansion needed for facial or neck resurfacing. Consequently, it is recommended that all contractures are released and wounds are healed prior to resurfacing neck and facial scars with tissue expanders. Tissue expansion of the neck can be used to either resurface neck scars or, alternatively, to resurface the lower two-thirds of the face. Expanders are placed in the supraplatysmal plane and in the neck the port is usually sutured in place superiorly. One should note that although expander placement is usually in close proximity to important structures in the

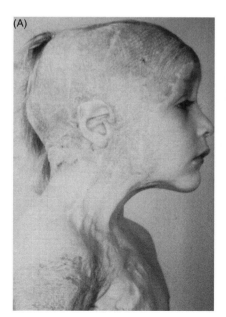
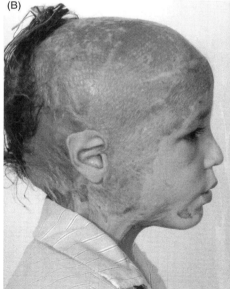
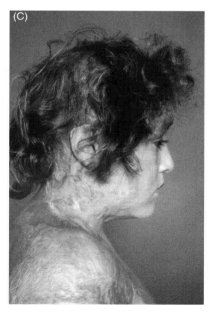

Figure 11.3 (A) Five-year-old white male with 75% burn alopecia (Type 1D). (B) Postoperative appearance after first-expansion covering of the occital region. (C) Total coverage after sequential expansion. Appearance 6 months after the last operation. [Reproduced with permission from McCauley et al. (40).]

neck, vascular compromise or respiratory distress has not been a problem.

Expansion of the head and neck of burn patients has been challenging (42,43). In theory, the resurfacing of the lower two-thirds of the face with normal tissue appears to be an ideal solution for a challenging problem. However, in practice accomplishing these goals may not be as straightforward. Even under ideal circumstances certain principles need to be followed. In order to ensure that the cervicomental angle is restored after flap advancement, expanders should be placed in the subcutaneous plane (33). Second, when resurfacing the face, rotation of the expanded flaps, not advancement, is necessary to minimize extrinsic eye ectropions or inferior displacement of the lip in these patients (33) (Fig. 11.4). If necessary, suspension sutures can be placed in the periosteum lateral orbital wall to avoid such problems (44).

C. Breasts

Breast reconstruction is an area where the initial use of tissue expanders became successful (31,45,46,71). However, its role in reconstruction of the burned breast has not received significant attention (47). In female patients with unilateral or bilateral loss of the nipple bud as a direct result of the burn injury, the breast may not develop. Under such circumstances, reconstruction of the affected breast may require expansion prior to the placement of a breast prosthesis. In young girls, the placement of tissue expanders under burned anterior chest wall scars may appear to be fraught with complications. Yet this may represent the only alternative if the latissimus dorsi myocutaneous flap is unavailable and inadequate soft tissue in the abdomen eliminates the transverse rectus myocutaneous (TRAM) flap as a choice for breast reconstruction. In unilateral

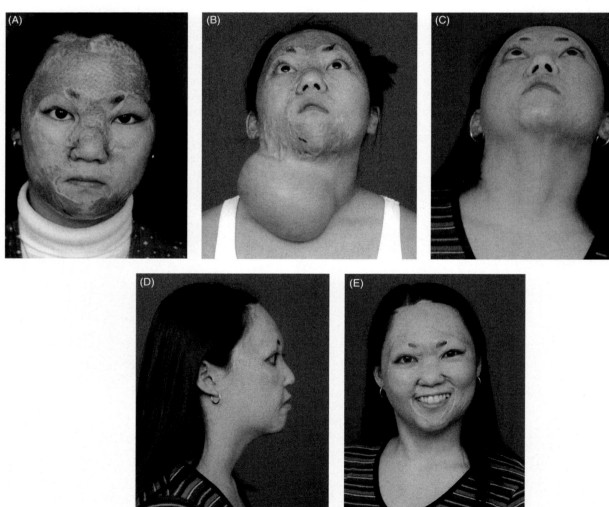

Figure 11.4   (A) Twelve-year-old oriental female with meshed grafts over forehead and right cheek regions has significant scarring of the burn injury. (B) Placement of a 500 cm³ tissue expander above the platysma muscle. (C) Excision of right cheek scars and resurfacing of the forehead unit with a full-thickness skin graft at 1 year. (D, E) Postoperative side and frontal views.

breast loss, the expander may be kept in place and gradually filled to keep up with the size of the contralateral developing breast. Alternatively, in the adult female patient, tissue expansion has been used to decrease the surface area of burn scars when contour has been altered (47,48).

D. Chest/Abdomen

Currently, insufficient data exists on the use of tissue expanders in this region. Stills et al. (49) reported a series of nine patients with excessive burn scars over the chest and abdomen that underwent expansion for correction. In this series, patients had a mean TBSA burn of 23.8% and all incisions were placed at the junction of the burn scar and unburned tissues. Expanders were placed at the level of the fascia. Complications occurred in 33% of the patients. These included expander extrusion and cellulitus. However, it is unclear as to whether the intended operative plans were completely successful.

Scarring of the abdominal wall has received some attention, especially in female patients with circumferential truncal burns. Previous studies have indicated that

pregnancy, a natural expansion process, is not interrupted or complicated by burn scars (50). In fact, some authors have utilized pregnancy as a natural expander to correct abdominal scarring in the postpartum period (51). More recently, preoperative pneumoperitoneum has been used for tissue expansion prior to the reconstruction of abdominal wall defects (52). Burns to the abdomen pose a special problem. Although serial excision of burn scars over the abdomen is possible, placement of tissue expanders to correction of abdominal scar is not ideal. In children, if expanders are placed above the rectus sheath, the lack of a rigid surface prevents ideal skin expansion since inward expansion also occurs. Although some expansion occurs outwardly, when compared to other parts of the body, this area is less then ideal. Expansion of burn scars over the back is more satisfying since expanders can be placed over a rigid surface (Fig. 11.5).

E. Upper Extremities

Documentation on the use of expanders in upper-extremity reconstruction is limited (53–57). The surgical techniques

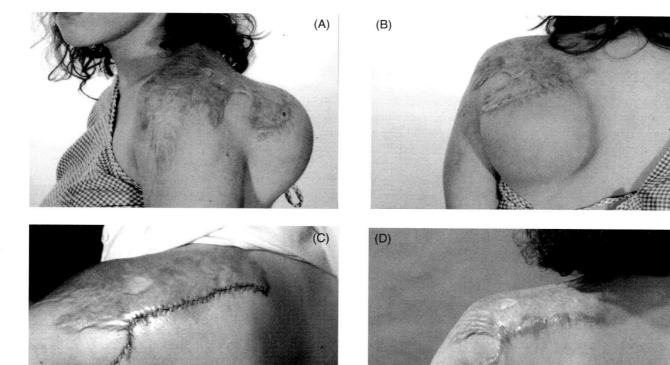

Figure 11.5 (A, B) Thirteen-year-old white female after overinflation of a 650 cm^3 tissue expander for correction of right shoulder and back scars. (C) Immediate postoperative view after partial removal of the scars, and resurfacing with the expanded flap. (D) Three-month follow-up showing some hypertrophy of the suture lines.

as well as the expansion schedule, results and long-term follow-up are scarce. In 1987, Marks et al. (32) reported their series of burn patients in whom tissue expansion was used for reconstruction. Of the 45 patients reviewed, only four underwent expansion of the upper extremity. However, it was felt that the subcutaneous placement of tissue expanders and a slower interval of inflation, 8–10 days, might prove to be efficacious. Later, Van Beek and Adson (55) published their series of 41 patients requiring reconstruction using 18 tissue expanders in the arms and hands. Although this series is also small, several points were made. First, this group noted that axial placement of multiple expanders is desirable. Secondly, the insertion of expanders through the smallest of incisions was felt to minimize wound-healing problems during the expansion process. Lastly, damage to major cutaneous nerves could be avoided by placing the expanders on top of them. Nevertheless, major complications occurred in 5 of the 11 patients (45%). Carneiro and Dichiara (56) believed that the high complication rate associated with upper-extremity expansion precluded the widespread use of expanders in the upper extremity. Consequently, they developed protocols for patient selection. All patients in this series had wounds which did not exceed 30% of the arm circumference. Twelve patients, employing 20 expanders over a 2-year period, were reviewed. Similar to Van Beek and Adson (55), Carneiro and Dichiara (56) inserted expanders through small incisions, used multiple expanders, and started expansion on postoperative days 10–14. In addition, they used low-profile expanders of limited size and injected only a maximum of 20 cc per visit. Overfilling of the expander was not done. Interestingly enough, there were no extrusions, infections, or tissue necrosis. However, 20% of their patients developed transient neuropathies. Subsequent studies by Aubert et al. (57) documented the safety and efficiency of expansion in the upper extremity.

The use of tissue expanders to correct burns of the upper extremity has met with mixed results. Often the expanders are of limited size because of availability of the surrounding normal tissue. In addition, the resulting postsurgical scar has a tendency to hypertrophy. The complication rate, here, appears to be higher when compared to other parts of the body.

F. Lower Extremities

The use of tissue expansion in the lower extremities has received significant attention (58–65). In the mid-1980s, Rees et al. (66) used a tissue expander to successfully resurface scar over a traumatic below-the-knee amputation. This technique preserved the length of the stump and provided stable, sensate coverage. Cole et al. (58) confirmed the safety and efficacy of lower-extremity stump

resurfacing with expanded flaps in his series of six patients, five of whom were children. Watier et al. (59) also confirmed the findings by Rees et al. (66) in his series of patients who required the use of expanded skin to resurface unstable scars in below-the-knee amputation. In 1987, Manders et al. (60) reported their series of 15 patients undergoing 16 expansions in the lower extremity. Four of these patients required excision of unstable scar or skin grafts. All expanders were placed in the subcutaneous plane with expansion carried out 1–2 weeks postoperatively. The use of devices to measure intraluminal pressures was recommended. Patients with preinflation pressures of ≥40 mm were not recommended for further expansion. Although 10 of the 15 patients had excellent results, one-third (5/15) of the patients had poor results because reconstruction was not accomplished. Eighty percent of the patients, however, had complications. Complications included infections, wound dehiscence, and expander exposure. In a review of soft tissue expansion in the lower extremity, Fihlo et al. (61) made several observations: (1) soft tissue expansion in the lower extremities is well tolerated although infection and wound dehiscence are common and (2) the more proximal the expander is placed, that is, thighs and buttocks, the easier and less complication prone the expansion will be. More recently, several investigators have addressed the use of tissue expanders in lower-limb reconstruction in a larger series of patients (62,63). Vögelin et al. (62) reported the use of 37 expanders in the lower extremities of 34 patients. Thirty-three of the patients were noted to have painful or unstable scars or post-traumatic ulcers as an indication for expansion. The areas of expansion occurred in the proximal and distal thirds of the leg. The technique was successful in 67.6% of the patients. However, within this group, 44% of the patients had healing problems. Nearly 50% of these problems (7/15) were due to partial flap necrosis (62). Although Filho et al. (61) recommended the placement of the expander incision at the edge of the defect, Vögelin preferred placement of the incision in distant healthy tissues.

To date, one of the largest series of patients studied on the use of tissue expansion in the lower extremity is that of Casanova et al. (63). Over a 10-year period, they reported their experiences of skin expansion in 95 patients using 207 expanders in 103 operative procedures. The indications for expansion in 77 patients were the correction of cosmetic or skin disorders. Complications occurred in 19.4% of patients involving 10.6% of the prostheses. Forty-five percent of their major complications (8.7% of the patients) were problems with sepsis. Casanova recommended that success was more likely with the use of external valves to avoid extensive undermining of tissues and the use of radial incisions away from the defect to decrease wound-healing

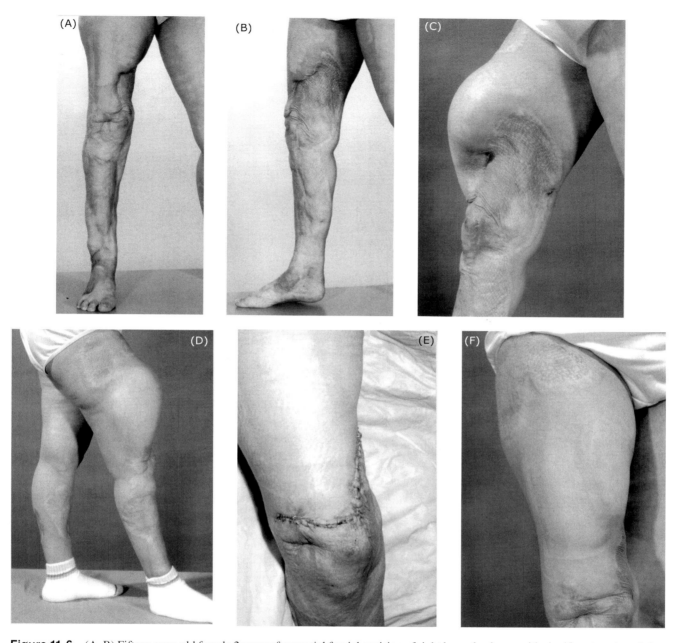

Figure 11.6 (A, B) Fifteen-year-old female 2 years after partial fascial excision of right lower leg burns with significant contour defect of distal medial thigh. (C, D) Placement of a 1200 cm³ tissue expander with full inflation. (E) Postoperative appearance after partial excision of the skin graft and medial advancement of the expanded flap. (F) Improvement in thigh contour 1 year later.

problems. Pandya et al. (64) in a comparative analysis of limb vs. nonlimb expansion, showed in a series of 88 patients that the completion of expansion in limb vs. nonlimb patients was similar (86% vs. 83%). However, complication rates were higher in the limb group (45%) vs. the nonlimb group (27%) (Figs. 11.6 and 11.7). Although no significant explanation is given for these difficulties, the 17% failure rate and 43% complication rate noted for expansion of the lower extremities

are consistent with those of other published investigators.

V. COMPLICATIONS OF TISSUE EXPANSION

Reports of complications in the use of tissue expansion are numerous. These reports are usually divided between

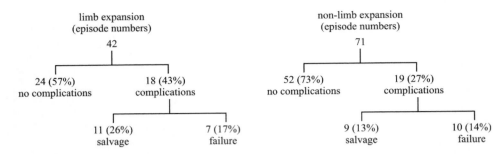

Figure 11.7 Complication rates of limb group vs. nonlimb group. [Reproduced with permission from Pandya et al. (64).]

those in which overall multisite expansion reviews are detailed vs. specific site reviews (i.e., scalp only). In 1984, Manders et al. (31) detailed his experience with 41 expanders in 35 patients as a multisite review. He defined complications as major or minor. Major complications of expansion were those which interrupted the expansion process (Table 11.2). Minor complications were defined as problems which were resolved without failure of the procedure (Table 11.3). In his review, 25% of patients had major complications requiring alterations in the treatment plan and 17% had minor problems,

Table 11.3 Minor Complications of Soft Tissue Expansion

Complications	No. of patients
1. Pain on expansion	3
2. Seroma and drainage after expander inflation	2
3. Dog-ears after advancement	1
4. Widening of scar with time	1

Note: Seventeen percent of expansions were attended by a minor complication.
Source: Reproduced with permission from Manders et al. (31).

Table 11.2 Major Complications of Soft Tissue Expansion

Complications	No. of patients
1. Infection	3
2. Expander exposure	5 (two more incipient exposures)
a. Dehiscence of incision	1
b. Erosion of envelope fold through skin	1 (two incipient)
c. Erosion of envelope or reservour through unadequate covering tissue	2
d. Manipulated by psychotic patients	1
3. Implant failure	1
a. Remote port connector	
b. Physician assembly may be faulty	
c. Injection port may lack proper back	1
d. Envelope may be perforated by needle	
4. Induced ischemia	1
a. Flaps may become ischemic when expanded	1 (recognized and no problem)
b. Irradiated tissue may not survive elevation	1

Note: Twenty-four percent of expansions were attended by a major complication.
Source: Reproduced with permission from Manders et al. (31).

Zellweger and Künzi (65) had similar problems with 5 of 21 patients requiring premature removal of the expander (22%). However, his most frequent minor complication was that of port leakage. Governa et al. (67) documented their experience in 157 patients with 262 expanders. Complete resurfacing of the intended area, however, was obtained in only 62% of the patients. Complications occurred in 27.9% of the expanders. However, 41% of these problems could not be solved and may be classified as major complications (12.6%). Although it is important to note expander complications, the number of patients who experience major complications is more important. This study alludes to only 10 failures in 157 patients.

In a retrospective review of 346 expanders in 132 patients, Pitanguy addressed the issue of re-expansion noted in 42 patients. Although the overall complication rate is low (7.5), it is unclear whether repeat expansions are associated with increased complication rates (2). In 1998, Pisarski et al. (68) shed a different light on multisite expansion studies by detailing their complication rates over two separate time periods. Refinements in techniques, protocols, and surgeon maturity, when all sites are included, reduced complication rates from 30% to 18%. To date, it appears that the overall complication rate for tissue expansion is around 15–20% in spite of advances in techniques and strict protocol procedures.

The number of site-specific studies lends crucial insight into complications associated with the expansion of different regions in the body. Scalp expansion for correction of burn alopecia is well documented (32,40,41). As noted in both scalp expansion reviews as well as multisite studies, the use of tissue expanders for the correction of burn alopecia has revolutionized our thinking as to the correction of this problem (2,31,39,65,67). Of major concern, here, is flap advancement to maintain proper orientation of the hair follicles. Whether or not these wounds are drained does not seem to affect the major complication rate of 12–20%.

In the face and neck region, excluding the scalp, expansion for the correction of facial and neck burn scars is challenging. Antoyshyn et al. (42) in a multisite study, reported an overall complication rate of 43% with the cheek and neck having the highest complication rate of 69%. Neale et al. (44) also experienced high complication rates of nearly 30%. More importantly, however, the long-term follow-up of patients who completed expansion in the head and neck was not uniformly pleasing. They, subsequently, alerted the surgical world to the pitfalls and limitations of this procedure. McCauley and Owiesy (69) presented their series on facial reconstruction using tissue expanders (Fig. 11.4). Although the major complication rate was 16.3%, improvement in facial aesthetics was dramatic. However, as noted by Neale, even small improvements in the reduction of facial scars can have a significant effect on the psychological well-being of these patients.

The use of expanders in the extremities is well documented (55,56,61–63). Regardless of protocols and various techniques, complication rates remain high (Table 11.4). In the upper extremity, complication rates range from 20% to 45%. In the lower extremity, a review of published series has shown complication rates to be as high as 19–45%. Even with adjustments in techniques, paraincisional vs. remote incisions and internal vs. external ports, complication rates remain high (Table 11.5).

It is clear that the use of tissue expanders to correct problems associated with burn scars will be accompanied by significant complication rates, regardless of the specific

Table 11.4 Tissue Expansion in the Limbs

Study	n	Complications (%)	Failures (%)
Manders et al.	35	42	16
Manders et al.	16	70	
Vogelin et al.	34	44	32
Mackinnon and Dellon	8	25	25
Antonyshyn et al.	76	40	17
Zoltie et al.	76	24	12
Cole et al.	6	3	0
Pandya	42	43	17

Source: Reproduced with permission from Pandya et al. (64).

site. It appears that the areas most prone to major complications include the facial neck regions and the extremities. For many patients who experience these problems, the light at the end of the tunnel may not shine as brightly. However, in spite of these problems the overwhelming majority of patients complete the expansion process with excellent results.

VI. CONCLUSIONS

Tissue expanders have reinforced their position in the armamentarium of reconstructive surgery, bringing with it new perspectives. The techniques have been refined, and although complication rates have become less, nonetheless, they remain high. The advantages of this technique are numerous: excellent color and texture match, and minimal donor site morbidity. The disadvantages are well known and include a protracted time period for completion of the expansion process, and a significant complication rate. All patients who are victims of trauma, especially burn injury, want to look and function at their best. Tissue expansion in certain patients offers the chance to replace unstable and unsightly scars with normal adjacent tissue. None of our current reconstructive

Table 11.5 Complications of Tissue Expansion in the Lower Limbs

Authors	No. of cases	No. of prostheses	Mean no. of prostheses per patient	Complication rate (%)	Rate of major complications (%)
Manders et al. (1988)	16	24	1.5	80	47
Jackson et al. (1987)	4	6	1.5	—	25
Antonyshyn et al. (1988)	6	6	1	50	33
Joss et al. (1990)	22			0	0
Esposito et al. (1991)	11	18	1.6	63	45
Meland et al. (1992)	11	21	1.9	30	30
Vögelin et al. (1995)	34	37	1.1	77	68
Wieslander et al. (1996)	5	9	1.8	0	0

Source: Modified with permission from Casanova et al. (63).

techniques offers this advantage. As we continue to refine our approach to certain problems using tissue expansion, it is important to communicate to our patients that although the process may be long and complicated, the end results can be exceptional. Our acceptance of the numerous problems associated with tissue expansion is a testament to the power of this unique reconstructive technique.

REFERENCES

1. Saszki G, Jurkiewicz MJ, Krizk TJ, Mathes S, Ariyan S. In: Tissue Expansion. Plastic Surgery, Principles and Practice. St Louis: Mosby, 1990:1608.
2. Pitanguy I, Gontijo de Amorim NF, Radwanski HN, Lintz JE. Repeated expansion in burn sequela. Burns 2002; 28:494–499.
3. Codivilla A. On a means of lengthening the muscle and tissues in the lower limbs which are shortened and highly deformity. Am J Orthop Surg 1905; 2:353–369.
4. Putti V. Operative lengthening of the femur. J Am Med Assoc 1921; 77:937.
5. Newmann CG. The expansion of an area of skin by progressive distention of a subcutaneous balloon. Plast Reconstr Surg 1957; 19:124–130.
6. Radovan C. Tissue expansion in soft tissue reconstruction. Plast Reconstr Surg 1984; 74:491–492.
7. Austad ED, Pasyk KA, McClatchy KD, Cherry GW. Histomophologic evaluation of guinea pig skin and soft tissue expansion. Plast Reconstr Surg 1982; 70:704–710.
8. Austad ED, Thomas SV, Pasyk KA. Tissue expansion: divided or loan? Plast Reconstr Surg 1986; 78:63–67.
9. Paysk KA, Argenta LC, Austad ED. Histopathology of human expanded skin. Clin Plast Surg 1987; 14:435–445.
10. Paysk KA, Argenta LC, Hassett C. Quantitative analysis of the thickness of human skin and subcutaneous tissue following controlled expansion with a silicone implant. Plast Reconstr Surg 1988; 81:516–523.
11. Pasyk KA, Austad ED, McClatchey KD, Cherry GW. Electron microscopic evaluation of guinea pig skin and soft tissues "expanded" with a self-inflating silicone implant. Plast Reconstr Surg 1982; 70:37–45.
12. Argenta LC, Marks MW, Pasyk KA. Advances in tissue expansion. Clin Plast Surg 1985; 12:159–171.
13. Cherry GW, Austed ED, Pasyk KA, McClatchey KD, Romich RL. Increased survival and vascularity of random pattern skin slaps evaluated in controlled, expanded skin. Plast Reconstr Surg 1983; 72:680–685.
14. Sasaki GH, Pang CY. Pathophysiology of skin flaps raised on expanded skin. Plast Reconstr Surg 1984; 74:59–65.
15. Llantieri LA, Martin-Garcia N, Wechslar, Mitrofaroff M, Rauloy Barueh JP. Vascular endothelial growth factor expressure in expanded tissues: a possible mechanism of anglogenesus in tissue expansion. Plast Reconstr Surg 1998; 101:392–398.
16. Squier CA. The stretching of mouse skin *in vitro*: effect on epidermal proliferation and thickness. J Invest Dermatol 1980; 68:74–78.
17. Takei T, Mills I, Katsuyuki A, Sumpo BE. Molecular basis for tissue expansion: clinical implementation for the surgeon. Plast Reconstr Surg 1998; 101:247–258.
18. Gibney RT. Tissue Expansion in Reconstructive Surgery. Las Vegas: American Society of Plastic Surgery, 1984.
19. Manders EK, Graham WO, Schendon MJ, Davis TS. Skin expansion to eliminate large scalp defects. Ann Plast Surg 1984; 12:305–312.
20. Brohmann GF, Huber J. Effects of different shaped tissue expanders on translomal pressure, oxygen tension, histopathologic changes and skin expansion. Plast Reconstr Surg 1985; 70:731–736.
21. Duits EHA, Molenzan J, Van Rappaed. The modeling of skin expanders. Plast Reconstr Surg 1989; 83:362–365.
22. Van Rappard JHA, Molenaan J, Van Door N, Sonneveld GS, Borghouts JMH. Surface area increase in tissue expansion. Plast Reconstr Surg 1988; 82:833–837.
23. Jackson IT, Sharpe DT, Polley J, Costanzo C, Rosenberg L. Use of external reservoirs in tissue expansion. Plast Reconstr Surg 1987; 80:266–273.
24. Lozano S, Drucker M. Use of tissue expanders with external ports. Ann Plast Surg 2000; 44:14–17.
25. Meland NB, Loessin SJ, Thimson D, Jackson IT. Tissue expansion in the extremities using external reservoirs. Ann Plast Surg 1992; 29:36–39.
26. Friedman RM, Ingram AE, Rohnch RJ et al. Risk factors for complications in pediatric tissue expansion. Plast Reconstr Surg 1996; 98:1242–1246.
27. Pietila JP, Nordstrom REA, Virkkunen PJ, Voutilzinen PEJ, Rintala AE. Accelerated tissue expansion with the overfilling technique. Plast Reconstr Surg 1988; 81:204–207.
28. Goldstein RD, Schuler SH. Methlene blue: a simple adjunct to aid in soft tissue expansion. Plast Reconstr Surg 1986; 180:452.
29. Hudson DA. Maximizing the use of expanded flaps. Br J Plast Surg 2003; 56:784–790.
30. Austad E, Rose G. A self-inflating tissue expander. Plast Reconst Surg 1982; 70:588–594.
31. Manders EK, Schenden MJ, Ferrey JA, Hetzler OT, Davis TS, Grahm WP. Soft tissue expansion: concepts and complications. Plast Reconstr Surg 1984; 74:493–507.
32. Marks M. Argenta LC, Thornton JW. Burn management: the role of tissue expansion. Clin Plast Surg 1987; 14:453–548.
33. MacLennon SE, Corcoran JF, Neale, HW. Tissue expansion in head and neck burn reconstruction. Clin Plast Surg 2000; 27:121–132.
34. Huang TT, Larson DL, Lewis SR. Burn alopecia. Plast Reconstr Surg 1977; 60:762–767.
35. Ortichochea M. Four flap scalp reconstruction technique. Br J Plast Surg 1971; 24:184–188.
36. Ortichochea M. New three flap scalp reconstruction technique. Br J Plast Surg 1967; 20:159–171.
37. Juri J. The use of parieto–occipital flaps in the treatment of baldness. Plast Reconstr Surg 1975; 55:456–460.
38. Juri J, Juri C. Aesthetic aspects of reconstructive scalp surgery. Clin Plast Surg 1981; 8:243–254.
39. Felman G. Post-thermal burn alopecia and its treatment using extensive horizontal scalp reduction in combination with a juri flap. Plast Reconstr Surg 1994; 93:1268–1272.

40. McCauley RL, Oliphant JR, Robson MC. Tissue expansion in the correction of burn alopecia; classification and methods of correction. Ann Plast Surg 1990; 25:103–115.

41. Buhrer DP, Huang TT, Yee HD. Treatment of burn alopecia with tissue expansion in children. Plast Reconstr Surg 1988; 82:840–845.

42. Antonyshyn O, Gruss JS, Zucker R, MacKinnon SE. Tissue expansion in head and neck reconstruction. Plast Reconstr Surg 1988; 82:58–68.

43. Argenta LC, Watanobe MJ, Grabb WC. The use of tissue expansion in head and neck reconstruction. Ann Plast Surg 1983; 11:31–37.

44. Neale HW, Kurtzman, Goh KBC, Billmire DA, Yakuboff KP, Wanden G. Tissue expanders in the lower face and anterior neck in pediatric burn patients; limitations and pitfalls. Plast Reconstr Surg 1993; 91:624–631.

45. Lapin R, Dani E, Hutchin H et al. Primary breast reconstruction following mastectomy using skin expander prosthesis. Breast 1980; 6:97–100.

46. Hafezi F, Boddouhi N, Nouh AH. Reconstruction of the burned breast. Ann Burn Fire Disaster 2002; 15:1–5.

47. Castello PR, Garro L, Majera D, Mirelis E, Sanchez-Olaso A, Barros J. Immediate breast reconstruction in two stages using anatomic tissue expansions. Scan J Plast Reconstr Surg Hand Surg 2000; 34:167–171.

48. Loss M, Infanger M, Künzi W, Meyer VE. The burned female breast: a report of four cases. Burns 2002; 28:601–605.

49. Still J, Craft-Coffman B, Law E. Use of pedicled flaps and tissue expanders to reconstruct burn scars of the skin of the anterior abdomen and chest. Ann Plast Surg 1998; 40(3):229–238.

50. McCauley RL, Stenberg BA, Phillips LG, Blackwell SJ, Robson MC. Long-term assessment of the effects of circumferential truncal burns in pediatric patients on subsequent pregnancies. J Burn Care Rehabil 1991; 12(1):51–53.

51. Del Frari B, Pülzl P, Schoeller T, Widschwendter M, Weschselberger G. Pregnancy as a tissue expander in the correction of scar deformity. Am J Obstet Gynecol 2004; 190:579–580.

52. Braye FM, Preton P, Caillot JL. Preoperative pneumoperitoneum used for tissue expansion before abdominal wall reconstruction. Ann Plast Surg 2003; 50(6):649–652.

53. Morgan RF, Edgerton MT. Tissue expansion in reconstructive hand surgery: case report. J Hand Surg 1985; 10A:754–757.

54. Mackinnon SE, Gruss JS. Soft tissue expander in upper limb surgery. J Hand Surg 1985; 10A:749–754.

55. Van Beek AL, Adson MH. Tissue expansion in the upper extremity. Clin Plast Surg 1987; 14(3):535–542.

56. Carneiro R, Dichiara J. A protocol for tissue expansion in upper extremity reconstruction. J Hand Surg 1991; 16A:147–151.

57. Aubert JP. Paulhe P. Magalon G. Skin expansion in the upper limb. Ann Chir Plast Esthét 1993; 38(1):34–40.

58. Cole WG, Bennett CS, Perks AGV, McManamny DS, Barnett JS. Tissue expansion in the lower limbs of children and young adults. J Bone Joint Surg 1990; 78B(4):578–580.

59. Waiter E, Georgieu N, Manise O, Husson JL, Pailheret JP. Use of tissue expansion in revision of unhealed below-knee amputation stumps. Scand J Plast Reconstr Hand Surg 2001; 35:193–196.

60. Manders EK, Oaks TE, Au VK, Wong RKM, Furrey JA, Davis TS, Graham III WP. Soft-tissue expansion in the lower extremities. Plast Reconstr Surg 1988; 81(2):208–217.

61. Filho PTB, Neves RI, Gemperli R, Kaweski S, Kahler SH, Banducci DR, Manders EK. Soft-tissue expansion in lower extremity reconstruction. Clin Plast Surg 1991; 18(3):593–599.

62. Vögelin E, de Roche R, Lüscher NJ. Is soft tissue expansion in lower limb reconstruction a legitimate option? Br J Plast Surg 1995; 48:579–582.

63. Casanova D, Bali D, Bardot J, Legre R, Magalon G. Tissue expansion of the lower limb: complications in a cohort of 103 cases. Br J Plast Surg 2001; 54:310–316.

64. Pandya AN, Vadodaria S, Coleman DJ. Tissue expansion in the limbs: a comparative analysis of limb and non-limb sites. Br J Plast Surg 2002; 55:302–306.

65. Zellweger G, Künzi W. Tissue expanders in reconstruction of burn sequelea. Ann Plast Surg 1991; 26:380–388.

66. Rees RS, Nanney LB, Fleming P, Cary A. Tissue expansion: its role in traumatic below-knee amputations. Plast Reconstr Surg 1986; 77(1):133–137.

67. Governa M, Bortolani A, Beghini D, Barisoni D. Skin expansion in burn sequelea: results and complications. Acta Chir Plast 1996; 38(4):147–153.

68. Pisarski GP, Mertens D, Warden GD, Neal HW. Tissue expander complications in the pediatric burn patient. Plast Reconstr Surg 1998; 102(4):1008–1012.

69. McCauley RL, Owiesy F. Aesthetic reconstruction of facial burns in expanded cervicofacial flaps. Proc Am Burn Assoc 2001; 22:91.

70. Neale HW, High RM, Billmire DA, Carey JP, Smith D, Warden G. Complications of controlled tissue expansion in the pediatric burn patient. Plast Reconstr Surg 1988; 82:840–845.

71. Radovan C. Breast reconstruction after mastectomy using the temporary expander. Plast Reconstr Surg 1982; 69:195–208.

12

Management of Pigmentation Changes in Burn Patients

PREMA DHANRAJ

Christian Medical College & Hospital, Vellore, Tamil Nadu, India

ROBERT L. McCAULEY

University of Texas Medical Branch and Shriners Hospital for Children—Galveston Unit, Galveston, Texas, USA

I. INTRODUCTION

With advances in the management of acute burns, the survival rates following extensive burns have increased. However, even with early wound closure, the end result of such injuries is a scar (1,2). Burn scars remain a lasting reminder of the insult for both the patient and the outside world (3,4). Scarring is further complicated by the limited availability of local tissue in patients who have survived major total body surface area burns. In addition, poor color match often complicates the

functional and aesthetic disfigurement associated with these injuries (5). Hence, the challenges in the burn care begin to highlight issues related to functional rehabilitation and quality of life (6,7). Currently, the goals of treatment are no longer mere survival, but the return of the patient to a meaningful and productive life. Consequently, management of the burn wound and its impact on pigmentation changes and scarring becomes a more focused issue.

With current technology, reconstructive surgeons can alter appearance and lessen the scarring associated with severe burns. Yet, in spite of aesthetic unit restoration for facial burns, the regular use of postoperative splinting, pressure garments, and silicone conformers and an emphasis on physical appearance, patients are still often left with scars and pigmentation differences as a constant reminder of a devastating injury (8–11). These issues may impact quality of life issues in a society that places such tremendous emphasis on physical beauty.

The psychological effects of visible scars has a significant impact on recovery from burn injuries (12–14). Since burns in other parts of the body have less impact on the patient's social and psychological behavior, a more focused outlook on improving the facial appearance of patients with visible scars is of paramount importance (15–17).

Pigmentation changes are common sequelae of burn injury. The pathophysiology of most pigmentation changes is not well understood. However, some studies have shown that scar tissue laid down after healing by secondary intention provides a barrier to both the transfer of melanin to keratinocytes and melanocyte migration (18). This makes reconstruction of burn patients more difficult. It has been noted that most burn injuries, particularly deep partial-thickness and full-thickness burns, when allowed to heal by secondary intention, leave behind not only significant problems with contracture but also pigmentation changes (19–21). Pigmentation differences can be either hyperpigmentation or hypopigmentation. Although these pigmentary changes improve with time, most often hypopigmentation persists, especially in areas such as head and neck, hands, wrist, and feet.

Skin pigmentation is due to melanin synthesized by melanocytes. Nordlund (22) studied the biology of pigmentation and noted that the color of the skin is determined by the quality, distribution, and type of the melanin in the epidermis. Willier et al. (23) in 1921 were the first to observe that melanocyte was the only cell to synthesize melanin and was present in the basal layer of the epidermis. Breathnach (24) described the functional component of epidermal melanin unit where melanin gets transferred to keratinocytes. This whole process he referred to as epidermal melanin unit.

Fitzpatrick and Szabo (25) discussed the morphogenesis of melanosomes and the four processes that occur during the melanin pigmentation in man. An understanding of these four processes, the formation, melanization, transfer, and degradation of melanosomes, provides a sound basis for the type of influence an agent can have at these different stages. The influence can either stimulate or inhibit melanocyte function. The factors which affect the pigmentation can be either local destruction of melanocytes or inhibition of their function.

In deep burns, damage to deeper layers of epidermis results in hypopigmentation due to destruction of melanocytes (26). The ability to repigment depends on the migration of melanocytes either from adjacent normal skin or from hair follicles. This process is possible if the hypopigmented area is very small. On the other hand, if the hypopigmented area is large, it is very unlikely to repigment. Breathnach (24) studied human scars at the second and third weeks following excisional wounds. He noted that the peripheral scar areas had reduced numbers of melanocytes, whereas the central areas had a complete absence of these cells. The resultant hypopigmentation is, therefore, permanent and causes severe disability, particularly in dark-skinned individuals. Other factors responsible for hypopigmentation are the absence of hair follicles in burned areas. This also leads to a reduced number of melanocytes resulting in permanent hypopigmentation. Although temporary improvement can be achieved by the use of camouflage creams, permanent treatment requires replacement of scarred tissue with normal pigmented skin.

Repigmentation occurs by a process of "pigment spread phenomenon" where melanocytes migrate from a pigmented area into the surrounding nonpigmented area (27–34). Falabella (35) presumed this process to be related to the ability of melanocytes to migrate from the graft into the hypopigmented skin. He referred to the process as the "melanocyte migration theory." Onur and Atabay (36) also based their treatment of hypopigmentation on this melanocyte migration theory by using split-thickness skin grafts.

Hyperpigmentation is occasionally seen following superficial burns. This occurs mainly due to the inflammatory process. Nordlund (22) reported that postinflammatory hyperpigmentation occurs for two reasons. The first is due to the dropping of pigments from epidermis into dermis, where they are ingested by dermal macrophages. Such a condition he called as "dermal melanosis." The second process occurs because of increased melanocyte activity following inflammation. He also discussed the management of postinflammatory hyperpigmentation based on whether they were caused by either epidermal or dermal hyperpigmentation.

As noted, hyperpigmentation is also seen in both split-thickness skin grafts and the donor site (37). This is attributed to both overactive melanocytes and altered melanocyte control following reinnervation of the skin graft. Hyperpigmentation of burned skin and skin grafts can also be due to melanin darkening, melanin migration, and melanin formation. Melanin darkening occurs within a few minutes after exposure to sunlight. Postinflammatory pigmentation seen in burns is due to melanin migration which occurs several days after exposure to sunlight.

Erythematous red immature scars seen after the burn injuries are the result of a complex sequence of events. If an injury is of sufficient depth to involve the reticular portion of dermis, the formation of a hypertrophic scar is likely. These scars are characterized by a reddened elevated hard mass of tissue. Studies by Dierickx and

Goldman (38) have shown that the immature scars have increased vascularization due to angiogenesis. Also, as scars mature, the angiogenesis process regresses resulting in fading of the red color. Clearly, the changes in pigmentation and our inability to control color changes compromises even the best of reconstructive efforts.

II. PATHOPHYSIOLOGY

Gilchrest and Goldwyn (39) studied the process of pigmentation and melanin metabolism extensively and reported human skin to have four pigments. Melanin which is brown or black is present in the basal layer of the epidermis. The yellow pigment of carotene is found in the dermis and in the keratinocytes of the epidermis. Oxygenated hemoglobin, which is red, is present in the dermal capillaries. Reduced hemoglobin, which is blue in color, is in the dermal venules (19,31). All four pigments contribute to the color of the skin. However, melanin is responsible not only for determining skin color, but also for protecting the skin from ultraviolet (UV) light (40).

The color of the skin is determined by the quantity and distribution of the melanin in the epidermis, the process of melanin synthesis, and the location of the melanin in the skin (22,41,42). The more superficial the melanin pigment, the darker its appearance. A thick layer of superficial melanin absorbs light and appears black. There are two types of melanin. Eumelanin, which is brown or black in color and synthesized from tyrosine, and pheomelanin, which is red is synthesized from tyrosine and cysteine. The total quantity and ratio of eumelanin to pheomelanin in the epidermal cells are responsible for the hue and color of the skin.

Melanin synthesis requires tyrosinase and tyrosine, which is found in the melanocyte. The enzyme tyrosinase converts tyrosine to dihydroxyphenalalanine (DOPA) and then DOPA to DOPA quinone and finally to melanin. UV light can also cause this conversion without tyrosinase. The melanoblast is a precursor to the mature melanocyte and is derived from the neural crest. It migrates from neural crest into the dermis and then into the basal layer of epidermis. Melanoblasts appear in the dermis and the melanocytes in the epidermis.

Melanosomes are membrane organelles seen in the cytoplasm of the melanocyte. Konrad and Wolff (37) studied the size and the distribution of melanosomes in both dark-skinned and light-skinned individuals. They observed that melanosomes were found to be larger in dark-skinned people, were transferred individually, and offer more protection against UV light. In fair-complexioned individuals, the melanosomes were smaller, were transferred in groups by a membrane, and provided lesser protection against UV light.

Table 12.1 Pigmentation Changes in Fitzpatrick Skin Types

Skin type	Color	Responses to sun
1	White	Always burn, never tan
2	White	Usually burn, tan with difficulty
3	White	Sometimes mild burn, tan average
4	Moderate brown	Rarely burn, tan with ease
5	Dark brown	Very rarely burn, tan very easily
6	Black	Never burn, tan very easily

Source: Reprinted with permission from Fitzpatrick (44).

Biosynthesis of melanin was studied extensively by Lerner (43) and Fitzpatrick in 1950. Fitzpatrick (44) classified skin into six types based on color and response to sunlight. This classification scheme has been very useful in predicting responses to a number of surgical procedures. Pigmentation changes occur least in Fitzpatrick skin types 1 and 2. However, pigmentation changes are frequent in Fitzpatrick skin types 4–6 (Table 12.1).

III. HISTOLOGY

Taki et al. (18) reported the histological findings of the depigmented, repigmented, and skin graft specimens. Hematoxylin and eosin staining and DOPA reaction showed that depigmented skin to have marked thickening of all layers with sparse amounts of melanin pigment in the basal cells. The scar tissue caused by deep partial- and full-thickness burns had no DOPA-positive melanocytes, whereas the repigmented skin showed dense granular melanin pigmentation in the basal cells. The skin after grafting showed a normal number of DOPA-positive melanocytes. The depigmented skin also showed no hair follicles. They concluded that deep partial-thickness and full-thickness burns which caused hypopigmentation would not respond to oral psoralen, sunlight exposure or topical administration of steroids. Only, autografting would return pigmentation. Kahn and Cohen (21) from their experience also believe that hypopigmented scar tissue had either an absent or a decreased concentration of hair follicles. Since hair follicles are the major source of melanocytes, surgical treatment is an option to repigment these regions.

IV. TREATMENT

A. Hyperpigmentation Following Superficial Burns

Management of pigmentation changes following burns has always been a challenge for plastic surgeons. Skin care following burns begins as soon as all the raw surfaces have been healed. Following superficial burns, pinpoint brown color pigment is seen in the newly healed skin due to melanocyte migration (45,46). Avoidance of sunlight exposure for six months or longer has been recommended after wound healing to avoid development of permanent hyperpigmentation (12,47). In view of the variable delays in the return of melanocytes, long periods of photoprotection appear warranted. Use of hats, appropriate clothing, timing of outdoor activities, and cosmetically effective topical sunscreen are recommended. If pigmentation is mainly epidermal, it may fade to a great extent over 6 months to several years (21). But, if hyperpigmentation is due to dermal melanosis, then it will persist. The treatment for pigmentation differences is long, often requiring 6–12 months.

de Chalain et al. (48) discussed pigmentation changes which occur after superficial burn injury (Figs. 12.1 and 12.2). They grouped the patients according to Fitzpatrick skin type based on skin color and response to sun exposure. They believed that in the early phase of healing, the typical superficial burn wound is hyperemic, but relatively hypopigmented. This changes over time. Burn injuries are likely to repigment within 1–3 years depending on skin color and sun responsiveness as well as the degree of UV light exposure. Boochai and Mutou

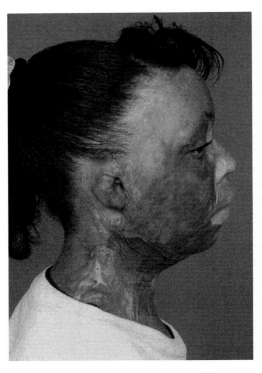

Figure 12.2 (See color insert) Ten-year-old black female with cheek hyperpigmentation after partial-thickness flame burns; note: hyperpigmentation of grafts after application to the right side of the neck.

(49) attribute hyperpigmentation to sun exposure and race. Ship and Weiss (50) reported few pigmentation problems with a regimen of strict sun protection for at least 6 months after dermabrasion. They concluded that skin color and UV exposure are both determining factors in the pigmentary response to a partial-thickness skin injury. However, several treatment options are available.

B. Nonsurgical Methods

1. Chemical Depigmentation by Hydroquinone

Hydroquinone is a hydroxy phenolic chemical used as a depigmenting agent in bleaching creams. It inhibits the conversion of tyrosine to DOPA and DOPA to melanin by inhibiting the enzyme tyrosinase. Hydroquinone is also known to cause both the degradation of melanosomes and the destruction of melanocytes. Thus, reversible depigmentation may occur on short-term application. However, irreversible depigmentation after prolonged application is attributed to the death of the melanocytes (42).

Grimes and Stockton (51) studied darker ethnic groups using hydroquinone in bleaching creams. When used alone, the efficacy of hydroquinone depends on its concentration. As the concentration increases, the efficacy also increases to a certain point. The problem is that skin

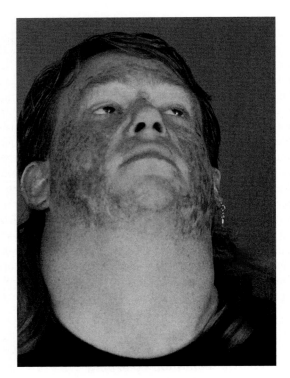

Figure 12.1 (See color insert) Fifteen-year-old white male status postsuperficial partial-thickness burns with facial hyperpigmentation.

irritation becomes more prominent. It is also noted that higher concentration does not produce good results (52). Hydroquinone in combination with other chemical products such as tretinoin has more therapeutic effect than hydroquinone alone. Tretinoin acts by improving epidermal penetration and increasing keratinocyte proliferation. The addition of steroids has the capacity to decrease the irritation effect of hydroquinone and is helpful in obtaining good results.

A combination of 4% hydroquinone, 0.05% retinoic acid, and 0.25% triamcinolone acetonide in a cream base results in depigmentation when applied twice daily for 6 weeks. Steroids also block tyrosinase when applied with 4% hydroquinone. Thus, the effectiveness is much more than what is achieved when hydroquinone is applied alone. Retin-A used in combination with steroid and hydroquinone enhances the desquamation of keratinocytes containing melanin (22,53). At 3 weeks, studies have shown that there is diminution in the number of melanosomes and in the number of actively functioning melanocytes. Consequently, this appears to be a safe agent for treating hyperpigmentation changes in skin grafts. The downside is that it causes contact dermatitis, postinflammatory pigmentation changes, nail bleaching, and permanent depigmentation. Hydroquinone can be used alone or in combination with other agents.

2. Chemical Peels

Chemical peels, also known as chemexfoliation or dermapeeling, is the application of a chemical agent to the skin resulting in partial destruction of the epidermis and dermis with subsequent regeneration (54,55). The result is the smoothing of surface irregularities and alterations in skin pigmentation. Their utilization in burn patients may not be applicable since these patients have few epidermal appendages for reepithelialization. Regardless, caution should also be exercised when peeling Fitzpatrick types 4–6 skin. Thick and oily skin responds less favorably and has a greater tendency to develop hyperpigmentation. Men, due to thicker skin, do not respond as well as women (29,56). Depending on the depth of penetration produced when they are applied, peeling agents are divided into superficial, medium, and deep. The most commonly used agents are phenol and trichloroacetic acid (TCA) (57,58).

3. Topical Sunscreens

A sunscreen is a photoprotective agent designed to reduce the effects of UV radiation from the sun. It acts by absorption, reflection, or scattering of solar rays. Upon application, sunscreens act as filters and inhibit the penetration of UV rays (UVR) to the cells of epidermis and dermis and thereby reduce pigmentation changes.

The other photoprotecting measures are clothing and sun avoidance. A commonly used sunscreen is para amino benzoic acid (PABA). The most common measure of sunscreen effectiveness is a sun protection factor (SPF) of 15 or greater (59). Sunscreens should be applied once a day in the morning to give protection against the sun which lasts the entire day (60). The benefits are numerous. The amount of actinic keratosis is reduced after its application. Sunscreen should be applied 15–30 min before actual solar exposure and then frequently reapplied while in the sun for sustained protection (61).

Sunscreens are classified into physical and chemical. Physical sunscreens are opaque and act by reflection and scattering UV rays. The various ingredients are zinc oxide, talc, titanium dioxide, and petrolatum (62). The advantages of physical sunscreens are that they are visible and easy to see when applied, give an excellent coverage against UV alpha and beta rays, and rarely cause allergy. The disadvantage is that because of their opaque qualities, these agents are noticeable, and can rub off easily. Chemical sunscreens contain agents to absorb UVR. They act as filters and inhibit penetration of UVR to epidermis and dermis. The most common agent used is PABA and its esters. The esters lower the potential for allergic reactions. SPF of 15 is adequate for lesser amount of sun exposure and SPF of >30 for a full day of exposure in summer months (63). These agents bind to the horny layer of the epidermis and have a protective action against sunlight for 3–4 days. They can be incorporated into lotions, creams, gels, and cosmetic formulations. The disadvantages of chemical sunscreens are twofold. PABA can cause contact dermatitis and may stain clothing.

4. Freezing

In 1988, Nordlund et al. (22) used freezing as a method to reduce the hyperpigmented color of skin. This concept is based on the fact that the cold sensitive melanocytes are destroyed. The therapeutic use of liquid nitrogen can result in a temporary or permanent loss of pigmentation in the treatment site. However, caution should be used when treating darker skin (22). In addition, the treatment of large areas is not only dangerous but also impractical.

5. Cosmetic Therapy

Cosmetic camouflage is the application of special makeup to conceal scars and pigmentation changes and other imperfections of the skin (64,65). It is a therapy to alleviate the suffering of those who have been disfigured and, until now, had little choice as to how to camouflage pigmentation differences. Although the benefits of cosmetic camouflage are numerous, its use has not been given a high level of priority in the rehabilitation of the burned patients. The products used by the medical makeup specialist have no gender or racial limitation (Figs. 12.3 and 12.4). They are durable and can be used successfully to camouflage lesions all over the body. However, correct cosmetic selection and proper application are very important to avoid the mask-like appearance (66,67).

There are many brands of cosmetics. All have the same goal of concealing pigmentation scars. It is easy to camouflage any size of the pigmented scars, but it is the texture of the scar which is difficult to conceal. Rough scars are more

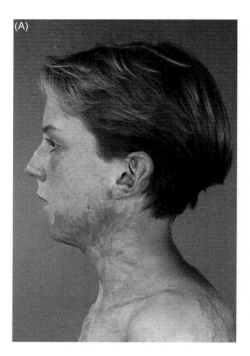

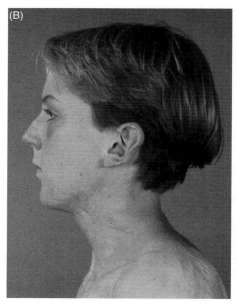

Figure 12.4 (See color insert) (A) Fourteen-year-old white male with hyperpigmentation of chin and neck. (B) After corrective makeup to improve appearance.

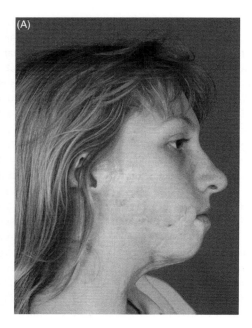

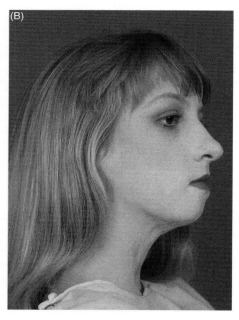

Figure 12.3 (See color insert) (A) Fifteen-year-old white female with areas of hyperpigmentation and hypopigmentation. (B) After corrective makeup to conceal imperfections.

difficult because of the irregular surface. Such scars are best camouflaged with darker shade pigment. But, if there is a depressed scar, then a pigment of lighter shade than the surrounding skin is used to even the surface.

Camouflage techniques can be used either to conceal completely or to blend pigments. Complete concealment is a method wherein the makeup extends beyond the lesion to involve normal skin. Pigment blending is a method that involves selecting a cream that matches the foundation. Selection of foundation depends on the patients' natural skin color. The use of a complimentary color can help mask a particular skin problem. For example, a green base is used for red or hypertrophic scars and a yellow base is used for white or hypopigmented scars (68) (Figs. 12.4 and 12.5). Both bases are used as counter balance correctors. Either can be applied under the foundation to match individual skin tones. Color blending is one of the keys to the successful use of makeup to camouflage scars.

A trained therapist with clinical knowledge and therapeutic skills not only helps patients to achieve a positive self-image but also helps reduce fears about cosmetic camouflage and educates them in the daily application of makeup. A medical makeup specialist may work as an adjunct to a physician's practice and communicates with the medical personnel to determine the patient's cosmetic needs. They should possess sensitivity and nurturing qualities to understand and fulfill patients' needs (69). A good cosmetic should have the following characteristics. It should be natural looking, opaque, easy to apply, waterproof, long lasting and fragrance free, and available for use by all skin types. In addition, it should be hypoallergenic and noncarcinogenic (70,71). The different types

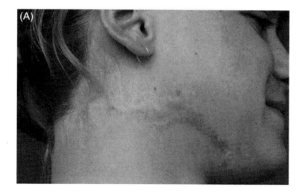

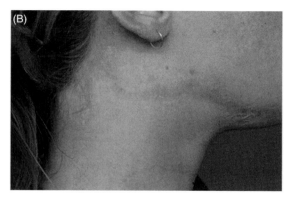

Figure 12.5 (**See color insert**) (A) Mature but red hyperpigmented cheek scar. (B) Green base for camouflage of red scars.

of camouflage makeup available are foundation, regular cosmetics, and corrective cosmetics (72).

Foundation is used to cover slight imperfections and gives excellent coverage with a velvety look. Pigments in the foundation are based on actual skin tones. This enables the person to perfectly match skin tones (73). It not only camouflages pigmentation changes, but also acts as a physical sunscreen protector. It is applied to the entire face and is available in the form of a cake, cream, stick, and lotion. Foundation is suitable for all skin types (Figs. 12.6 and 12.7). There are four basic facial foundations—oil based, water based, oil free, and water free. Oil based products are designed for dry skin and create a moist feeling of the skin. Water based foundations are generally used for normal skin. Oil free foundations are used for oily skin, but they tend to leave the skin feeling dry. Water free foundations are waterproof with a high concentration of pigment yielding an opaque character to camouflage lesions better than the other types of foundations. Unfortunately, a regular foundation cannot conceal burn scars, which is why corrective cosmetics were developed.

Corrective cosmetics contain a higher concentration of pigments. They are waterproof, lightweight, and comfortable. These are most effective when applied over pigmented areas and are available in the form of a cream. The technique of application is very important in order to achieve the goal of natural long-lasting color matching (65,74–76). However, unlike the foundation type of cosmetics, the corrective type is used to camouflage primarily over the lesion. The advantage of corrective cosmetics is that they are available in many shades. Occasionally, the blending of several shades achieves the best results. However, it is important to remember that as with all cosmetics, less is better than more (77).

Setting powder is translucent and essential to prevent smearing and the rubbing off of the corrective cosmetics thus allowing corrective cosmetics to have a long-lasting effect. The treated areas are thus water proof and rub resistant (75). Facial powder is applied after application of makeup to provide smoothness to the skin. It also absorbs oil and perspiration. It is available in compact form and in three shades, that is, light, medium, and dark. It imparts a matte finish to the face. Face powder not only improves sun protection qualities but also allows facial products to remain in place. It may require reapplication throughout the day.

Regular cosmetics are nonopaque and do not conceal scars and pigmentation. However, these are used along with the camouflage makeup to add color and enhance beauty. Blush adds vitality to the cheeks, lipstick adds color to the lips, and eye makeup is also used for enhancement (66). Every patient should understand the types of cosmetics available and be encouraged to use them. The knowledge of cosmetics can help each patient improve their social and emotional security. Although cosmetics

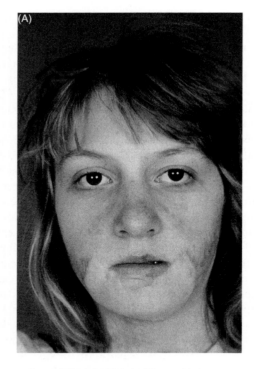

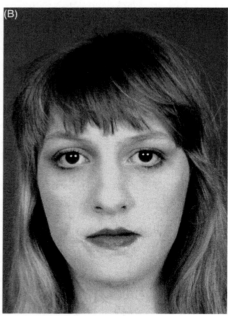

Figure 12.6 (**See color insert**) (A) Sixteen-year-old white female before corrective cosmetics with hyperpigmented scars. (B) Sixteen-year-old female after application of corrective cosmetics to even out skin tones.

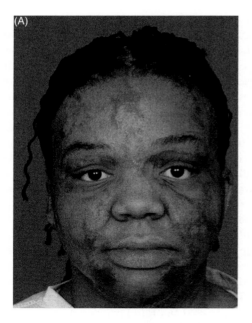

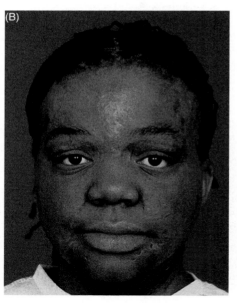

Figure 12.7 (**See color insert**) (A) Fourteen-year-old black female with hyperpigmented areas over facial region before corrective makeup. (B) Same patient after minimal application of corrective cosmetics.

are mainly used by women, they are available for use by men and children to camouflage scars and pigmentation changes (Figs. 12.8 and 12.9). Women use cosmetics daily to enhance their physical appearance. It is important that these camouflage techniques fit the patient's lifestyle (71).

Men, due to obvious disadvantages such as facial hair, tend not to use camouflage techniques. Makeup for men requires a more intricate approach, and if properly motivated and instructed, male patients become comfortable using these topical aids. Makeup in children, on the other hand, should be limited to as little as possible to maintain the appearance of a normal child. In reality, here, less is better.

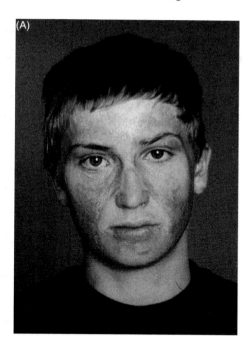

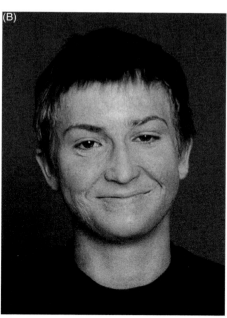

Figure 12.8 (**See color insert**) (A) Sixteen-year-old white male with facial hypopigmentation. (B) Same patient after corrective makeup.

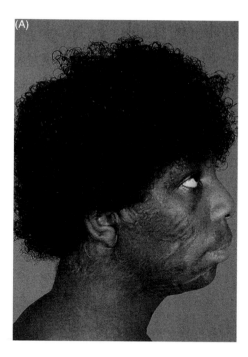

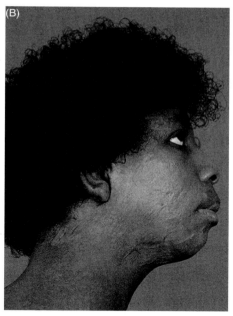

Figure 12.9 (**See color insert**) (A) Seventeen-year-old black female with hyperpigmented burn scars over facial region. (B) Same patient with corrective makeup.

V. SURGICAL THERAPY

A. Primary Excision

1. Grafts

If the lesion is very small, the hyperpigmented scar can be excised and the wound closed primarily. Moderate-size scars can be serially excised when the surrounding tissue is normal and elastic. Local advancement and rotation flaps can also be used when sufficient surrounding skin permits the procedure. The goal is elimination of the hyperpigmented regions with as little scarring as possible (78).

The excision of pigmented scars and resurfacing with skin grafts is risky. Improvement to appearance may not be guaranteed. Takao and Iso (79) noted that excision and resurfacing of defects with split-thickness skin grafts have unfavorable results due to contour deformity and donor site morbidity (79). Needless to say, postgraft hyperpigmentation is still possible.

Dermabrasion is the surgical process by which the superficial layers of the skin are removed by sanding and using motor driven dermabrader with a diamond or conical burr. It is used to abrade scars with irregular surfaces in an attempt to produce a more even surface. This process removes the epidermis and superficial dermis at and above the level of the papillary dermis. Paul Kurtin in New York first introduced the concept of dermabrasion about 50 years ago. Norman Orentreich and Jim Burke further refined his technique. Tom Alt introduced the diamond fraize and John Yarborough introduced the wire brush. Dermabrasion has been shown to be a powerful resurfacing treatment in scar management (80,81). The advantage of dermabrasion is that the depth of abrasion is controllable and that it gives a uniform surface with pleasing results, particularly in the aesthetic facial units. The disadvantages include possible color mismatch. Another common complication can be postdermabrasion milia.

B. Treatment of Hyperpigmentation of Skin Grafts

Lagrot et al. (82) in 1960 believed that factors such as exposure to the sun, in addition to hormonal factors, increased pigmentation in free grafts. Lorengo also supported the hypothesis of Lerner that there is a relationship between reinnervation of the grafts and hyperpigmentation since cutaneous nerve endings can have excessive production of melanin.

Hyperpigmentation seen after application of grafts occurs sometimes in spite of careful selection of donor site. The pigmentation changes which occur constitute a major aesthetic problem. Tsukada (83) in his studies on pigmentation of skin grafts found that keratinocytes of hyperpigmented skin grafts have increased numbers of large, deeply pigmented melanosomes when compared to the skin grafts which did not hyperpigment. Other factors responsible for pigmentation changes in these grafts are due to alterations in melanocyte control following the reinnervation of grafts. He concluded that it is best to treat hyperpigmented patches once the graft is fully reinnervated.

Hyperpigmentation of the grafted skin may also be due to several other factors, namely solar exposure, racial predisposition, and graft contraction (63). Conway and Sedar (84) suggested that contraction of the graft resulted in a closer approximation of the melanin particles within it (84). Tsukada (83) found that hyperpigmentation was also due to an excessive, overactive, and persistent accumulation of the melanin content in these grafts. He suggested that this may result from altered melanocyte control following reinnervation. The coloration of a skin graft appears to be regulated not only by the melanogenesis but also by unknown effects from reinnervation of the graft. It has been known that split-thickness skin grafts have a greater tendency to develop abnormal pigmentation than full-thickness skin grafts.

When split-thickness skin grafts are reharvested from a donor site, hyperpigmentation of the second graft may be less. Multiple graft harvests seem to prevent melanin hyperpigmentation of the graft as the amount of melanin pigment is thought to be less than in the normal skin (38,48). However, de-epithelization skin grafts have not been ideal compared to the decolorized previous donor area (85). It is unclear as to whether hyperpigmented skin grafts treated with dermabrasion with or without overgrafting are of benefit.

C. Treatment of Hypopigmentation Changes

Considering that the epidermis damaged in burn injuries results in destruction of melanocytes, hypopigmentation is a phenomenon seen less than hyperpigmentation. However, when present, particularly in patients of color, hypopigmentation is physically striking. To addressing this problem there are nonsurgical options and surgical options. The surgical methods in treating hypopigmented areas are similar to those outlined in the management of hyperpigmentation and will not be reiterated. However, the concept of dermabrasion and overgrafting will be discussed.

1. Nonsurgical Options

Micropigmentation (Tattooing)

Tattooing in medical terminology is defined as a process of permanent deposition of color fast pigment into the skin. The traditional tattoo was first started by Japanese in the 17th century and was known as painting or body decoration. Medical tattooing dates back to 1835 when it was used for congenital purple plaques. Although the popular decorative tattooing is often completed in one session, the medical tattoo requires more skill and, occasionally, multiple sessions to achieve a natural shade. Medical tattooing is time consuming but the results are remarkable (28,36,54,86,87). The practice of medical tattoos was first popularized by van der Velden who learned this technique from the traditional Japanese master Horiken in the early 1980s. Since then, van der Velden and others have studied its medical and cosmetic aspects (88–90). In 1984, van der Velden refined the art of tattooing when he applied this technique to treat hypopigmented areas in burn patients. Multiple sessions were required as compared to the popular decorative tattooing which was often completed in one session. Tattooing provides a safe and reliable alternative method of repigmenting hypopigmented areas. The current system consists of an electric tattooing machine with a cluster of 3–18 needles set for a depth and maximum speed. Nonallergenic iron oxide pigment is tattooed into the skin by means of a high-speed reciprocating drill. This apparatus consists of a main unit to which a hand piece equipped with a needle holder tip and a foot pedal to activate the hand piece can be plugged in. The area to be tattooed is marked. The depth of needle penetration can be adjusted from 1 to 1.75 mm. The cluster of needles are dipped into the pigment and with traction of the skin the needle penetrates at 45° angle. At this setting the pigment penetrates to the level of the dermis. Gentle up and down motion is repeated until a layer of pigment gets deposited in the skin. The force applied depends on the firmness and thickness of the skin being tattooed. A dry gauze is used to wipe away the excess pigment and also to see the uniformity of the pigment during the procedure. The pigments used are inert, colorfast, and remain in the skin permanently. The mixture of pigment contains iron oxide in a glycerol and alcohol base. Color selection is made by a color chart preoperatively. A color darker than the natural skin tone is sometimes recommended to minimize the need for repeating the treatment as pigments may fade over time. Tattooing is applicable in treating facial hypopigmented lesions or tattooing of the nipple complex. The advantage is that when color blending is addressed, tattooing has little contrast with the surrounding skin. Loss of some pigment usually occurs, with maximum fading noted by 6 weeks. The depth of pigment implantation depends on the type of skin and requires different amounts of force to achieve pigment implantation. Tattooing does not cause infections, allergy, or cyst formation. It provides a reliable method of repigmentation with very little demarcation between the zones of treatment and normal skin. The disadvantages, however, are to be noted. Hyperpigmentation due to poor selection of pigments and, as noted, repeat procedures due to fading of pigments are common.

Natural Dyes

Natow (91) described henna as one of the oldest cosmetic product used as a coloring agent for hair. It is also used as one of the components in a variety of shampoos and conditioners. This form of coloring is used extensively by various communities to color their skin for important ceremonies. Henna is available in a greenish powder form made from the leaves of the *Lawsonia alba* (19). It is mixed with water to form a paste. The paste is applied to the skin and hair. It is a nonpermanent dye that leaves a light brown discoloration for about 4–6 weeks. Variation in pigmentation can be achieved by altering the length of time the pigment remains in contact with the skin. However, Gupta et al. (92) have noted hypersensitivity and pigment fading after 4–6 weeks.

Topical Solutions

Rayner (64) used topical solution of dihydroxy acetone and potassium permanganate (1:10,000) solution for temporary improvement of hypopigmented lesions. Since this solution pigments only the epidermal keratin, it sheds from the epidermis within a 7-day time period. He found these agents to provide only temporary improvement. Gilchrest and Goldwyn (39) used methoxsalen 1% solution in combination with UV light exposure for moderate repigmentation. This solution is to be applied topically 20 min prior to UV light exposure on alternative days for 2–6 months. Repigmentation was noted in hypopigmented areas. In addition to this treatment, he also suggested the application of a sunscreen, 5% PABA ointment, prior to natural sunlight exposure to prevent sunburn. Fitzpatrick and Szabo (25) reported the stimulatory effect of methoxsalen on epidermal melanogenesis. Patients treated with methoxsalen and UV light had moderate repigmentation. New pigmentation was noted at the periphery and small brown spots within the hypopigmented region. He also felt that the safety of these medications justifies their use in an appropriate clinical setting. To date, there are no extensive studies utilizing these agents in burn patients.

Oral Psoralens

Grimes (93) suggested that oral psoralens might be worthwhile in the treatment of very small hypopigmented scars and hair follicles nearby. Psoralens repigments hypopigmented skin by inducing the migration of melanocytes from normally pigmented hair follicles and by increasing melanogenesis. Repigmentation is a slow process and requires a protected period of treatment. Psoralens should be taken 1–2 hours prior to UV-A exposure. Twice weekly treatment is given until repigmentation occurs.

VI. SURGICAL TREATMENT

The surgical treatment of hypopigmentation in some areas parallels that in the management of hyperpigmented scars. Excision and resurfacing of the area with either split thickness skin grafts or full-thickness skin grafts often leads to improvement (Fig. 12.10). However, some areas differ.

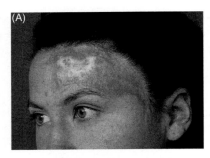

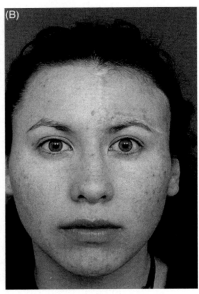

Figure 12.10 **(See color insert)** (A) Fifteen-year-old Hispanic female with forehead hypopigmentation with peripheral hyperpigmentation after partial-thickness burn injury. (B) Nine months after excision and grafting of half of the forehead with a full-thickness skin graft; color match not perfect but improved over preoperative appearance; no corrective makeup used.

A. Grafts

Billingham and Silvers (94) showed that pigmentation can result from the migration of melanoblasts and melanocytes from pigmented grafts into the surrounding hypopigmented areas in the guinea pig. Falabella (47) showed a similar form of pigmentation when he used epidermis obtained by suction and referred it as an "extension of pigment". Similarly, Orentreich and Selmanowitz (32) showed that punch grafts transferred to a hypopigmented area produced a halo of pigment around the grafted piece of skin, referred to as "pigment spread phenomenon."

The minigraft method is based on the ability of melanocytes to migrate centrifugally from grafts into hypopigmented skin to produce pigmentation. It is used for small hypopigmented burn areas. The advantage of this technique is minimal scarring in both the donor and the

recipient sites. It is a simple office procedure where grafts 1–2 mm in diameter of superficial split-thickness grafts can be taken. However, patchy pigmentation is common.

Punch grafts are full-thickness grafts and taken by using a punch to cut grafts about 4 mm in diameter down to fat. The hypopigmented recipient site into which the grafts would be transplanted was also prepared with a punch. Grafts retained their pigmentation and pigment spread was observed around the grafts to about three to four times the diameter of the grafts. Orentreich and Selmanowitz (32) implanted punch auto grafts from normally pigmented skin into hypopigmented skin and observed pigmentation around the grafts. This technique was further refined by Falabella (35) who reported 90–100% repigmentation in his cases. However, large numbers of punch biopsy samples are required to cover sizable areas. The donor site may have a cobble stone appearance and harvesting and implanting is time consuming. Patchy pigmentation requires further surgical intervention.

Hypopigmentation may be treated with dermabrasion and overgrafting. Dermabrasion is an abrasive procedure to remove the epidermis and superficial dermis resulting in a smoothing of contour irregularities. A very thin split-thickness skin graft is harvested and applied to the dermabraded bed and immobilized with dressing (95,96). The dressing is usually taken down on the fifth postoperative day. The donor site heals in a week. The final scars on the recipient areas are usually smooth and donor site morbidity is minimal. Hypopigmentation is usually corrected. However, the procedure can be repeated several times if needed. Kahn and Cohen (21) and Grover and Morgan (19) have shown that inclusion cysts may develop between 2 and 6 weeks after the procedure. Stephens (81) has shown that pretreatment with topical tretinoin cream for 4–6 weeks decreases the incidence of postdermabrasion milia. Grover and Morgan (19) have discussed the difficulties of this technique, particularly in the head and neck region, where a precise color match is required. The edges of graft and the normal surrounding skin are distinct in making this method less suitable for facial treatment. To overcome this problem, Harashina et al. (97), utilized the technique of chip grafting based on the ability of melanocytes to migrate and repigment skin. With this technique, a small split-thickness skin graft is taken. It is passed through the skin graft mesher twice and subsequently cut into very small pieces. The resulting chip, which looks like mud, is spread evenly over the dermabraded area and covered with nonadherent ointment gauze. It has the advantage in that a wide area can be grafted from a small donor site. In addition, the borderline between the normal skin and the chip skin may be less conspicuous. Donor deformity is rare because of the thin split-thickness grafts which

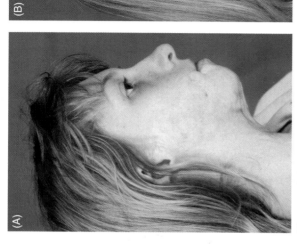

Figure 12.1 Fifteen-year-old white male status postsuperficial partial-thickness burns with facial hyperpigmentation.

Figure 12.2 Ten-year-old black female with cheek hyperpigmentation after partial-thickness flame burns; note: hyperpigmentation of grafts after application to the right side of the neck.

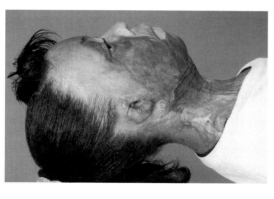

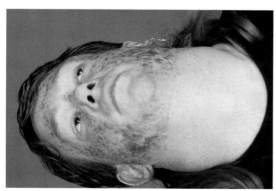

Figure 12.3 (A) Fifteen-year-old white female with areas of hyperpigmentation and hypopigmentation. (B) After corrective makeup to conceal imperfections.

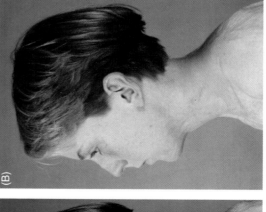

Figure 12.4 (A) Fourteen-year-old white male with hyperpigmentation of chin and neck. (B) After corrective makeup to improve appearance.

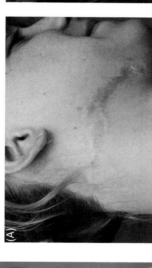

Figure 12.5 (A) Mature but red hyperpigmented cheek scar. (B) Green base for camouflage of red scars.

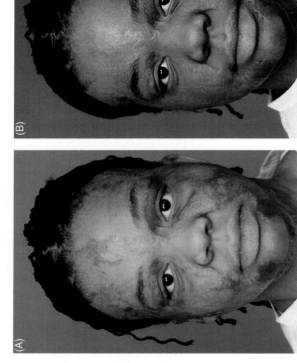

Figure 12.6 (A) Sixteen-year-old white female before corrective cosmetics with hyperpigmented scars. (B) Sixteen-year-old female after application of corrective cosmetics to even out skin tones.

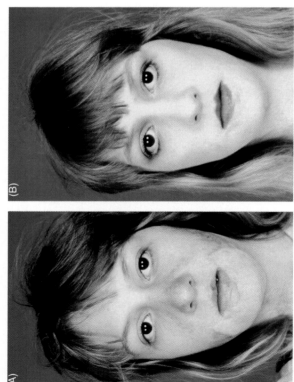

Figure 12.7 (A) Fourteen-year-old black female with hyperpigmented areas over facial region before corrective makeup. (B) Same patient after minimal application of corrective cosmetics.

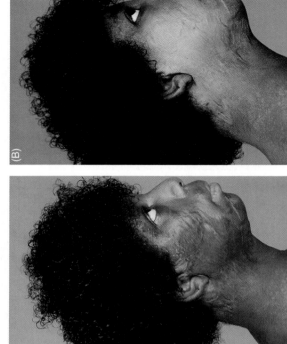

Figure 12.8 (A) Sixteen-year-old white male with facial hypopigmentation. (B) Same patient after corrective makeup.

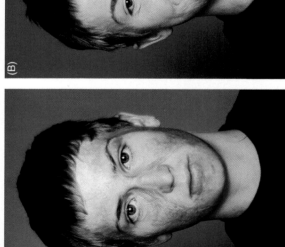

Figure 12.9 (A) Seventeen-year-old black female with hyperpigmented burn scars over facial region. (B) Same patient with corrective makeup.

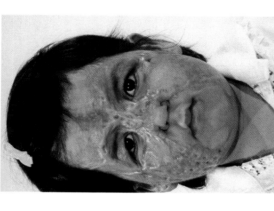

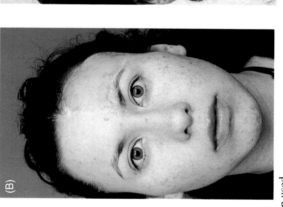

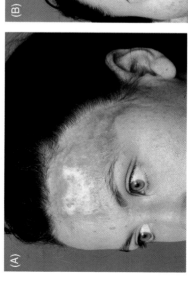

Figure 12.10 (A) Fifteen-year-old Hispanic female with forehead hypopigmentation with peripheral hyperpigmentation after partial-thickness burn injury. (B) Nine months after excision and grafting of half of the forehead with a full-thickness skin graft; color match not perfect but improved over preoperative appearance; no corrective makeup used.

Figure 12.11 Five-year-old Hispanic female with immature red hypertrophic scars.

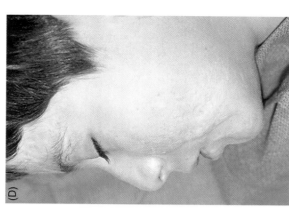

Figure 14.1 V-beam PDL system.

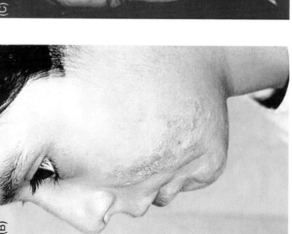

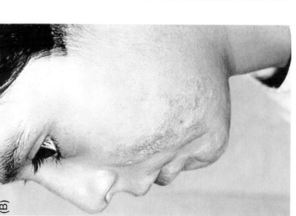

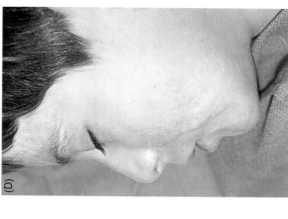

Figure 14.2 (A) Patient who sustained facial burn 18 months ago. (B) Note improved appearance after four treatments with V-beam PDL system. (C) Note further improvement after V-beam laser. (D) Further improvement noted.

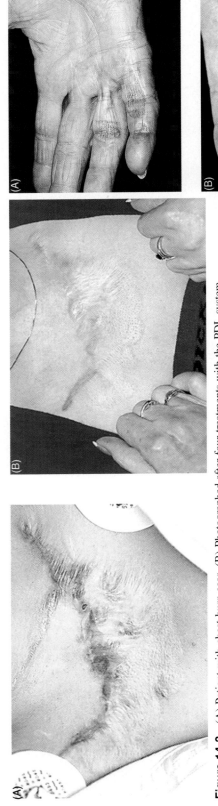

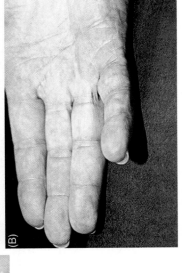

Figure 14.3 (A) Patient with chest burn scar. (B) Photographed after four treatments with the PDL system.

Figure 14.4 (A) Patient with hand scars following burn 1-year ago. (B) After three treatments with V-beam PDL system, the scars are softer and more pliable. The patient also reported less hypersensitivity.

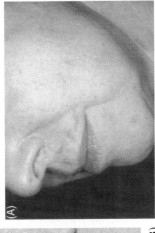

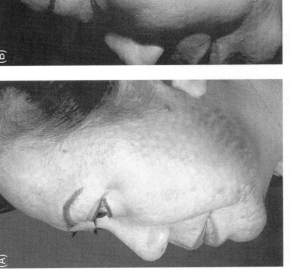

Figure 14.5 (A) Patient 1-year after burn complication of CO₂ laser treatment. (B) Note improved color and texture following two treatments with V-beam PDL system.

Figure 14.6 (A) Patient who suffered burns after treatment with CO₂ laser 1-year ago. (B) After one treatment with V-beam PDL system, there is improved color and pliability.

need be only one-third to one-fifth the size of the recipient site. Final scars are reportedly even and smooth. This technique is very useful in the treatment of facial hypo-pigmented patches.

Falabella (47) and Koga et al. (98), have reported repig-mentation of the skin in vitiligo patients using autologous epidermis by suction blister method. Kiistala (99), in 1968, used the suction blister device for separating the epi-dermis from the dermis. Flabella, in 1971, in his original article, used the tops of suction blisters for treatment of depigmented skin including burns. In 1988, Koga, using a modification of this procedure, removed a blister induced by a combination of methoxsalen plus UV-A. Three days prior to surgery red donor site is also blistered. This system is used to create negative pressure that will blister the epidermis between the basal cell membrane with melanocytes and the basement membrane. The advantage of epidermal grafts is the total absence of scar-ring in both donor and recipient sites. The dermis remains unharmed. No anesthesia is required. In addition, the grafted area gives a lighter appearance as the stratum corneum becomes detached once the graft has taken well. The disadvantage is the limitation of areas for gener-ating suction blister though abdomen and thighs are often used. Substantial time is required to perform the pro-cedure and restricted activity is recommended. The pro-cedure is complicated and the delicacy of handling flimsy epidermal sheets makes it even more difficult. The pigment spread is not uniform and the lack of aesthetic is a major complaint.

Brysk et al. (29), have used cultured cells from pigmen-ted skin to repigment hypopigmented skin in vitiligo patients. Experiments have been tried by Lobuono and Shatin (100) where the transplantation of melanocytes from the normal skin was cultured and applied over affected areas after dermabrasion, with good results (101). The technique of melanocyte culture and grafting has shown promising results in the management of vitiligo. But its value in the treatment of burn hypopigmented areas has yet to be established.

For completeness, it should be mentioned that lasers have also been used to address hypopigmentation. The carbon dioxide laser assisted dermabrasion and overgraft-ing has been described by Acikel et al. (87), with good results. However, the procedure is time consuming and costs are high. However, a smooth, bloodless surface can be obtained in a very short period of time.

VII. TREATMENT OF IMMATURE HYPERTROPHIC RED SCARS

Erythematous hypertrophic burn scars represent a most challenging aspect in the treatment of burn patients

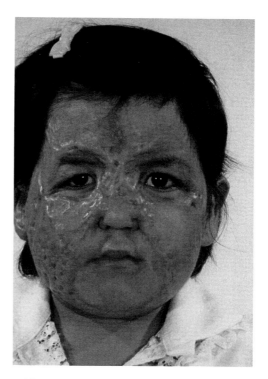

Figure 12.11 **(See color insert)** Five-year-old Hispanic female with immature red hypertrophic scars.

(Fig. 12.11). These scars are a consequence of injury to the reticular portion of the dermis. Many factors are known to contribute to its development. Baur et al. (102) in 1976, suggested pressure therapy to reduce the blood flow to the scar tissue. He also noticed α_2 globulin which is a collagenase inhibitor in these scars. Page et al. (103) in 1983 suggested that it was possible that the vascular changes could be the primary factor in scar maturation. They manipulated the blood supply to scars by applying pressure sufficient to occlude capillary circu-lation. Leung et al. (104) in 1989, described the increased microvasculature with few intercommunications to be responsible for erythematous burn scars. Alster et al. (105) in 1993, discussed the mechanism of wound healing and collagen metabolism and reported that erythe-matous scars were due to a prolongation of angiogenesis and slow capillary regression during the formation of gran-ulation tissue. Dierickx et al. (38) in 1995, also noted that the scar telangiectasias produced the persistently red color noted in immature scars. The different approaches to flatten and lighten burn hypertrophic scars is beyond the scope of this chapter. However, numerous treatments have been proposed. Among them are surgical excision, radiotherapy, intralesional injections, dermabrasion, skin graft, topical retinoids, silicone injections, pressure dres-sings, and laser treatment (106,107).

VIII. CONCLUSION

The options for the management of pigmentation changes in burn patients are extensive. Both surgical and nonsurgical options are less than ideal and not always reliable. In the absence of distortions or irregular surfaces, patients may wish for the proper use of corrective makeup to blend scars. This is a reasonable requirement, which need not fall into the "last resort" category. The well-being of burn patients will often hinge on the appearance of burn scars. The techniques described are designed to minimize such problems. As we continue to advance in the treatment of pigmentation changes in burns, a combination of old principles combined with innovative techniques may lead to perfection in the resolution of these problems.

REFERENCES

1. McCauley RL, Hollyoak M. Medical therapy and surgical approach to the burn scar. In: Herndon DN, ed. Total Burn Care. Philadelphia: W.B. Saunders, 1996:473–478.
2. McCauley RL, Robson MC, Herndon DN, Evans B, Blakeney PE. Longitudinal evaluation of a burned child. In: Herndon DN, ed. Total Burn Care. Philadelphia: W.B. Saunders, 1996:479–484.
3. Janzekovic Z. A new concept in the early excision and immediate grafting of burns. J Trauma 1970; 10:1103–1108.
4. Lyle WG, McCauley RL, Robson MC. Reconstruction of the head and neck. In: Herndon DN, ed. Total Burn Care. Philadelphia: W.B. Saunders, 1996:492–498.
5. Rose EH. Aesthetic restoration of the severely disfigured face in burn victims: a comprehensive strategy. Plast Reconstr Surg 1995; 96:1573–1585; discussion 1586–1577.
6. Blakeney PE, Meyer WJ. Psychosocial recovery of burned patients and reintegration into society. In: Herndon DN, ed. Total Burn Care. Philadelphia: W.B. Saunders, 1996:556.
7. Robson MC. Reconstruction of the burned face, neck and scalp. In: Bostwick JA, ed. The Art and Science of Burn Care. Rockville: Aspen Publishers, Inc., 1987:373–383.
8. Bernstein NR. Medical tragedies in facial burn disfigurement. Psych Ann 1976; 6:28–49.
9. Carr-Collins JA. Pressure techniques for the prevention of hypertrophic scars. Clin Plast Surg 1993; 19:733–743.
10. Robson MC. Overview of burn reconstruction. In: Herndon DN, ed. Total Burn Care. Philadelphia: W.B. Saunders, 1996:485–491.
11. Warden GD. Outpatient care of thermal injuries. Surg Clin North Am 1987; 67:147–157.
12. Bernstein NR. Emotional Care of the Facially Burned and Disfigured. Boston: Little, Brown & Co., 1976.
13. Berscheid E, Gangestad S. The social psychological implications of facial physical attractiveness. Clin Plast Surg 1982; 9:289–296.
14. Blumenfield M, Schoeps M. Reintegrating the healed burned adult into society: psychological problems and solutions. Clin Plast Surg 1992; 19:599–605.
15. Graham JA, Kligman AM. Cosmetic therapy for the patient with facial disfigurement. Ear Nose Throat J 1987; 66.
16. Guzick SS. Clinical camouflage: a burn survivor's case study. Dermatol Nurs 1993; 5:118–120, 130.
17. Sawyer MG, Minde K, Zuker R. The burned child—scarred for life? A study of the psychosocial impact of a burn injury at different developmental stages. Burns Incl Therm Inj 1983; 9:205–213.
18. Taki T, Kozuka S, Izawa Y, Usuda T, Hiramatsu M, Matsuda T, Yokoo K, Fukaya Y, Tsubone M, Aoki J. Surgical treatment of skin depigmentation caused by burn injuries. J Dermatol Surg Oncol 1985; 11:1218–1221.
19. Grover R, Morgan BD. Management of hypopigmentation following burn injury. Burns 1996; 22:627–630.
20. Halder RM, Pham HN, Breadon JY, Johnson BA. Micropigmentation for the treatment of vitiligo. J Dermatol Surg Oncol 1989; 15:1092–1098.
21. Kahn AM, Cohen MJ. Treatment for depigmentation following burn injuries. Burns 1996; 22:552–554.
22. Norlund JJ. Post inflammatory hyperpigmentation. Dermatol Clin 1988; 6:185.
23. Willier BH. The control of hair and feather pigmentation as revealed by grafting melanophores in the embryo. Ann Surg 1942; 116:598.
24. Breathnach AS. Melanocytes in early regenerated human epidermis. J Invest Dermatol 1960; 35:245.
25. Fitzpatrick TB, Szabo G. The melanocyte: cytology and cytochemistry. J Invest Dermatol 1959; 32:197–209.
26. Pele NJ, Norlund JJ. Pigmentary changes in the skin. Clin Plast Surg 1993; 20:1.
27. Barker DE. Pigment migration following "z" plasty. Plast Reconstr Surg 1947; 4:384.
28. Barker DE. Pigment changes in experimental whole thickness skin grafts. Arch Pathol 1947; 44:163.
29. Brysk MM, Newton RC, Rajaraman S, Plott T, Barlow E, Bell T, Penn P, Smith EB. Repigmentation of vitiliginous skin by cultured cells. Pigment Cell Res 1989; 2:202–207.
30. Falabella R. Repigmentation of leukoderma by autologous epidermal grafting. J Dermatol Surg Oncol 1984; 10:136–144.
31. Morgan JE, Gilchrest B, Goldwyn RM. Skin pigmentation. Current concepts and relevance to plastic surgery. Plast Reconstr Surg 1975; 56:617–628.
32. Orentreich N, Selmanowitz VJ. Autograft repigmentation of leukoderma. Arch Dermatol 1992; 105:734.
33. Selmanowitz VJ. Pigmentary correction of piebaldism by autografts. II. Pathomechanism and pigment spread in piebaldism. Cutis 1979; 24:66–71, 73.
34. Selmanowitz VJ, Rabinowitz AD, Orentreich N, Wenk E. Pigmentary correction of piebaldism by autografts. I. Procedures and clinical findings. J Dermatol Surg Oncol 1977; 3:615–622.
35. Falabella R. Treatment of localized vitiligo by autologous minigrafting. Arch Dermatol 1988; 124:1649–1655.

36. Onur Erol O, Atabay K. The treatment of burn scar hypopigmentation and surface irregularity by dermabrasion and thin skin grafting. Plast Reconstr Surg 1990; 85:754–758.

37. Konrad K, Wolff K. Hyperpigmentation, melanosome size, and distribution patterns of melanosomes. Arch Dermatol 1973; 107:853–860.

38. Dierickx C, Goldman MP, Fitzpatrick RE. Laser treatment of erythematous/hypertrophic and pigmented scars in 26 patients. Plast Reconstr Surg 1995; 95:84–90; discussion 91–82.

39. Gilchrest BA, Goldwyn RM. Topical chemotherapy of pigment abnormalities in surgical patients. Plast Reconstr Surg 1981; 67:435–439.

40. Kaidbey KH, Kligman AM. Sunburn protection by longwave ultraviolet radiation-induced pigmentation. Arch Dermatol 1978; 114:46–48.

41. Fitzpatrick TB, Seiji M, Mc GA. Melanin pigmentation. N Engl J Med 1961; 265:430–434.

42. Jimbow K, Obata H, Pathak MA, Fitzpatrick TB. Mechanism of depigmentation by hydroquinone. J Invest Dermatol 1974; 62:436–449.

43. Lerner AB. Physiol Rev 1950; 30.

44. Fitzpatrick TB. The validity and practicality of sun reactive skin types 1 through V1. Arch Dermatol 1998; 124:869.

45. Coleman WP III. Dermal peels. Dermatol Clin 2001; 19:405–411.

46. Mir Y, Mir L. The problem of pigmentation in the cutaneous graft. Br J Plast Surg 1961; 14:303.

47. Falabella R. Epidermal grafting. An original technique and its application in achromic and granulating areas. Arch Dermatol 1971; 104:592–600.

48. de Chalain TM, Tang C, Thomson HG. Burn area color changes after superficial burns in childhood: can they be predicted? J Burn Care Rehabil 1998; 19:39–49.

49. Boochai K, Mutou YM. Complications after dermabrasion in Asians. Plast Reconstr Surg 1961; 27:412.

50. Ship AG, Weiss PR. Pigmentation after dermabrasion: an avoidable complication. Plast Reconstr Surg 1985; 75:528–532.

51. Grimes PE, Stockton T. Pigmentary disorders in black. Dermatol Clin 1998.

52. Perez-Bernal A, Munoz-Perez MA, Camacho F. Management of facial hyperpigmentation. Am J Clin Dermatol 2000; 1:261–268.

53. Kahn AM, Cohen MJ, Kaplan L. Treatment for depigmentation resulting from burn injuries. J Burn Care Rehabil 1991; 12:468–473.

54. Baker TJ, Stuzin JM. Chemical peeling and dermabrasion. In: McCarthy JG, ed. Plastic Surgery. Philadelphia: W.B. Saunders, 1990:748.

55. Behl PN. Treatment of vitilgo with homologous: thin Thiersch's skin grafts. Curr Med Pract 1964; 8:218.

56. Brody HJ. Complications of chemical resurfacing. Dermatol Clin 2001; 19:427–438, vii–viii.

57. Glogan RG, Matarrasso SL. Chemical peel TCA and phenol. Dermatol Clin 1995; 13:2.

58. Monheit GD. Medium-depth chemical peels. Dermatol Clin 2001; 19:413–425.

59. Luftman DB, Lowe NJ, Moy RL. Sunscreens. Update and review. J Dermatol Surg Oncol 1991; 17:744–746.

60. O'Donoghue MN. Sunscreen. The ultimate cosmetic. Dermatol Clin 1991; 9:99–104.

61. Scherschun L, Lim HW. Photoprotection by sunscreens. Am J Clin Dermatol 2001; 2:131–134.

62. Lowe NJ. Sunscreens and the prevention of skin aging. J Dermatol Surg Oncol 1990; 16:936–938.

63. Margolis RJ, Dover JS, Polla LL, Watanabe S, Shea CR, Hruza GJ, Parrish JA, Anderson RR. Visible action spectrum for melanin-specific selective photothermolysis. Lasers Surg Med 1989; 9:389–397.

64. Rayner VL. Camouflage therapy. Dermatol Clin 1995; 13:467–472.

65. Roberts NC. Corrective cosmetics—need, evaluation and use. Cutis 1988; 41:439–441.

66. O'Donoghue MN. Cosmetics for the elderly. Dermatol Clin 1991; 9:29–34.

67. Sattenspiel SL. The use of cosmetics in facial plastic surgery. Ear Nose Throat J 1987; 66:19–23.

68. Natow AJ. Corrective cosmetics. Cutis 1985; 36:123–124.

69. Lazar AP, Lazar P. An overview of cosmetics. Ear Nose Throat J 1987; 66:6–8.

70. Grimes PE, Davis LT. Cosmetics in blacks. Dermatol Clin 1991; 9:53–68.

71. Westmore MG. Make-up as an adjunct and aid to the practice of dermatology. Dermatol Clin 1991; 9:81–88.

72. O'Donoghue MN. Clinical uses and effects of cosmetics. Ear Nose Throat J 1987; 66:9–11.

73. Draelos ZD. Colored facial cosmetics. Dermatol Clin 2000; 18:621–631.

74. Roberts C. The corrective cover or camouflage clinic. Ear Nose Throat J 1989:68.

75. Roberts FL, Forget BM. Application techniques for corrective and camouflage cosmetics. Ear Nose Throat J 1987; 66:12–18.

76. Roberts NC. Uses and abuses of cosmetics. Ear Nose Throat J 1987; 66:4–5.

77. Norlund JJ, Wright C. Letter to the editor-corrective cover or camouflage clinic. Ear Nose Throat J 1989; 68:480.

78. Converse JM, McCarthy JG, Dobrkovsky M. Facial burns. In: Reconstructive Plastic Surgery. 2nd ed. Philadelphia: W.B. Saunders, 1977:1595.

79. Takao H, Iso R. The treatment of leukoderma after burns by a combination of dermabrasion and "chip" skin grafting. Br J Plast Surg 1985; 38:301.

80. Kahn AM, Cohen MJ. Vitiligo: treatment by dermabrasion and epithelial sheet grafting. J Am Acad Dermatol 1995; 33:646–648.

81. Stephens DR. Scars and scar revision. In: Grotting JG, ed. Reoperative, Aesthetic and Reconstructive Plastic Surgery, 1995:73.

82. Lagrot F, Antoine G, Bensoussan H. Survey on the pigmentation of cutaneous grafts. Ann Chir Plast 1960; 5:19–21.

83. Tsukada S. The melanocytes and melanin in human skin autografts. Plast Reconstr Surg 1974; 53:200–207.

84. Conway H, Sedar J. Report of the loss of pigment in full thickness autoplastic skin grafts in the mouse. Plast Reconstr Surg 1956; 18:30.

85. Lopez-Mas J, Ortiz-Monasterio F, Viale De Gonzalez M, Olmedo A. Skin graft pigmentation. A new approach to prevention. Plast Reconstr Surg 1972; 49:18–21.

86. Abergel RP, Meeker CA, Dwyer RM, Lesavoy MA, Uitto J. Nonthermal effects of ND:YAG laser on biological functions of human skin fibroblasts in culture. Lasers Surg Med 1984; 3:279–284.

87. Acikel C, Ulkur E, Guler MM. Treatment of burn scar depigmentation by carbon dioxide laser-assisted dermabrasion and thin skin grafting. Plast Reconstr Surg 2000; 105:1973–1978.

88. Thomson HG, Wright AM. Surgical tattooing of the port-wine stain. Operative technique, results, and critique. Plast Reconstr Surg 1971; 48:113–120.

89. van der Velden EM, Baruchin AM, Jairath D, Oostrom CA, Ijsselmuiden OE. Dermatography: a method for permanent repigmentation of achromic burn scars. Burns 1995; 21:304–307.

90. van der Velden EM, de Jong BD, van der Walle HB, Stolz E, Naafs B. Cosmetic tattooing as a treatment of port-wine stains. Int J Dermatol 1993; 32:372–375.

91. Natow AJ. Henna. Cutis 1986; 38:21.

92. Gupta BN, Mathur AK, Agarwal C, Singh A. Contact sensitivity to henna. Contact Dermatitis 1986; 15:303–304.

93. Grimes PE. Vitiligo. An overview of therapeutic approaches. Dermatol Clin 1993; 11:325–338.

94. Billingham RE, Silvers WK. Studies on the migratory behavior of melanocytes in guinea pig skin. J Exp Med 1970; 131:101–117.

95. Harmon CB. Dermabrasion. Dermatol Clin 2001; 19:439–442.

96. Kahn AM, Cohen MJ, Kaplan L, Highton A. Vitiligo: treatment by dermabrasion and epithelial sheet grafting—a preliminary report. J Am Acad Dermatol 1993; 28:773–774.

97. Harashina T, Iso R. The treatment of leukoderma after burns by a combination of dermabrasion and chip skin grafting. Br J Plast Surg 1985; 38:301.

98. Koga M. Epidermal grafting using the tops of suction blisters in the treatment of vitiligo. Arch Dermatol 1988; 124:1656.

99. Kiistala U. Suction blister device for separation of viable epidermis from dermis. J Invest Dermatol 1968; 50:129–137.

100. Lobuono P, Shatin H. Transplantation of hair bulbs and melanocytes into leukodermic scars. J Dermatol Surg 1976; 2:53–55.

101. Stoner ML, Wood FM. The treatment of hypopigmented lesions with cultured epithelial autograft. J Burn Care Rehabil 2000; 21:50–54.

102. Baur PS, Larson DL, Stacey TR, Barratt GF, Dobrkovsky M. Ultrastructural analysis of pressure-treated human hypertrophic scars. J Trauma 1976; 16:958–967.

103. Page RE, Robertson GA, Pethgrew NM. Microcirculation in hypertrophic burn scars. Burns 1983; 10:64.

104. Leung KS, Sher A, Clark JA, Cheng JC, Leung PC. Microcirculation in hypertrophic scars after burn injury. J Burn Care Rehabil 1989; 10:436–444.

105. Alster TS, Kurban AK, Grove GL, Grove MJ, Tan OT. Alteration of argon laser-induced scars by the pulsed dye laser. Lasers Surg Med 1993; 13:368–373.

106. Henning JPH, Roskam Y, Gemert V. Treatment of keloids and hypertrophic scars with an argon laser. Lasers Surg Med 1986; 6:72–75.

107. Anderson RR, Parrish JA. Microvasculature can be selectively damaged using dye lasers: a basic theory and experimental evidence in human skin. Lasers Surg Med 1981; 1:263–276.

13

The Etiology and Management of Hypertrophic Scars and Keloids Following Thermal Injury

EDWARD E. TREDGET, PAUL G. SCOTT, AZIZ GHAHARY

University of Alberta, Edmonton, Alberta, Canada

I. INTRODUCTION

Keloids and hypertrophic scars (HSc) that occur following burns or other trauma are a unique form of human dermal fibroproliferative disorders (FPD) which can also affect other tissues and organs in the body (1). By definition, keloids occur in individuals with a familial predisposition, enlarge and extend beyond the margins of the original wounds and rarely regress (Fig. 13.1). HSc are raised, erythematous, pruritic, fibrous lesions which typically

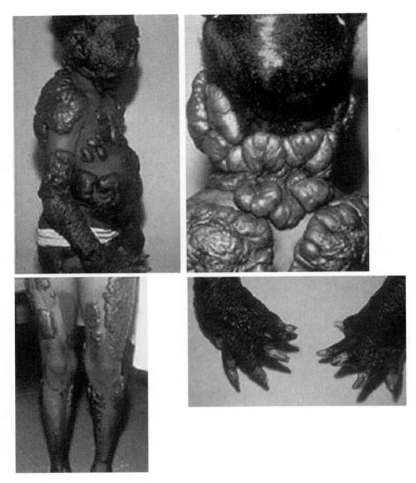

Figure 13.1 A 12-year-old black child with severe keloids following a scald injury. (Reprinted from Scott PG et al. Biological basis of hypertrophic scarring. Adv Structural Biol 1994; 3:157, with permission from Elsevier Science.)

remain within the confines of the original wound and usually undergo at least partial spontaneous resolution over widely varying time courses and are often associated with contractures of the healing tissues (Fig. 13.2). The development of contractures is by definition the pathologic shortening of scar tissue resulting in deformities as opposed to wound contraction that occurs in an open wound with the positive outcome of reducing the wound surface area. These disorders represent aberrations in the fundamental processes of wound healing which include cell migration and proliferation, inflammation, modulation and secretion of cytokines and extracellular matrix (ECM) proteins, and finally, remodeling of the newly synthesized matrix. Conceptually, it is the goal of individuals caring for wounds to facilitate regeneration of the injured skin and associated structures; however, at present adult mammalian healing occurs by the formation of scar, characterized by a disordered architecture, which in the case of HSc and keloids is also associated with excessive deposition of ECM proteins (Fig. 13.3).

II. PATHOGENESIS OF HYPERTROPHIC SCAR, KELOIDS, AND CONTRACTURES

A. Histopathology and Ultrastructure

While there is considerable variability, compounded by such factors as age of the scar and site of sampling, there are nevertheless commonly observed features that may be considered pathognomonic for HSc. Grossly, the scars are raised, erythematous, and hard to the touch. They usually contain cigar-shaped or branching accretions of dense connective tissue which may be up to 2 cm long and have been termed "nodules" (2). The epidermis in HSc is often much thicker than that overlying normal dermis and lacks rete ridges (Fig. 13.4). Beneath this thickened epidermis there may be a narrow zone of parallel-fibered collagen, but deep within the nodules the collagen consists mostly of thin, poorly defined fibers, often arranged in a whorl-like pattern. This organization is in marked contrast to that in normal dermis, which is made up mainly of thick

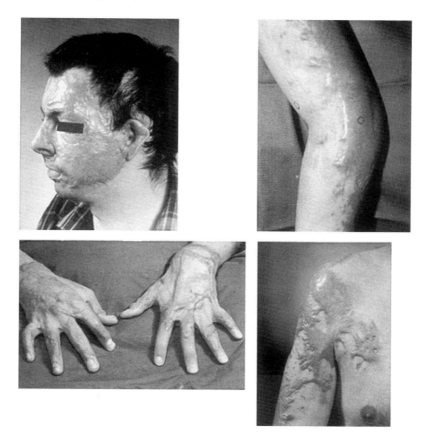

Figure 13.2 Hypertrophic scarring in a 34-year-old caucasian man 8 months following a 60% total body surface area burn involving the face, upper extremities, and hands. (Reprinted from Scott PG et al. Biological basis of hypertrophic scarring. Adv Structural Biol 1994; 3:157, with permission from Elsevier Science.)

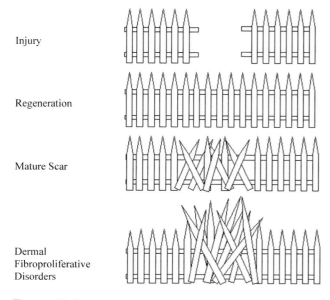

Figure 13.3 Repair of dermal injury is analogous to reconstruction of a picket fence postinjury. [Reprinted from Tredget et al. (1), with permission from Elsevier Science.]

collagen fibers and fiber-bundles, many of which run parallel to the surface. In nodules present in the deep dermis there may again be a narrow zone of parallel fibers, giving the impression that the abnormal structure is almost completely encapsulated in normal tissue. Mature postburn scars (many of which may have at one time been hypertrophic) show coarser collagen fibers, and some fiber-bundles, many oriented parallel to the surface, but these are often not as well organized as those in normal, uninjured dermis. In the electron microscope, the collagen fibrils are found to be narrower (most common diameter $\sim$60 nm) than those in normal dermis ($\sim$100 nm), and more widely separated by amorphous interfibrillar matrix (2). While the collagen fibrils of normal dermis are circular or ovoid in cross-section, those in hypertrophic scar are often irregular and angular (3). Recent information on the structure and properties of the extracellular matrix proteoglycans allows rationalization of some of these observations (see following text).

The main cell type within HSc is the fibroblast, with smaller numbers of infiltrated lymphocytes, Langerhans cells, macrophages, and mast cells. The mast cell load is

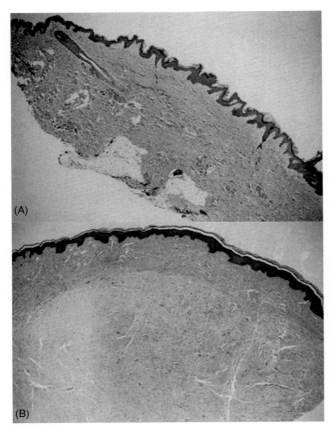

Figure 13.4 Hematoxylin and eosin staining of sections from (A) normal human skin and (B) a hypertrophic scar containing a nodule (original magnification ×10). [Reprinted from Scott PG et al. Molecular and cellular aspects of fibrosis following thermal injury. In: Thermal Injuries. Hand Clin 2000; 16(2): 271–287, with permission from Elsevier Science.]

significantly (four fold) higher than that in normal dermis, probably accounting after the degranulation triggered by dermal injury for the pruritis commonly experienced by recovering burn patients (4,5). Conflicting descriptions of the cellularity of HSc have been presented, some authors considering them to be relatively acellular, at least within the nodules, and others that they are hypercellular (6). This disagreement probably reflects variability in scar age and sampling. Our own data indicate that HSc sampled within 3–24 months after burn injury have twice the density of fibroblasts as normal dermis or mature scar (7). This includes a proportion of myofibroblasts, characterized by an indented nuclear envelope and prominent subcortical stress fibers consisting of actin and associated proteins (8). Myofibroblasts, detected by staining for alpha-smooth muscle actin, are especially prominent within the centers of the nodules of HSc where "degenerating" fibroblasts were earlier described and associated with the onset of scar resolution (9,10). A consensus seems to be emerging that the myofibroblast

represents a terminally differentiated preapoptotic cell (see following text for a discussion on apoptosis).

B. Macromolecular Composition of the Extracellular Matrix

In a fibrous connective tissue like dermis the mechanical integrity and ultimate tensile strength are conferred by the collagen fibrils with the sulfated glycosaminoglycan chains of hyaluronic acid and the proteoglycans providing resilience and resistance to compression by virtue of their contribution to tissue osmotic pressure. Other components include elastin fibers, cell-adhesive (and antiadhesive) glycoproteins such as fibronectin and tenascin, and serum proteins. While an increased collagen content is usually considered the hallmark of fibrosis and HSc is commonly classified as a FPD, it should be noted that the proportion of collagen on a dry weight basis is actually ~30% lower than in normal dermis or mature scar (11) (Fig. 13.5). This is because there are much larger increases in the noncollagen components such as fibronectin and the proteoglycans. Nevertheless, since the dermis is grossly thickened in HSc, the collagen content per unit surface area is increased.

The collagen in postburn HSc is primarily of the same genetic type (I) as that in normal dermis but with higher proportions of type III (~33%) and type V (6,12,13). Type III collagen usually makes up ~10–15% of collagen in adult dermis and more in fetal dermis. The persistently

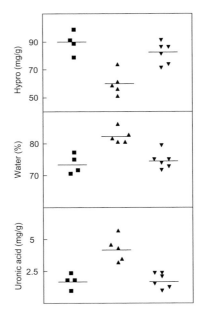

Figure 13.5 Scattergrams of the hydroxyproline, water, and uronic acid contents of normal skin (■), hypertrophic scar (▲), and mature scar (▼). [Reprinted from Scott et al. (11), with permission from Elsevier Science.]

high level of type III collagen in hypertrophic scar reflects the immaturity of the scar tissue.

The content of uronic acids, one of the monosaccharides making up the repeating disaccharides characteristic of the glycosaminoglycans (GAGs) hyaluronic acid (HA), chondroitin sulfate (CS), and dermatan sulfate (DS), is increased about 2.4-fold in HSc relative to normal dermis or mature scar (11) [Fig. 13.6(A)]. Not surprisingly, since the GAGs are largely responsible for the water-holding capacity of connective tissues, HSc are hyperhydrated, although only by ~12% (11,14). Swelling of connective tissues is normally limited by the collagen fibers, therefore this disproportionate increase in GAGs over water content is probably responsible for the greater turgor of the HSc tissue.

With the exception of HA, all GAGs occur as covalently attached side-chains on proteoglycans (PGs). These ubiquitous ECM components influence many processes and properties of connective tissues, including collagen fibril morphology and assembly, cell–matrix interactions and cell metabolic activity. The most abundant proteoglycan in normal dermis is decorin, accounting for most of the dermatan sulfate and ~0.4% of the dry weight of the tissue (11) (Fig. 13.6). Decorin is primarily or exclusively associated with the surfaces of the collagen fibrils in a regular array (15). It appears to be expressed early and abundantly in normally healing wounds, but is found in HSc at only ~25% of the level in normal dermis or mature postburn scar (11,16). There is considerable evidence to support a role for decorin in the regulation of collagen fibril diameters and in the lateral alignment of fibrils to form fibers and fiber-bundles (17,18). In the decorin-null mouse, collagen fibrils in the skin are angular in cross-section, as are those in HSc, and variable in diameter, presumably because of the lack of the PG, which normally defines the fibril surface and controls its properties (2,19). Decorin can also act as a negative regulator of the fibrogenic growth factor transforming growth factor-beta (TGF-beta) (see following text) (20).

The increased concentration of GAGs in HSc is largely a consequence of the approximately six-fold elevated levels of a versican-like large CS-PG and biglycan—a second DS-PG related to decorin, but normally present in only small amounts in adult dermis (11). The large CS-PG probably occupies an equivalent position within the microarchitecture of HSc connective tissue to that in fibrocartilage, that is, between the collagen fibrils where it exerts osmotic pressure that tends to expand the collagenous meshwork (21) [Fig. 13.6(B)]. At the light microscope level there is a striking reciprocity in immunohistochemical staining for decorin and for the CS-PG in HSc (18). The very considerable increase in this PG accounts

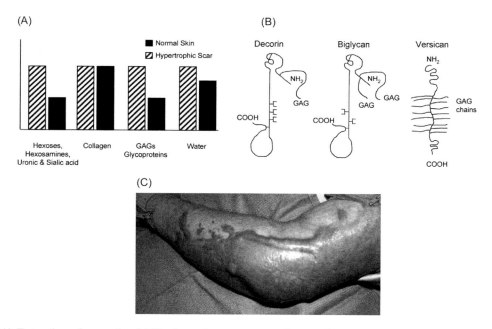

Figure 13.6 (A) Extraction of normal and HSc tissue demonstrates an increased water content in HSc relative to normal. This is probably caused, in part, by the hydrophilic sugar chains associated with the GAG (stippled bar = hypertrophic scar; black bar = normal skin). (B) Decorin and biglycan are small proteoglycans with one and two dermatan sulphate sugar chains, respectively. Versican is a large proteoglycan with as many as 30 sugar chains, thereby contributing significant rigidity to HSc because of its hydrophilic properties (not drawn to scale). (C) The expulsion of water from HSc is depicted visually over this burn patient's elbow immediately following the removal of his silicone gel sheet and pressure garments. This expulsion of water is reversed rapidly if pressure is not maintained because of the continued presence of the GAG sugar chains that attract the water back into the region. [Reprinted from Tredget et al. (1), with permission from Elsevier Science.]

for the early observation of increased staining for CS and reduced staining for DS within the nodules of HSc (22). The distribution of biglycan in normal tissues has been described as primarily pericellular rather than fibril-associated, as is the decorin. In HSc, biglycan appears to be mostly associated with the collagen of the ECM, rather than with the cells (18,23). What effect it might have on collagen organization or properties is not known.

III. ETIOLOGY OF DERMAL FIBROSIS FOLLOWING THERMAL INJURY

A. Hypertrophic Scar Fibroblasts

Although limitations exist in extrapolating *in vitro* data to account for the clinical findings in FPD, fibroblasts obtained from postburn HSc often display altered behavior which might have been anticipated from tissue properties, for example, increased synthesis of collagen, at least in some cell strains and transforming growth factor-beta and decreased synthesis of decorin, collagenase, and nitric oxide (24–29) (Table 13.1). These observations support the idea that the composition and properties of HSc tissue are determined by the activity of a phenotypically distinct strain (or strains) of fibroblast. How this putative cell selection operates within the healing wound is not yet known, although two general mechanisms might be suggested: the first that proliferation of certain fibroblast subpopulations is triggered by fibrogenic cytokines (see following text), and the second that the thermal injury itself selectively destroys a proportion of the cells, for example, those in the more superficial dermis. In this case the fibroblasts repopulating the wound might derive mainly from superficial fascia or deep dermis, and therefore display a distinct phenotype. In support of this suggestion is the observation that fibroblasts cultured from reticular dermis synthesize less decorin than do those from papillary dermis (30).

Table 13.1 Unique Features of Fibroblasts from Hypertrophic Scar (HSc) Dermis Compared with Site Matched Normal Dermal Fibroblasts from the Same Patient

	Hypertrophic scar	Reference
Proliferation rate	35.4 h (HSc) vs. 36.2 h (normal) $n = 5$ (ns)	
Collagen synthesis	↑ in 50–70%	31
Intracellular degradation	↔	32
Collagenase activity	↓ ↓ ↓	27
Nitric oxide production	↓ ↓	34
Decorin synthesis	↓ ↓	11,18
TGF-β production	↑ ↑	33

B. Fibroblast Proliferation and the Possible Failure of Apoptosis

A simple and obvious hypothesis to explain the development of HSc, but one not supported by most studies on cultured fibroblasts, is that there has been selection of cells with an intrinsically higher rate of proliferation. Unchanged or slightly longer doubling times have been reported for HSc compared to normal dermal fibroblasts (35–37). The use of tritiated thymidine to label cells actively synthesizing DNA led Oku et al. (38) to conclude that most fibroblasts in HSc are dormant, but that there is a small population of more rapidly proliferating cells. It is difficult to reconcile the reported higher rate of labeling of HSc fibroblasts with bromodeoxyuridine with the lower directly measured population doubling times (25,35–37), other than by suggesting that the former technique emphasizes the contribution of a small and atypical subpopulation of cells. The regulation of cell proliferation in the tissue is almost certainly under the control of cytokines such as TGF-beta (see following text).

The conversion of granulation tissue into normal scar, or of HSc into mature scar, is accompanied by a large decrease in the density of fibroblasts, about two-fold in our own experience (7,39) (Fig. 13.7).

Much of this loss of cells is believed to occur through programmed cell death ("apoptosis"), rather than by simple necrosis, presumably with the advantage that the local inflammatory response is less (40). Not surprisingly, there have been several attempts to correlate apoptosis, or rather its delay, with the persistence of HSc, although a direct connection remains to be established. Whether a cell will survive or undergo apoptosis is determined by a complex and incompletely understood balance between the actions of proapoptotic cell surface receptors of the Fas or "tumour necrosis factor (TNF) superfamily," leading to activation of an intracellular proteolytic cascade involving the caspases such as interleukin 1 beta-converting enzyme (ICE) and the action of apoptosis-inhibiting protooncogene products such as Bcl-2 protein [see Ref. (41) for a brief review]. In the present context it has been reported that peripheral blood mononuclear cells from burn patients showed elevated production of Bcl-2 protein, while fibroblasts cultured from the scars of these patients showed reduced staining for Fas and ICE (42). TNFs are produced by activated macrophages and many other cell types can kill cells by inducing both necrosis and apoptosis (43,44). Castagnoli et al. (45) have reported that a reduced proportion of the infiltrating cells in HSc stain for TNF-alpha, compared to those in normal scar. It would be tempting to speculate that a consequential lower level of TNF-alpha in the tissue leads to a reduced rate of apoptosis but the situation is complicated since TNF-receptor I also activates the NF-kappa B pathway which is

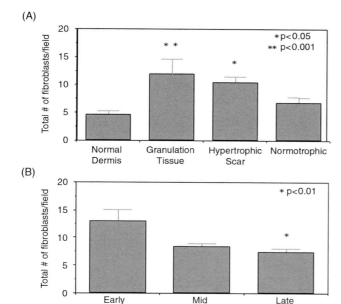

Figure 13.7 The total number of fibroblasts per high-power field differs between various types of wound healing and returns to a more normal level as the scar matures from 10 randomly sampled fields. Panel A depicts the total numbers of fibroblasts in granulation tissue and HSc relative to normal dermis (12.0 ± 2.6 and 10.5 ± 1.0 vs. 4.7 ± 0.5). Normotrophic scar did not differ significantly from normal dermis (6.8 ± 0.9). Panel B depicts the gradual reduction in total number of fibroblasts as a function of time, where early scar is 0–4 months postburn (13.1 ± 2.0) ($n = 5$), mid is 5–18 months (8.5 ± 0.4) ($n = 25$), and late is 19–30 months (7.6 ± 0.5) ($n = 20$). [Reprinted from Nedelec et al. (39), with permission from Elsevier Science.]

linked to cell survival (46). Nitric oxide is another factor which has been found to have both pro- and antiapoptotic activity, depending on the type of cell studied and other less well-understood factors (47). Fibroblasts cultured from HSc synthesize less nitric oxide than do normal dermal fibroblasts and the tissue shows less intense immunohistochemical staining for nitric oxide synthases (29). Interestingly, TNF-alpha is a potent inducer of nitric oxide synthesis by macrophages (48).

C. Circulating Peripheral Blood Fibrocytes

Recently, it has been recognized the bone marrow-derived circulating peripheral blood cells or fibrocytes possess the typical antigen presenting and immunologic features of lymphocytes, but are capable of entering wounds and sites of injured tissues where they appear to contribute matrix formation through the synthesis of type I collagen, fibronectin, and various integrins (49). In burn patients, the number of circulating fibrocytes is increased as compared to normal

uninjured volunteers, and the differentiation and proliferation appears to be strongly influenced by the fibrogenic cytokine, transforming growth factor (TGF)-alpha which has already been identified to be elevated in the serum of burn patients who suffer increased amounts of HSc (50).

IV. WOUND CONTRACTION FOLLOWING THERMAL INJURY

Wound contraction after thermal injury begins as a beneficial process in that it facilitates earlier wound closure by reducing the surface area of the original wound, albeit to a much greater extent in animals than in humans. However, the continuation of contraction beyond the point at which re-epithelialization occurs (scar contraction) leads to significant clinical morbidity due to the development of joint contractures, functional loss, delayed return to work, and poor cosmetic results (51).

At a molecular and cellular level, myofibroblasts have been proposed as a subtype of fibroblasts that are responsible for contraction in healing wounds. The myofibroblast was initially defined as a specialized mesenchymal cell found in granulation tissue that exhibited morphologic and biochemical features of both a fibroblast and a smooth muscle cell (52). The term "myofibroblast" was coined when it was shown that strips of granulation tissue contracted *in vitro* when treated with smooth muscle stimulants. Electron microscopic analysis revealed that the myofibroblast possessed an extensive cytoplasmic fibrillar system (stress fibers), undulations of the nuclear membrane, abundant endoplasmic reticulum, and peripheral attachment sites reminiscent of hemidesmosomes. Thus, the myofibroblast was proposed as the fibroblast, which becomes modified into a smooth muscle-like cell and contracts the ECM to which it is attached, by traction. Using a monoclonal antibody which specifically recognized the alpha-smooth muscle isoform of actin (SMA), which is also expressed in vascular cells, myofibroblasts have been shown to express increased amounts of alpha-SMA, rather than beta and gamma-cytoplasmic actin isoforms, which are characteristically expressed by normal fibroblasts. Expression of alpha-SMA in fibroblasts has therefore come to define a myofibroblast.

Using an *in vitro* assay in which fibroblasts suspended in a collagen gel attach to the fibrils causing progressive contraction of the gel over time [the fibroblast-populated collagen lattice (FPCL)], Arora and McCulloch (53) were able to demonstrate that increased contractility correlated with higher concentrations of alpha-SMA expression in several primary cell strains. However, substantial variability exists among fibroblast strains (54). Comparisons between the contractility of normal fibroblasts and those derived from HSc or keloids have demonstrated increased contractility or no difference. This variability may be attributable to the source of normal fibroblasts used as controls.

An alternative theory of contraction proposes that fibroblasts exert a traction force generated by the continual extension and retraction of filipodia in a treadmill fashion, rather than by progressive shortening of their cytoskeleton (55). This theory is supported by the observations that stress fibers are not essential for motility and that cellular motility is associated with a more diffuse distribution of actin and myosin, which is most consistent with continuous rearrangement of the cytoskeleton. The microfilaments that do form remain stationary as the nuclear region moves toward the anterior focal contacts and then decays, coupled with continual recycling of disassembled cortical actin to the dorsal lamellipodia.

Several pieces of evidence also argue against the role of the myofibroblast as the contractile cell in tissue. It has been demonstrated that myofibroblasts are prominent *in vivo* in the presence of mechanical tension even in the absence of wounding, suggesting that there may be a feedback mechanism from the extracellular environment which induces the myofibroblast phenotype, rather than the myofibroblast specifically influencing the ECM (56). Also, Leavitt et al. (57) have demonstrated that transformed cell strains expressing alpha-SMA, phenotypically exhibited greater contact inhibition and lower invasive and motility capabilities (features required of fibroblasts during wound healing and contractile situations), as compared to others lacking alpha-SMA expression, further questioning the correlation of alpha-SMA expression and wound contraction.

Recently, Ehrlich and Rudolph have proposed that the myofibroblast appears following the termination of dynamic contraction and locomotion, thereby maintaining a static equilibrium that is established within the tissue (6,9). Interestingly, examination of the time-course of wound healing has shown that alpha-SMA is maximally expressed at 12–15 days, which correlates with the end of the most actively contractile period. In addition, myofibroblasts are associated with open wound healing and the closure of wounds using tissue flaps reduces contraction and the number of cells through the induction of apoptosis or programmed cell death. Thus, it appears that alpha-SMA expression correlates more with the termination of a proliferative/migrational phase and delineates a terminally differentiated cell.

Finally, components of the ECM itself appear to alter the ability of fibroblasts to contract. Increased concentration of type III collagen in the FPCL leads to an increase in the rate of contraction, whereas the presence of decorin inhibits lattice contraction, conditions recognized in HSc *in vivo* (59). Stimulation of lattice contraction has also been induced by the addition of TGF-beta and platelet derived growth factor (PDGF) to the FPCL.

Thus, "normal" fibroblasts appear fully capable of wound contraction if the appropriate ECM components and cytokine signals are present.

V. FIBROGENIC CYTOKINES

Many, if not all of the interrelated processes involved in wound healing are under the control of a set of locally secreted and acting "growth factors" or "cytokines." Some of these factors have multiple overlapping biologic activities, such as their influence on chemotaxis, cytoskeletal structure, and the expression of a wide variety of genes (60,61). Major cytokines involved in wound healing can be divided into three categories based on their activities (proinflammatory, fibrogenic, and antifibrogenic) with some functions overlapping (62). For example, interleukin-1alpha (IL-1alpha), IL-1beta, IL-6, IL-8, and TNF-alpha are important in the proinflammatory phase of wound healing, while TGF-beta 1 and IL-1 are both proinflammatory and fibrogenic factors (Fig. 13.8). Others such as the interferons (IFN-alpha, beta and gamma) are considered to be antifibrogenic factors because they inhibit fibroblast proliferation and ECM production. The therapeutic potential of the interferons will be discussed later. Six well-characterized human growth factors: epidermal growth factor (EGF), TGF-beta 1, TGF-beta, fibroblast growth factor (FGF), insulin-like growth factor (IGF)-1, and PDGF, were evaluated by topical application on skin wounds in swine (63). Of these, TGF-beta 1 was the only one that produced a marked tissue response and enhanced inflammation. While the literature suggests that many of the extracellular mediators play prominent roles during wound healing by affecting fibroblast growth

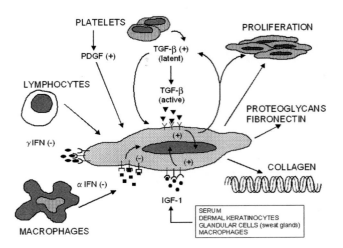

Figure 13.8 The fibrogenic and antifibrogenic factors that modulate fibroblast function during wound healing. [Reprinted from Scott PG et al. Molecular and Cellular Aspects of Fibrosis following Thermal Injury. In: Thermal Injuries. Hand Clin 2000; 16(2):271–287, with permission from Elsevier Science.]

and metabolism, only a few of these growth factors, such as TGF-beta 1, IGF-1 and PDGF, have the ability to trigger the proliferation of fibroblasts directly and/or stimulate the production of connective tissue (46,64). Of these IGF-1 and TGF-beta 1 seem to persist into the final stages of healing (31,66). We have recently found a greater expression of TGF-beta 1 and IGF-1 in postburn HSc tissue relative to normal tissue obtained from the same patients (64,65). Therefore, we concentrate here on these two prominent fibrogenic factors.

A. Transforming Growth Factor-beta 1

TGF-beta 1 is a multifunctional cytokine that influences many important physiological processes such as cellular proliferation and differentiation (66). It is secreted as a latent high molecular weight complex (LTGF-beta), consisting of a 25 kDa dimeric mature protein with 112 amino acids in each subunit and the dimeric N-terminal precursor peptide known as latency associated peptide (LAP) (67). TGF-beta 1 is a member of a large family of proteins including five TGF-beta isoforms (TGF-beta 1–5), the inhibins, activins, and mullerian inhibiting substance. TGF-beta isoforms share 70–80% sequence identity. The sequences of the mature, proteolytically processed forms of each member are highly conserved between species (68). TGF-beta 1–3 have been found in mammals and their tissue-specific differential expression may have important biological consequences [reviewed in Ref. (69)]. In a number of cell types, such as fibroblasts, platelets, and bone cells, the latent TGF-beta 1 complex also contains a covalently associated 125–205 kDa glycoprotein termed the latent TGF-beta binding protein (LTBP). Latent TGF-beta 1 produced by some osteoblast-like cells and recombinant TGF-beta 1 synthesized by Chinese hamster ovary cells is not associated with this binding protein (70,71). Although the functional significance of the various forms of latent TGF-beta 1 has not been elucidated, it is believed that disruption of the latent complex, either by conformational changes induced by binding to another component or by complete dissociation of the LAP, results in activation (71,72).

TGF-beta 1 is a potent chemoattractant for monocytes and fibroblasts (73,74). Both TGF-beta 1 and IGF-1 can stimulate the synthesis and deposition of various ECM proteins important in differentiation, morphogenesis, and wound healing (68,75,76). TGF-beta 1 stimulates fibroblasts to synthesize collagen, fibronectin, and GAGs, downregulates decorin synthesis while upregulating production of versican and biglycan, enhances neovascularization, stimulates collagen production in normal human dermal fibroblasts and modulates production of a variety of proteinases and their inhibitors (64,68,77–81). Subcutaneous injection of TGF-beta 1 into newborn mice stimulates granulation tissue formation and accelerates healing of incisional wounds in rats (68,82). All these effects and evidence implicating it in other fibrotic conditions point to its probable involvement in the pathogenesis of HSc [reviewed in Ref. (69).]

A number of transgenic models of wound healing where TGF-beta is expressed in a constitutively active form and under the direction of various keratin promoters have demonstrated that TGF-beta inhibits re-epithelialization *in vivo* and likely contributes to dermal fibrosis. In our own experience, TGF-beta 1 expressed under the control of the keratin 14 promoter (a basal keratin active in mature keratinocytes) increased TGF-beta protein expression and activity in the epidermis and dermis, inhibited epithelialization and delayed heal before the slowly healing wound developed fibrotic features in the dermis either in response to open excisional wounds or following laser induced thermal injury (83,84).

B. Connective Tissue Growth Factor

Connective tissue growth factor (CTGF) is a mitogenic protein, which is immunologically related to PDGF (85). It is secreted by fibroblasts after treatment with TGF-beta and is coordinately expressed with TGF-beta in several fibrotic conditions (although there does not appear to be evidence directly relating to postburn hypertrophic scars) (86,87). These observations suggest that CTGF is a downstream mediator of the action of TGF-beta in connective tissue where it stimulates proliferation of fibroblasts and synthesis of ECM (88). The range of cell types responding to CTGF is much more restricted than that for TGF-beta and it has no activity against epithelial or immune cells, for example, suggesting that it may be a more suitable target for the selective control of connective tissue metabolism in FPD (88).

C. Insulin-Like Growth Factor-1

IGF-1 mediates the actions of growth hormone on many tissues and also plays a role in wound healing through its effects on dermal fibroblasts (89). IGF-1 is mitogenic for fibroblasts and endothelial cells and stimulates collagen production by osteoblasts (90,91). Although IGF-1 was initially identified in serum and found to be produced in the liver, subsequent studies have revealed its expression in most tissues examined (90). Like TGF-beta 1, IGF-1 is expressed locally in response to tissue injury and its expression is increased in parallel to the formation of granulation tissue between weeks 1 and 5 after injury (92–94). In regenerating skeletal muscle and arterial injuries, increased mRNA for IGF-1 was detected within 24 h after injury (92,95). As for TGF-beta 1, IGF-1 stimulates collagen production in human lung fibroblasts, bovine fetal growth-plate chondrocytes, and human dermal fibroblasts (75,76,96). It stimulates DNA synthesis, replication of isolated epiphyseal growth-plate chondrocytes, induction of GAGs, and incorporation of radiolabeled proline into collagen by these cells (97,98). Interestingly, IGF-1 reduces the level of collagenase mRNA and collagenase activity secreted by dermal fibroblasts (27). We recently found greater expression of TGF-beta 1 and IGF-1 in postburn HSc tissue compared to normal dermis from the same patients (99). Similar results have been reported in other fibrotic conditions including scleroderma, hepatic, intraocular, and pulmonary fibroses (100). Takeda et al. (101) provided evidence that the excessive accumulation of collagen in patients with systemic sclerosis is due to differential expression of collagen and collagenase by fibroblasts.

While the actions of IGF-1 *in vitro* are impressive, the source(s) of IGF-1 is (are) not well described in normal and fibrotic human tissues. In normal skin, IGF-1 is restricted to the cells of epidermal, sweat, and sebaceous glands; therefore, it is unlikely that fibroblasts in the dermis will normally have access to IGF-1 (102). However, in healing burn wounds, these structures are disrupted and residual glandular cells migrating toward the wound surface to form the epithelial layer secrete IGF-1 in close proximity to dermal fibroblasts, thus contributing to the development of postburn HSc. These glandular epithelial cells have other important functions besides production of sebum and sweat including production of IL-8, a cytokine with chemotactic activity for neutrophils (103). Thus, dermal appendages appear to contribute growth factors including IGF-1, which are mitogenic and fribogenic and contribute to the development of postburn HSc.

D.   Interactions of IGF-1 and TGF-beta 1

Activated platelets and macrophages release IGF-1 and TGF-beta 1 at the site of injury and these growth factors are detectable in tissue and in wound chambers (90,104–106). Fibroblasts, which are the primary source of ECM, synthesize both TGF-beta 1 and IGF-1 and respond to these growth factors (107). Okazaki et al. demonstrated that TGF-beta markedly increases IGF-1 expression in osteoblast-like cells and we recently reported that IGF-1 stimulates the production of TGF-beta 1 through an increased rate of gene transcription (108,109). These findings suggest that IGF-1 in wound fluid is likely to function as a TGF-beta 1 stimulating factor.

Because IGF-1 binding proteins (IGFBPs) modulate the biological activity of IGF-1, the effects of both IGF-1 and TGF-beta 1 on the expression of these binding proteins have recently been studied in different cell types. TGF-beta 1 increased IGFBP-2 and IGFBP-3 in alveolar epithelial cells and Hs578T breast cancer cells (110). IGFBP-3, which is considered to be the main binding protein associated with IGF-1 in the blood and tissue, has been reported to mediate the antiproliferative effects of TGF-beta 1 on human breast cancer cells (111).

E.   The Role of the Th1/Th2 Paradigm After Burn Injury

Over the past decade, considerable evidence has emerged to suggest that T helper cells (CD4+) are major immunoregulators which mediate their function by the production of cytokines after activation by macrophages, Langerhans cells, or other antigen presenting cells (APCs) in the context of a major histocompatibility complex molecule which binds to the T cell receptor (TCR) (112–114). Mosmann defined two murine subsets of CD4+ cells which produce distinct groups of cytokines: Th1 clones, which express IL-2, IFN-gamma, and TNF-alpha, as well as IgG_2a isotype antibodies, and are principally mediators of cell mediated immunity and defense against intracellular pathogens and Th2 clones, which express IL-4, IL-5, and IL-10, and are associated with antibody mediated immunity, IgE and IgG_1 production, eosinophilia, and mast cell production [reviewed in Refs. (114–117)]. Although both cell types are thought to arise from a common precursor, the presence of IL-4 in the early stages of T cell stimulation leads to strong polarization of T cells toward the Th2 phenotype and secretion of high levels of IL-4 upon restimulation (118). IL-4 along with IL-10 inhibits the synthesis of IFN-gamma and other Th-1 cytokines (119). IL-12 is very effective in inducing IFN-gamma, but is inhibited by Th2 cytokines, IL-4, and IL-10 and also strongly by TGF-beta (120,121). Both Langerhans cells (113) and keratinocytes (112) function as APCs in the skin capable of inducing differentiation *in vitro* to both Th1 and Th2 or Th2 only clones, strongly supporting the importance of T helper cell immunoregulation of healing in the skin. Considerable evidence exists to suggest that the murine patterns of cytokine production occur in humans, and are involved in the pathogenesis of a number of human disorders including systemic lupus erythematosus (122), systemic scleroderma (123), atopic dermatitis (124), protozoal and fungal infections including leprosy (125), leischmaniasis (126), and schistosomiasis (127).

In a murine model of burn injury, Hunt et al. (128) demonstrated a depletion in splenic T helper cells (CD4), an increase in cytotoxic T-lymphocyte response associated with reduced IL-2 and IFN-gamma production as well as increased IL-5 cytokine production, thus a Th2 polarized response. Studies of immune function in burn patients during the early acute or open wound stages of burn injury have well documented the deficiency of IL-2, a Th1 cytokine (129). In both an animal model of burn injury and subsequently in burn patients, increased IL-4 mRNA and protein have been documented (128). With the development of techniques to allow for intracellular staining of CD4+ lymphocytes (130,131), Zedler et al. (132,133) examined burn patients in the early phase of injury up to 7 days postburn and found significant upregulation of IL-4 and reduction in IFN-gamma. In a larger series of burn patients, again examined only during the first month postburn, Faist et al. (134) also found significant reductions in IFN-gamma which were predictive of those patients who died from sepsis and multiple organ failure due to burn injury. Unfortunately, IFN-gamma therapy in these severely ill patients did not protect them from infections, or decrease the mortality from infections in the early phase of burn injury (42).

By developing a method of cryopreservation of peripheral blood monocytes (PBMC), we have been able to extend the period of observation of the intracellular cytokine profile from the first few days of burn injury as described earlier, to as late as 13 months postinjury in 17 burn patients to date, well into the period when many surviving patients demonstrate significant HSc. Significant reductions in IFN-gamma are present and persist at least to 6 months postinjury are associated with three- to fourfold increases in IL-4 in patients who develop HSc postburn injury. This is similar to the findings of Shi et al. (135) in an animal model of liver injury, where mice with a Th2 response had severe hepatic fibrosis, whereas Th1 responding animals developed minimal fibrosis.

VI. TREATMENT OF HYPERTROPHIC SCAR, KELOIDS, AND CONTRACTURES

Currently, treatment of FPD including keloids and HSc remains time consuming, expensive, and with few consistently successful approaches, which results in many proposed methods of care and few standardized treatment regimes. Surgical excision of HSc and keloids without adjuvant therapy is associated with a high rate of recurrence (136). One of the difficulties in the assessment of new therapies is that immediately following re-epithelization the healed skin may be flat and soft, although red, but it thickens over time with a resulting increase in total volume. The time at which the volume peaks depends on the patient, location, and conservative intervention, making it difficult to assess how much worse the scar would have become without the treatment intervention or whether it was already at a point in time where it was resolving on its own (Figs. 13.9 and 13.10).

A. Prevention of Dermal Fibroproliferative Disorders

As illustrated in Fig. 13.10, HSc becomes apparent weeks or months after re-epithelialization of the injured dermis and continues to increase in size before undergoing

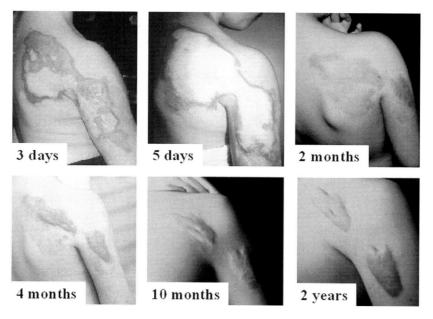

Figure 13.9 Serial documentation of a scald burn in a 10-year-old girl, which illustrates that after prolonged inflammation and delayed wound healing HSc often results despite pressure therapy. [From Tredget et al. (1).]

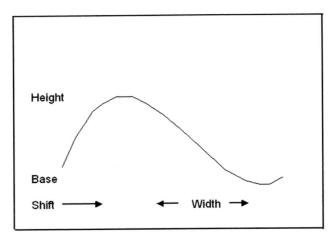

Measures

Figure 13.10 Mathematic modeling of serial measurements of HSc volume in eight patients over time revealed that immediately following re-epithelialization, scars are flat and supple. They gradually increase in height, thereby increasing the total volume of the scar. The time taken to reach the peak height, the ultimate extent to which the total volume increases, and the time required for the scar to flatten and mature (the slope of the line) are extremely variable among patients. Assessment of treatment interventions is complicated as it may be initiated at any point in the development or resolution of scar formation. [Reprinted from Tredget et al. (1), with permission from Elsevier Science.]

spontaneous remodeling, often to an incomplete or unacceptable extent. Keloids increase in volume at a rate often predicted by the extent of inflammation associated with the original injury, may undergo periods of slowed growth or stability, but rarely regress. Because HSc will spontaneously regress over time, it becomes very important to distinguish them from keloids, so that appropriate treatment modalities can be individualized to specific lesions based on their predicted cellular behavior, extent and location of involvement, and social factors which will influence the patients ability to comply with a wide range of therapies.

A family history of keloids, previous exuberant response to injury, prolonged inflammation at the site of injury, and anatomic location of injury to the shoulders, anterior chest, neck, upper arms, and cheeks may be predictive of fibroproliferative lesions of significant extent. Unfortunately, no HLA-A or HLA-B tissue antigen associations have been consistently found among patients with keloids or HSc, nor has an autosomal or sex-linked pattern of inheritance been established. However, most keloids occur in patients between the ages of 10 and 30 and a strong sex hormonal influence has been found with a predisposition of keloids to develop during puberty and pregnancy with reports of softening and flattening of lesions with menopause and advancing age (seventh and eighth decades) (59).

Wound tension is an important critical factor in skin and wound closure, which can be reduced by planning surgical incisions and reconstruction along lines of relaxed skin tension. Autocrine production of fibrogenic growth factors after activation of cells in matrix appears to occur by the transmission of ECM forces to the cell membrane through cell surface adhesion molecules including integrins before it is transmitted intracellularly via focal adhesion complexes. Subsequently, alterations in the intracellular cytoskeleton can increase nuclear gene transcription of TGF-beta and other cytokine and matrix protein genes leading to abnormal matrix production (137).

Another factor of high predictive value for the development of dermal fibrosis is the persistence of chronic inflammation in wounds. We and others have found that burn wounds in the deep dermis which required prolonged periods for healing had a very high rate of developing HSc independent of the patient's age, sex, and racial background. Thus, timing of wound closure for burns within 2–3 weeks has become an important prerequisite in minimizing HSc, particularly in important cosmetic regions such as the face (51,138) and in mobile skin of the hands and joints.

Similarly, persistent or exaggerated inflammation from infection is a known trigger for keloids (Fig. 13.1). Cellulitis of the scalp, acne vulgaris, acne conglobata, hidradenitis suppurativa, pilonidal cysts, and foreign body reactions as well as folliculitis, pyoderma, vaccinia, and varicella have been associated with the development of keloids (139). Bacterial endotoxin has been shown to induce the production of TGF-beta by immune cells in wounds, which may be one of the mechanisms leading to fibrosis (140).

B. Conservative Therapy for Keloids, Hypertrophic Scar, and Contractures

Conservative management of HSc and contractures includes the use of pressure garments, silicone gel sheets, conformers, transparent facemasks, serial casting, and splints. Custom fabricated pressure garments are commonly used and are supplied by several companies based on individual patient measurements. Pressure therapy begins as soon as re-epithelialization occurs and garments should be ideally worn 24 h/day, until scar maturation is evident (141). Although the optimum pressure required for effect is unknown, the recommended level is greater than 25 mmHg; however, good clinical results have been reported with levels as low as 5–15 mmHg (142). The molecular and cellular basis for the success of pressure therapy is not known but the creation of a hypoxic environment may reduce fibroblast proliferation and reduce collagen synthesis (143) by occlusion of small vessels within the scar (144). These authors also noted that interstitial spaces between collagen fibrils in HSc were virtually absent following treatment with continuous pressure and there was a decrease in the number of nodules, with a more parallel orientation of collagen relative to the epidermis and an increase in collagen fiber bundle formation. Also reduction in the mast cell population in HSc occurred following pressure therapy (145). Finally, a recent controlled study of burns patients treated with and without elastic pressure garments has suggested that no statistically significant benefit could be determined for the use of this approach to warrant the considerable cost, inconvenience, and side effects which includes obstructive sleep apnea, patient discomfort, and wound breakdown under pressure spots (138,146). However, the lack of documentation of patient compliance, measurements of pressure achieved, control of anatomical site, surgical intervention, and wound complications, as well as the limited number of patients studied suggest that further re-examination is required before the results can be more generally accepted. Recently, studies are emerging in which more objective measures of scar assessment using instruments to measure erythema and melanin (147), elastic recoil of the skin and dermal compliance (148) and thickness (149), as well as improved clinical scar scoring systems continue to be unable to demonstrate significant improvements of scar modulation with pressure garments in well-controlled trials. These studies, however, are still in their preliminary stages (150).

The use of silicone gel sheets was introduced as an alternative form of treatment and has been successful with HSc, keloids (55,151,152), and contractures (153). Gel sheets can be worn as long as 24 h/day, with particular attention paid to hygiene to avoid the development of contact dermatitis (154). Silicone gel may exert its effects by increasing the temperature of the scar, thereby enhancing the activity of collagenase, which is known to increase several fold over 1° or 2° of body temperature (155). Such increases in temperature are typical following silicone gel treatment and have been documented in burn patients with HSc (156). Other effects of silicone gel such as increased pressure, lowered oxygen tension, or occlusion may be less important. Hydration of the stratum corneum and direct release of low-molecular weight silicone fluid into the scar are other possible modes of action (157); however, silicone does not appear to enter scar tissues (158).

Silastic conformers can be used as independent inserts in conjunction with pressure garments to supplement pressure in concave regions (159) or embedded within a supporting matrix (160) or as an adhesive dressing as a primary treatment (161).

Transparent face masks (162) are an alternative means to achieve optimal pressure and conformity for the treatment of HSc and contractures following facial burns and are more readily accepted by patients as they provide an easier transition and are more socially acceptable due to the exposure of facial features in public (138).

Currently, serial casting has become the most effective conservative form of treatment for reducing burn scar contractures (163,164), although static serial splinting and dynamic splinting continue to be extensively utilized (165).

C. Intralesional Corticosteriods

Intralesional injection of triamcinolone alone or combined with other therapies for the control of local discomfort and flattening of the scars has been found to be associated with a 50% response rate in keloids over 5 years (166) with another study reporting a recurrence rate of 5 of 56 keloids over 4 years. Although various guidelines exist for preparations, dosage, and administration, one approach employs varying concentrations (10, 20, 30, or 40 mg/mL) in different lesions or areas of the same lesion to establish the minimum effective dosage for subsequent treatments usually at 3–4 week intervals. Such therapy is likely to be effective by inhibiting transcription of certain matrix protein genes [including beta 1 (1) and beta 1 (III) procollagen, fibronectin, TGF-beta, and other cytokines] as well as reducing alpha-2 macroglobulin synthesis, a known inhibitor of collagenase activity (167). A common complication of corticosteriod injections is pain at the site of injection, which can be averted by topical anesthesia and/or regional injections of local anesthetic around the scars to be injected (168). Other adverse side effects include scar or subcutaneous tissue atrophy, telangiectasia, necrosis, ulceration, and cushingoid habitus. Local pigmentation and atrophy can be minimized by confining the injection to the scar and maintaining the steroid concentration below 5 mg/mL. Various delivery systems exist including spring or CO_2-powered devices, but most commonly luer-locked syringes with 25- to 30-guage needle are employed aiming to place the injection 0.5 cm apart and into the bulk of the lesion. Systemic effects are avoided by timing injections greater than every 4 weeks after which therapeutic effects should be apparent.

Cryotherapy has been reported as a preliminary adjunct prior to corticosteroids for localized HSc and keloids to facilitate penetration of the steroid with the lesions, but by itself varying results have been achieved, most successfully in newly formed lesions with multiple treatments (169,170).

Recently, calcium channel blockers (verapamil) or calmodulin inhibitors (trifluoperazine) have been injected into HSc and keloids which failed to respond to corticosteroids, in an attempt to activate collagenase synthesis in the lesions through the alterations in fibroblast morphology which are known to induce collagenase gene transcription (171). Although beneficial effects were found in three of five treated patients, the approach entailed few if any side effects with a maximum intralesional injection of 2 mL (2.5 mg/mL) in an attempt to achieve 100–500-μmol/L in the scar.

Antimetabolite medications including topical fluorouracil and intralesional bleomycin have been found to be effective in small clinical trials and appear to have nonspecific antiproliferative and antiinflammatory effects which are incompletely understood (172,173).

D. Surgical Therapy

Recurrence rates for simple surgical excision of keloids and HSc alone vary from 50% to 80% (174). Attempts to resurface with skin grafts have a reported recurrence rate of 59%, but half of the keloid patients treated developed new lesions in the donor site (136,175). However, beneficial effects of surgical excision of keloids have occurred with narrow-based (<1 cm) pedunculated lesions and when surgical procedures are combined with local flaps to reduce wound tension and adjunctive therapy. Such adjuncts include local steroid therapy in the margins of the wound and monthly injections thereafter. The more common earlobe keloid often is treated by local excision of the lesion and intraoperative steroids followed by pressure therapy using a variety of earring pressure devices (176). During surgical excision of HSc and keloids, care must be taken to remove all sources of residual inflammation which occurs with trapped hair follicles, epithelial cysts, sinus tracts, and infected pilosebaceous units which may be a source of fibrogenic growth factors. Surgical reconstruction should be designed to minimize tissue trauma and wound tension while avoiding dead space,

foreign material, hematoma, and infection. Reorientation of scars parallel to lines of relaxed skin tension should be an integral part of preoperative planning.

Intramarginal excision of HSc and keloids has been proposed as a useful surgical technique to minimize recurrence of lesions which have failed nonoperative surgical therapy. Similar approaches maintaining remnants of keloid epithelium have been proposed but objective trials of this approach are lacking.

Radiation therapy in the form of photons, electrons, and interstitial therapy has been employed as a measure to control proliferative lesions in the skin usually following surgical therapy. Darzi et al. (174) provided a 10-year follow up of 65 patients treated with beta radiation alone, pre- and postoperative radiation and surgery followed by beta radiation, and steroid injection alone. Eleven percent of lesions reduced with radiation alone, whereas radiation combined with surgical therapy yielded a 75% reduction in lesions with no benefit to preoperative radiotherapy. Intralesional triamcinolone produced complete flattening in 64% of patients in this trial. Recognition of the beneficial postoperative effects has been reported by others also; however, malignant transformation of radiation treated keloids has been reported limiting its usefulness particularly in young individuals who are at higher risk of difficult to measure late sequelae (52,165,177–179) (Fig. 13.11).

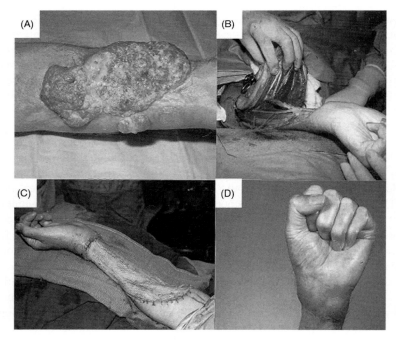

Figure 13.11 (A) Squamous cell carcinoma of the upper extremity 30 years after spontaneous healing of thermal injury of the upper extremity and radiation therapy for the management of severe hypertrophic scarring. The tumor was removed at the level of the superficial flexor muscles of the forearm (B) and the arm was resurfaced with a split-thickness autograft (C), resulting in stable wound coverage with good hand function (D). [Reprinted from Tredget et al. Management of the acutely burned upper extremity. In: Thermal Injuries. Hand Clin 2000; 16(2):187–203, with permission from Elsevier Science.]

E. Surgical Therapy of Contractures

Although most contractures are effectively treated by a combined program of pressure therapy, serial casting, and/or splinting, surgical release is necessary for refractory lesions or for contractures which are physically impossible to treat conservatively based on location or by exposure of vital structures, for example eyelid ectropion. Surgical incision across the line of tension must be followed by wound closure to minimize recurrence. Split-thickness skin grafts are less effective than full-thickness grafts which are in turn less effective than flaps of local or distant tissues (180) (Fig. 13.12). Control of contraction appears closely related to elements of the dermis, as the use of keratinocyte sheets has been associated with rates of contraction which resemble those in uncovered wounds (181). To date, pharmacologic control of contraction with inhibitors of smooth muscle or cortisone have been unrewarding or impractical; however, newer antifibrotic growth factors may provide novel therapeutic modalities in the future (50).

Recently, Integra® artificial dermis has become the first dermal substitute available for reconstructive surgery. Although experience with the material is required for effective usage, it represents another new method to treat severe HSc and possibly keloids. Many small studies and case reports support its utility as illustrated in Fig. 13.13; however, larger studies, cost effectiveness and comparison to other methods has to be completed. Recently, objective measures of quality of tissue regeneration after Integra™ reconstruction would suggest that dermal compliance and elastic recoil is better that scar or split-thickness skin graft reconstruction (182,183).

F. Laser Therapy of HSc and Keloids

Recently, Alster (184) has described the use of 585 nm flash lamp pulsed dye lasers for selective photothermolysis of vascular endothelial cells in HSc. Fifty-seven to eighty-three percent improvement in surface texture measurements and clinical criteria with one or two treatments

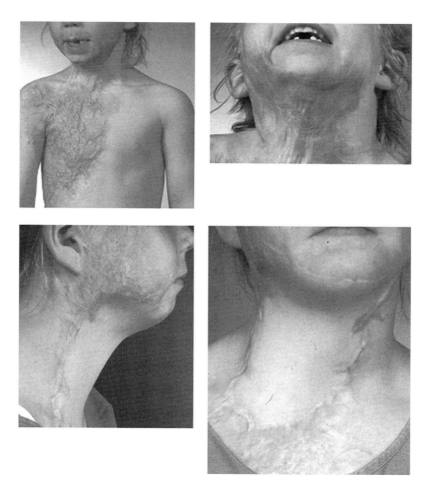

Figure 13.12 Control of burn wound contractures in the neck of a 9-year-old girl treated with a previously tissue expanded radial forearm free flap. [From Tredget et al. (1).]

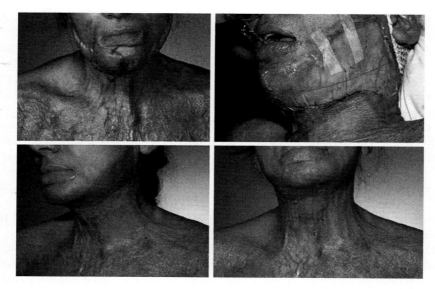

Figure 13.13 Treatment of an east-Indian patient who developed severe scarring of the face and neck (A) and right upper extremity (B) after suffering a 50% burn injury using the artificial dermal matrix Integra®, prior to surgery, 3 weeks after placement of Integra, and 3 months following second stage thin split thickness donor site coverage.

was claimed with similar results reported by Dierickx et al. (185). In a nonrandomized study of portions of median sternotomy scar halves, symptomatic improvement resembled that previously described. However, Sheridan et al. (186) failed to find significant benefit from pulsed dye laser therapy in HSc in burn patients. Further, carefully designed randomized trials investigating multiple unanswered questions including the role of combination laser therapy and the most appropriate timing after injury and scar formation are indicated (184).

VII. NEW PHARMACOTHERAPIES FOR HYPERTROPHIC SCARRING

A. Antifibrotic Factors: IFN-alpha2b and IFN-gamma

The experimental therapies discussed here are of two broad types: those using pleiotropic cytokines such as the IFNs, which may be expected to affect several cell types and their associated processes, and those targeted to specific components of the pathology, such as the excessive collagen synthesis or impaired collagen degradation. The IFNs have been quite extensively investigated in the clinic and will receive most attention here, but other possible therapies suggested by insights into the pathogenesis of HSc obtained primarily or exclusively from studies *in vitro* will also be discussed.

Antifibrogenic cytokines include the IFN family and consist of type I IFNs that include IFN-alpha and IFN-beta, which are produced by leukocytes and fibroblasts,

respectively, and type II IFN or IFN-gamma which is produced by T-lymphocytes. Type I and type II IFNs bind to destruct high-affinity receptors, present on most cell types, which are each associated with two tyrosine kinases from the Janus family of kinases (187). These kinases phosphorylate cytoplasmic signal transduction proteins, which bind to *cis*-acting elements, thereby enhancing or inhibiting the transcription rate of various genes. For fibroblasts, this in turn results in a decrease in the rate of proliferation and a reduced rate of synthesis of collagen and fibronectin.

The reduction of protein synthesis is of particular interest in fibroproliferative disorders, where abnormally high amounts of ECM protein production are characteristic. *In vitro* IFN-alpha and gamma have been shown to reduce the synthesis of collagen by normal and HSc fibroblasts (32,188). The reduction of mRNA for type I and III collagen by IFN may be partially accounted for by a reduction in the stability of the message, as well as a downregulation of nuclear factor 1, which is a procollagen gene-activating transcription factor (189). The downregulation of nuclear factor 1 may account for the delay in maximal inhibition of collagen production. However, in addition to decreasing the level of type I collagen mRNA, exposure to IFN-alpha2b led to a reduction in posttranslational hydroxylation and an increase in the proportion of newly synthesized collagen which undergoes intracellular degradation. Fibronectin production by HSc and patient-matched normal dermal fibroblasts has also been shown to be reduced by IFN-alpha2b (102). Importantly, IFN-alpha2b differs from IFN-gamma by increasing mRNA and collagenase activity, whereas IFN-gamma decreases collagenase

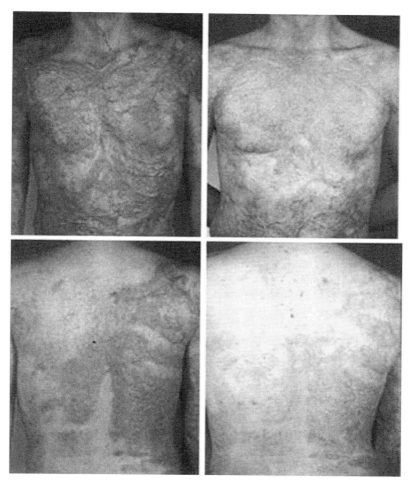

Figure 13.14 HSc maturation of a 45-year-old male who suffered a 40% TBSA burn and developed severe HSc of face chest back and upper extremities prior to systemic IFN-α2b, 3 months and 6 months postinjury. (Reprinted from Tredget et al. (50) with permission from Williams & Wilkins.)

activity. IFN-alpha2b, IFN-beta, and IFN-gamma have also been shown to reduce the rate and extent of FPCL contraction, which may act through a reduction in beta and gamma-cytoplasmic actin production or alterations in the functional interactions of actin microfilaments and their associated proteins (136).

Using murine wound healing models, Granstein et al. (190) were able to demonstrate *in vivo* that IFN-gamma decreased local wound erythema, neutrophil infiltration and collagen deposition and inhibited the fibrotic reaction to implanted foreign bodies (191). Intralesional injections of IFN-alpha2b into a keloid resulted in a gradual reduction in size, as did IFN-gamma when injected into keloids, HSc, and Dupytrens disease nodules. McCauley et al. (192) have suggested that keloid patients have deficient systemic production of IFN-alpha and IFN-gamma, which may contribute to the development of these lesions and provide a theoretical basis for the provision.

As discussed earlier, alterations in ECM components are believed to be responsible for the undesirable physical properties of fibrotic scar tissue. We have found that expression of mRNA for several ECM macromolecules is altered in fibroblasts derived from HSc, compared to normal cells obtained from the same patients. The differential synthesis of collagen and collagenase in postburn HSc appears to be one of the main reasons for the excessive accumulation of collagen. The interferons have been found to normalize the expression of ECM proteins by dermal fibroblasts derived from fibrotic tissue. IFN-gamma is secreted by activated T-lymphocytes, whereas IFN-alpha and -beta are the products of leukocytes and fibroblasts, respectively (193). Several *in vitro* studies have shown both IFN-gamma and IFN-alpha2b to reduce the expression of type I and to a lesser extent type III procollagen mRNA in dermal fibroblasts (50,65). We have further shown that IFN-alpha2b increases the expression of collagenase by dermal fibroblasts, whereas IFN-gamma does not (62). This suggests that IFN-alpha2b could have some advantages over IFN-gamma for the treatment of FPD, such as postburn HSc. Animal studies have shown that IFN-alpha2b can modulate wound healing *in vivo* (194). Some preliminary clinical trials using IFNs in patients with keloid and postburn HSc have been reported. Keloid patients treated with IFN-alpha2b demonstrated only limited improvement over nontreated patients (195,196) but early trials in postburn HSc patients seem promising (50). Systemic administration of IFN-alpha2b was associated with reduction in elevated levels of serum TGF-beta and plasma histamine levels. In addition, HSc tissues demonstrated earlier reduction in the elevated levels of mRNA for TGF-beta with IFN therapy, which was due in part to a reduction in the autocrine production of TGF-beta by fibroblasts present in the tissues (33). In patients treated with IFN-alpha2b at doses mimicking the initiating regimes for hepatitis B patients, visible improvement in scar maturation is possible as well as more objective evidence such as reduction in scar volume, improvement in scar rating, together with normalization of elevated histamine and TGF-beta in the systemic circulation (Figs. 13.12 and 13.13). However, larger numbers of patients in double-blinded randomized trials are required to establish systemic cytokine therapy for severe FPD such as HSc and keloids. Such trials have begun for systemic sclerosis, pulmonary fibrosis, and postburn HSc.

However, there are practical drawbacks to the systemic or intralesional administration of IFN-alpha2b. First, systemic administration is not suitable for children due to the necessity for frequent intradermal or intralesional injections. Second, in our clinical trial five of nine patients treated with IFN-alpha2b experienced flu-like symptoms including fatigue, nausea, headache, and low-grade fever (5). Finally, large quantities of IFN-alpha2b are required making treatment moderately expensive. Normally, topical administration of IFN-alpha2b in solution is not effective because the free cytokine does not penetrate the epidermis efficiently. Topical application of liposome-associated IFN-alpha2b could circumvent many of these problems, including the adverse side-effects because the quantity required should be significantly less (thousands of units rather than millions) than when administered systemically. Liposomes with IFN-alpha have been used successfully for treatment of cutaneous herpes simplex in guinea pigs (197). Liposome-associated IFN-alpha2b retains its effectiveness in modulating collagen synthesis by cultured fibroblasts (198) and in skin wounds in guinea pigs (117).

B. Other Antagonists of TGF-beta

The absence of decorin from healing burn wounds (11) could have profound implications for the development of HSc, both because of its role in promoting normal fibrous tissue architecture (18) and because it may function as a natural regulator (antagonist) of TGF-beta (20). Since mature postburn scars contain normal amounts of this proteroglycan (11) and stain strongly for TGF-beta (18), and since it is massively re-expressed in HSc starting about 12 months after injury (7), decorin could be suggested as a therapy, if suitable delivery vehicles for the protein itself or its gene can be devised. Both intramuscular injection (100) and synthesis from an expression vector (199) have been demonstrated to be effective in counteracting the fibrotic changes mediated by TGF-beta1 in experimental glomerulonephritis in rats.

The latency-associated peptide of the small latent TGF-beta complex carries three N-linked oligosaccharides, two of which have mannose-6-phosphate (M6P) residues (200). These mediate the attachment of TGF-beta1 to the M6P/IGF-II receptor (M6P/IGF-II) (201). The activation of latent TGF-beta1 in cocultures of bovine aortic endothelial and smooth muscle cells can be blocked by M6P, presumably by interfering with this association (201). Although the precise mechanism by which binding to the M6P/IGF-II receptor promotes activation of TGF-beta is not known, these observations have stimulated interest in the use of M6P to prevent scarring (202).

Other pharmacologic agents developed and applied initially following a different rationale may exert some of their activity directly or indirectly through effects on TGF-beta expression or activity. Tranilast [*N*-(3,4-dimethoxycinnamoyl) anthranilic acid], an anti-allergic drug that has been applied to the treatment of HSc and keloids (203), can inhibit the release of TGF-beta1 and other cytokines from human monocytes/macrophages (204). A cross-linked mixture of type I collagen and polyvinylpyrrolidone ("Fibroquel"), injected intralesionally into HSc, reduced immunostaining of the treated tissue for IL-1beta, TNF-alpha, and PDGF and secretion of TGF-beta1 and PDGF by fibroblasts cultured from it (205).

C. Modulators of Fibroblast-Mediated ECM Metabolism

Various strategies have been proposed, and some tested in the clinic, to increase the rate of turnover of the scar collagen through increased secretion of collagenase by the fibroblasts. These include treatment with PG E1 and SM-10906 (the synthetic analog of PGI) (206,207), relaxin (208), and calcium channel blockers such as verapamil (209). Presumably acting by a completely different mechanism, is putrescine ("Fibrostat"), an inhibitor of the transglutaminase-mediated cross-linking of type III collagen that has been tested with some apparent success in the clinic (210).

VIII. SUMMARY

The pathogenesis of HSc following thermal injury remains a complex and incompletely understood process, but recent investigations into the composition of the tissue itself, the activities of the scar fibroblasts and the effects of various cytokines and growth factors, have all contributed to the emergence of an increasingly clear picture. Although it may be considered just one example of a broad range of FPDs which afflict many different organs, often in response to diverse environmental insults, the nature of the burn injury and the special properties of skin probably play important roles in promoting the development of this especially troublesome variety of excessive connective tissue. This knowledge has provided the rationale for a number of experimental therapies that, individually or in some combination, may augment or one day supplant the more commonly employed surgical or physical treatments.

REFERENCES

1. Tredget EE, Nedelec B, Scott PG, Ghahary A. Hypertrophic scars, keloids, and contractures. The cellular and molecular basis for therapy. Surg Clin North Am 1997; 77(3):701–730.
2. Linares HA, Kischer CW, Dobrkovsky M, Larson DL. The histiotypic organization of the hypertrophic scar in humans. J Invest Dermatol 1972; 59(4):323–331.
3. Kischer CW. Collagen and dermal patterns in the hypertrophic scar. Anat Rec 1974; 179(1):137–145.
4. Kischer CW. Fibroblasts of the hypertrophic scar, mature scar and normal skin: a study by scanning and transmission electron microscopy. Tex Rep Biol Med 1974; 32(3–4):699–709.
5. Tredget EE, Shen YJ, Forsyth N, Smith C, Scott P, Ghahary A. Regulation of collagen synthesis and mRNA levels in normal and hypertrophic scar fibroblasts in vitro by interferon alpha-2b. Wound Repair Regen 1993; 1:156–165.
6. Ehrlich HP, White BS. The identification of alpha A and alpha B collagen chains in hypertrophic scar. Exp Mol Pathol 1981; 34(1):1–8.
7. Sayani K, Dodd CM, Nedelec B, Shen YJ, Ghahary A, Tredget EE, Scott PG. Delayed appearance of decorin in healing burn scars. Histopathology 2000; 36(3):262–272.
8. Baur PS, Larson DL, Stacey TR. The observation of myofibroblasts in hypertrophic scars. Surg Gynecol Obstet 1975; 141(1):22–26.
9. Ehrlich HP, Desmouliere A, Diegelmann RF, Cohen IK, Compton CC, Garner WL, Kapanci Y, Gabbiani G. Morphological and immunochemical differences between keloid and hypertrophic scar. Am J Pathol 1994; 145(1):105–113.
10. Kischer CW, Bailey JF. The mast cell in hypertrophic scars. Tex Rep Biol Med 1972; 30(4):327–338.
11. Scott PG, Dodd CM, Tredget EE, Ghahary A, Rahemtulla F. Chemical characterization and quantification of proteoglycans in human post-burn hypertrophic and mature scars. Clin Sci (Lond) 1996; 90(5):417–425.
12. Hayakawa T, Hashimoto Y, Myokei Y, Aoyama H, Izawa Y. Changes in type of collagen during the development of human post-burn hypertrophic scars. Clin Chim Acta 1979; 93(1):119–125.
13. Bailey AJ, Bazin S, Sims TJ, Le Lous M, Nicoletis C, Delaunay A. Characterization of the collagen of human hypertrophic and normal scars. Biochim Biophys Acta 1975; 405(2):412–421.
14. Ogston A. Chemistry and Molecular Biology of the Intracellular Matrix. New York: Academic Press, 1970.
15. Scott J. Proteoglycan-fibillar collagen interactions in tissues: dermatan sulphate proteoglycan as a tissue organizer. In: Scott J, ed. Dermatan Sulphate Proteoglycans: Chemistry, Biology, Chemical Pathology. London: Portland Press, 1993:65.
16. Yeo TK, Brown L, Dvorak HF. Alterations in proteoglycan synthesis common to healing wounds and tumors. Am J Pathol 1991; 138(6):1437–1450.
17. Kuc IM, Scott PG. Increased diameters of collagen fibrils precipitated in vitro in the presence of decorin from various connective tissues. Connect Tissue Res 1997; 36(4):287–296.
18. Scott PG, Dodd CM, Tredget EE, Ghahary A, Rahemtulla F. Immunohistochemical localization of the proteoglycans decorin, biglycan and versican and transforming growth factor-beta in human post-burn hypertrophic and mature scars. Histopathology 1995; 26(5):423–431.
19. Danielson KG, Baribault H, Holmes DF, Graham H, Kadler KE, Iozzo RV. Targeted disruption of decorin leads to abnormal collagen fibril morphology and skin fragility. J Cell Biol 1997; 136(3):729–743.
20. Yamaguchi Y, Mann DM, Ruoslahti E. Negative regulation of transforming growth factor-beta by the proteoglycan decorin. Nature 1990; 346(6281):281–284.
21. Kuc IM, Scott PG. Ultrastructure of the bovine temporomandibular joint disc. Arch Oral Biol 1994; 39(1):57–61.
22. Shetlar MR, Shetlar CL. The hypertrophic scar: location of glycosaminoglycans within scars. Burns 1977; 4:14–29.
23. Bianco P, Fisher LW, Young MF, Termine JD, Robey PG. Expression and localization of the two small proteoglycans biglycan and decorin in developing human skeletal and non-skeletal tissues. J Histochem Cytochem 1990; 38(11):1549–1563.
24. Ghahary A, Pannu R, Tredget EE. Fibrogenic and antifibrogenic factors regulating the extracellular matrix in wound repair. In: Malhotra SK, ed. Advances in Structural Biology. London: JAI Press, 1996:197–232.
25. Zhou LJ, Inoue M, Ono I, Kaneko F. The mode of action of prostaglandin (PG) I1 analog, SM-10906, on fibroblasts of hypertrophic scars is similar to PGE1 in its potential

role of preventing scar formation. Exp Dermatol 1997; 6(6):314–320.

26. Scott PG, Ghahary A, Chambers M, Tredget EE. Biological basis of hypertrophic scarring. In: Malhotra SK, ed. Advances in Structural Biology. London: JAI Press Inc, 1994:157–201.

27. Ghahary A, Shen YJ, Nedelec B, Scott PG, Tredget EE. Interferons gamma and alpha-2b differntially regulate the expression of collagenase and tissue inhibitor of metalloproteinase-1 messenger RNA in humans hypertrophic and normal dermal fibroblasts. Wound Repair Regen 1995; 3:176–184.

28. Arakawa M, Hatamochi A, Mori Y, Mori K, Ueki H, Moriguchi T. Reduced collagenase gene expression in fibroblasts from hypertrophic scar tissue. Br J Dermatol 1996; 134(5):863–868.

29. Wang R, Ghahary A, Shen YJ, Scott PG, Tredget EE. Nitric oxide synthase expression and nitric oxide production are reduced in hypertrophic scar tissue and fibroblasts. J Invest Dermatol 1997; 108(4):438–444.

30. Schonherr E, Beavan LA, Hausser H, Kresse H, Culp LA. Differences in decorin expression by papillary and reticular fibroblasts in vivo and in vitro. Biochem J 1993; 290(Pt 3):893–899.

31. Ghahary A, Scott PG, Malhotra S et al. Differential expression of type I and type III procollagen mRNA in human hypertrophic burn fibroblasts. Biomed Lett 1992; 47:169–184.

32. Tredget EE, Forsyth N, Uji-Friedland A, Chambers M, Ghahary A, Scott PG, Hogg AM, Burke JF. Gas chromatography-mass spectrometry determination of 18O2 in 18O-labelled 4-hydroxyproline for measurement of collagen synthesis and intracellular degradation. J Chromatogr 1993; 612(1):7–19.

33. Tredget EE, Wang R, Shen Q, Scott PG, Ghahary A. Transforming growth factor-beta mRNA and protein in hypertrophic scar tissues and fibroblasts: antagonism by IFN-alpha and IFN-gamma in vitro and in vivo. J Interferon Cytokine Res 2000; 20(2):143–151.

34. Wang R, Ghahary A, Shen YJ, Scott PG, Tredget EE. Human dermal fibroblasts produce nitric oxide and express both constitutive and inducible nitric oxide synthase isoforms. J Invest Dermatol 1996; 106(3):419–427.

35. Savage K, Swann DA. A comparison of glycosaminoglycan synthesis by human fibroblasts from normal skin, normal scar, and hypertrophic scar. J Invest Dermatol 1985; 84(6):521–526.

36. Scott PG, Dodd CM, Ghahary A, Shen YJ, Tredget EE. Fibroblasts from post-burn hypertrophic scar tissue synthesize less decorin than normal dermal fibroblasts. Clin Sci (Lond) 1998; 94(5):541–547.

37. Kischer CW, Wagner HN Jr, Pindur J, Holubec H, Jones M, Ulreich JB, Scuderi P. Increased fibronectin production by cell lines from hypertrophic scar and keloid. Connect Tissue Res 1989; 23(4):279–288.

38. Oku T, Takigawa M, Fukamizu H, Inoue K, Yamada M. Growth kinetics of fibroblasts derived from normal skin and hypertrophic scar. Acta Derm Venereol 1987; 67(6):526–528.

39. Nedelec B, Shankowsky H, Scott PG, Ghahary A, Tredget EE. Myofibroblasts and apoptosis in human hypertrophic scars: the effect of interferon-alpha2b. Surgery 2001; 130(5):798–808.

40. Desmouliere A, Redard M, Darby I, Gabbiani G. Apoptosis mediates the decrease in cellularity during the transition between granulation tissue and scar. Am J Pathol 1995; 146(1):56–66.

41. Orrenius S. Apoptosis: molecular mechanisms and implications for human disease. J Intern Med 1995; 237(6):529–536.

42. Wassermann RJ, Polo M, Smith P, Wang X, Ko F, Robson MC. Differential production of apoptosis-modulating proteins in patients with hypertrophic burn scar. J Surg Res 1998; 75(1):74–80.

43. Meager A. Cytokines. Englewood Cliffs, NJ: Prentice-Hall, 1991.

44. Laster SM, Wood JG, Gooding LR. Tumor necrosis factor can induce both apoptic and necrotic forms of cell lysis. J Immunol 1988; 141(8):2629–2634.

45. Castagnoli C, Stella M, Berthod C, Magliacani G, Richiardi PM. TNF production and hypertrophic scarring. Cell Immunol 1993; 147(1):51–63.

46. Schultz GS, White M, Mitchell R, Brown G, Lynch J, Twardzik DR, Todaro GJ. Epithelial wound healing enhanced by transforming growth factor-alpha and vaccinia growth factor. Science 1987; 235(4786):350–352.

47. Brune B, von Knethen A, Sandau KB. Nitric oxide and its role in apoptosis. Eur J Pharmacol 1998; 351(3): 261–272.

48. Albina JE, Cui S, Mateo RB, Reichner JS. Nitric oxide-mediated apoptosis in murine peritoneal macrophages. J Immunol 1993; 150(11):5080–5085.

49. Chesney J, Bucala R. Peripheral blood fibrocytes: mesenchymal precursor cells and the pathogenesis of fibrosis. Curr Rheumatol Rep 2000; 2(6):501–505.

50. Tredget EE, Shankowsky HA, Pannu R, Nedelec B, Iwashina T, Gharary A, Taerum TV, Scott PG. Transforming growth factor-beta in thermally injured patients with hypertrophic scars: effects of interferon alpha-2b. Plast Reconstr Surg 1998; 102(5):1317–1328; discussion 1329–1330.

51. Engrav LH, Covey MH, Dutcher KD, Heimbach DM, Walkinshaw MD, Marvin JA. Impairment, time out of school, and time off from work after burns. Plast Reconstr Surg 1987; 79(6):927–934.

52. Enhamre A, Hammar H. Treatment of keloids with excision and postoperative X-ray irradiation. Dermatologica 1983; 167(2):90–93.

53. Arora PD, McCulloch CA. Dependence of collagen remodeling on alpha-smooth muscle actin expression by fibroblasts. J Cell Physiol 1994; 159(1):161–175.

54. Fakhrai H, Dorigo O, Shawler DL, Lin H, Mercola D, Black KL, Royston I, Sobol RE. Eradication of established intracranial rat gliomas by transforming growth factor beta antisense gene therapy. Proc Natl Acad Sci USA 1996; 93(7):2909–2914.

55. Farquhar J. Silicone gel and hypertrophic scar formation: a literature review. Can J Occup Ther 1992; 59:78.

56. Squier CA. The effect of stretching on formation of myo-fibroblasts in mouse skin. Cell Tissue Res 1981; 220(2):325–335.

57. Leavitt J, Gunning P, Kedes L, Jariwalla R. Smooth muscle alpha-action is a transformation-sensitive marker for mouse NIH 3T3 and Rat-2 cells. Nature 1985; 316(6031):840–842.

58. Ferguson MW. Skin wound healing: transforming growth factor beta antagonists decrease scarring and improve quality. J Interferon Res 1994; 14(5):303–304.

59. Ford LC, King DF, Lagasse LD, Newcomer V. Increased androgen binding in keloids: a preliminary communication. J Dermatol Surg Oncol 1983; 9(7):545–547.

60. Kovacs EJ. Fibrogenic cytokines: the role of immune mediators in the development of scar tissue. Immunol Today 1991; 12(1):17–23.

61. Baird A, Mormede P, Bohlen P. Immunoreactive fibroblast growth factor in cells of peritoneal exudate suggests its identity with macrophage-derived growth factor. Biochem Biophys Res Commun 1985; 126(1):358–364.

62. Kovacs EJ, DiPietro LA. Fibrogenic cytokines and connective tissue production. FASEB J 1994; 8(11):854–861.

63. Lynch SE, Colvin RB, Antoniades HN. Growth factors in wound healing. Single and synergistic effects on partial thickness porcine skin wounds. J Clin Invest 1989; 84(2):640–646.

64. Sporn MB, Roberts AB, Wakefield LM, de Crombrugghe B. Some recent advances in the chemistry and biology of transforming growth factor-beta. J Cell Biol 1987; 105(3):1039–1045.

65. Ghahary A, Shen YJ, Nedelec B, Scott PG, Tredget EE. Enhanced expression of mRNA for insulin-like growth factor-1 in post-burn hypertrophic scar tissue and its fibrogenic role by dermal fibroblasts. Mol Cell Biochem 1995; 148(1):25–32.

66. Sporn MB, Roberts AB, Wakefield LM, Assoian RK. Transforming growth factor-beta: biological function and chemical structure. Science 1986; 233(4763):532–534.

67. Tsuji T, Okada F, Yamaguchi K, Nakamura T. Molecular cloning of the large subunit of transforming growth factor type beta masking protein and expression of the mRNA in various rat tissues. Proc Natl Acad Sci USA 1990; 87(22):8835–8839.

68. Roberts AB. Peptide Growth Factors and Their Receptors. New York: Springer-Verlag, 1990.

69. Ghahary A, Shen YJ, Nedelec B, Wang R, Scott PG, Tredget EE. Collagenase production is lower in post-burn hypertrophic scar fibroblasts than in normal fibroblasts and is reduced by insulin-like growth factor-1. J Invest Dermatol 1996; 106(3):476–481.

70. Moren A, Olofsson A, Stenman G, Stenman G, Sahlin P, Kanzaki T, Claesson-Welsh L, ten Dijke P, Miyazono L, Heldin CH. Identification and characterization of LTBP-2, a novel latent transforming growth factor-beta-binding protein. J Biol Chem 1994; 269(51):32469–32478.

71. Dallas SL, Park-Snyder S, Miyazono K, Twardzik D, Mundy GR, Bonewald LF. Characterization and autoregulation of latent transforming growth factor beta (TGF beta) complexes in osteoblast-like cell lines. Production of a latent complex lacking the latent TGF beta-binding protein. J Biol Chem 1994; 269(9):6815–6821.

72. Kanzaki T, Olofsson A, Moren A, Wernstedt C, Hellman U, Miyazono K, Claesson-Welsh L, Heldin CH. TGF-beta 1 binding protein: a component of the large latent complex of TGF-beta 1 with multiple repeat sequences. Cell 1990; 61(6):1051–1061.

73. Wakefield LM, Smith DM, Masui T, Harris CC, Sporn MB. Distribution and modulation of the cellular receptor for transforming growth factor-beta. J Cell Biol 1987; 105(2):965–975.

74. Postlethwaite AE, Keski-Oja J, Moses HL, Kang AH. Stimulation of the chemotactic migration of human fibroblasts by transforming growth factor beta. J Exp Med 1987; 165(1):251–256.

75. Hill DJ, Logan A, McGarry M, De Sousa D. Control of protein and matrix-molecule synthesis in isolated ovine fetal growth-plate chondrocytes by the interactions of basic fibroblast growth factor, insulin-like growth factors-I and -II, insulin and transforming growth factor-beta 1. J Endocrinol 1992; 133(3):363–373.

76. Goldstein RH, Poliks CF, Pilch PF, Smith BD, Fine A. Stimulation of collagen formation by insulin and insulin-like growth factor I in cultures of human lung fibroblasts. Endocrinology 1989; 124(2):964–970.

77. Ignotz RA, Massague J. Transforming growth factor-beta stimulates the expression of fibronectin and collagen and their incorporation into the extracellular matrix. J Biol Chem 1986; 261(9):4337–4345.

78. Kahari VM, Hakkinen L, Westermarck J, Larjava H. Differential regulation of decorin and biglycan gene expression by dexamethasone and retinoic acid in cultured human skin fibroblasts. J Invest Dermatol 1995; 104(4):503–508.

79. Varga J, Rosenbloom J, Jimenez SA. Transforming growth factor beta (TGF beta) causes a persistent increase in steady-state amounts of type I and type III collagen and fibronectin mRNAs in normal human dermal fibroblasts. Biochem J 1987; 247(3):597–604.

80. Overall CM, Wrana JL, Sodek J. Transforming growth factor-beta regulation of collagenase, 72 kDa-progelatinase, TIMP and PAI-1 expression in rat bone cell populations and human fibroblasts. Connect Tissue Res 1989; 20(1–4):289–294.

81. Edwards DR, Murphy G, Reynolds JJ, Whitham SE, Docherty AJ, Angel P, Health JK. Transforming growth factor beta modulates the expression of collagenase and metalloproteinase inhibitor. EMBO J 1987; 6(7):1899–1904.

82. Mustoe TA, Pierce GF, Thomason A, Gramates P, Sporn MB, Deuel TF. Accelerated healing of incisional wounds in rats induced by transforming growth factor-beta. Science 1987; 237(4820):1333–1336.

83. Yang L, Qiu CX, Ludlow A, Ferguson MW, Brunner G. Active transforming growth factor-beta in wound repair: determination using a new assay. Am J Pathol 1999; 154(1):105–111.

84. Yang L, Chan T, Demare J, Iwashina T, Gharary A, Scott PG, Tredget EE. Healing of burn wounds in transgenic mice overexpressing transforming growth factor-beta 1 in the epidermis. Am J Pathol 2001; 159(6):2147–2157.

85. Bradham DM, Igarashi A, Potter RL, Grotendorst GR. Connective tissue growth factor: a cysteine-rich mitogen secreted by human vascular endothelial cells is related to the SRC-induced immediate early gene product CEF-10. J Cell Biol 1991; 114(6):1285–1294.

86. Igarashi A, Nashiro K, Kikuchi K, Sato S, Ihn H, Fujimoto M, Grotendorst GR, Takehara K. Connective tissue growth factor gene expression in tissue sections from localized scleroderma, keloid, and other fibrotic skin disorders. J Invest Dermatol 1996; 106(4):729–733.

87. Igarashi A, Okochi H, Bradham DM, Grotendorst GR. Regulation of connective tissue growth factor gene expression in human skin fibroblasts and during wound repair. Mol Biol Cell 1993; 4(6):637–645.

88. Grotendorst G, Grotendorst C, Gilman T. Production of growth factors (PDGF and TGF-beta1) at the site of tissue repair. Symposium on Tissue Repair. Growth Factors and Other Aspects of Wound Healing. New York: Liss AR, 1988.

89. Jones JI, Clemmons DR. Insulin-like growth factors and their binding proteins: biological actions. Endocr Rev 1995; 16(1):3–34.

90. Spencer EM, Skover G, Hunt TK. Somatomedins: do they play a pivotal role in wound healing? Prog Clin Biol Res 1988; 266:103–116.

91. McCarthy TL, Centrella M, Canalis E. Regulatory effects of insulin-like growth factors I and II on bone collagen synthesis in rat calvarial cultures. Endocrinology 1989; 124(1):301–309.

92. Edwall D, Schalling M, Jennische E, Norstedt G. Induction of insulin-like growth factor I messenger ribonucleic acid during regeneration of rat skeletal muscle. Endocrinology 1989; 124(2):820–825.

93. Blatti SP, Foster DN, Ranganathan G, Moses HL, Getz MJ. Induction of fibronectin gene transcription and mRNA is a primary response to growth-factor stimulation of AKR-2B cells. Proc Natl Acad Sci USA 1988; 85(4):1119–1123.

94. Steenfos HH, Jansson JO. Gene expression of insulin-like growth factor-I and IGF-I receptor during wound healing in rats. Eur J Surg 1992; 158(6–7):327–331.

95. Hansson HA, Jennische E, Skottner A. Regenerating endothelial cells express insulin-like growth factor-I immunoreactivity after arterial injury. Cell Tissue Res 1987; 250(3):499–505.

96. Bird JL, Tyler JA. Dexamethasone potentiates the stimulatory effect of insulin-like growth factor-I on collagen production in cultured human fibroblasts. J Endocrinol 1994; 142(3):571–579.

97. O'Keefe RJ, Puzas JE, Brand JS, Rosier RN. Effects of transforming growth factor-beta on matrix synthesis by chick growth plate chondrocytes. Endocrinology 1988; 122(6):2953–2961.

98. Makower AM, Wroblewski J, Pawlowski A. Effects of IGF-I, rGH, FGF, EGF and NCS on DNA-synthesis, cell proliferation and morphology of chondrocytes isolated from rat rib growth cartilage. Cell Biol Int Rep 1989; 13(3):259–270.

99. Ghahary A, Shen YJ, Scott PG, Gong Y, Tredget EE. Enhanced expression of mRNA for transforming growth factor-beta, type I and type III procollagen in human post-burn hypertrophic scar tissues. J Lab Clin Med 1993; 122(4):465–473.

100. Border WA, Noble NA. TGF-beta in kidney fibrosis: a target for gene therapy. Kidney Int 1997; 51(5):1388–1396.

101. Takeda K, Hatamochi A, Ueki H, Nakata M, Oishi Y. Decreased collagenase expression in cultured systemic sclerosis fibroblasts. J Invest Dermatol 1994; 103(3):359–363.

102. Ghahary A, Shen YJ, Scott PG, Tredget EE. Expression of fibronectin mRNA in hypertrophic and normal dermal tissues and in vitro regulation by interferon alpha-2b. Wound Repair Regen 1993; 1:166–174.

103. Jones AP, Webb LM, Anderson AO, Leonard EJ, Rot A. Normal human sweat contains interleukin-8. J Leukoc Biol 1995; 57(3):434–437.

104. Karey KP, Marquardt H, Sirbasku DA. Human platelet-derived mitogens. I. Identification of insulinlike growth factors I and II by purification and N alpha amino acid sequence analysis. Blood 1989; 74(3):1084–1092.

105. Nagaoka I, Trapnell BC, Crystal RG. Regulation of insulin-like growth factor I gene expression in the human macrophage-like cell line U937. J Clin Invest 1990; 85(2):448–455.

106. Grotendorst GR. Connective tissue growth factor: a mediator of TGF-beta action on fibroblasts. Cytokine Growth Factor Rev 1997; 8(3):171–179.

107. Barreca A, De Luca M, Del Monte P, Bondanza S, Damonte G, Cariola G, DiMarco E, Giordano G, Cancedda R, Minuto F. In vitro paracrine regulation of human keratinocyte growth by fibroblast-derived insulin-like growth factors. J Cell Physiol 1992; 151(2):262–268.

108. Okazaki R, Durham SK, Riggs BL, Conover CA. Transforming growth factor-beta and forskolin increase all classes of insulin-like growth factor-I transcripts in normal human osteoblast-like cells. Biochem Biophys Res Commun 1995; 207(3):963–970.

109. Ghahary A, Shen YJ, Wang R, Scott PG, Tredget EE. Expression and localization of insulin-like growth factor-1 in normal and post-burn hypertrophic scar tissue in human. Mol Cell Biochem 1998; 183(1–2):1–9.

110. Oh Y, Muller HL, Ng L, Rosenfeld RG. Transforming growth factor-beta-induced cell growth inhibition in human breast cancer cells is mediated through insulin-like growth factor-binding protein-3 action. J Biol Chem 1995; 270(23):13589–13592.

111. Cazals V, Mouhieddine B, Maitre B, LeBouc Y, Chadelat K, Brady JS, Clement A. Insulin-like growth factors, their binding proteins, and transforming growth factor-beta 1 in oxidant-arrested lung alveolar epithelial cells. J Biol Chem 1994; 269(19):14111–14117.

112. Goodman RE, Nestle F, Naidu YM, Green JM, Thompson CB, Nickoloff BJ, Turka LA. Keratinocyte-

derived T cell costimulation induces preferential production of IL-2 and IL-4 but not IFN-gamma. J Immunol 1994; 152(11):5189–5198.

113. Hauser C. The interaction between Langerhans cells and CD4+ T cells. J Dermatol 1992; 19(11):722–725.

114. Romagnani S. Development of Th 1- or Th 2-dominated immune responses: what about the polarizing signals? Int J Clin Lab Res 1996; 26(2):83–98.

115. Mosmann TR, Coffman RL. TH1 and TH2 cells: different patterns of lymphokine secretion lead to different functional properties. Annu Rev Immunol 1989; 7:145–173.

116. Mosmann TR, Cherwinski H, Bond MW, Giedlin MA, Coffman RL. Two types of murine helper T cell clone. I. Definition according to profiles of lymphokine activities and secreted proteins. J Immunol 1986; 136(7):2348–2357.

117. Takeuchi M, Tredget EE, Scott PG, Kilani RT, Ghahary A. The antifibrogenic effects of liposome-encapsulated IFN-alpha2b cream on skin wounds. J Interferon Cytokine Res 1999; 19(12):1413–1419.

118. Kelly JL, O'Suilleabhain CB, Soberg CC, Mannick JA, Lederer JA. Severe injury triggers antigen-specific T-helper cell dysfunction. Shock 1999; 12(1):39–45.

119. Seder RA, Germain RN, Linsley PS, Paul WE. CD28-mediated costimulation of interleukin 2 (IL-2) production plays a critical role in T cell priming for IL-4 and interferon gamma production. J Exp Med 1994; 179(1):299–304.

120. Fiorentino DF, Bond MW, Mosmann TR. Two types of mouse T helper cell. IV. Th2 clones secrete a factor that inhibits cytokine production by Th1 clones. J Exp Med 1989; 170(6):2081–2095.

121. Trinchieri G, Gerosa F. Immunoregulation by interleukin-12. J Leukoc Biol 1996; 59(4):505–511.

122. Fargeas C, Wu CY, Nakajima T, Cox D, Nutman T, Delespesse G. Differential effect of transforming growth factor beta on the synthesis of Th1- and Th2-like lymphokines by human T lymphocytes. Eur J Immunol 1992; 22(8):2173–2176.

123. Caligaris-Cappio F, Bertero MT, Converso M, Stacchini A, Vinante F, Romagnani S, Pizzolo G. Circulating levels of soluble CD30, a marker of cells producing Th2-type cytokines, are increased in patients with systemic lupus erythematosus and correlate with disease activity. Clin Exp Rheumatol 1995; 13(3):339–343.

124. Needleman BW, Wigley FM, Stair RW. Interleukin-1, interleukin-2, interleukin-4, interleukin-6, tumor necrosis factor alpha, and interferon-gamma levels in sera from patients with scleroderma. Arthritis Rheum 1992; 35(1):67–72.

125. Robinson DS, Kay AB. Role of Th1 and Th2 cells in human allergic disorders. Chem Immunol 1996; 63:187–203.

126. Barral A, Teixeira M, Reis P, Vinhas V, Costa J, Lessa H, Bittencourt AL, Reed S, Carvalho EM, Barral-Netto M. Transforming growth factor-beta in human cutaneous leishmaniasis. Am J Pathol 1995; 147(4):947–954.

127. Swihart K, Fruth U, Messmer N, Hug K, Behin R, Huang S, Del Giudice G, Aguet M, Louis JA. Mice from a genetically resistant background lacking the interferon gamma receptor are susceptible to infection with Leishmania major but mount a polarized T helper cell 1-type CD4+ T cell response. J Exp Med 1995; 181(3):961–971.

128. Hunt JP, Hunter CT, Brownstein MR, Giannopoulos A, Hultman CS, deSerres S, Bracey L, Frelinger J, Meyer AA. The effector component of the cytotoxic T-lymphocyte response has a biphasic pattern after burn injury. J Surg Res 1998; 80(2):243–251.

129. Williams ME, Caspar P, Oswald I, Sharma HK, Pankewycz O, Sher A, James SL. Vaccination routes that fail to elicit protective immunity against Schistosoma mansoni induce the production of TGF-beta, which down-regulates macrophage antiparasitic activity. J Immunol 1995; 154(9):4693–4700.

130. O'Sullivan ST, Lederer JA, Horgan AF, Chin DH, Mannick JA, Rodrick ML. Major injury leads to predominance of the T helper-2 lymphocyte phenotype and diminished interleukin-12 production associated with decreased resistance to infection. Ann Surg 1995; 222(4):482–490; discussion 490–492.

131. Horgan AF, Mendez MV, O'Riordain DS, Holzheimer RG, Mannick JA, Rodrick ML. Altered gene transcription after burn injury results in depressed T-lymphocyte activation. Ann Surg 1994; 220(3):342–351; discussion 351–352.

132. Zedler S, Faist E, Ostermeier B, von Donnersmarck GH, Schildberg FW. Postburn constitutional changes in T-cell reactivity occur in CD8+ rather than in CD4+ cells. J Trauma 1997; 42(5):872–880; discussion 880–881.

133. Zedler S, Bone RC, Baue AE, von Donnersmarck GH, Faist E. T-cell reactivity and its predictive role in immunosuppression after burns. Crit Care Med 1999; 27(1):66–72.

134. Faist E, Mewes A, Strasser T, Walz A, Alkan S, Baker C, Ertel W, Heberer G. Alteration of monocyte function following major injury. Arch Surg 1988; 123(3):287–292.

135. Shi Z, Wakil AE, Rockey DC. Strain-specific differences in mouse hepatic wound healing are mediated by divergent T helper cytokine responses. Proc Natl Acad Sci USA 1997; 94(20):10663–10668.

136. Da Costa J. Modern Surgery. Philadelphia: W.B. Saunders, 1931.

137. Varedi M, Tredget EE, Scott PG, Shen YJ, Ghahary A. Alteration in cell morphology triggers transforming growth factor-beta 1, collagenase, and tissue inhibitor of metalloproteinases-I expression in normal and hypertrophic scar fibroblasts. J Invest Dermatol 1995; 104(1):118–123.

138. Fraulin FO, Illmayer SJ, Tredget EE. Assessment of cosmetic and functional results of conservative versus surgical management of facial burns. J Burn Care Rehabil 1996; 17(1):19–29.

139. Murray JC. Keloids and hypertrophic scars. Clin Dermatol 1994; 12(1):27–37.

140. Assoian RK, Komoriya A, Meyers CA, Miller DM, Sporn MB. Transforming growth factor-beta in human platelets. Identification of a major storage site, purification, and characterization. J Biol Chem 1983; 258(11):7155–7160.

141. Larson DL, Abston S, Willis B, Linares H, Dobrkovsky M, Evans EB, Lewis SR. Contracture and scar formation in the burn patient. Clin Plast Surg 1974; 1(4):653–656.

142. Cheng JC, Evans JH, Leung KS, Clark JA, Choy TT, Leung PC. Pressure therapy in the treatment of post-burn hypertrophic scar—a critical look into its usefulness and fallacies by pressure monitoring. Burns Incl Therm Inj 1984; 10(3):154–163.

143. Kischer CW, Shetlar MR, Shetlar CL. Alteration of hypertrophic scars induced by mechanical pressure. Arch Dermatol 1975; 111(1):60–64.

144. Kischer CW, Shetlar MR. Microvasculature in hypertrophic scars and the effects of pressure. J Trauma 1979; 19(10):757–764.

145. Kischer CW, Bunce H III, Shetlah MR. Mast cell analyses in hypertrophic scars, hypertrophic scars treated with pressure and mature scars. J Invest Dermatol 1978; 70(6):355–357.

146. Chang P, Laubenthal KN, Lewis RW II, Rosenquist MD, Lindley-Smith P, Kealey GP. Prospective, randomized study of the efficacy of pressure garment therapy in patients with burns. J Burn Care Rehabil 1995; 16(5):473–475.

147. Clarys P, Alewaeters K, Lambrecht R, Barel AO. Skin color measurements: comparison between three instruments: the Chromameter®, the DermaSpectrometer® and the Mexameter®. Skin Res Technol 2000; 6(4):230–238.

148. Fong SS, Hung LK, Cheng JC. The cutometer and ultrasonography in the assessment of postburn hypertrophic scar—a preliminary study. Burns 1997; 23(suppl 1):S12–S18.

149. Hambleton J, Shakespeare PG, Pratt BJ. The progress of hypertrophic scars monitored by ultrasound measurements of thickness. Burns 1992; 18(4):301–307.

150. Moore LM. Effectiveness of custom pressure garments a prospective trial within wounds and with verified pressure. 11th Quadrennial Congress of the International Society for Burn Injuries, Seattle, WA, 2002.

151. Sproat JE, Dalcin A, Weitauer N, Roberts RS. Hypertrophic sternal scars: silicone gel sheet versus Kenalog injection treatment. Plast Reconstr Surg 1992; 90(6):988–992.

152. Gold MH. A controlled clinical trial of topical silicone gel sheeting in the treatment of hypertrophic scars and keloids. J Am Acad Dermatol 1994; 30(3):506–507.

153. Wessling N, Ehleben CM, Chapman V, May SR, Still JM Jr. Evidence that use of a silicone gel sheet increases range of motion over burn wound contractures. J Burn Care Rehabil 1985; 6(6):503–505.

154. Quinn KJ. Silicone gel in scar treatment. Burns Incl Therm Inj 1987; 13(suppl):S33–S40.

155. Lee R, Doong H. Control of matrix production during tissue repair. In: Lee RC, Mustoe TA, Siebert J, eds. Advances in Wound Healing and Tissue Repair. Chicago: World Medical Press, 1993.

156. Musgrave MA, Umraw N, Fish JS, Gomez M, Cartotto RC. The effect of silicone gel sheets on perfusion of hypertrophic burn scars. J Burn Care Rehabil 2002; 23(3):208–214.

157. Quinn KJ, Evans JH, Courtney JM, Gaylor JD, Reid WH. Non-pressure treatment of hypertrophic scars. Burns Incl Therm Inj 1985; 12(2):102–108.

158. Ahn ST, Monafo WW, Mustoe TA. Topical silicone gel: a new treatment for hypertrophic scars. Surgery 1989; 106(4):781–786; discussion 786–787.

159. Carr-Collins JA. Pressure techniques for the prevention of hypertrophic scar. Clin Plast Surg 1992; 19(3):733–743.

160. Van den Kerchhove E, Boeckx W, Kochuyt A. Silicone patches as a supplement for pressure therapy to control hypertrophic scarring. J Burn Care Rehabil 1991; 12(4):361–369.

161. Davey RB, Wallis KA, Bowering K. Adhesive contact media—an update on graft fixation and burn scar management. Burns 1991; 17(4):313–319.

162. Rivers EA, Strate RG, Solem LD. The transparent face mask. Am J Occup Ther 1979; 33(2):108–113.

163. Ridgway CL, Daugherty MB, Warden GD. Serial casting as a technique to correct burn scar contractures. A case report. J Burn Care Rehabil 1991; 12(1):67–72.

164. Bennett GB, Helm P, Purdue GF, Hunt JL. Serial casting: a method for treating burn contractures. J Burn Care Rehabil 1989; 10(6):543–545.

165. Leman CJ. Splints and accessories following burn reconstruction. Clin Plast Surg 1992; 19(3):721–731.

166. Kiil J. Keloids treated with topical injections of triamcinolone acetonide (kenalog). Immediate and long-term results. Scand J Plast Reconstr Surg 1977; 11(2):169–172.

167. Cohen IK, Diegelmann RF, Bryant CP. Alpha globulin collagenase inhibitors in keloid and hypertrophic scar. Surg Forum 1975; 26:61–62.

168. Pittet B, Rubbia-Brandt L, Desmouliere A, Sappino AP, Roggero P, Guerret S, Grimaud JA, Lacher R, Montandon D, Gabbiani G. Effect of gamma-interferon on the clinical and biologic evolution of hypertrophic scars and Dupuytren's disease: an open pilot study. Plast Reconstr Surg 1994; 93(6):1224–1235.

169. Rusciani L, Rossi G, Bono R. Use of cryotherapy in the treatment of keloids. J Dermatol Surg Oncol 1993; 19(6):529–534.

170. Ceilley RI, Babin RW. The combined use of cryosurgery and intralesional injections of suspensions of fluorinated adrenocorticosteroids for reducing keloids and hypertrophic scars. J Dermatol Surg Oncol 1979; 5(1):54–56.

171. Lee RC, Doong H, Jellema AF. The response of burn scars to intralesional verapamil. Report of five cases. Arch Surg 1994; 129(1):107–111.

172. Espana A, Solano T, Quintanilla E. Bleomycin in the treatment of keloids and hypertrophic scars by multiple needle punctures. Dermatol Surg 2001; 27(1):23–37.

173. Uppal RS, Khan U, Kakar S, Talas G, Chapman P, McGrouther AD. The effects of a single dose of 5-fluorouracil on keloid scars: a clinical trial of timed wound irrigation after extralesional excision. Plast Reconstr Surg 2001; 108(5):1218–1224.

174. Darzi MA, Chowdri NA, Kaul SK, Khan M. Evaluation of various methods of treating keloids and hypertrophic scars: a 10-year follow-up study. Br J Plast Surg 1992; 45(5):374–379.

175. Apfelberg DB, Maser MR, Lash H. The use of epidermis over a keloid as an autograft after resection of the keloid. J Dermatol Surg 1976; 2(5):409–411.

176. Rauscher GE, Kolmer WL. Treatment of recurrent earlobe keloids. Cutis 1986; 37(1):67–68.

177. Horton CE, Crawford J, Oakey RS. Malignant change in keloids. Plast Reconstr Surg 1953; 12(1):86–89.

178. Sloan DF, Brown RD, Wells CH, Hilton JG. Tissue gases in human hypertrophic burn scars. Plast Reconstr Surg 1978; 61(3):431–436.

179. Levy DS, Salter MM, Roth RE. Postoperative irradiation in the prevention of keloids. Am J Roentgenol 1976; 127(3):509–510.

180. Feldman J. Reconstruction of the burned face in children. In: Serafin D, Georgiade N, eds. Pediatric Plastic Surgery. St. Louis: CV Mosby, 1984.

181. Williamson JS, Snelling CF, Clugston P, Macdonald IB, Germann E. Cultured epithelial autograft: five years of clinical experience with twenty-eight patients. J Trauma 1995; 39(2):309–319.

182. Mozingo DW. Comparison of the biomechanical properties of burns grafted with conventional split thickness skin vs. Integra artificial skin. 11th Quadrennial Congress of the International Society for Burn Injuries, Seattle, WA, 2002.

183. Moiemen NS, Staiano JJ, Ojeh NO, Thway Y, Frame JD. Reconstructive surgery with a dermal regeneration template: clinical and histologic study. Plast Reconstr Surg 2001; 108(1):93–103.

184. Alster T. Laser treatment of scars. In: Pulser Lasers Aesthetic and Medical Cutaneous Application. Boston: Department of Continuing Medical Education, 1996.

185. Dierickx C, Goldman MP, Fitzpatrick RE. Laser treatment of erythematous/hypertrophic and pigmented scars in 26 patients. Plast Reconstr Surg 1995; 95(1):84–90; discussion 91–92.

186. Sheridan RL, MacMillan K, Donelan M, Choucair R, Grevelink J, Petras L, Lydon M, Tompkins R. Tunable dye laser neovessel ablation as an adjunct to the management of hypertrophic scarring in burned children: pilot trial to establish safety. J Burn Care Rehabil 1997; 18(4):317–320.

187. Kalvakolanu DV, Borden EC. An overview of the interferon system: signal transduction and mechanisms of action. Cancer Invest 1996; 14(1):25–53.

188. Harrop AR, Ghahary A, Scott PG, Forsyth N, Uji-Friedland A, Tredget EE. Regulation of collagen synthesis and mRNA expression in normal and hypertrophic scar fibroblasts in vitro by interferon-gamma. J Surg Res 1995; 58(5):471–477.

189. Duncan MR, Hasan A, Berman B. Pentoxifylline, pentifylline, and interferons decrease type I and III procollagen mRNA levels in dermal fibroblasts: evidence for

190. Granstein RD, Flotte TJ, Amento EP. Interferons and collagen production. J Invest Dermatol 1990; 95(suppl 6):75S–80S.

191. Dans MJ, Isseroff R. Inhibition of collagen lattice contraction by pentoxifylline and interferon-alpha, -beta, and -gamma. J Invest Dermatol 1994; 102(1):118–121.

192. McCauley RL, Chopra V, Li YY, Herndon DN, Robson MC. Altered cytokine production in black patients with keloids. J Clin Immunol 1992; 12(4):300–308.

193. Sen GC, Lengyel P. The interferon system. A bird's eye view of its biochemistry. J Biol Chem 1992; 267(8):5017–5020.

194. Nedelec B, Shen YJ, Ghahary A, Scott PG, Tredget EE. The effect of interferon alpha 2b on the expression of cytoskeletal proteins in an in vitro model of wound contraction. J Lab Clin Med 1995; 126(5):474–484.

195. Wong TW, Chiu HC, Yip KM. Intralesional interferon alpha-2b has no effect in the treatment of keloids. Br J Dermatol 1994; 130(5):683–685.

196. al-Khawajah MM. Failure of interferon-alpha 2b in the treatment of mature keloids. Int J Dermatol 1996; 35(7):515–517.

197. Weiner N, Williams N, Birch G, Ramachandran C, Shipman C Jr, Flynn G. Topical delivery of liposomally encapsulated interferon evaluated in a cutaneous herpes guinea pig model. Antimicrob Agents Chemother 1989; 33(8):1217–1221.

198. Telasky C, Tredget EE, Shen Q, Khorramizadeh MR, Iwashina T, Scott PG, Ghahary A. IFN-alpha2b suppresses the fibrogenic effects of insulin-like growth factor-1 in dermal fibroblasts. J Interferon Cytokine Res 1998; 18(8):571–577.

199. Isaka Y, Brees DK, Ikegaya K, Kaneda Y, Imai E, Noble NA, Border WA. Gene therapy by skeletal muscle expression of decorin prevents fibrotic disease in rat kidney. Nat Med 1996; 2(4):418–423.

200. Purchio AF, Cooper JA, Brunner AM, Lioubin MN, Gentry LE, Kovacina KS, Roth RA, Marquardt H. Identification of mannose 6-phosphate in two asparagine-linked sugar chains of recombinant transforming growth factor-beta 1 precursor. J Biol Chem 1988; 263(28):14211–14215.

201. Dennis PA, Rifkin DB. Cellular activation of latent transforming growth factor beta requires binding to the cation-independent mannose 6-phosphate/insulin-like growth factor type II receptor. Proc Natl Acad Sci USA 1991; 88(2):580–584.

202. MacCallion R, Fergusonn M. Fetal wound healing and the development of antiscarring therapies for adult wound healing. In: Clark R, ed. The Molecular and Cellular Biology of Wound Repair. New York: Plenum Press, 1996.

203. Shigeki S, Murakami T, Yata N, Ikuta Y. Treatment of keloid and hypertrophic scars by iontophoretic transdermal delivery of tranilast. Scand J Plast Reconstr Surg Hand Surg 1997; 31(2):151–158.

204. Suzawa H, Kikuchi S, Arai N, Koda A. The mechanism involved in the inhibitory action of tranilast on collagen biosynthesis of keloid fibroblasts. Jpn J Pharmacol 1992; 60(2):91–96.

205. Krotzsch-Gomez FE, Furuzawa-Carballeda J, Reyes-Marquez R, Quiroz-Hernandez E, Diaz de Leon L. Cytokine expression is downregulated by collagen-polyvinylpyrrolidone in hypertrophic scars. J Invest Dermatol 1998; 111(5):828–834.

206. Zhou LJ, Inoue M, Gunji H, Ono I, Kaneko F. Effects of prostaglandin E1 on cultured dermal fibroblasts from normal and hypertrophic scarred skin. J Dermatol Sci 1997; 14(3):217–224.

207. Zhou LJ, Ono I, Kaneko F. Role of transforming growth factor-beta 1 in fibroblasts derived from normal and hypertrophic scarred skin. Arch Dermatol Res 1997; 289(11):646–652.

208. Unemori EN, Pickford LB, Salles AL, Piercy CE, Grove BH, Erikson ME, Amento EP. Relaxin induces an extracellular matrix-degrading phenotype in human lung fibroblasts in vitro and inhibits lung fibrosis in a murine model in vivo. J Clin Invest 1996; 98(12): 2739–2745.

209. Doong H, Dissanayake S, Gowrishankar TR, LaBarbera MC, Lee RC. The 1996 Lindberg Award. Calcium antagonists alter cell shape and induce pro-collagenase synthesis in keloid and normal human dermal fibroblasts. J Burn Care Rehabil 1996; 17(6 Pt 1): 497–514.

210. Dolynchuk KN, Ziesmann M, Serletti JM. Topical putrescine (Fibrostat) in treatment of hypertrophic scars: phase II study. Plast Reconstr Surg 1996; 97(1):117–123; discussion 124–125.

14

Lasers in the Treatment of Postburn Scars

ANGELO CAPOZZI, HUGH L. VU, ALBERT K. OH, SUZANNE L. KILMER
Shriners Hospital for Children, Sacramento, and University of California, Davis, California, USA

I. INTRODUCTION

Postburn scarring represents a significant clinical problem due to both the number of patients who develop scars and the notoriously difficult treatment of these scars. These scars can limit social interaction, negatively impact self-esteem, and adversely affect daily activities. Because thermally induced scars are typically recalcitrant to treatment owing to their proliferative nature, their appropriate management remains a challenge.

The treatment of burn scars includes a multitude of chemical, physical, and surgical options, and ranges from conservative modalities such as steroid injections, pressure garments, and application of silicone gel sheets, to more invasive measures including cryotherapy, radiation, and/or excision.

Intralesional injection of corticosteroids has been a standard modality for the treatment of hypertrophic scarring in nonburn injuries (1–3). However, burn scars are usually much larger and may involve a large body surface area with distortion of multiple aesthetic subunits, making injection of the entire scar impractical. In addition to the pain associated with intralesional injection, corticosteroids can also induce skin atrophy, telangiectasias, and

dyspigmentation (3). The use of pressure garments and silicone gel sheeting or hydrocolloid dressing is essential in postburn scar management, but the results are delayed and may be variable (4–6). In addition, scar pigmentation and elevation are often not changed (7).

Cryotherapy has been used by some centers in the management of hypertrophic scars and keloids (8,9). Results, however, are varied and some groups have reported no benefit from the use of cryotherapy (10,11). Adjuvant radiotherapy following surgical scar excision has been used for many years in the management of hypertrophic scars and keloids (12–14). However, the large size of postburn scars, as well as age, pregnancy, risk of malignancy, and side effects such as pigment changes, erythema, telangiectasias, and atrophy may all limit the use of radiation in burn scar management. Surgical excision of scar tissue with primary scar revision or immediate skin grafting can result in improved function and range of motion. However, scar recurrence is common and final cosmesis is often less than desirable.

Beginning in the early 1980s, lasers have been used in an attempt to eradicate scars. Vaporization lasers which target water molecules, such as the carbon dioxide (CO_2), argon, and neodynium:yttrium-aluminum-garnet

(Nd:YAG), were initially used, but often led to immediate scar recurrence (15–17). In 1994, Alster (18) reported improvement in hypertrophic scar quality after treatment with the pulsed dye laser (PDL), which targets oxyhemoglobin. This particular laser has been used extensively in the management of vascular lesions such as port-wine stains (19–21). Scar flattening as well as a reduction in scar erythema has been noted after hypertrophic scars were treated with PDL (18).

Currently, there is no consensus as to which is the "best" laser for the treatment of burn scars. Although the preference leans toward PDL systems, an array of vascular-specific lasers are being used and potentially show improvement in burn scars. This chapter will describe current laser modalities in treating postburn scarring.

II. SCAR FORMATION IN BURNS

The color, size, and shape of the burn scar are determined by local cellular and humoral responses. Thermal injury immediately induces the body's wound healing response. These wound repair events can be grouped into three overlapping phases: inflammation, regeneration, and remodeling (22). The inflammatory phase shows minimal clinical consequences in smaller burns, but can produce devastating and lethal systemic sequelae in burns >25% total body surface area (TBSA). This phase is responsible for the large amount of fluid resuscitation needed during the first 24 h postburn injury. The inflammatory phase is followed by granulation tissue formation that consists of neovascularization accompanied by a dense population of macrophages and fibroblasts. Several months postburn injury, the wound will progress into the remodeling, phase in which there is reduction in the number and the activity of fibroblasts and vascularity accompanied by deposition, remodeling, and rearrangement of collagen. Collagen remodeling during scar formation is dependent on the balance between collagen synthesis and degradation.

Burn injury produces various types of scars, ranging from atrophy to erythema, hypertrophy, and keloid formation. Hypertrophic and erythematous scar formation occurs commonly after burn injury. Patients with greater skin pigmentation have a higher likelihood of hypertrophic scar formation. Hypertrophic scarring is likely to develop when collagen synthesis prevails over catabolism during the remodeling phase of wound healing. In addition, hypertrophic scars tend to occur in areas of high tension or motion, that is, flexor surfaces such as joints and abdomen and are limited by the boundary of the wound.

zOn the other hand, keloid scars are not limited by the wound boundary and tend to grow beyond the area of initial injury. This initial size of injury is often irrelevant and cannot be used to predict the formation of keloids.

Minor injuries may produce very large lesions. Keloid scars are independent of motion or tension and have a high predilection for earlobes, shoulders, and presternal skin (23).

III. LASER TYPES AND MECHANICS

Problems with postburn scars can be divided into two main components: hypertrophy and erythema. To specifically treat burn scarring, the laser device must deliver a potent effect that will reduce both the thickness and the redness of the scar. In addition, patients with burn scars will often complain of itching or pruritis (24).

Currently, there is no definitive data to show which is the "best" laser for the treatment of burn scars. Although the preference is currently leaning toward PDL systems, an array of vascular-specific lasers are being used and can potentially produce better results in the management of burn scars. The following is a list of laser systems for treating cutaneous vascular lesions that may have use in the treatment of burn scars.

A. Argon Laser

The argon laser was one of the first lasers used in the treatment of hypertrophic scars and keloids (3). This laser emits light at six wavelengths from 458 to 514 nm, with 80% of its emission at 488 and 534.4 nm. When used for

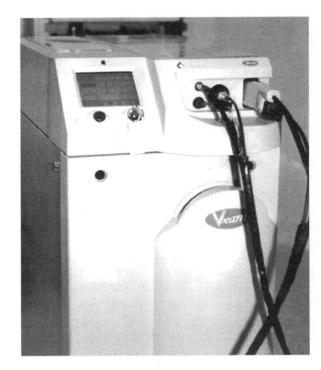

Figure 14.1   **(See color insert)** V-beam PDL system.

vascular lesions, 75% of patients can expect good to excellent results. However, it is a continuous wave laser and therefore may deposit more heat, resulting in a moderate risk of hypertrophic scarring, especially in children (4–23%). Results of studies from argon laser treatment of hypertrophic scar and keloids have been mixed (16,25,26). In addition, recurrence rates have been high (27). This laser is rarely used today.

B. Nd:YAG Laser

The original Nd:YAG laser has been reported to have benefits in the treatment of selected cutaneous pigmented lesions (28). Because of nonspecific blood and tissue interaction at this wavelength, however, the depth of thermal injury is as deep as 5–8 mm. Its usefulness is limited to those lesions having a thick bulky mass. It also has a higher risk of hypertrophic scarring (27). A more recent modification of this laser has reduced the wavelength to 532 nm, making it potentially more useful in treating scar pigmentation without the high incidence of hypertrophic scar recurrence (29).

C. Copper Vapor and Copper Bromide Lasers

This laser system has a wavelength of 578 nm which is in the hemoglobin absorption peak. However, a single pulse mode may not deliver enough energy to heat a vascular lesion to an efficacious temperature. Therefore, it must use a train of pulses, thus losing the capability to minimize collateral injury (30). These systems have a much higher risk for scarring and are not commonly used today.

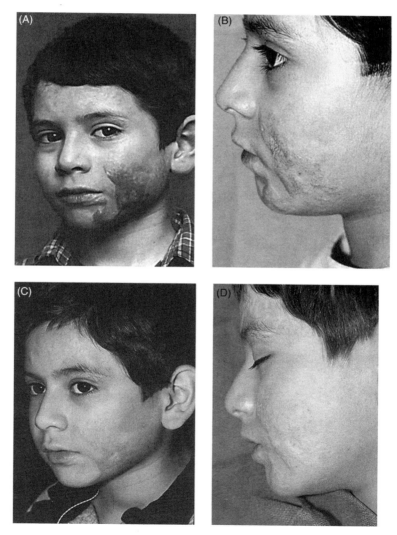

Figure 14.2 **(See color insert)** (A) Patient who sustained facial burn 18 months ago. (B) Note improved appearance after four treatments with V-beam PDL system. (C) Note further improvement after V-beam laser. (D) Further improvement noted.

D. Flashlamp-Pumped PDL

This laser has shown the most promising results with hypertrophic scars and keloids (18,23,24,31–33). PDL systems have also been used in the treatment of other scars and in the prophylactic treatment of deep burn wounds to prevent hypertrophic scarring with some success (34–36). PDL systems have more specific absorption characteristics for intravascular oxyhemoglobin (HbO_2), the treatment target. Although the original model had a wavelength of 577 nm, the next model had a wavelength of 585 nm and some current models have wavelengths up to 595 nm. These wavelengths are selectively absorbed by HbO_2 in red blood cells. The epidermal cells are spared, especially if a cooling system is employed. The pulse duration was originally kept much shorter than the time necessary to allow heat to spread from the treated target to the surrounding tissue. This minimized collateral damage to adjacent tissues, but often caused purpura due to vessel rupture. Newer models now have longer pulse widths that better match vessel size, but pulse width may not be as important for scar remodeling.

E. Tuneable Dye Laser

Another approach to treatment of vascular lesions has been the meticulous tracing of vessels using a 100 μm spot size at 577 nm wavelength generated by an argon-pumped tunable dye laser. This laser is similar to the PDL, but with a finer control of spot size. Although there is a 5% rate of hypertrophic scarring, some investigators found this technique to be very safe and effective in both adults and children (37,38). This laser also has good potential for the treatment of burn scars.

F. V-Beam PDL System

This laser is a long pulse-duration 595 nm PDL system (Fig. 14.1) which we have been using at Shriners Hospitals for Children of Northern California for postburn scars. Primarily used for vascular lesions, especially those resistant to other laser systems (39), the V-Beam PDL system appears to improve the hypertrophy and redness of burn scars with limited discomfort for the patient (Figs. 14.2 and 14.3). In addition, it can decrease the pruritis and

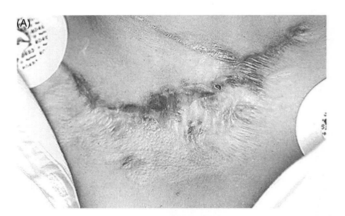

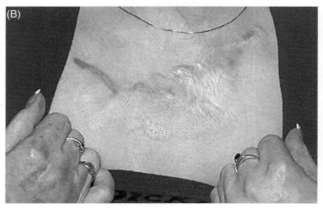

Figure 14.3 **(See color insert)** (A) Patient with chest burn scar. (B) Photographed after four treatments with the PDL system.

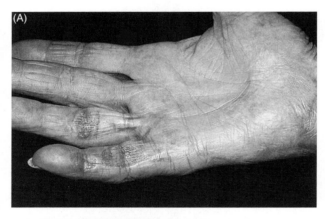

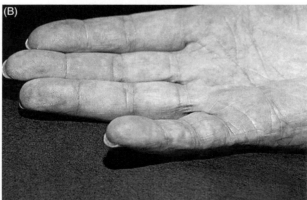

Figure 14.4 **(See color insert)** (A) Patient with hand scars following burn 1-year ago. (B) After three treatments with V-beam PDL system, the scars are softer and more pliable. The patient also reported less hypersensitivity.

tightness often associated with burn scars. Following treatment, scars often become more pliable and patients have enhanced range of motion. Patients also report less skin hypersensitivity to touch as well (Fig. 14.4).

Cosmesis can be improved as smooth and regular lined scars become softer and more irregular, thereby not attracting unwanted attention. The V-Beam PDL system

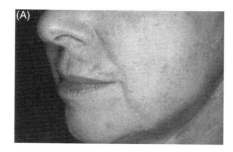

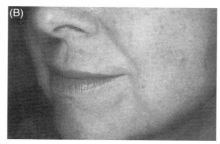

Figure 14.6 **(See color insert)** (A) Patient who suffered burns after treatment with CO_2 laser 1-year ago. (B) After one treatment with V-beam PDL system, there is improved color and pliability.

has been used to treat CO_2 laser scars with good results (Figs. 14.5 and 14.6). Although the mechanism of action remains to be fully elucidated, several theories exist including a relative hypoxia induced by the laser's vascular specificity, an alteration in the ratio of types I and III collagen, the dissociation of disulfide bonds with rearrangement of collagen, and the relative increase in mast cells noted in laser treated scars which may modulate fibroblastic growth and other factors (3,23,31).

IV. SUMMARY

Lasers appear to have potential in the treatment of postburn scars. Results to date seem to indicate that the PDL systems appear to be the best modality for softening, increasing pliability, and decreasing hypersensitivity of burn scars. PDL systems also improve cosmesis by decreasing erythema, flattening scars, and promoting return of more normal skin markings. Confirmation of these results will require larger studies.

REFERENCES

1. Griffith VH. The treatment of keloids with triamcinolone acetonide. Plast Reconstr Surg 1966; 38:202–208.
2. Ketchum LD, Robinson DW, Masters FW. Follow-up on treatment of hypertrophic scars and keloids with triamcinolone. Plast Reconstr Surg 1971; 48:256–259.
3. Alster TS, West TB. Treatment of scars: a review. Ann Plast Surg 1997; 39:418–432.

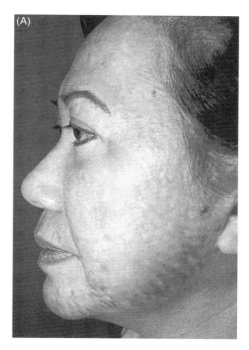

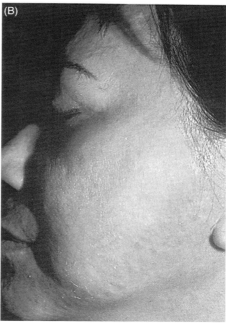

Figure 14.5 **(See color insert)** (A) Patient 1-year after burn complication of CO_2 laser treatment. (B) Note improved color and texture following two treatments with V-beam PDL system.

4. Borgognoni L. Biological effects of silicone gel sheeting. Wound Repair Regen 2002; 10(2):118–121.

5. Quinn KJ, Evans JH, Courtney JM, Gaylor JD, Reid WH. Non-pressure treatment of hypertrophic scars. Burns Incl Therm Inj 1985; 12:102–108.

6. Ahn ST, Monafo WW, Mustoe TA. Topical silicone get: a new treatment for hypertrophic scars. Surgery 1989; 106:781–786.

7. Phillips TJ, Gerstein AD, Lordan V. A randomized controlled trial of hydrocolloid dressing in the treatment of hypertrophic scars and keloids. Dermatol Surg 1996; 22:775–778.

8. Rusciani L, Rosse G, Bono R. Use of cryotherapy in the treatment of keloids. J Dermatol Surg Oncol 1993; 19:529–534.

9. Zouboulis CC, Blume U, Buttner P, Orfanos CE. Outcome of cryosurgery in keloids and hypertrophic scars. Arch Dermatol 1993; 129:1146–1151.

10. Muti E, Ponzio E. Cryotherapy in the treatment of keloids. Ann Plast Surg 1983; 11:227–232.

11. Shepherd JP, Dawber RF. The response of keloids scars to cryotherapy. Plast Reconstr Surg 1982; 70:677–682.

12. Borok TL, Bray M, Sinclair I, Plafker J, LaBirth L, Rollins C. Role of ionizing irradiation for 393 keloids. Int J Radiat Oncol Biol Phys 1988; 15:865–870.

13. Enhamre A, Hammar H. Treatment of keloids with excision and post-operative X-ray irradiation. Dermatologica 1983; 167:90–93.

14. Ragoowansi R, Cornes PGS, Moss AL, Glees JP. Treatment of keloids by surgical excision and immediate postoperative single-fraction radiotherapy. Plast Reconstr Surg 2003; 111:1853–1859.

15. Apfelberg D, Maser M, White D. Failure of carbon dioxide laser excision of keloids. Lasers Surg Med 1989; 9:382–388.

16. Hulsbergen-Henning JP, Roskam Y, van Gemert MJ. Treatment of keloids and hypertorphic scars with an argon laser. Lasers Surg Med 1986; 6:72–75.

17. Sherman R, Rosenfeld H. Experience with the Nd:YAG laser in the treatment of keloid scars. Ann Plast Surg 1988; 21:231–235.

18. Alster T. Improvement of erythematous and hypertrophic scars by the 585 nm flashlamp pumped pulsed dye laser. Ann Plast Surg 1994; 32:186–190.

19. Anderson RR, Parrish JA. Selective photothermolysis: precise microsurgery by selective absorption of pulsed radiation. Science 1983; 220:521–527.

20. Ashinoff R, Geronemus, R. Capillary hemangiomas and treatment with the flash lamp-pumped pulsed dye laser. Arch Dermatol 1991; 127:202–205.

21. Ashinoff R, Geronemus R. Treatment of a port-wine stain in a black patient with the pulsed dye laser. J Dermatol Surg Oncol 1992; 18:147–148.

22. Glat PM, Longaker MT. Wound healing. In: Aston SJ, Beasley RW, Thorne CHM, eds. Plastic Surgery. Philadelphia: Lippincott, 1997:3–12.

23. Alster T. Laser treatment of hypertrophic scars, keloids and striae. Dermatol Clin 1997; 15:419–429.

24. Allison K, Kiernan M, Waters R, Clement R. Pulsed dye laser treatment of burn scars. Alleviation or irritation? Burns 2003; 29:207–213.

25. Apfelberg DB, Maser MR, Lash H, White D, Weston J. Preliminary results of argon and carbon dioxide laser treatment of keloid scars. Lasers Surg Med 1984; 4:283–290.

26. Ginsbach G, Kohnel W. The treatment of hypertrophic scars and keloids by argon-laser: clinical data and morphologic findings. Plast Surg Forum 1978; 1:61–67.

27. Grossman MC, Kauvar ANB, Geronemus RG. Cutaneous laser surgery. In: Aston SJ, Beasley RW, Thorne CHM, eds. Plastic Surgery. Philadelphia: Lippincott, 1997:205–219.

28. Lask GP, Glassberg E. Neodymium:yttrium-alluminum-garnet laser for the treatment of cutaneous lesions. Clin Dermatol 1995; 13:81–86.

29. Bowes LE, Nouri K, Berman B, Jimenez G, Pardo R, Rodriguez L, Spencer JM. Treatment of pigmented hypertrophic scars with the 585 nm pulsed dye laser and the 532 nm frequency-doubled Nd:YAG laser in the q-switched and variable pulse modes: a comparative study. Dermatol Surg 2002; 28:714–719.

30. Haedersdal M, Therkildsen P, Bech-Thomsen N, Poulsen T, Wulf HC. Side effects from dermatological laser treatment related to UV exposure and epidermal thickness: a murine experiment with the copper vapor laser. Lasers Surg Med 1997; 20(3):233–241.

31. Dierickx C, Goldman M, Fitzpatrick R. Laser treatment of erythematous and hypertrophic and pigmented scars in 26 patients. Plast Reconstr Surg 1995; 95:84–90.

32. Alster T, Williams C. Treatment of keloid sternotomy scars with 585 nm flashlamp-pumped pulsed dye laser. Lancet 1995; 345:1198–2000.

33. Manuskiatti W, Fitzpatrick R. Treatment response of keloidal and hypertrophic sternotomy scars. Arch Dermatol 2002; 138:1149–1155.

34. Alster T, Kurban A, Grove G, Grove M, Tan O. Alteration of argon induced scars by the pulsed dye laser. Lasers Surg Med 1993; 13:368–373.

35. Alster T, McMeekin T. Improvement of facial acne scars by the 585 nm flashlamp-pumped pulsed dye laser. J Am Acad Dermatol 1996; 35:79–81.

36. Liew S, Murison M, Dickson W. Prophylactic treatment of deep dermal burn scars to prevent hypertrophic scarring using the pulsed dye laser: a preliminary study. Ann Plast Surg 2002; 49:472–475.

37. Gaston P, Humzah M, Quaba A. The pulsed tuneable dye laser as an aid in the management of postburn scarring. Burns 1996; 22:203–205.

38. Raine C, Al-Nakib K, Quaba AA. A role for lasers in the treatment of pigmented skin grafts. Burns 1997; 23:641–644.

39. Laube S, Taibjee S, Lanigan SW. Treatment of resistant port wine stains with the V-beam pulsed dye laser. Lasers Surg Med 2003; 33:282–287.

15

Evaluation of the Burned Face

MARC FUNKE, MARCUS SPIES, PETER M. VOGT
Medizinische Hochschule Hannover, Hannover, Germany

I. INTRODUCTION

According to recent literature 25–50% of all severe burns involve the head and neck region. Burns in this region represent some of the most challenging problems in plastic surgery. The urgency felt to reconstruct the burned face is mainly due to the severe deformities with functional impairment. This results in gross visual abnormalities and enormous psychological problems of the patients. In addition, facial burns in children may be associated with a high risk of facial growth inhibition and subsequent loss of function.

The vast majority of burn deformities resulting in functional problems typically seen in past decades can be eliminated by proper acute care and a treatment strategy, which includes short- and long-term goals for each patient. Acute care is aimed at survival and wound coverage. Reconstruction involves both short-term and long-term goals. Short-term goals are the restoration of the patient's range of motion and his functional abilities. Long-term goals include multiple reconstructive procedures aiming at the best feasible reintegration into society in combination with psychological counseling and therapy to compensate for the functional loss associated with burns.

Good surgical practice is always a major key to burn reconstruction. This means choosing the best operation at the best time for the patient. To achieve this goal, the patient has to take part in the decision making process and the planning of the procedure. The patient must fully understand and accept the surgical objectives. In addition, patients must not only be fully aware of the limitations of facial reconstruction, but also must accept them. There are no miracles in plastic surgery. An open discussion between the surgeon and the patient, relative to the objectives, the plans, and the limitations of each procedure, helps to minimize postoperative discontent.

The timing of reconstruction may be difficult, as complete scar maturation is preferred prior to reconstruction. However, immediate or early reconstructive procedures may be necessary to prevent functional restrictions in activities of daily living or correct rapidly progressive and disabling deformities. If the reconstructive strategy includes waiting for full scar maturation, therapy with pressure garment or silicone sheeting may be a good technique to assist scar maturation.

II. ACUTE TRAUMA: OPERATIVE VS. CONSERVATIVE THERAPY AND PREVENTION OF SECONDARY DEFORMITIES

A. Principles and Other Considerations

The individual body image defines one of the most important aspects of personal identity. Today's society expects a perfect appearance without any stigma. According to contemporary lifestyle magazines, a perfect body and appearance are presented as a fundamental condition for a successful social and business career. Burns patients may lose this basic qualification. The reintegration of patients into society may be hampered by both aesthetic and functional deficits.

Burn reconstruction of facial deformities is a very delicate part of the patient's rehabilitation. Hiding severe deformities by using casual or elegant clothing is not possible. On a daily basis, the patient and his environment are confronted with the consequences of the burn trauma and its painful and unappealing scars. The lack of total acceptance, combined with the often aggressive reactions by peers, urges the patient with facial burns to press his surgeon for early reconstructive procedures, hoping to get rid of the traumatizing facial scars.

Before planning any surgical procedure, a detailed examination and evaluation of the patterns of deformity has to be performed to obtain a reliable and well-documented status quo ante. Depending on the clinical evaluation, an inventory of short- and long-term goals should be specified and a specific therapy program should be established.

Burn reconstruction begins with the acute admission for burn trauma. Urgent procedures have to be performed within hours after admission to preserve important functional structures, such as exposed bone, cartilage, vessels, joints, or corneas. In the rehabilitation phase of treatment, multiple-staged procedures have to be performed to improve function. With completed scar maturation at 12–18 months after burn injury, definite reconstructive procedures need to be planned according to the patient's priorities.

Scar maturation is essential to obtain good surgical and aesthetic results in head and neck reconstruction. Only in a few cases will scar maturation with time allow for significant improvement of scars by softening and return to normal coloration, texture, and contour. Unfortunately, these cases are rare. To date, no means exist to predict the outcome in any individual patient. However, typical areas requiring monitoring for future demand of surgical correction can be identified in most patients, such as the eyelids, commissures, and neck. To accelerate scar maturation and control hypertrophic burn scar formation, conservative therapy attempts including pressure garments and silicone sheeting have proven to be therapeutic options. There are a number of nonoperative techniques available to influence the healing of burn scars or to improve local skin properties for subsequent surgery. The continuous use of compression after facial burns have reepithelialized reduces the tendency to develop hypertrophic scars. Such scars are aesthetically unattractive and may cause facial distortions by producing scar contractures. A number of technical advances in this area have been developed in the last few years. The use of pressure garments is the mainstay of these therapeutic strategies. However, often temporary garments or elastic wraps are used until custom-made garments can be fitted. An accurate measurement and custom fit are an essential part of this pressure therapy and special experience is needed to provide a correct fitting for individual problem zones. A crucial part of compression therapy is to motivate the patient and achieve sufficient cooperation to continuously wear the pressure garments. Constant follow-up is necessary to ensure that the garments remain in a proper state of repair and that their fit is continuously adjusted to maintain adequate compression. In addition, a variety of thermoplastic materials are used to produce rigid, custom-molded facemasks. These masks provide sufficient pressure on healing areas and hypertrophic scars. Transparent material eases direct inspection of the underlying skin (1,2).

Other useful nonoperative techniques to at least partially influence facial scar formation is the use of topical pharmacological agents, such as the use of topical vitamin E and topical or intralesional injection of steroids. Concentrated vitamin E oil and 0.025% Triamcinolone are used in topical preparations. If topical use does not affect scar formation, 0.1% Triamcinolone solution may be injected into multiple sites of the scar. However, signs of improvements may not be seen for at least a few weeks or months (3). Time and repetitive compression massages are further methods of nonoperative treatment of postburn facial scaring.

Although physical and pharmacological agents hasten scar maturation, there is sometimes not enough time to wait for final scar development. In certain high-priority areas of the face, contracture and hypertrophic scar formation require early surgical attention. These high-priority areas include upper and lower eyelids, nostrils, upper and lower lips, and the neck. Prolonged contractures of the eyelids may lead to chronic conjunctivitis and expose the cornea to chronic irritation, leading to corneal ulceration. Failure to relieve lip contractures hampers eating and drinking by restricting lip closure and retention of liquid or solid foods. If allowed to persist too long, lip contractures may alter the finely balanced muscular system of tongue and lip, leading to impairment of bite occlusion.

B. Scalp

The special anatomic features of the skull and scalp explain the special considerations to observe when treating injuries of the scalp. Unlike most other body areas, there is only a thin and delicate soft tissue coverage of the head region. The differing blood supply of the involved tissues is characterized by two different arterial systems. The blood supply of the scalp is maintained through the arterial systems of the carotid and vertebral arteries, whereas diploe and meningeal vessels supply the skull.

Current literature reports up to 25% incidence of scalp burns in relation to the number of total burns. The injuries of increased depth and involved area are more likely in children (4). Besides the thermal tissue damage, additional secondary scalp defects may occur with scar contractures and skin graft donor areas. This may occur with harvest of thick split-thickness skin grafts and lead to alopecia of different grades (5).

In the acute management of scalp burns, nonoperative therapy remains the treatment strategy that is most often used. The primary goal is the preservation of viable hair follicles to allow regeneration of scalp skin. This does not preclude necessary tangential debridement as regeneration may occur from deep hair follicles.

With deeper partial- and full-thickness injuries, complete debridement may be necessary. Further treatment strategy depends on the extent of calvarial involvement (6,7). If viable periosteum is present, the defect may be covered by primary autologous skin grafts or temporary allograft coverage and subsequent autografting. Small defects with involvement of the external table of the calvarial may be covered by local rotation or transposition flaps. With larger areas of involvement, direct flap coverage with or without superficial debridement of necrotic bone may not be possible. A safe and efficient strategy

consists of superficial debridement of the external table by a rotating burr followed by primary or delayed autografting (8,9). Extensive bone defects or full-thickness calvarial burns with potential involvement of meninges or brain may significantly modify the therapeutic course. Additional diagnostic tests such as CT or MRI scans may be warranted. However rare, the management of calvarial burns is widely discussed. Some authors claim that the calvarial bone, even if nonviable, is a better coverage of the dural cavity than any of the potential substitutes. There are case reports of bone regeneration and revitalization in long-term follow-up (10). Once the decision is made to leave nonviable calvarial bone in place, early flap coverage is mandatory. If the defect is too large for local flap coverage, microvascular free flaps may be needed.

The "deluxe" blood supply of the scalp allows the creation of large local skin flaps. Using axial pattern flaps, local transposition flaps of extreme dimension are possible as described earlier (11,12). The delay of these larger flaps can add an additional safety valve to ensure successful survival. If local flaps fail to cover extensive and deep defects, microvascular free-tissue transfer may be needed (13). Several options, such as different muscle or myofasciocutaneus flaps, may be adopted according to local needs. The omental free flap is another viable option, although it requires laparatomy, which may expose the patient to additional risks (14).

With acute burn care of scalp injuries, the attention of the surgeon should focus on the preservation of as much hair-bearing scalp as possible. Any efforts toward secondary reconstruction are lengthy. Surgical alternatives often are not complete or cosmetically satisfying. If local transposition flaps are not feasible, the use of primary skin grafts on a viable wound bed is advisable. Small defects, then, may undergo serial excision in the reconstructive postburn period to correct burn alopecia. With the inherent contraction, the split-thickness skin grafts may shrink the size of the defect by up to 30% during the wound-healing period. Every area of viable scalp should be preserved, even if restoration of a hair-bearing scalp appears not possible.

Scalp burns with exposure of calvarial bone may present special treatment problems. With intact calvarial periosteum, any further manipulation should be avoided and a thin split-thickness skin grafts will suffice to cover the defect. With nonviable periosteum or nonviable outer plate of the calvarial burn, the lamina externa should be debrided until vascularized diploe is exposed to support a split-thickness skin graft. Whether skin grafts are performed as immediate or delayed procedures may not be of any importance. Under proper and aseptic management infectious complications are rare (9).

Some authors report that nonviable calvarial bone, if it remains in place and is covered with vascularized tissue, may regenerate (10). Therefore, nonviable calvarial bone may provide sufficient mechanical protection to the underlying brain. With the improved resolution of CT and MRI scans, craniotomy may be rarely needed to explore the damage to underlying dural or cerebral structures. Removal of necrotic calvarial bone and subsequent skin grafting onto the dura are problematic but may be addressed, if necessary, by using decellularized human dermis (Alloderm®) as additional reinforcement (15,16). However, the resulting contour defect is difficult to correct. Subsequent cranioplasty is necessary to provide aesthetic reconstruction and protective support to the cerebral structures. With any additional incision line, the surgeon should bear in mind the future planning of further reconstruction using local flaps and tissue expansion.

C. Face

The treatment of facial burns is rather complex, as any subunit of the face has to be recognized and evaluated separately. According to the literature, burns involve the face in 45–55% of all burn victims. Depending on the severity of the burn, therapy consists of cooling and soothing dressings (first-degree burn), local antimicrobials or synthetic coverages (superficial second degree), or operative debridement, surgical excision, and grafting (deep second degree, third degree).

The decision for surgical treatment of facial burns and its timing are continuously debated. Early excision and grafting within the first few days after burn injury appear to improve the metabolic and the wound-healing responses. Others argue that only wounds failing to heal within 2 weeks should be excised and grafted. This concept is especially valuable in facial burns. The high potential for regeneration of the facial skin may lead to spontaneous healing of many facial burn wounds. Thus, large areas of otherwise excised facial skin may regenerate and should have been preserved. With clear demarcation, local isolated areas may be excised and grafted. Initial coverage may be achieved by using distant skin graft donor areas; so, local, aesthetically more valuable skin areas (scalp, neck, supraclavicular region) may be preserved for later functional and aesthetic reconstructive procedures. Local flaps or serial excision also should be postponed until later reconstruction (3).

After complete wound coverage is achieved, measures to improve scar quality should be included in the therapeutic plan. Significant improvement of scar quality and aesthetic outcome may be achieved by compression therapy. These issues have to be discussed with the patient and tailored to his special needs. Facial masks may be manufactured using elastic fabric with or without local pressure inserts over regions with high risk of scar hypertrophy. Other options include the use of special three-dimensionally molded silicone or plastic facemasks fixed with elastic straps. Regardless of the type of compression system, the adequacy of pressure has to be continuously monitored and adapted to the changing needs of the individual patient (1–3).

During the acute phase of burn treatment, aggressive excision and grafting should be avoided as it often results in the loss of already limited skin donor areas. These areas may be of crucial importance during future reconstructive efforts. Until scar maturation is complete, reconstructive procedures should be kept to a minimum. Procedures to correct functional impairments, however, may be necessary. If large areas of the face require excision and resurfacing with skin grafts, large unmeshed split-thickness skin graft sheets are applied horizontally. In contrast to the former techniques of placing skin graft into the individual facial subunits, this technique reduces hypertrophic scar formation at the border of the sheets and reduces the prominent borders of the facial subunits [Fig. 15.1(A)]. However, facial compression masks are indispensable to achieve a cosmetically appealing appearance. With the described technique and subsequent compression therapy, the healed skin will behave in a similar fashion as that of the original skin regarding skin folds and further characteristics.

D. Ears

Involvement of one or both ears is frequently seen with facial burns. Due to the thin and very delicate skin coverage of the ear, the resistance to thermal injury is minimal, leading to a high risk of skin defects and subsequent exposure of ear cartilage. Desiccation and infection of perichondrium and cartilage, respectively, may cause further tissue necrosis and the resulting defects can lead to serious deformations (17).

Prevention of ear cartilage infection is paramount, as the therapy of an established infection is difficult and most often futile (18). Local application of mafenide acetate and frequent dressing changes, local debridement, and local flap coverage of exposed cartilage may prevent and contain the infection. To avoid ear cartilage infections, local debridement and temporary coverage with vascularized tissue may be necessary. If these methods fail to achieve coverage of the ear cartilage, the cartilage may be excised and subcutaneously implanted as a unit to another body area. At a later time point the cartilage may be repositioned as a free-cartilage transplant (17). Any reconstruction of partially or completely damaged ears requires intensive preoperative discussions with the patient. Depending on the expectations and the cooperation of the patient, a great number of

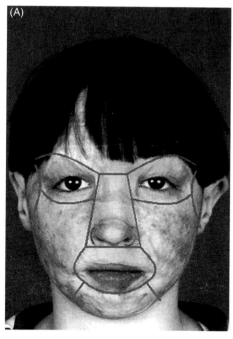

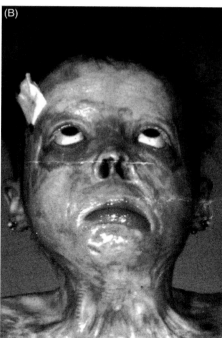

Figure 15.1 (A) Aesthetic units of the face. (B) Scarring of facial burns leads to distortion of aesthetic subunits and impaired facial mimics. In severe burns, additional functional problems such as oral incompetence or eyelid closure may occur.

reconstructive techniques available must be adapted to the patient's individual needs.

As noted, the major challenge in the care of ear burns is the constant risk of cartilage infection and tissue loss.

Once there is structural damage, further reconstructive efforts become increasingly difficult. All operative procedures are more complex and not always successful. Starting with the acute treatment phase, care should be taken to protect the ear cartilage. Due to its thin skin and soft tissue coverage lacking a subcutaneous layer, the risk of exposure of the cartilage is relatively high. However, this may not be immediately recognized and thus may lead to delayed diagnosis of the local infection. In this situation, the smoldering local infection and subsequent loss of cartilage are difficult to handle.

E. Eyelids and Eyebrows

The likelihood to suffer from eye damage by a facial burn has to be considered relatively high. Besides damage to the upper and/or lower eyelids, the main risk is a laceration of the cornea, which may lead to blindness of the injured eye. The risk of corneal injury increases with explosions, flash burns, or chemical injuries. Fortunately, patients with facial flame burns or scalds show a lower incidence of corneal lacerations. The primary reason for this is a functioning blink reflex. Accordingly, in these cases serious injuries are seen in the eyelid region.

An exact clinical evaluation of the eyes and the eye region is mandatory following a facial injury, no matter what the cause. As time between trauma and clinical examination increases, so does edema in the orbital and periorbital tissues. As this conditions worsens, an adequate evaluation becomes difficult. A basic exam by an experienced ophthalmologist upon admission is advisable, to obtain a correct clinical status and to initiate appropriate ophthalmological care.

In case of extensive soft tissue damage to the eyelids and subsequent exposure of the cornea, several possibilities of temporary coverage remain. However, the simplest solution of an eye patch with antibiotic ointment may be difficult to use in case of extensive facial burns. A commonly used coverage is a temporary tarsorrhaphy using silicone tubes assisting with approximation of the upper and lower eyelids. Critics of this technique argue that it is difficult to achieve the approximation of upper and lower eyelids, especially as any movement of the eyeball results in intermittent exposure of the cornea. The applied sutures may also damage the lid margins. With increased edema in the orbital and periorbital tissues, the suture may even cut through. Consequently, satisfying future reconstruction may be rendered difficult, if not impossible. An alternative is the development of a conjunctival flap to cover the cornea. An additional split-thickness skin graft may be necessary to increase mechanical stability (19).

During the early phase of burn, the operative therapy of eyelid injuries should be restricted to excision and grafting of full-thickness injuries as necessary. Definitive reconstruction should be performed at a later stage, when scars have matured. The eyelid's function and its aesthetic significance often require further sequential reconstructive procedures. Correction of ectropions, reconstruction of the medial or lateral canthal areas, as well as eyebrow reconstruction will only be successful if scars have matured and future scar traction can be avoided.

Inadequate treatment of exposed corneal segments will have disastrous effects. This situation being unrecognized will lead to desiccation and ulceration of the cornea. Alternately, bacterial superinfection (most often by *Pseudomonas aeruginosa*) can also develop. An initial eye examination by an experienced ophthalmologist is, therefore, necessary and should be a standard procedure in the evaluation of patients with facial burns.

The development of an ectropion, especially in the lower lid region, is very difficult to alter with the present elastic and contractive forces. An abundantly measured skin graft and adequate postoperative compression therapy may show some effect on the imminent scar contraction. Primary operative correction in the medial or lateral canthal region should be avoided, as postoperative scarring and contracture will be lessened with postburn scar maturation. Vital parts of the eyebrows should be preserved whenever feasible.

Reconstruction of eyebrows, until recently, has been less than satisfactory. Composite grafts can be unreliable and predicled scalp flaps are not aesthetically pleasing in women. Recently, Berrera has shown that the use of micrografts (one to two hair follicles) and minigrafts (two to four hair follicles) is ideal for such reconstruction.

F. Nose

The prominent position, the structure, form, and function of the nose lead to increased exposure with facial burns and may be associated with impairment of respiratory function. Full-thickness burns may directly damage the cartilage scaffold of the nose. Indirect damages occur with infected superficial burns. The most common indirect damages to the nose occur during intensive care treatment. Malpositioning of nasogastric tubes or pressure from endotracheal tubes placed through the nose can lead to local necrosis of soft tissue and cartilage.

Superficial burns of the nose will readily heal under daily dressing changes and topical antimicrobials, such as Silvadene™ or Sulfamylon™. These burns will heal without scar. However, hyperpigmentation or hypopigmentation may be found frequently. The principal goal in the acute care is to preserve as much local tissue as possible. This implies a very cautious and restrictive debridement and may include skin grafting of exposed nasal cartilage to prevent desiccation and infection. Local

infections, nasal chondritis or perichondritis will lead to cartilage necrosis and serious deformation of the nose (17).

Before attempting further reconstructive procedures, complete wound healing and scar maturation should occur. During this time, pressure masks and nasal splints may be useful to prevent hypertrophic scarring. Stenosis of the nostrils may be avoided or minimized with the use of customized splints. If significant stenosis occurs, burn scar release and resurfacing with skin graft followed by subsequent nasal splinting, may be sufficient. The extent of the procedures necessary to reconstruct the residual defects may vary. In case of scar contractures, simple burn scar release and Z-plasties may be sufficient. The correction of a nasal ectropion may require resurfacing with local flaps and skin grafts. Subtotal soft tissue defects require extensive flaps for complete nose reconstruction (17).

The nose is the central aesthetic feature of the face. Early, aggressive debridement will increase the defect and most likely destroy soft tissue which could be used for future reconstruction (17). Initially, conservative treatment seems advisable. Needless to say, during the acute phase of injury, all due care should be taken to avoid further damage by tubes and other manipulations. Suture fixation of enteral and tracheal tubes should be avoided, as the secondary damages can be immense. Such scarring deformities are usually restricted to necrosis of the nasal area. Immediate and subsequent splinting is the most important prophylactic measure to avoid stenosis of the nostrils. Once early intervention has been missed, scar formation will result in significant restriction of nasal ventilation. Any future corrections are very difficult to implement and will require prolonged wearing of nasal splints.

G. Lips and Mouth

After wound closure during the acute phase of treatment, subsequent care relies on oral splints to prevent formation of tight burn scars and microstomia (2). Prefabricated splints are commercially available, but often splints have to be adjusted or custom made to suit the individual patient. The splints should be worn continuously and removed only for food intake and oral hygiene. As most splints are uncomfortable and unappealing to wear, sufficient compliance, especially in young children, is often difficult to achieve. Attempts to clarify the benefits to the patient may be worthwhile (20,21). However, if the subsequent deformity is severe, early burn scar release or corrections may have to be undertaken. Indications for this include problems in obtaining sufficient oral hygiene, or planned dental procedures (22).

Early operative management of oral and perioral burns is rarely necessary. Once complete wound healing and scar maturation have been achieved under continuous wearing of oral splints, most defects will need no further operative treatment. However, omitting the use of splints might lead to serious contractures and very severe microstomia. It appears advisable to carry out any corrective procedures at later time points (21,23,24).

Reconstruction of perioral and oral burns requires special attention. Primary reconstruction during the acute phase seems not very promising as constant movement of lips and tongue and their continuous contact with saliva and food may increase the risk of local infections. Consequently, a more conservative approach with initial stages of injury will result in secondary wound healing with an increased likelihood of hypertrophic scarring and scar contractures. Eversion of oral mucosa and impairment of oral closure or opening due to burn scars are common problems. In extensive facial burns, microstomia will result from scar contractures. Electrical injury to the mouth, mostly found in toddlers, needs special attention, as extensive local soft tissue damage especially at the oral commissure will lead to contractures and microstomia.

Scar formation and the resulting contraction of burn scars in the upper lip-nasal unit, often lead to shortening or bulging of the upper lip. Local burn scar release and skin grafting may help to restore normal lip function and closure. Deformities of the lower lip often result from additional sternomental scar formation and contractures. Combined neck and lower lip scar release may be necessary to obtain satisfying results.

H. Neck

Similar to other events in the the acute burn stage, therapy for oral–perioral burns and neck burns should rely preferentially on splinting. In the acute phase, excision and split-thickness skin grafting may be necessary. However, adequate splinting and compression may minimize mentosternal contracture and achieve a long-term benefit. The grotesque deformation occurring without sufficient therapy will be very difficult and expensive to correct and most often leads to additional secondary problems.

The formation of a mentosternal contracture is a common sequela of full-thickness burns which, fortunately, has decreased over time. The development and use of custom-made splints could reduce the incidence of these grotesque scar contractures and the resulting functional deficits. Frequent problems seen include oral incompetence with salivation, dental damage, incomplete occlusion, recurrent folliculitis, and serious difficulties in perioperative airway management.

The incidence of these contractures was further reduced with the advent of early excision and grafting. However, this does not reduce the need for adequate splinting (2).

Significant neck contractures can still be found in patients with extensive burns. Intensive care related measures, such as central lines and tracheostomies, may impede proper and efficacious splinting. Most often, however, the compliance of patients in wearing these neck splints decreases enormously after hospital discharge. Operative corrections have to be adjusted according to the extent and orientation of neck contractures (3).

I. Prevention of Secondary Problems

In acute burn care, burn surgeons are facing an inherent dilemma. On the one hand, the extent and depth of the burned skin require surgical debridement and early coverage and on the other, this will undoubtedly induce irreversible damage. The face with its differentiated facial expressions, the features of eyes, nose, mouth, and ears form individual are identifying characteristics of the patient. Due to the difficulties in hiding the facial scars, patients with facial burns often are socially stigmatized and often may withdraw from public view.

Therapy and rehabilitation have to be properly planned to achieve the optimal reconstruction aiming to restore most features and specific characteristics of the patient's face while, simultaneously, attaining unrestricted function. This goal may not be reached in many cases. However, every attempt should be made to come close to this ideal.

For the exact planning of the therapeutic efforts, the following suggestions may be useful. The major unsolved problem in burn care is uncontrolled scar formation. This in turn determines the future course of rehabilitation and the outcome of reconstructive endeavors. When questioned about the most desired reconstructive surgery, most burn survivors will ask for scar release, reduction, or removal. Scar formation and maturation is a process that takes its due time. Therefore, reconstructive procedures aiming at achieving definitive restoration may be less than optimal during this time period. However, there are limitations to the number of corrective procedures that may be undertaken. The limited resources of local tissue have to be used diligently, as further repeated corrections are problematic (3).

The initiation of definitive reconstruction of the burn face should, therefore, be delayed until scar maturation is complete. Early or immediate reconstruction, however, may be necessary in case of progressing deformity or severe functional problems, such as in case of severe ectropion of the eyelids, where the defect has to be restored to avoid further damage to the eye. To avoid further problems during scar formation and maturation, coverage should be attempted using abundant tissue for reconstruction of the defect. This will reduce local tension and decrease scar hypertrophy. Adequate splinting and compression therapy should follow after surgery. In acute injury of the face, primary closure of defects is preferred. However, in most cases, defects may have to be covered with skin grafts or local flaps. For primary coverage, the use of skin grafts is the simplest procedure and should be favored. Thus, local and regional flaps may be still available for definite future reconstruction. For facial subunits, special issues may apply.

III. RECONSTRUCTIVE CONSIDERATIONS AND PLANNING

A. Functional Deficits

In some areas of the burned face, secondary reconstruction of hypertrophic scars and contractures are of high priority. Areas such as the upper and lower eye lids, upper and lower lip, and neck will need early and continuous evaluations during the recovery period. Functional impairments will be recognized and corrected early, thus preventing permanent severe damage to functional structures. In these situations early correction, including complete reconstruction, may be advisable, although this may cause further problems in the later course.

1. Eyelids

Even with all initial attempts to prevent the postoperative formation of eyelid ectropion, such as early use of skin grafts, the risk cannot be completely eliminated. Every damage and abnormality of the eyelid leads to impairment of the eye's function and protection, with resultant secondary problems. Corrections of ectropions of the upper and lower eyelids will, in most cases, be achieved by the use of skin grafts. Local flaps present alternative techniques for eyelid reconstruction, although rarely used. The important principle in the operative treatment is complete excision of the scar and overcorrecting with skin grafts. With each procedure, only one lid should be corrected in each eye. Otherwise, the needed overcorrection is difficult to achieve. Also the need for medial or lateral canthopexy makes restriction to one lid per eye advisable (19). Suitable donor areas for skin grafts may be found in the retroauricular region of the upper inner arm for the lower eyelid, and for split-thickness skin grafts to the upper eyelids, skin may be harvested from the supraclavicular region. An additional, temporary tarsorrhaphy may be advisable until complete healing of the skin graft has occurred.

2. Lips

Treatment of upper and lower lip burns can be summarized in three steps. Initial therapy includes the use of custom fit of oral splints to avoid severe damage. However, in rare cases it may be necessary to perform a corrective procedure within 2–3 weeks after injury without waiting for complete scar maturation. The most common problem here is microstomia. As complete opening and closure of the mouth depend on the symmetry and functional integrity of both commissures, scars in this area will cause significant impairment. Most reconstructive techniques use variations of oral mucosa flaps or Z-plasties (20,23). With an additional ectropion of the lower lip, a burn scar release and an overcorrecting skin graft should be used to eliminate pre-operative scar tension.

3. Neck

In spite of intensified splinting during the acute phase therapy, vertical scar bands may develop in neck burns and lead to later neck contractures [Fig. 15.1(B)]. Minor scar bands may be corrected with Z-plasties, by interposing normal tissue with scar tissue into a horizontal orientation. Major scar bands need increased surgical efforts. The severe immediate and long-term effects of a neck contracture will socially and functionally debilitate the patient. Therefore, a concise plan of reconstruction should be formed early. Whenever possible, waiting for scar maturation is advisable. The use of faciocutaneous flaps, either random or axial-patterned, may be necessary in late reconstruction of the neck. The supraclavicular island flap has been described to address this issue (3,25).

Tissue expanders for neck reconstruction may be used without a problem, if placed in a supraplastysmal plane (26). Expanders in the cervical region have been performed without significant problems. In the cervical position, expander inflation does compress the underlying structures such as the jugular vein, carotid artery, thyroid, trachea, and esophagus but without clinical significance. Distant transposition flaps or free flaps are rarely indicated in neck defects.

The most frequently used technique to correct extensive burn scars is scar excision followed by full-thickness skin grafts or split-thickness skin grafts (3). Complete excision of the scar bands is necessary to achieve the maximum correction of neck contractures in burn patients. With limited donor sites in severely burned patients, full-thickness skin grafts may not be available. Here, split-thickness skin grafts are utilized. Overcorrection may be desirable with all skin grafts. The tendency of grafts to contract is much higher in split-thickness grafts. After the take of split-thickness skin grafts, customized splints should be applied to prevent head and neck movements until the skin grafts have matured to prevent a recurrent contracture (1,2).

B. Aesthetic Reconstruction

The final aesthetic reconstruction of the burned face is the product of a long series of operative procedures. If the outcome of early-stage procedures is optimal, only small corrections are necessary to perfect the final details. Upon completion of early reconstructive procedures, patients may request additional operations to further correct the remaining aesthetic units. With complete scar maturation, a final reconstruction of the ear or the nose-facial features can now be undertaken. In addition, reconstruction of ears, eyebrows, nasal deformities and the upper lip nasal unit can be addressed. The major guideline for therapy planning in this reconstruction stage is communication with the patient. The patient assists in determining the focus of his reconstructive needs. The surgeon has to advise and help the patient to reach an informed decision about the proposed operations and their expected outcome (Fig. 15.2).

C. Decision Making

Burn reconstruction is characterized by the use of different operative strategies in one patient. The primary goal is to achieve early and complete burn wound closure without scar deformities and contractures. Additional goals are the correction of soft tissue defects and functional impairment. Individualized postoperative treatment with splints and compression garments is of utmost importance. The early concept of treatment goals is the basic measure to avoid secondary complications. Treatment goals are realized in a sequential order, first restoring active and passive function followed by aesthetic reconstruction. When these goals are combined in a single operative setting, patient satisfaction improves. The techniques used for reconstruction follow a hierarchical order starting from simple procedures leading to more complex and resource intensive procedures. Burn scar excision followed by primary closure of the wound is the simplest and easiest possible corrective procedure. The preformed free flap is a more complex procedure limited to special situations. Every technique used, includes specific advantages and disadvantages, which need to be considered.

As previously mentioned, primary closure may be the simplest and fastest reconstructive procedure after removal of burned tissue. However, this may only be used in small defects, when the burn is surrounded by healthy normal tissue, which may be sufficiently mobilized to facilitate primary closure. With undue tension on wound edges, the reconstructive goal will not be achieved and the scar will tend to hypertrophy. Z-plasties are double opposing transposition skin flaps. They are a surgical option to correct a burn scar contracture by lengthening and reorienting the contracted scar. The methods, however, depend on sufficient tissue being available laterally from the respective scar. By understanding the basic principles of Z-plasties, this reliable procedure is frequently used in the reconstruction of burn scar contractures, closure of skin defects, or redirection of scar lines.

Once the burn areas are too extensive for excision and primary closure or closure using Z-plasties, skin grafting is the next available step in the sequence of reconstructive procedures. After excision of large burn scars or contractures, wound edges will often retract resulting in a large tissue defect. Closure of these defects is performed in an easy, sufficient, and safe manner by full-thickness skin grafts or split-thickness skin grafts. Although the choice of the type of skin graft may depend on individual experience, several suggestions may guide the use of skin transplants. Split-thickness skin grafts are suited for closure of larger defect areas. A thin skin graft usually results in greater take and requires a less optimal wound bed. However, STSGs will contract more easily and the cosmetic appearance may be unsatisfactory and completely different from the donor and/or recipient areas. Full thickness skin grafts will achieve aesthetically the most appealing results. However, disadvantages include a limited availability and the creation of an additional scar. The size of the skin graft is limited by the need for primary closure of the donor defect. In addition, full-thickness skin grafts require an optimal wound bed with high vascularity and low bacterial contamination. Once full take has been achieved, full-thickness skin grafts will provide a high-quality substitute for the original skin cover by similar properties of skin color and texture. In contrast, full-thickness skin grafts, contract less and thus achieve their final outcome earlier.

Composite grafts may be necessary with extensive tissue defects, including skin and underlying supporting tissue, such as in reconstruction of the nose. Total or partial loss of alar cartilage may be replaced by an appropriately sized composite graft from the ear. However, the use of composite grafts is limited. They are basically free grafts without a defined blood supply and depend on an optimal wound bed to support the graft. This also

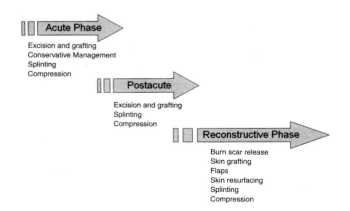

Figure 15.2 Facial burns—sequence of therapeutic options to prevent long-term sequelae.

limits the size up to which a composite graft may be safely transplanted. A size of 0.5 cm × 0.5 cm × 0.5 cm will nearly always result in take of the composite graft. Besides subtle surgical technique during graft harvest and wound bed preparation, stable graft fixation must be achieved to obtain a good take rate. Local compression bandages or tie-over dressings are of use to provide fixation of grafts on the wound bed. This prevents fluid or hematoma retention underneath the skin grafts, improves neovascularization, and provides perfect alignment with the underlying surface.

In situations where skin grafts will not be available or not be sufficient to cover the defect, flap coverage may be necessary. Exposed bone without periosteal coverage, uncovered tendons, and open joint will not support a skin graft, and hence require definite flap coverage. Flap also may be necessary in the reconstruction of contour irregularities after extensive soft tissue defects or to cover prominent bone. The flaps used include fasciocutaneous random pattern or axial pattern flaps and musculocutaneous flaps. Free flaps are rarely used in special situations. Tissue expansion is a valuable tool in facial reconstruction and may be used for correction of burn alopezia, neck contracture release, and resurfacing of the jaw line. Tissue expansion supplies tissue of similar color, thickness, and texture. However, exact planning is necessary to achieve the required amount of tissue. Advantages include the often limited availability of an unburned local skin area for expander implantation. The need for several procedures and the prolonged period of expansion and the associated aesthetic distortion and disfiguration will put additional stress on the patient.

D. Skin Match

The reconstructive surgeon is facing yet another additional problem. For reconstruction of the burned face, donor skin has to be of high quality. Locally, the donor skin should provide matching texture, color, thickness, and hair growth. Donor areas fulfilling all these requirements are rare. Thus, regions of lesser quality may have to be used. This is especially true in cases of large total body surface area burns where donor sites are limited. A skin graft taken from a donor site close to the reconstructed area generally shows a closer match of skin properties.

The areas of choice for the reconstruction of facial burns are the retroauricular region, the neck, and the supraclavicular region, and less frequently the upper arm or the upper thoracic areas. In case these areas are not available, donor sites with minimal hair growth and areas with minimal color mismatch should be chosen. A color mismatch of lighter skin graft areas will always be apparent on a normally tanned face. Similarly, the porous skin taken from the thigh will always be prominently visible

when used in facial reconstruction. The unique properties of facial skin with its fine structure, thin subcutaneous layer, and high elasticity can only be insufficiently replaced. If extended areas of burned facial skin have to be covered, then the whole aesthetic region should be covered with skin grafts of the best available quality. Lacking those, every effort should be undertaken to cover multiple aesthetic subunits in one session. The best results will be achieved by using large-sized skin grafts on the excised facial burn wound without patch working. Skin graft borders and sutures should be placed in inconspicuous regions of the face. By taking maximum-size skin grafts and placing them in transverse orientation across the face, two or three skin graft sheets will be sufficient to achieve complete coverage and efficient reconstruction. A major advantage of this approach is the resulting minimal scarring in the central face. Suture lines and graft borders may be placed laterally into the hair-bearing temporal region or the lateral frontal region. The resulting horizontal suture line can be relatively well hidden in the periocular or perioral facial submits. The long-term results of this technical approach are surprising, as over time, facial wrinkling occurs similar to the original facial feature. The restoration of facial expression is greatly enhanced in comparison to a restoration oriented toward individual facial subunits, the resulting increased scarring, and the mask-like appearance. A similar approach may be used in full-thickness skin grafts or with cervico-pectoral fasciocutaneous flaps. The need for primary closure of the donor sites, however, restricts the use of full-thickness skin grafts to smaller areas comprising several facial subunits. The use of cervico-pectoral flaps will require primary and secondary thinning of the flap to reduce the contour mismatch between donor area and the recipient facial region.

E. Compression Therapy

Treatment of burn scars is a time-consuming and tedious process. It requires strenuous efforts of both patient and surgeon, and often yields only insufficient results. A principal element of postburn scar treatment is compression therapy. External compression as a means to affect scar maturation has been investigated and introduced into clinical practice during the last decades. During this time several improvements have been achieved, such as the availability of custom-made compression garments or custom-made splints. The exact fit of compression garments is of utmost importance for achieving the desired results. A loose fit of garments will not be able to provide sufficient compression on burn scars; a tight fit might result in pressure related skin lacerations or vascular compromise. Bearing in mind that compression therapy of scars is a dynamic process, continuous monitoring of scars and the compression used is necessary. In the initial period, garments may have to be modified and altered frequently; torn garments have to be replaced, as they will not provide the desired effects. Achieving sufficient patient compliance may pose an additional problem to the treating burn team. Perfectly fitting and well-maintained compression garments will improve patient compliance. Suboptimal fit with the resulting pain or scar tenderness will most certainly lead to a significant delay in effective scar therapy. In extensive burn scars, equal distribution of pressure will be difficult to achieve. On the irregularly shaped body surface this can only be provided by the use of custom-made silicone elastomer inlays in the fabricated garments. In addition to local pressure, silicone elastomer itself shows positive effect by softening the scar tissue. The underlying mechanism for this phenomenon is still under investigation. Risks of long-standing compression therapy have been described as delayed development of the mandible, loss of the anatomic architecture of the palmar arch, or thoracic deformities.

F. Artificial Skin Coverage

The loss of the epidermal and dermal skin layer significantly endangers survival of a burn victim. The skin functions as barrier against fluid and protein loss, or to prevent the invasion of microbial organisms over large wound surfaces. Until now, grafting of the patient's own skin remains the best means to replace damaged and lost skin areas. However, extensive burns limit the area of donor sites available and alternative skin coverage materials need to be considered during the acute treatment period. During the last decades, significant progress has been achieved in the development of artificial skin coverage materials. The materials introduced into clinical use can be differentiated as temporary and permanent skin coverage materials.

1. Temporary Skin Coverage Materials

Human amnion is being used for coverage of clean superficial burns or skin graft donor areas. After burn wound excision, it may be used as temporary cover until sufficient autologous skin grafts are available. Amnion has been used as fresh, cryo-preserved or as devitalized, glycerol treated product. Major advantages include the easy and fast procurement and its large availability also in underdeveloped countries. The major disadvantage is the potential risk of viral contamination and the risk of HIV and hepatitis transmission, which may be minimized, but not completely excluded, by donor screening and additional glycerol treatment of amnion. These issues currently limit the clinical use of amnion.

Pig skin has been established as temporary coverage material over several years. Its procurement and preparation are easy and can be performed in an industrialized fashion. Pig skin may be ordered as sheets or as mesh grafts. It is available as fresh, refrigerated, cryo-preserved, or glycerol treated skin. Pig xenografts will adhere to a clean wound, thus improving pain relief and wound healing. However, pig skin will not be vascularized and dermal elements will not be integrated into the regenerated skin. Transmission of viral vectors seems to be an issue of minor importance. Bacterial contamination may be decreased by using additional local antiseptics, such as Dakins solution or silver-nitrate solution.

Human cadaveric donor skin may be used in a similar fashion as pig skin for the temporary coverage of excised burn wounds. It will be partially vascularized and may even be partially integrated into the neo skin. As temporary cover, it stimulates local growth factor production and granular tissue formation. However, procurement is restricted to accredited tissue and skin banks. Guidelines set by the American Association of Tissue Banks (AATB) significantly reduce the risk of viral and bacterial transmission. Allografts are supplied by AATB accredited institutions or the Euro skin bank as fresh, cryo-preserved, or glycerol-preserved sheet or meshed skin grafts.

Synthetic, semipermeable membranes are commercially available for temporary wound coverage. They provide sufficient barrier function to prevent wound desiccation or bacterial contamination. They also reduce pain. These, mostly one or bilayered, membranes are used for superficial burn wound dressings or coverage of skin graft donor sites. As most of these membranes are effective occlusive wound dressings, usage on a contaminated wound will result in bacterial infection of the burn wound. Recently, synthetic membranes have been used in combination with viable allogenic cell grafts (usually allogenic neonatal fibroblast). In addition to its barrier function, the membrane acts as a carrier of viable cells which, in turn, will express and stimulate local growth factor production.

2. Permanent Skin Coverage

The culture of epidermal autografts (CEA) has been established as a useful tool in burn surgery. However, the initial expectations have not been fufilled. The possibility to culture large areas of epidermal skin grafts from small available donor sites is appealing. However, with increasing use and long-term follow-up, significant drawbacks became apparent. In addition to enormous financial costs, CEA show a significantly decreased healing potential and are delicate and vulerable requiring later secondary autografting. In extensive burns with minimally available donor sites, however, CEA may offer a valuable opportunity to achieve wound coverage.

The clinical problems seen with cultures of epidermal autografts led to the finding that an intact dermal layer is important to provide supple and resistant skin coverage with diminished scarring. A synthetic acellular dermal matrix substitute is available as Integra®. It consists of a matrix of glycosaminoglycans and collagen fibers, covered by a semipermeable silicone layer. After initial temporary coverage of the excised burn wound, the dermal matrix layer is vascularized and can be grafted with a thin autograft. Major disadvantages are the increased risk of secondary infection and the cost of the product. Another approach to the restoration of the dermal matrix is the use of cryo-preserved cadaveric dermal autografts, which are subsequently covered by thin autografts. The combination of the aforementioned techniques appears to be a logical consequence. All research focused on this goal demonstrated impressive results in animal experiments. However, reliable clinical data are still missing.

IV. FUTURE PERSPECTIVES

Additional techniques, such as genetic modifications of keratinocytes may enhance wound healing by optimizing the local wound environment. Cells are engineered to overexpress growth factors, such as PDGF, IGF-1, EGF, KGF, or others. This approach opens the field to various modifications of the above mentioned techniques, biological and synthetic skin coverage materials. Donor site wound healing may be improved and fastened. Various combinations of tissue engineered skin substitutes may be improved. The ideal solution, however, of a permanent and complete skin substitute, which can be applied after initial excision of the burn wound and will heal completely without the need of regrafting, requires further research. The combination of tissue engineering techniques and genetic modification of cells activated during the wound healing sequence may finally solve the problems related to a surgeon's dream of complete restoration of the lost tissue.

REFERENCES

1. Rivers EA, Strate RG, Solem LD. The transparent face-mask. Am J Occup Ther 1979; 33:108–113.
2. Jordan RB, Daher J, Wasil K. Splints and scar management for acute and reconstructive burn care. Clin Plast Surg 2000; 27:71–85.
3. Remensnyder JP, Donelan MB. Reconstruction of the head and neck. In: Herndon, ed. Total Burn Care. 2nd ed Philadelphia: WB Saunders, 2002:656–689.
4. Hunt J, Purdue G, Spicer T. Management of full thickness burns of the scalp and skull. Arch Surg 1983; 118:621–625.
5. Huang TT, Larson DL, Lewis SR. Burn alopecia. Plast Reconstr Surg 1977; 60:763–767.
6. Ranev D, Shindarsky B. Operative treatment of deep burns of the scalp. Brit J Plast Surg 1969; 12:309–312.
7. Harrison SH. Exposure of the skull from burns. Br J Plast Surg 1952; 4:279.
8. Sheridan RL, Choucair RJ, Donclan MB. Management of massive calvarial exposure in young children. J Burn Care Rehabil 1998; 19:29–32.
9. Spies M, McCauley RL, Mudge BR, Herndon DN. Management of acute calvarial burns in children. J Trauma 2003; 54(4):765–769.
10. Fried M, Rosenberg B, Tuchman I, Ben-Hur N, Yardeni P, Sternberg N, Golan J. Electrical burn injury of the scalp—bone regrowth following application of latissimus dorsi free flap to the area. Burns 1991; 17:338.
11. Orticochea M. New three-flap reconstruction technique. Br J Plast Surg 1971; 24:184–188.
12. Jurkiewicz MJ, Hill HL. Open wounds of the scalp: an account of methods of repair. J Trauma 1981; 21:769–778.
13. Silverberg B, Banis JC, Verdi GD, Acland RD. Microvascular reconstruction after electrical and deep thermal injury. J Trauma 1986; 26:128–134.
14. Losken A, Carlson GW, Culbertson JH, Scott Hultmann C, Kumar AV, Jones GE, Bostwick J III, Jurkiewicz MJ. Omental free flap reconstruction in complex head and neck deformities. Head Neck 2002; 24:326–331.
15. Barret JP, Dziewulski P, McCauley RL, Herndon DN, Desai MH. Dural reconstruction of a class IV calvarial burn with decellularized human dermis. Burns 1999; 25:459–462.
16. Groenevelt F, van Trier AJ, Khouw YL. The use of allografts in the management of exposed calvarial electrical wounds of the skull. Ann NY Acad Sci 1999; 888:109–112.
17. Bernard SL. Reconstruction of the burned nose and ear. Clin Plast Surg 2000; 27:97–112.
18. Skedros DG, Goldfarb IW, Slater H. Chondritis of the burned ear: a review. Ear Nose Throat J 1992; 71:359–362.
19. Achauer BM, Adair SR. Acute and reconstructive management of the burned eyelid. Clin Plast Surg 2000; 27:87–96.
20. Pensler JM, Rosenthal A. Reconstruction of the oral commissure after an electrical burn. J Burn Care Rehabil 1990; 11:50–53.
21. Silverglade D, Ruberg RL. Nonsurgical management of burns to the lips and commissures. Clin Plast Surg 1986; 13:87–94.
22. Ortiz-Monasterio F, Factor R. Early definitive treatment of electric burns of the mouth. Plast Reconstr Surg 1980; 65:169–176.
23. Leake JE, Curtin JW. Electrical burns of the mouth in children. Clin Plast Surg 1984; 11:669–683.
24. Dado DV, Polley W, Kernahan DA. Splinting of oral commissure electrical burns in children. J Pediatr 1985; 107:92–95.
25. Pallua N, Machens HG, Rennekampff O, Becker M, Berger A. The fasciocutaneous supraclavicular artery island flap for releasing postburn mentosternal contractures. Plast Reconstr Surg 1997; 99(7):1878–1884.
26. MacLennan SE, Corcoran JF, Neale HW. Tissue expansion in head and neck burn reconstruction. Clin Plast Surg 2000; 27:121–132.

16

Reconstruction of the Burned Scalp

ENRIQUE GARAVITO

Shriners Hospital for Children, Mexico Unit and School of Medicine, Anahuac University, Mexico, Mexico

ROBERT L. McCAULEY

University of Texas Medical Branch and Shriners Hospital for Children—Galveston Unit, Galveston, Texas, USA

JACOBO VERBITZKY

Shriners Hospital for Children, Mexico Unit, Mexico

I. INTRODUCTION

Burns to the hair-bearing scalp can not only be life threatening but may also impair overall aesthetics. The defects are not easily hidden. In patients with 80% total body surface area (TBSA burns), scalp involvement was noted in 32% of the patients. These injuries can be classified into two groups; those which are pure soft tissue injuries and scalp burns which involve the calvarium. Pure soft tissue injuries can either be partial-thickness burns or full-thickness burns without the involvement of the periosteum. One should bear in mind that even partial-thickness thermal burns, which heal secondarily, can cause alopecia by injuring the hair follicles. Third-degree burns cause deep scalp destruction that often requires a skin graft for coverage if the periosteum is intact.

Scalp burns, which involve the skull, are managed differently. The outer table is protected by the periosteum. Once necrosis of the outer table is noted, we face a different set of problems. Depending on the size and depth of the defect, various options are available for either immediate or delayed coverage. Full-thickness scalp injuries with calvarial involvement have been a topic of continuous discussion for burn surgeons. Harrison (1) devised a classification scheme that allows us to adjust treatment plans based on the depth of the injury. (Table 16.1). Three scenarios occur when we evaluate patients with scalp burns involving the calvarium. First, these patients may

Table 16.1 Harrison Classification of Skull Burns

Type I	Total skin loss with intact pericranium
Type II	Total skin loss with involvement of pericranuim
Type III	Total skin loss with involvement of outer table
Type IV	Total skin loss with involvement of both plates of the skull

Source: Adapted with permission from Harrison (1).

have a devascularized outer table in which debridement of the outer table is performed to access the diploe to achieve enough vascularity to close the wound with a split-thickness skin graft. Alternatively, if outer table debridement still produces a nonvascular wound, coverage with vascularized tissue is recommended. Last, if the initial patient assessment indicates a full-thickness calvarial injury, that is, exposed dura or skull fractures with CSF leaks, immediate coverage of the defect with a vascularized flap should be the primary operative procedure. Here, long-term follow-up of patients is crucial to determine if calvarial defects develop or persist in patient with obvious full-thickness loss. Habal (2) developed a classification system based on the size of the defect to predict the treatment options for patients who have defects. However, scalp injuries, with or without involvement of the calvarium, can present reconstructive challenges for plastic surgeons. As with acute burns in other parts of the body, the goals are to obtain early wound closure and restore aesthetic and functional integrity to the scalp and skull.

II. ACUTE BURN CARE

A. Soft Tissue Injuries Only

Soft tissue injuries in patients with large TBSA involvement of the head and neck can range from 25% to 45% (3,4). The scalp has been a popular donor site for coverage of a patient with large TBSA burns. However, controversy exists as to the incidence of complications associated with graft harvesting. Brou et al. (3) reported a 61% incidence of alopecia in patients with existing scalp burns in which skin grafts were subsequently harvested for wound closure. However, only a 2.2% incidence of alopecia is noted in patients without burns to the scalp that underwent harvesting of scalp grafts for closure of burn wounds (5).

The management of scalp burns acutely is the avoidance of pressure, cleansing, and the use of topical antimicrobial agents. In partial-thickness wounds, this management plan has been successful in achieving re-epithelialization. The development of folliculitis can protract the healing course and produce cicatricial alopecia. Scalp wounds that do not heal in 2 weeks, may

require skin grafts for closure (6). The management of burn alopecia is based on both the extent of the defect and its location.

B. Calvarial Involvement

In patients with thermal injuries, involvement of the outer table of the skull can be problematic. Debridement until the underlying diploe is reached is the classic approach. If a vascular surface is reached, then coverage with skin grafts is possible. Spies et al. (7) reported a comparison to burn patients with thermal injury that included Harrison Class III/IV injuries to burned children without calvarial burns. Patients with calvarial burns not only required more operations to achieve wound closure, but also had longer lengths of hospital stay (7). The overwhelming majority of patients were able to obtain wound closure by debridement of the outer table and coverage with split-thickness skin grafts (STSG). In patients in which outer table debridement produced an avascular wound, the use of scalp flaps has allowed closure up to nearly 50% of the hair-bearing scalp. However, free-tissue transfers may also be indicated (8).

III. RECONSTRUCTION

The long-term effect of burns to the scalp is cicatricial alopecia. The management of this problem depends on size of the defect, its location, and whether or not an underlying calvarial defect is present. A careful physical examination is essential. Areas of folliculitis may require systematic antibiotics or excision prior to definitive treatment of the alopecia. In patients with previous Harrison III or IV calvarial injuries, calvarial defects may be suspected. A 3-D CAT scan may be necessary to not only determine the extent and location of the defect, but to also plan operative correction.

A. Scalp Burns without Bony Involvement

1. Local Scalp Flaps

The majority of burns involving the scalp are in children. Scald burns or grease burns account for the majority of these injuries. Whether these injuries are partial-thickness defects, which heal secondary or deeper burns, which require skin grafts, alopecia is likely to be the final result. Prior to tissue expansion, Huang et al. (9) classified the extent of burn alopecia in children in an attempt to not only guide our surgical interventions, but also give us some expectations as to what to tell our patients (Table 16.2). Patients classified as Group A had alopecia that was <15% of the hair-bearing scalp; in Group B, the alopecia was >15% but <30% of the hair-bearing

Table 16.2 Classification and Sex Distribution of Burn Alopecia

			Male	Female	Total
Group A	(<15%)	Adults	3	2	51
		Children	29	17	
Group B	(16–30%)	Adults	6	0	36
		Children	11	19	
Group C	(31–60%)	Adults	1	0	19
		Children	10	8	
Group D	(>61%)	Adults	4	1	11
		Children	3	3	

Source: Adapted with permission from Huang (2).

scalp; in Group C, the alopecia was >30% but <50% of the hair-bearing scalp; in Group D, the alopecia was >50% of the scalp. Using this classification system, scar excision can remove alopecia segments up to 15% of the hair-bearing scalp. Currently, if complete excision of the alopecia segment can be carried out in three or less operations, this approach is still preferred by many surgeons. If more operations are deemed necessary, alternative approaches are available.

In 1968, Orticochea (10) published the four-flap technique for coverage of moderate-size scalp defects. In 1972, this technique was modified to a three-limb flap design for correction of scalp defects (11). Although the exact extent of hair bearing flap coverage achieved is not clear. Although coverage of moderate-sized scalp defects can be achieved with these techniques, increased blood loss and excessive scaring from the multiple scalp flaps can be problematic (12). The flaps may not cover large alopecia segments. Later, Juri (13) developed the mono-pedicled scalp flap for coverage of segmental areas of alopecia. This flap was particularly useful in the re-creation of the frontal hairline. However, these flaps did not solve the problem of total correction of large alopecia segments. In recent years, the Juri flap has been used in combination with scalp reduction surgery or expanded prior to transfer (14,15). In order to minimize excision scarring and blood loss, the lateral scalp flap was developed for coverage of the frontal hairline. This flap differed from the Juri flap in that it required no delay and the donor site could be easily closed. However, this flap could only reach the midpoint of the frontal hairline (16).

Barrera (17) has shown that micrografts (one to two hair follicles) and minigrafts (three to four hair follicles) are useful with the corrections of burn alopecia. In a series of 32 burn patients, he successfully corrected large alopecia segments with excellent outcomes. The successful application and survival of micrografts and minigrafts in burn scar is believed to be a function of their very low metabolic rate. Neeedless to say, the use of micrografts in

extremely large areas of alopecia is not only labor intensive, but also costly. However, the use of tissue expansion for the closure of large areas of burn alopecia has given our patients yet another option for improving scalp aesthetics.

2. Tissue Expansion

The historical aspects of soft tissue expansion have been previously discussed. However, it suffices to say that tissue expansion is the result of a constant mechanical stress load that leads to tissue regeneration (18,19). Although the initial medical application of this concept occurred with bone, pure soft tissue expansion occurred in 1956 by Neumann (20). However, this concept remained dormant for another 20 years. The subsequent explosive rediscovery of soft tissue expansion has been applied to nearly every aspect of reconstruction today (20). The histologic features of tissue expansion are well known (25). Briefly, the epidermis becomes thicker with most of the mitotic activity occurring in the stratum spongiosum (24). The dermis thins out with the greatest amount of thinning occurring in the papillary dermis (25). The molecular basis for this phenomenon appears to be the activation of various signal transduction pathways induced by mechanical strain. The activation of a numbers of growth factors for epithelial and connective tissue growth may be responsible for this tissue regeneration (19).

In 1976, Radavan (26) popularized the concept of tissue expansion. Simultaneously, Austed et al. (27) presented his laboratory and clinical experience (27). This technique in the reconstruction of burn alopecia has rapidly become the gold standard by which other techniques are judged, in spite of complication rates of ~15–20% (28,29). In 1990, McCauley et al. (29) classified burn alopecia based on the extent of the defect and the pattern of alopecia and as a template for which reconstructive efforts may be designed. (Table 16.3). Patients with type 1A or 1B burn alopecia can be corrected with a single expansion, although

Table 16.3 Classification of Burn Alopecia

Type I	Single alopecia segment
	A <25% of the hair-bearing scalp
	B 25–50% of the hair-bearing scalp
	C 50–75% of the hair-bearing scalp
	D >75% of the hair-bearing scalp
Type II	Multiple alopecia segments amendable to tissue expansion placement
Type III	Patchy burn alopecia not amendable to tissue expansion
Type IV	Total alopecia

Source: Adapted with permission from McCauley RL. Correction of burn alopecia. In: Herndon DN, ed. Total Burn Care. Philadelphia: W.B. Saunders, 1996:449–502.

overinflation may be necessary. Patients with type 1C and 1D burn alopecia may require multiple expanders either together or sequentially to correct these large areas of alopecia. Patients with type IIA or IIB alopecia may also be corrected with a single expansion. However, patients with type IIC and IID alopecia require intricate flap designs to correct the problem. Sasaki (30) emphasized the importance of preoperative planning in these patients since the size of the expander and subsequent flap movement may affect the final aesthetic result (Fig. 16.1). The size of the expander, the shape of the expander, and the size and location of the scalp defect, all play an important role in achieving a satisfactory result. The placement of tissue expanders in the subgaleal plane is routine. The use of perioperative antibiotics is also commonplace. Incisions can be placed at the junction of the hair-bearing skin and the alopecia segment. Alternatively, radial and remote incisions have also been utilized. The adjustments are at the discretion of the surgeon since currently no studies exist comparing these two techniques for exposure rates or infection rates. Once the dimensions of the dissected pocket have been maximized, an expander is selected with dimensions 1.0–2.0 cm smaller than the pocket size. The use of integrated ports vs. remote ports is based on surgical preference and the experience of the physician injecting the expander. The person injecting the expander may not be the operative surgeon. Prior to the placement of the expander, the device is checked for leaks. Submergence in saline with air injected is routine to look for air leaks.

Alternatively, the use of methylene blue has also been recommended (31). Once the wounds are closed, sterile saline is injected into the expander, filling it as much as possible without placing undue tension on the skin flaps or the incision line. Usually 10–20% of the expander volume can be injected. Sutures are left in place for 2 weeks and expansion is then started. Saline is injected on a weekly or biweekly basis. The volume of saline injected is a function of patient discomfort and flap elasticity. Usually 10% of the volume per week is adequate to insure complete inflation of the expander within 3 months. Should capillary refill become a problem during the expansion process or the patient complains of pain, a 23-gauge needle is used to remove saline from the expander to correct these problems. Once expansion is completed, the length of flap advancement is calculated by measuring the dome of the expanded scalp flap and subtracting its base width. Prior to removal of the expander, advancement and/or rotation of the expanded scalp flap is decided based on the extent of the defect and the subsequent orientation of the hair follicles (Figs. 16.2 and 16.3). Intraoperatively, scalloping of the skull is usually noted, especially in children. However, the skull appears to remodel itself after removal of the expander. Postoperatively, this contour defect in the skull may be noted. After advancement or rotation of the expanded scalp flap, intraoperative capsulotomy has been described as a method to increase flap length. The amount gained in the length of the expanded flap is not well documented. In addition, increased bleeding and damage to the overlying vessels is always a risk.

Complications of tissue expansion are divided into major vs. minor (32). Major complications have been reported that are as low as 3% and as high as 44% (29,32–34). Major complications are defined as those that interrupt the expansion process such that the

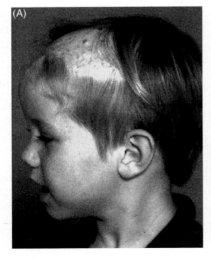 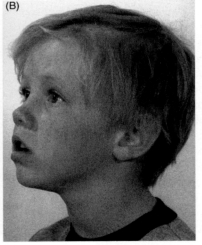

Figure 16.1 (A) Six-year-old male with Type 1A burn alopecia. (B) Postoperative view 6 months later. (Reprinted with permission from McCauley RL. Correction of burn alopecia. In: Herndon DN, ed. Total Burn Care. Philadelphia: W.B. Saunders, 1996:499–502.)

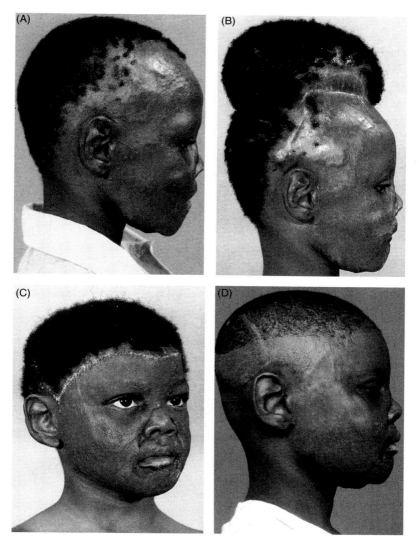

Figure 16.2 (A) Seven-year-old male with Type 1B burn alopecia. (B) Complete inflation of a 500 cc tissue expander. (C) One week after correction of alopecia with a single flap advancement. (D) Follow-up 1 year later.

preoperative plan cannot be achieved. Such complications as infections, flap necrosis, implant exposure, or wound dehiscence. MacLennon et al. (35) have documented that with proper protocols and patient selection, their rate of major complications decreased from 22% to 12% (35). Minor complications have been described as those in which there is poor patient compliance, intolerance of the saline injections to fill the expander and alterations in the initial surgical plan secondary to incomplete coverage. Rates for minor complications vary from 17% to 40% (32,34). Several unique complications of tissue expansion have been noted such as calvarial erosion and traumatic extrusions (36,37).

B. Scalp Burns with Involvement of the Skull

Although soft tissue burns to the scalp represent significant challenges in acute management and subsequent reconstruction, burns that also involve the skull are not only life threatening problems but also present different challenges (38–41). Involvement of the outer table or deeper structures (Harrison III and IV injuries) is of particular concern. The method for closure of these defects varies depending on the cause of injury, the size of the defect, and the availability of healthy local tissue. Approaches for the correction of this problem include partial or complete debridement of the necrotic bone with immediate

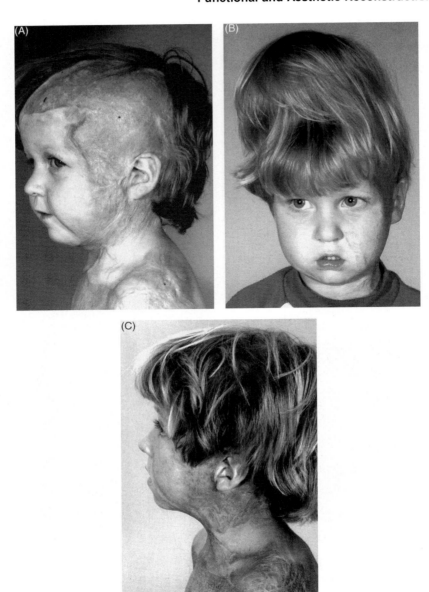

Figure 16.3 (A) Type 1C burn alopecia. (B) Complete inflation of a 800 cc tissue expander. (C) Three-year follow-up after correction of alopecia.

or delayed auto graft coverage (7,39–41). Other options include immediate coverage with vascularized tissue. These flaps may be random, axial patterned flaps on microvascular free flaps (42,43).

1. Acute Care/Early Reconstruction

In evaluation of 27 patients with Harrison III and IV calvarial burns by Spies et al. (7), ∼75% of these injuries were secondary to thermal wounds and 25% were electrical injuries. Patients with calvarial burn usually have injuries to other the parts of the body. The respective TBSA

burns were of 47% and 23%. These patients are resuscitated using the Galveston formula of 5000 plus 2000 mL/m^2 TBSA lactated ringers solution over the initial 24 h. Treatment of the burned skull involved debridement of the calvarial bone using a high-speed drill to remove necrotic bone (6). Once a viable surface is reached, STSG are used for resurfacing of the skull. However, if graft take is poor, resurfacing of the defect with vascularized tissue is indicated (Fig. 16.4). Alternatively, if intraoperative examination reveals Harrison IV calvarial defect with exposed dura, immediate coverage with vascularized flaps is indicated (Fig. 16.5). The use

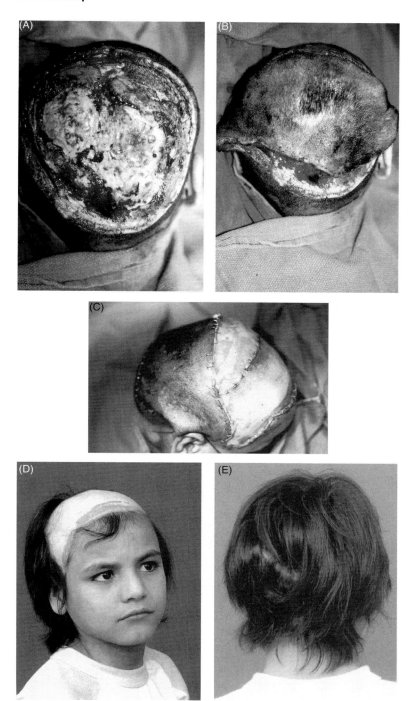

Figure 16.4 (A) Twelve-year-old male with Harrison III calvarial burn in the occipital region of the scalp. Unsuccessful graft take after debridement of outer table. Defect encompasses nearly 50% of the hair-bearing scalp. (B) Immediate mobilization of anterior scalp as a bipedicle visor flap for coverage of the defect. (C) Skin grafts placed over donor site of the flap anteriorly. (D) Six-month follow-up showing well-healed grafts anteriorly with preservation of hairline for future reconstruction. (E) Posterior view showing survival of the visor flap and subsequent hair growth.

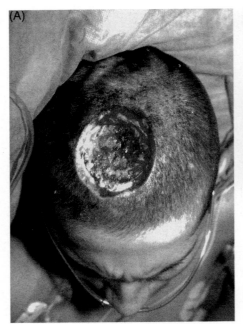
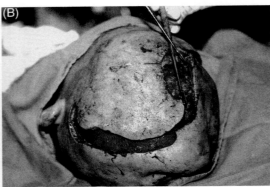
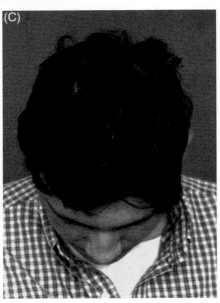

Figure 16.5 (A) Fifteen-year-old patient with a high-voltage electrical injury with 6 × 8 cm area of exposed but intact dura (Harrison IV burn). (B) Coverage with scalp rotation flap. (C) Stable coverage at 6 months after closure. [Reprinted with permission from Spies et al. (7).]

of tissue substitutes such as Alloderm® has also been reported to be successful in the management of Harrison IV calvarial defects (44). However, this is not routine. Wound closure was achieved in all cases. In the majority of patients, 23/27 (85%) wound closure was achieved with autografts. However, long-term follow-up revealed calvarial defects in 30% of these children. Involvement

of the calvarium tends to occur more often in electrical burns, although the defects tend to be smaller (7,45).

Principles in the delayed management of calvarial defects are straightforward. Stable soft tissue coverage of the scalp must be achieved prior to reconstuction of calvarial defects. Habal (2) believes that calvarial defects <2 cm in children will undergo osteoneogenesis and closure. Large defects or those in adults may require vascularized coverage prior to reconstruction with calvarial bone grafts.

IV. CONCLUSION

The management of patients with scalp burns is complex. Patients are divided into two groups: those with scalp burns only and those with involvement of the skull. Needless to say, management issues within these groups differ significantly. Subsequent reconstructive options are also different. The closure of scalp defects without calvarial involvement can be a less challenging issue. Small defects are closed primarily or with the use of micrografts. However, large segments of alopecia are addressed with tissue expansion, micrografts, or a combination of local flaps combined with these procedures. Although scalp expansion complications rates can be 15–20%, the results are uniformly successful and aesthetically pleasing. Alternatively, defects of the scalp with calvarial involvement are most challenging both in acute phase of injury and in subsequent reconstruction. Acutely, protection of the brain is of paramount importance. Wound closure can be obtained in all patients. However, even with successful wound closure, follow-up of these patients is crucial to determine subsequent development of full-thickness calvarial defects.

REFERENCES

1. Harrison SH. Exposure of the skull from burns. Br Plast Surg 1952; 4:279–292.
2. Habal M. Burns of the skull and scalp and their clinical management. In: McCauley RL, ed. Functional and Aesthetic Reconstruction of the Burn Patient. New York: Marcel Dekker, 2005.
3. Brou JA, Vu T, McCauley RL, Herndon DN, Desai MH, Rutan RL, Stenberg B, Phillips LG, Robson MC. The scalp as a donor site: revisited. J Trauma 1990; 30(5):579–581.
4. Burns BF, McCauley RL, Murphy FL, Robson MC. Reconstructive management of patients with >80% TBSA burns. Burns 1993; 19(5):429–433.
5. Barret JP, Dziewulski P, Wolf SE, Desai MH, Herndon DN. Outcome of scalp donor sites in 450 consecutive pediatric burn patients. Plast Reconstr Surg 1999; 103:1139–1142.
6. Vallis CP. Surgical management of cicatricial alopecia of the scalp. Clin Plast Surg 1982; 178–186.
7. Spies M, McCauley RL, Mudge BP, Herndon DN. Management of acute calvarial burns in children. J Trauma 2003; 54(4):765–769.
8. Worthen EF. Regenerations of the skull following a deep electrical burn. Plast Reconstr Surg 1971; 48:1–4.
9. Huang TT, Larson DL, Lewis SR. Burn alopecia. Plast Reconstr Surg 1977; 60:763–767.
10. Orticochea M. Four flap scalp reconstruction technique. Br J Plast Surg 1967; 20:159–171.
11. Orticochea M. New three flap scalp reconstructive technique. Br J Plast Surg 1971; 24:184–188.
12. Manders EK, Schendou MJ, Fussey JA, Helzler PT, Davis TS, Graham WP. Soft tissue expansion: concepts and complications. Plast Reconstr Surg 1984; 74:493–504.
13. Juri J. Use of parieto-occipital flaps in the surgical treatment of baldness. Plast Reconstr Surg 1975; 55:456.
14. Feldman G. Post-thermal burn alopecia and its treatment using extensive horizontal reduction in combination with a Juri flap. Plast Reconstr Surg 1994; 93:1268–1273.
15. Juri J, Juri C, Arufe HN. Use of rotation scalp flaps for the treatment of occipital baldness. Br J Plast Surg 1978; 61:23.
16. Elliot RA. Lateral scalp flaps for instant results in male patterned baldness. Plast Reconstr Surg 1977; 60:669.
17. Barrera A. The use of micrografts and minigrafts for the treatment of burn alopecia. Plast Reconstr Surg 1989; 103:581–589.
18. McCauley RL. Correction of burn alopecia. In: Herndon DN, ed. Total Burn Care. Philadelphia: W.B. Saunders, 1996:499–502.
19. Takei T, Mills I, Arai K, Sumpio BE. Molecular basis for tissue expansion: clinical implications for surgeons. Plast Reconstr Surg 1998; 102:247–258.
20. Neumann CG. The expansion of an area of skin by progressive distention of a subcutaneous balloon. Plast Reconstr Surg 1957; 19:124.
21. Cherry GW, Austed ED, Pasyk KA, McClatchey KD, Rorich RJ. Increased survival and vascularity of random pattern skin laps elevated in controlled, expanded skin. Plast Reconstr Surg 1982; 72:680–685.
22. Sasaki GH, Plang CY. Pathophysiology of skin flaps raised on expanded skin. Plast Reconstr Surg 1984; 79:59–65.
23. Lantieri LA, Martin-Garcia N, Wechsler J, Mitrofanoff M, Raulo Y, Bauch. Vascular endothelial growth factor expression in expanded tissue: a possible mechanism of angiogenesis in tissue expansion. Plast Reconstr Surg 1998; 101:392–398.
24. Pasyk KA, Argenta LC, Hasseh C. Quantitative analysis of the thickness of human skin and subcutaneous tissue following controlled expansion with a silicone implant. Plast Reconstr Surg 1988; 81:516.
25. Pasyk KA, Argenta LC, Austed ED. Histopathology of human expanded tissue. Clin Plast Surg 1987; 14:435–445.
26. Radavan C. Tissue expansion in soft tissue reconstruction. Plast Reconstr Surg 1984; 74:491.
27. Austed ED, Pasyk KA, McClatchey KD, Cherry GW. Histomorphometric evaluation of guinea pig skin and soft tissue after controlled tissue expansion. Plast Reconstr Surg 1982; 70:704–710.
28. Neale HW, High RM, Billmire DA, Carey JP, Smith D, Warden G. Complications of controlled tissue expansion in the pediatric burn patient. Plast Reconstr Surg 1988; 82:840–845.
29. McCauley RL, Oliphant JR, Robson MC. Tissue expansion in the correction of burn alopecia: classification and methods of correction. Ann Plast Surg 1990; 25:103–115.

30. Sasaki GH. Intraoperative sustained limited expansion (ISLE) as an intermediate reconstructive technique. Clin Plast Surg 1987; 14:563–571.

31. Goldstein RD, Schuler SH. Methylene blue: a simple adjunct to aid in soft tissue expansion. Plast Reconstr Surg 1986; 180:4522.

32. Manders EK, Schenden MJ, Furrey JA, Hetzler PT, Davis TS, Graham WP III. Soft tissue expansions concepts and complications. Plast Reconstr Surg 1984; 74:493–504.

33. Manders ED, Graham WP, Schendon MT, Davis TS. Skin expansion to eliminate large scalp defects. Ann Plast Surg 1984; 12:305–312.

34. Neale HW, High RM, Billmire DA, Carey JP, Smith D, Warden G. Complications of controlled soft tissue expansion in the pediatric burn patient. Plast Reconstr Surg 1988; 82:840–845.

35. MacLennon SE, Corcoran JF, Neale HW. Tissue expansion in head and neck burn reconstruction. Clin Plast Surg 2000; 27:121–132.

36. Hemmer KM, Marsh JL, Picker S. Calvarial erosion after scalp expansion. Ann Plast Surg 1987; 19:454–459.

37. Ortega MT, McCauley RL, Robson MC. Salvage of an avulsed expanded scalp flap to correct burn alopecia. South Med J 1990; 83(3):220–223.

38. Bizhko IP, Slesarenko SV. Operative treatment of deep burns to the scalp and skull. Burns 1992; 18:220–223.

39. Norkess T, Klebanovas J, Viksrain et al. Deep electrical burns of the calvarium: early or delayed reconstruction. Burns 1992; 18:220–223.

40. Sheridan RL, Choucair RJ, Donelan MB. Management of massive calvarial exposure in young children. J Burn Care Rehab 1998; 19:29–32.

41. Srivastava JL, Biswas G, Narayon RP, Goel A. Chronically exposed calvarium after electrical burns. Burns 1993; 19:138–141.

42. Fried M, Rosenberg B, Techman I, Benhur N, Yardeni P, Sternberg N, Golan J. Electrical burn injury of the scalp: bone regrowth following applications of latissimus dorsi free flap to the area. Burns 1991; 17:338–339.

43. Silverberg B, Banis JC, Verdi GD, Acland RD. Microvascular reconstruction after electrical and deep thermal injury. J Trauma 1986; 26:128–134.

44. Barret JP, Dziewulski P, McCauley RL, Herndon DN, Desai MH. Dura reconstruction of the class IV calvarial burns with decellularized human dermis. Burns 1999; 25:459–462.

45. Luce EA. Electrical burns. Clin Plast Surg 2000; 37(1):133–144.

17

Burns of the Skull and Scalp and Their Clinical Management

MUTAZ B. HABAL

Tampa Bay Craniofacial Center, Tampa, Florida, USA

I. INTRODUCTION

Burns of the skull and the scalp represent a major challenge to the treating surgeon. Though such injuries are rare, representing only $\sim 1-6\%$ of cases in our practice and that of others (1), they are devastating both in the resulting patient trauma and disfigurement and in the sequela that may follow unsuccessful attempts to cover, heal, and reconstruct the exposed, injured cranium. Throughout medical history, injuries resulting in loss of scalp and damage to the underlying cranium have been reported, and various strategies for treatment have been used (2,3). In the past, the reconstructive dilemma was a product of the lack of available surgical strategies, materials, or tools to produce coverage for the exposed skull. The location of this injury presented a singular difficulty: the lack of tissue to vascularize either the underlying or the overlying structures of exposed, burned skull, and to cover damaged, bare cranial bone successfully with skin graft.

Treatment of cranial burn injuries has developed gradually through time, and its success has built upon an increasing understanding of the anatomy of the affected region and the innovations of practitioners who have sought methods to restore their patients to function and health. It is important to acknowledge and discuss here the ingenuity of our surgical forefathers in treating these wounds.

II. HISTORICAL PERSPECTIVE

Surgeons throughout the history of medicine have had to possess the ability to be both innovative and aggressive when faced with a clinical problem, yet not jeopardize the patient's care or well-being by such strategies. Any discussion of calvarial burns should include this historical prospective, which is of great value to all contemporary surgeons. The reality that the surgeon must improvise a treatment plan, yet not compromise its subject still exists today in the operating room.

The following story is referred to in the first edition of the J.M. Converse textbook, *Plastic and Reconstructive Surgery 2*. In 1777, at Camp Lady Ambler in Holsten, TN, Dr. Patrick Vance treated a victim of the Cherokee Indian conflict who had "nearly the whole of his head skinned" in an Indian attack (3). The unfortunate patient's skull was "quite naked, and began to turn black" (2,3). Dr. Vance instructed the military physician stationed at the fort, Dr. James Robertson, to bore holes in the patient's skull as it began to blacken, going only so deep as to see "a reddish fluid appear" (3). This would allow "the flesh . . . to rise in these holes," which were to be spaced about an inch apart (3). The surgical instrument of choice was an awl, which was able to penetrate the skull and could also be used to remove the black scales of dead bone as granulation tissue appeared. These burr holes produced, in time, a good bed of granulation tissue that stopped the desiccation of the skull and provided a slow (sometimes 4 years before the defect would completely "cure up"), but often successful, method of coverage that became widespread during the conflicts with the American Indian: "This operation became . . . so common that there were persons in every fort who performed it" (3). The technique was attributed to an unnamed "French surgeon." Dr. Vance's inspiration for this technique appears to have been Augustin Belloste, a Parisian surgeon born in 1654, who wrote in 1696 of treating scalp avulsion by this method, and had also used it to treat combat injuries (3). This "most unique procedure" was used and reported on by Sneve (4) 1888 in the treatment of a severe cranial burn.

Of historical note, this form of treatment for exposed and injured skull resulted in an early understanding of the use of autologous bone grafts. Those initial findings form the basis for the evolution of the bone grafting procedures that are available to us today in the repair and reconstruction of cranial defects (5). Their ultimate sophistication is the process used today in bone engineering for the reconstruction of skull defects: using the basic elements of stem cells, a scaffold, and a carrier, for enhancing factors that contribute to the formation of new bone *de novo*. Other historic landmarks in the treatment of scalp and skull burns follow the course of innovations in the treatment for scalp avulsion. These include various methods of skin grafting, initiated by Netolitsky's use of full-thickness grafts to cover denuded skull, and the development of skin flaps by Gould, Gillies and Kilner, New and Erich, and Cahill and Caulfield. For a more in-depth account of the historical treatment of scalp loss see Kazanjian and Webster's (6) venerable article on treatment of scalp loss.

III. ANATOMICAL PERSPECTIVES

The ultrastructure of the anatomy of the skull and its two engulfing fasciae is well described in previous publications (5–7). It is essential to have a clear understanding of the layers of the skull, since they represent an important anatomical and physiologic system of protection, coverage, and biologic function for the central nervous system.

The scalp is the hair-bearing component and a last evolutionary remnant for protection of the head from environmental factors such as heat, solar radiation, and cold temperatures. The upper circulation does not follow the countercurrent mechanisms of the other parts of the biologic system. The scalp is arterially supplied from its periphery by four major vessels: the paired occipital arteries and the paired temporal arteries. Other vessels traverse the scalp from three dimensions. Topographic vascular flow from the front of the scalp anteriorly and via the cranial sinuses has an important function in disease processes. When there is an internal obstruction, the circulation may use this dormant, vestigial system. In spite of such rich blood supply, in our practice we still occasionally see necrotic skull with compromised vascular supply (5).

The second layer is the galia aponeurotica, which is an anatomical aponeurosis that connects the frontalis to the occipitalis muscles in the scalp. This unit is anatomically poorly vascularized, but its vascularity is adequate enough to support skin graft (8). The space on top and underneath is almost avascular, though there are vessels crossing the space to enhance the vascular communication. That component is, however, marginal (8).

The next layer of the skull is the pericranium, the periosteum of the skull, which is loosely attached to the cortex of the outer table except at the suture lines of the skull. The pericranium is a thin layer of connective tissue that envelops the neurocranium. It is a vascular, dynamic layer containing fibrous elements, fibrous tissue, nerves, and a rich vascular network. This layer is similar to the periosteum of long bone. It has been viewed as a supplier of new blood vessels to the osteogenic cells in the underlying bone (5,7). A good portion of the inner layer has active fibroblasts, which are useful in the formation of new bone in children and in the remodeling of bones in adults. The sinus pericranii act as arterials or venules that convey a two-way traffic in and out of the skull. This is an important concept for the understanding of disease processes of the skull and for understanding the physiology of the flaps used for skull coverage (6,7).

The osseous skull itself is composed of two layers, with empty space between them. This space increases as a person reaches adulthood. The thickness of the bony layers is also age-dependent: the older the patient, the thicker the skull. The skull's thickness is also site-dependent: different anatomical sites have different measures of thickness. There are also ethnical variations: certain races seem to have different configurations, and it has been speculated that these were influenced by physical environment and evolution.

The inner portion of the skull cap is lined with the dura matter, which is also the engulfing fibrous tissue fascia of the brain. The dura is vascular and takes skin graft well (9). However, this menengial layer is devoid of lymphatics, so that tumors may spread along the dura mater but very rarely can go through it. This is another natural protective mechanism against disease and neoplasms (5). The layers that engulf the skull are important units that will be referred to during discussions of the pathophysiology and the treatment of the calvarial burns.

A. Pathophysiology of the Burned Skull

The skull, with its thick soft tissue protection, comprises a difficult anatomical structure to be burned directly. For this reason, skull burns represent only ~1–6% of all burns (1,9,10). The majority of patients with burned skulls, ~70%, can now be managed clinically with few life-threatening problems. That leaves the reconstructive surgeon with a small but critical number of patients who need the intensive management provided by a burn unit that we have available to us today. These patients will be the focus of my discussion on care for burned scalps and skulls.

The burns of the head almost invariably involve the scalp (9). As discussed earlier, the scalp has good, sensate reflexive reaction to pain: even an infant or youngster will withdraw from a painful thermal source. Unless a human being is in a neurological or other altered state of consciousness such as coma, the thermal injury will not traverse the bone. Although thermal burns may heat the bone, it will not cause the thermal necrosis that is seen in the dermal burns. The patient with a burn injury limited to the scalp will require the same care as other dermal burns. There is usually adequate tissue for transfer or expansion to the area, or there is adequate vascularity for free-tissue transfer such as a graft (11).

The other form of more focused thermal injury is that of electrical burns. The entry and exit points generate a much higher degree of thermal damage, in which all the tissue levels traversed by the currents will be necrotic or charred. The brain may be affected and will need to be monitored physiologically (9). The skull area affected will become dead bone, acting only as a scaffold that may or may not be able to withstand physiological and environmental factors, and survive. Dead bone survival has fascinated both clinicians and scientists. This severely compromised bone will usually regenerate to living bone in children, but is less likely to do so in adults (7). In these situations, grafts may not be feasible because of compromise to the blood supply. Therefore, adjacent tissue transfer, expansion, and free flaps may be the only alternative available for the production of soft tissue coverage for the skull (10–12).

We can thus summarily point out that the patient condition that caused the thermal injury to the usually well-protected cranium, as well as the density of penetration,

the length of exposure, and the intensity of temperature or current will be the determining factors for the final degree of destruction of the skull. In all these circumstances, the skull should be considered as a closed vault that has sustained injury. All the contents in the vault were operational before the injury, and should remain so after the management, treatment, and reconstruction of the vault itself. As surgeons, we may be called upon to improvise, but we must work never to compromise function. We should follow the principle that we do not create a deformity to correct another one.

B. Types of Skull Wounds

In order to understand management protocols for the patient with a burn injury of the skull, it is necessary to review the classification of cranial thermal wounds according to their extent and location on the skull (13).

Type I: Wounds limited to the scalp and galea aponeurotica.

Type II: Wounds in which the bone is devascularized and exposed after removal of charred soft tissue. The outer table is necrotic based on clinical exam. Dead bone could be limited to the first table of the skull.

Type IIA: Critical size that is exposed is <2 cm.

Type IIB: Critical size defect of the exposed skull is >2 cm.

Type III: The full thickness of the skull is necrotic and the dura is exposed after removing the soft tissue, the defect is >2 cm

Type IV: The thermal injury extends to the dura and the brain. Portions of these structures have to be removed and replaced by transferred tissues.

This simple classification will help with two components of the management of burns. First, this classification system will help the surgeon in the initial evaluation process of the patient and in the assessment of the extent of the injuries. Second, initial classification of the injury is valuable in the eventual charting and assessment of bone healing and its outcome, so that there is a standard of comparison to assess.

In our practice we find that it is critical to assess the size of the defect in order to predict the outcome of bone healing. Bone loss <2 cm usually heals very well by its own regenerative processes, especially in children under 12 years of age (12,14). The process of regeneration is strongest at age 6 years, slowing down through the next 6 years until the age of 12 years. In adults, bone regeneration is unpredictable. Regeneration is dependent on the environmental factors of the individual patient and on the patient's physical status and internal milieu (9).

The ability of dead bone to heal occupies a major place in the understanding of the bone healing processes, particularly in the skull. From the time that surgeons first learned strategies for the reconstruction of skull defects with cadaver or animal bone, the process of bone healing became more thoroughly understood. Clinicians now know that bone can survive even when it is not vascularized by merely acting as a scaffold and protecting the underlying structures (4,14,15). In some cases, it may regenerate. For dead bone to survive, the anatomical site must be clean of debris and not grossly contaminated. The injured soft tissue must be cleaned and dead tissue debrided promptly before septic conditions set in, and before the necrotic bone starts to flake, changing the wound into a grossly contaminated site. These conditions are most often seen in electrical burns, where the thermal components are of a high level (16). The extent of the thermal injury should be assessed and also the extent of involvement of other anatomic sites. All these factors influence the eventual outcome and the degree of treatment needed or used. Consideration of the patient as a whole must be stressed, rather than a separate anatomic focus on the injured calvarial bone. You must treat the patient as well as the injury.

C. Diagnostics

The standard diagnostic tests are all applicable but may not be helpful in diagnosing the extent of the viability of the bone and the degree of the injury. A bone scan may shed some light, but in the initial phase of the injury there may be thrombosis of the interosseous vessels, which will alter the finding of the scan. Regular radiographs of the skull can be used as a baseline, as can computer generated axial scans. An electroencephalogram should be done, and also a magnetic resonance scan. The data collected can assist later on with evaluation of the disposition of all the involved bones. A change to a "ground glass" appearance or a change to higher or lower density of the involved bone will help the clinician in directing the management plans for the patient.

D. Treatment Modalities

In the treatment of the burned skull we follow the basic principles of plastic surgery: first, provide coverage as soon as possible without any compromise to the adjacent tissue or to the biological system as a whole. The following treatment modalities are practiced with all thermal injuries and apply, as well, to the scalp and the cranial bones (9,12,14,16).

1. Immediate treatment of the patient while in the acute phase, which may include debridement and temporary coverage.

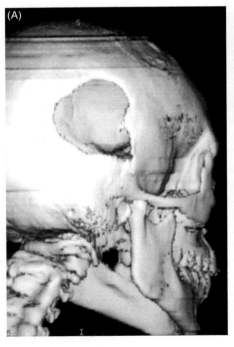 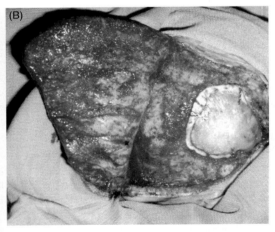

Figure 17.1   (A) Three-dimensional CAT scan of 17-year-old patient with a right sided parietal skull defect after an electrical burn to the scalp. (B) Intraoperative coverage using methylmethacrylate. (Reprinted with permission from McCauley RL, Barret JP. Electrical injuries. In: Erikson, ed. Plastic Surgery: Indications, Operations and Outcomes. St. Louis: Mosby, Inc., 2000:375–387.)

2. Delayed or elective treatment after the patient is stabilized, which may include permanent coverage in the form of grafts and flaps.
3. Reconstruction of the thermally injured defects to reconstitute the anatomical configurations.

Bone grafts and tissue expanders are used in reconstruction for patients in this and other stages of reconstruction.

These maneuvers have no limitation except the imagination of the operating surgeon and his team, and the ultimate well-being of the patient.

Skin grafting can include the use of three forms of grafts (8,9,16,17). Autografts are the most useful for temporary, as well as permanent, coverage. The major problem with these grafts is the limitation of supply, especially in extensively burned patients. The skin left for grafting may be limited and the surgeon may have to harvest the area more than one time. Such grafts should be taken as thin as possible to allow for good regeneration of the donor site. In smaller burns, that will not be a problem. However, the thinner the skin graft, the more scarring will be formed since the collagen bed in the dermis will be limited. The skull should have a blood supply from the pericranium or in the form of granulation tissue to allow for a good take of the skin graft. The other two types of grafts are allografts and xenografts. These are used only as temporary measures for coverage. These grafts will allow the healthy tissue bed below the burn to be covered early to preserve the underlying structures and prevent invasive infections in the wound (9,16).

The use of flaps is secondary in the immediate care for limited burns of the skull. In small-area electrical burns, adjacent tissue transfer in the form of full-thickness graft may be ideal as a primary procedure and as an immediate measure to cover the open site. The burned skull should be treated more aggressively to avoid any invasive infection with nosocomial bacteria into the underlying structures, since meningitis can be fatal in these situations. Meningitis can occur even in limited burns of the skull (9,14). Delayed treatment involves two components: the reconstruction of the bone and that of the soft tissue (5,12,14,16). Without stable soft tissue coverage, reconstruction of the bony defect cannot be done. Bone grafts will depend on the soft tissue for vascularization. Bone substitutes should not be used if there is any evidence of infection in the adjacent areas. Our preference is to use the calvarial reconstruction 6 months after all healing and only for protection of the adjacent central nervous system (Figs. 17.1 and 17.2).

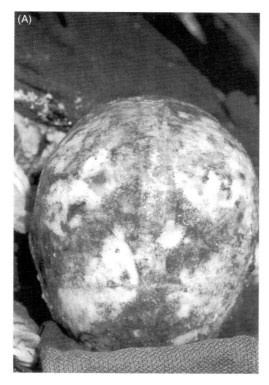
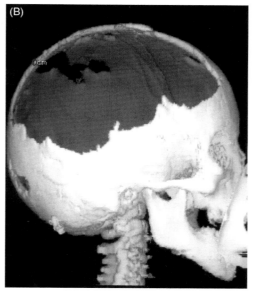

Figure 17.2 (A) Large thermal calvarial injury with debridement of the outer table and successful coverage with skin grafts. (B) Subsequent 3D CAT scan showing large calvarial defect. (Courtesy of R. L. McCauley.)

IV. CONCLUSION

Though rare, calvarial burns are devastating to the patient and sometime life-threatening. Through an understanding of the anatomy of the skull and scalp, and a clear, working knowledge of plastic surgery and burn care principals, the surgeon can do much to restore function, appearance, and health to the victims of these injuries.

REFERENCES

1. Spies M, McCauley RL, Mudge BP, Herndon DN. Management of acute aalvarial burns in children. J Trauma 2003; 54:765–769.
2. Converse JM. Plastic and Reconstructive Surgery. Vol. 2, 1st ed. Philadelphia: W.B. Saunders, 1964.
3. Strayer, LM. Augustin Belloste and the treatment of avulsions of the scalp. N Engl J Med 1939; 220:901–905.
4. Sneve H. Operation for re-covering the denuded cranium. Med News 1893; 62:239.
5. Habal MB, Reddi AH. Bone Graft and Bone Substitute. Philadelphia: W.B. Saunders, 1992:327–336.
6. Kazanjian VH, Webster RC. The treatment of extensive losses of the scalp. Plast Reconstr Surg 1946; 1:360–385.
7. Habal MB. Observations on the ultrastructure of the pericranium. Ann Plast Surg 1981; 6:6–7.
8. Molnar JA, DeFranzo AJ, Marks MW. Single-stage approach to skin grafting the exposed skull. Plast Reconstr Surg 2000; 105:174–177.
9. Barret JP, Dziewulski P, McCauley RL, Herndon DN, Desai MH. Dural reconstruction of a Class IV calvarial burn with decellularized human dermis. Burns 1999; 25:459–462.
10. Warrington SA, Wright CM, Team AS. Accidents and resulting injuries in premobile infants: data from the ALSPAC study. Arch Dis Child 85:104–107.
11. Bizhko IP, Sleszrenko SV. Operative treatment of deep burns to the scalp and skull. Burns 1992; 18:220–223.
12. Sheridan RL, Choucair RJ, Donelan MB. Management of massive calvarial exposure in young children. J Burn Care Rehabil 1998; 19:29–32.
13. Molnar JA, DeFranzo AJ, Marks MW. Single-stage approach to skin grafting the exposed skull. Plast Reconstr Surg 2000; 105(1):174–177.
14. Ioannides C, Fossion E, McGrouther AD. Reconstruction for large defects of the scalp and cranium. J Craniomaxillofac Surg 1999; 27:145–152.
15. Jackson D. Burns of bone: can these bones live? Burns 1993; 19:356–372.
16. Norkus T, Klebanovas J, Viksraitis S, Astrauskas T, Gelunas J, Rimkus R, Zobakas A. Deep electrical burns of the calvarium: early or delayed reconstruction? Burns 1998; 24:569–572.
17. Groenevelt F, van Trier AJ, Khouw YL. The use of allografts in the management of exposed calvarial electrical burn wounds of the skull. Ann NY Acad Sci 1999; 888:109–112.

18

Role of Micrografts and Minigrafts in Burn Reconstruction

ALFONSO BARRERA

Baylor College of Medicine, Houston, Texas, USA

I. ROLE OF MICROGRAFTS AND MINIGRAFTS IN BURN RECONSTRUCTION

Fujita from Japan first described the use of single-hair grafts to reconstruct the eyebrows in 1953 (1). This was the first mention of the use of micrografts since Tamura, also from Japan, reported transplanting single-hair grafts from the pubic area (2). It was another four decades before there was further experimentation with small grafts.

Various methods have been used for the treatment of burn alopecia, including scalp flaps, punch grafts, and tissue expansion. More recently, micrografts and minigrafts have been added to our armamentarium in burn reconstruction (3).

The idea of using micrografts and minigrafts to treat burn alopecia came to me after treating primarily patients with male pattern baldness; some of these patients had a bit of scarring from previous hair transplantation, I was impressed to see how they survived quite well on scar tissue, after seeing this I went on to try them on burn scar tissue and it worked; the technique is basically the same as that described for male pattern baldness (4–6).

Micrografts and minigrafts may be used to complement other reconstructive techniques to camouflage scars and cover areas of residual alopecia or as a sole technique of reconstruction. All techniques have advantages and disadvantages.

The main advantages that I see regarding the use of micrografts and minigrafts is the fact that with only one session a significant improvement occurs and after a second procedure a quite acceptable result is accomplished. It avoids altogether the worries about flaps ischemia, tip necrosis, or the possibility of tissue expander extrusion, with the added benefit of no expansion process. The disadvantages include the fact that the hair growth is not immediate, it takes 4–5 months to see an improvement, and about a year for the final result.

The fibrotic scar tissue that normally forms after burn injuries has a precarious blood supply and is not an optimal site for any type of graft. However, we have found that single- and double-hair follicular unit grafts (micrografts) and follicular unit grafts with three to four hairs (minigrafts), because of their small size, have a very low metabolic requirement, which allows them to survive in this hostile environment (Fig. 18.1).

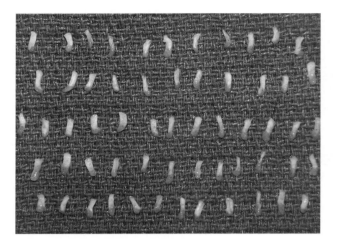

Figure 18.1 View of micro- and minigrafts ready for transplantation.

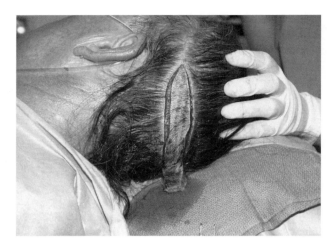

Figure 18.3 Donor site.

Transverse microscopic sections of the scalp show that hair grows in follicular units [Fig. 18.2(A) and 18.2(B)] this was demonstrated by Headington (7) in 1984. These follicular units are true physiological units and contain one, two, three, and up to four hairs, have their independent sebaceous glands, sweat glands, piloerector muscle, and neurovascular supply, being surrounded by a sheath of collagen. It is important to maintain the integrity of these units as much as possible. As long as we do not make grafts larger than a follicular unit, we avoid altogether the "plug look," the appearance of clumpiness.

Having seen these small grafts survive in patients with male pattern baldness who had scarred scalps from previous surgical procedures, I decided to try them in patients with burn alopecia. Their survival was better than expected. I believe that it is important to allow sufficient time for the scalp to heal, soften, and fully recover from

the insult of surgery or trauma before proceeding with hair transplantation in the case of burns I like to wait for a minimum of 6–8 months, ideally a year.

The procedure usually is performed in our office surgical suite after the patient is given a mild IV sedative and local anesthetic as described for the treatment of male pattern baldness; however, on the temporal or occipital areas, or in the case of restoring facial hair, there is a variation of technique as will be described later. On children the procedure is of course done under general anesthesia in the hospital.

It is not a matter of just getting the hair to grow, but getting it to look natural and aesthetically pleasing as well. We have learned that we can control to a significant degree the direction of hair growth from the grafts; this, of course, is a must. On the various areas of scalp, we should keep this in mind especially on the face (eyebrows, mustache, eyelashes).

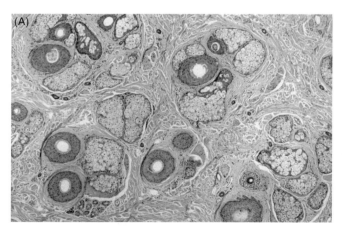

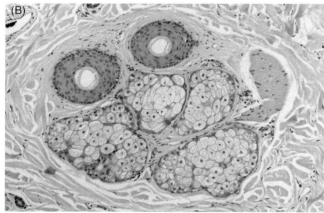

Figure 18.2 (A) Horizontal microscopic appearance of several follicular units. (B) Horizontal microscopic appearance of a two-hair follicular unit micrograft. Note the sebaceous glands, sweat glands, and piloerector muscle.

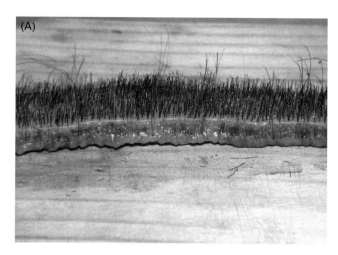
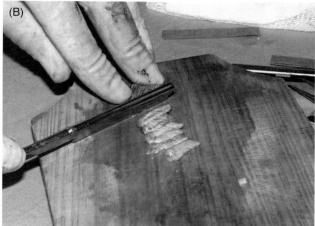

Figure 18.4 (A) View of donor ellipse. (B) Making 2 mm slices with a persona prep Blade on a Weck free graft blade handle.

A. Technique

1. Scalp Alopecia

With the patient under IV sedation in a supine position, a horizontal donor ellipse is harvested from the occipital area (Fig. 18.3). The patient's head is turned to the left for harvesting the right half of the donor ellipse (Fig. 18.4).

This piece of the ellipse is immediately dissected into 1.5–2.0 mm slivers by the surgeon and handed to the two assistants to prepare the micrografts and minigrafts. The surgeon then sutures the right half of the donor site and turns the patient's head to the right to repeat the process as two assistants dissect the grafts. As one harvests the donor ellipse the incisions are made precisely parallel to the hair follicles under 3.5 loupe magnification using a single blade (#10 Bard-Parker) (Fig. 18.5).

The donor site closure is done in a single layer with #3 "0" prolene (Fig. 18.6). The grafts are then transplanted by using a slit and insert technique as in the case of male pattern baldness without the need for dilators or punching out tissue at the recipient site (Fig. 18.7).

These slits are made in the front 5.0 mm of the hairline with a 22.5 sharpoint blade, and posterior to that with Feather #11 blades, then the grafts are inserted with jewelers forceps.

2. Facial Hair Loss

Fortunately, micrografts and minigrafts grow anywhere including the face and thus are useful for restoring the eyebrows, mustache, and beard. However, since the consistency of the skin is softer and more elastic than the scalp, the surgeon will encounter more problems with grafts popping out when transplanting these areas (facial areas) (Fig. 18.8).

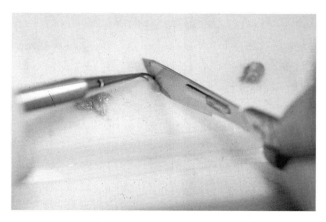

Figure 18.5 Micrografts dissection with a #10 Bard Parker blade.

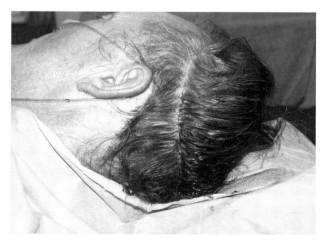

Figure 18.6 Donor site close with a 3 "0" Prolene simple running suture with a few interrupted ones.

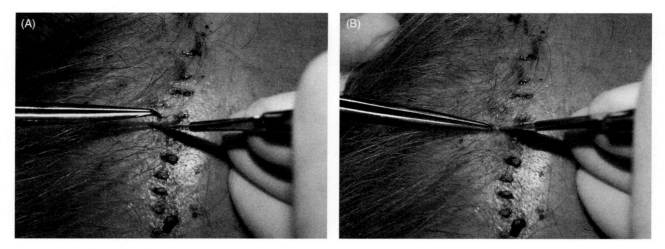

Figure 18.7   (A) Insertion of grafts; a slit is made into which the graft is then introduced. (B) The graft in position and being held in place by the tip of the blade as the jewelers forceps come out.

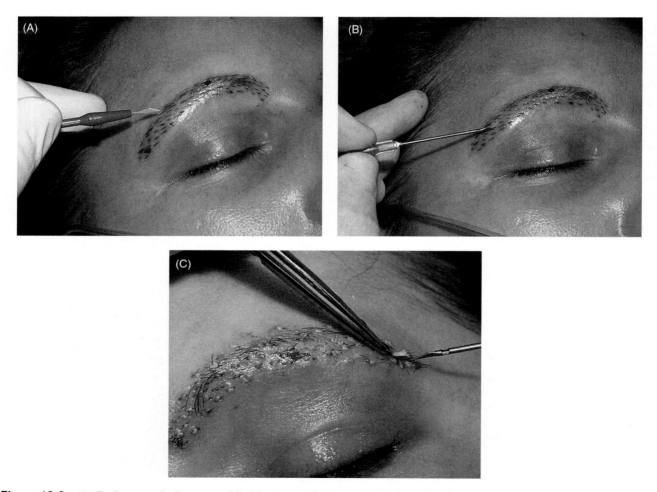

Figure 18.8   (A) Eyebrows and other areas of facial hair are a little more difficult, as there is a bit more popping out (of grafts) as they are being inserted. To minimize that problem, we may make the slits in a preliminary fashion and then insert the grafts. Here, we see the slits being made with a 22.5 Sharpoint. (B) Here, we see an 18-gauge NoKor needle which may be used alone instead of a 22.5 Sharpoint blade, or to dilate the slits made by the Sharpoint blade. (C) Eyebrow micrografts inserted, using the 18-gauge NoKor needle.

My experience in restoring the eyebrows, mustache, or beard has shown that it is best to make most or all of the slits initially and insert the grafts later to minimize this problem. In addition, the grafts can be packed more densely. The same combination of IV sedation and local anesthesia followed by tumescent infiltration is used as in scalp transplantation. However, I use 1:50,000 epinephrine to ensure optimal hemostasis. If the procedure is minor, local anesthesia alone may be used, if the patient prefers. In these cases the patient is sedated in the same manner as described for treatment of male pattern baldness.

For the eyebrows or mustache, a smaller donor strip is needed. Generally, the grafts are harvested from a small donor ellipse from the occipital area posterior to the mastoid prominence or horizontally from the midoccipital area as in male pattern baldness cases. The graft dissection is done as in cases of male pattern baldness.

The donor strip measures 3.0 × 0.5 cm depending on the donor density. A strip of this size strip will usually yield 100–120 micrografts. In the case of the eyebrows the slits are made with a No. 22.5 sharp point blade that is angled laterally and upward following the direction of the natural eyebrows. The only variable when transplanting mustaches is that the direction of the slits follows the natural direction of the hair growth, which is usually in a caudal direction. The slit and insert technique is employed using an 18-gauge NoKor needle which acts as a dilator.

For dressings, I generally use one or two layers of Adaptic, trimmed squares of 4 × 4 in. gauze, and 0.5 in.

SteriStrips or hypoallergic paper tape (Micropore). The hair transplanted to the face will have the characteristics of scalp hair and will thus need to be trimmed frequently. Axillary or pubic hair can also be used but they require a larger donor ellipse since these areas normally have less hair density.

II. CASE 1

A 56-year-old man with third-degree burns to the upper body including his face and scalp, due to a propane vapor explosion, had undergone multiple surgical procedures including skin grafts and scalp flaps bilaterally (Case 18.1). There was residual burn scalp alopecia at the middle. The area was very thin, fibrotic, and right over bone. The bilateral temporoparietal flaps were a bit low (anterior) and blunting to match the natural contour of a mature hairline. The plan was to do some 1500 micro- and minigrafts in the first session and then possibly another 800–1000 later to further increase the density and enhance the result. I suggested while at it, to resect part of those flaps to provide a slight fronto-temporal recession recycling the hair of those resections into micro- and minigrafts. The patient did not want to have fronto-temporal recessions, so that was not done.

The patient underwent a total of 2300 micro- and minigrafts in two sessions. Interestingly, the thin fibrotic area of the anterior scalp at the middle not only proved to be an acceptable recipient, it also gained thickness.

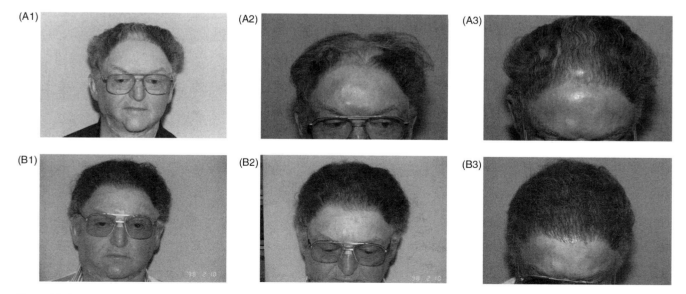

Case 18.1 A 56-year-old man with severe third-degree burns including the face and scalp. (A) Before and (B) 1 year after two mega sessions of micro- and minigrafts (total of 2300 grafts). See text for full description.

I believe that happened due to the fact that the follicular unit micro- and minigrafts have their adnexal appendices such as the sebaceous glands and sweat glands, which may well contribute along with the hair itself to add thickness to the recipient area of the scalp. It looks and feels healthier.

III. CASE 2

This was a 10-year-old boy from Saudi Arabia with severe third-degree burns on most of his body including the face and part of the scalp (Case 18.2). This patient sustained a large total body surface burn as a result of a housefire. Unfortunately, he has lost both lower extremities and the distal forearm of the right upper extremity. The only

hand he has is adversely disabled also. He had many surgical procedures back home where they did multiple scalp grafts (too thick) resulting in further alopecia and abnormal facial hair growth (at the grafted areas) and more recently has had additional work done here in the United States. He was referred to me to address primarily the eyebrows and scalp alopecia. Unfortunately, he has very limited donor hair and judging from the male pattern baldness his father has, and based on additional family history, he will very likely will lose most of what little hair he has on the top of his head. My plan was to restore the right eyebrow, the right anterior temporal hairline, which at the very least would help to frame his face, and some micro- and minigrafts if available on the top of the head to improve his appearance and self-esteem. One session of 705 micro- and minigrafts was performed. He is

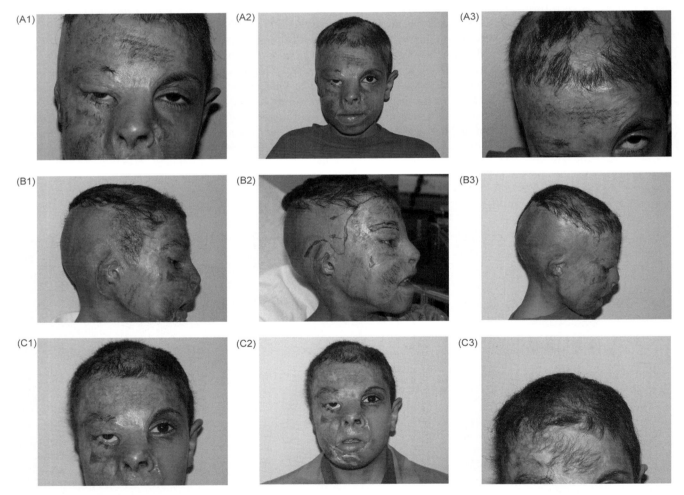

Case 18.2 A 10-year-old boy with severe third-degree burns to ∼90% body surface area. He had limited donor areas, the main objective was to restore the right eyebrow, right temporal hairline, and anterior top hairline. He received 705 grafts. (A) Before surgery, (B) surgical planning, and (C) after surgery. See text for full description.

scheduled for a second session of another 700 grafts ~1 year after the first procedure. I concentrated on the right eyebrow, anterior right temple, and anterior hairline on the top of the head (vertex).

IV.   CASE 3

A 10-year-old boy with residual scarring alopecia after multiple reconstructive procedures using tissue expanders, which were required after the removal of a large congenital lesion of the scalp and not a burn helps to illustrate how

we can deal with residual alopecia after tissue expansion reconstruction (Case 18.3). Additionally, this illustrates how we can also manage linear scars of the scalps that can result after scalp incisions, flaps, or scalp closures after expansion.

The photos shown are after only one session of 973 micro- and minigrafts. It was performed in my office surgical suite under IV sedation and local anesthesia; even though he is a kid, he was brave and cooperative, eliminating the need for general anesthesia normally needed in this age group. A year later, he underwent a second session of 923 grafts to further improve the

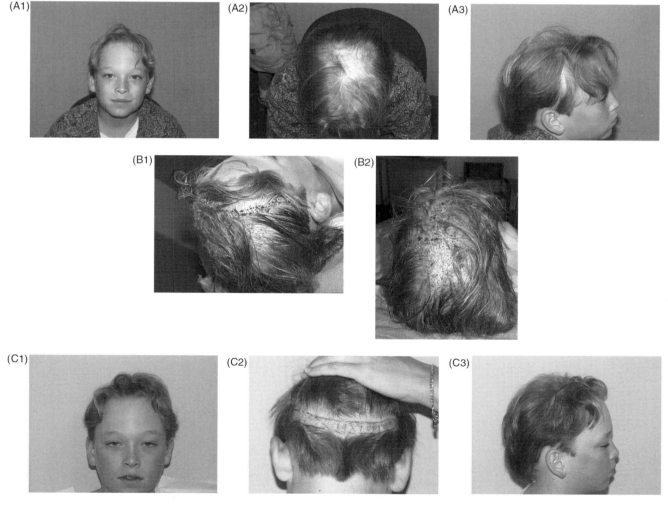

Case 18.3   A 10-year-old boy with residual scarring alopecia secondary to excision of a large congenital scalp skin; lesion and multiple reconstructive procedures using tissue expanders. This interesting case illustrates how in cases of tissue expansion reconstruction significant improvement can be accomplished with the use of micro- and minigrafts to correct such residual areas and hair loss along scalp scars. He had a single session of 973 micro- and minigrafts to the top of the head and right temporal scar. (A) Before surgery, (B) donor site, and (C) after surgery. See text for full description.

result. The photos of the latter were not available at the time of this publication (after the second session).

REFERENCES

1. Fujita K. Reconstruction of eyebrows. La Lepro 1953; 22:364.
2. Tamura H. Pubic hair transplantation. Jpn J Dermatol 1943; 53:76.
3. Barrera A. The use of micrographs and minigrafts for the treatment of burn alopecia. Plast Reconstr Surg 1999; 103:581–584.
4. Barrera A. Micrograft and minigraft megasession hair transplantation: review of 100 consecutive cases. Aesthetic Surg J 1997; 17(3):165–169.
5. Barrera A. Micrograft and minigraft megasession hair transplantation results after a single session. Plast Reconstr Surg 1997; 100(6):1524–1530.
6. Barrera A. Refinements in hair transplantation: micro and minigraft megasession. Perspect Plast Surg 1998; 11(1):53–70.
7. Headington JT. Transverse microscopic anatomy of the human scalp. Arch Dermatol 1984; 120:449.

19

Reconstruction of Burned Eyelids

BRIAN WONG
University of Texas Medical Branch, Galveston, Texas, USA

ROBERT L. McCAULEY
University of Texas Medical Branch and Shriners Hospital for Children—Galveston Unit, Galveston, Texas, USA

I. INTRODUCTION

The face is frequently involved in burn injury. Estimates range from 10% to 22% (1–4). It is estimated that injuries to the eyelid vary from 15% to 67% (5,6). Flame and flash burns appear to be the most common cause of eyelid burns. However, acid and alkali burns are occasionally noted. It is believed that 5–20% of all industrial eye injuries are caused by chemical irritants (7). Acid burns usually are self-limiting whereas alkaline burns can cause extensive tissue damage. Complications associated with chemical burns include destruction of the cornea as well as symblepharon and epithelial and/or stromal ulceration. Adhesions to the conjunctiva can be prevented by mechanical disruption of the adhesions using a specially made glass rod on a daily basis (8,9).

Thermal burns to the eyelids and the resultant injuries are usually superficial. However, full-thickness eyelid injuries are associated with high complication rates such as corneal ulcerations, exposure keratitis, and conjunctivitis (3). Here, aggressive treatment is warranted in order to decrease the incidence of subsequent complications (3,8). Release of eyelid burns with or without a tarsorrhaphy remains controversial. Corneal protection, however it is achieved, is of paramount importance. Regardless of the depth of injury corneal exposure and subsequent blindness must not occur.

Although an in-depth review of corneal injuries is not the focus of this chapter, they deserve to be mentioned. Burns to the cornea are quite unusual. Because of the rapid blink reflex and Bell's phenomenon, these injuries are usually not seen (7,8). Yet there have been reports of contact thermal injuries to the cornea from a number of unusual sources (8,10,11). Most such injuries are superficial and rarely involve the corneal epithelium. In other countries such injuries may be more common. The offending agent is usually boiling fluids. In 89% of these cases, the injuries are usually limited to the corneal epithelium. Debridement of the epithelium, antibiotic ointment, and patching resolves the problem in 80% of the cases (12).

II. ANATOMY

Placement of skin grafts is the primary treatment for eyelid burns as it is for other parts of the body in patients with large total body surface area (TBSA) burns. However, understanding the nuances of eyelid anatomy is of the utmost importance to restore the proper function of the eyelids, as well as to optimize their cosmesis. Special consideration is required in preparing eyelid recipient sites and in placement of the skin grafts. For example, to prevent persistent or recurrent cicatricial lid retraction, the depth of the burn will determine the surgical dissection plane. Damage to structures in the eyelid margin (eyelashes, meibomian glands, mucocutaneous margin) will also complicate eyelid reconstruction. Attention to the nasolacrimal system, especially the punctum, canaliculus, and nasolacrimal sac, must be emphasized since early identification and treatment may avert more invasive procedures in the future.

A. Eyelid Margin

There are four important landmarks in the eyelid margin, which are the same in the upper and lower eyelids. Beginning posterior (near globe) to anterior, the mucocutaneous margin is first, followed by the meibomian gland orifices, gray line, and lash line. The mucocutaneous margin marks the end of the nonkeratinized conjunctiva epithelium and the beginning of the keratinized eyelid epithelium. The meibomian gland orifices number approximately 40 in the upper lid and 20 in the lower lid. The gray line is the end of the pretarsal orbicularis oculi muscle, called the muscle of Riolan. Three or four rows of upper lid eyelashes and one or two rows of lower lid eyelashes

emanate approximately where the eyelid skin turns 90° from horizontal to vertical. The cilia begin just lateral to the puncta and end at the lateral canthus (Fig. 19.1) (13).

Burns of the eyelid margin may cause significant irritation of the eye. Kalish et al. (9) reported scorched eyelash particles falling into the conjunctival fornix causing a foreign body sensation. To help prevent ocular discomfort, they recommend trimming burned eyelashes.

If a significant number of meibomian orifices are scarred, then the lipid layer of the tear film may be reduced enough to cause dry eye. The lipid layer functions to help reduce evaporation of the tears from the cornea. Lubrication of the eye may require artificial tear drops and ointments.

Metaplastic skin changes causing keratinization at the mucocutaneous junction will cause ocular irritation. Keratin acts as an abrasive against the cornea, resulting in epithelial breakdown. Excision of the abnormally keratinized tissue is indicated with replacement by conjunctival autograft, amniotic membrane, or oral mucous membrane. If a donor site is available, the authors prefer using conjunctival autograft as this tissue more exactly replaces the tissue which was altered or lost.

1. Eyelid

The eyelids serve as the primary coverage for the eyeball and disperse the tear film over the cornea. If retracted from cicatricial changes due to a burn injury, proper anatomical reconstruction is imperative to protect the globe from the risk of exposure keratopathy.

In the primary open position, the upper eyelid margin rests 2 mm below the superior limbus. Its peak is just

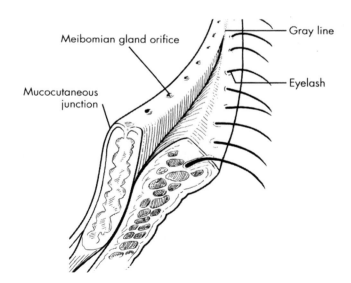

Figure 19.1 From posterior (near globe) to anterior, the eyelid margin landmarkers are the mucocutaneous junction, the meibomian gland orifices, the gray line, and the eyelashes. [Reprinted with permission from Nerad (13).]

nasal to the center of the pupil. The lower eyelid margin rests at the border of the inferior limbus. Its lowest point is below the lateral limbus. The vertical lid fissure is 9–10 mm measured from upper to lower mucocutaneous margins. The horizontal lid fissure is 30 mm with the lateral canthus slightly higher than the medial canthus. The structure which gives the eyelid its structural support is the tarsus. The upper and lower tarsi are made up of dense fibrous connective tissue measuring 10 and 4 mm in height, respectively. The tarsi are 25 mm in length and 1 mm thick. A floppy eyelid, which may roll out or in, will occur without a normal tarsus. Therefore, it must be reconstructed with an appropriate tissue substitute if damaged by burns. The meibomian glands lie vertically within the tarsus. The superior margin of the upper tarsus is a useful landmark to help differentiate between the upper and lower halves of the eyelid. Below the superior margin, beginning anterior to posterior, is the skin, pretarsal orbicularis oculi muscle, levator aponeurosis, tarsus, and conjunctiva. Above the superior margin and below the orbital rim is the skin, preseptal orbicularis oculi muscle, orbital septum, preaponeurotic fat, levator aponeurosis, Muller's muscle, and conjunctiva (Fig. 19.2) (14).

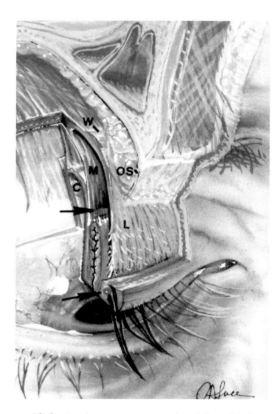

Figure 19.2 L: levator aponeurosis; OS: orbital septum; W: superior transverse ligament of Whitnall; M: Muller's muscle; C: conjunctive; upper arrow: peripheral arterial arcade. [Reprinted with permission from Zide and Jelks (14).]

Burns of the upper eyelid causing cicatricial ectropion may be the most damaging to the eye. Even with an excellent Bell's phenomenon, the retracted upper eyelid may not cover the eye well enough to prevent exposure keratopathy. Bell's phenomenon is the upward movement of the globe with eyelid closure. It serves as a protective mechanism for the cornea in cases of incomplete closure of the upper eyelid or lagophthalmos.

2. Skin

The horizontal eyelid crease of the upper eyelid is usually 7–8 mm in men and 9–10 mm in women. The crease is formed by attachment of the levator aponeurosis fibers into the orbicularis oculi and skin below its fusion with the orbital septum. An eyelid fold overhanging the crease is seen because the skin above the crease is only loosely attached to the underlying tissue, whereas skin below the crease is more adherent to the deeper tissue (15).

3. Orbicularis Oculi Muscles (Eyelid Protractors)

The orbicularis oculi muscles are the protractors of the eyelid and serve to close the eyelids. The orbicularis muscles are divided into three divisions: orbital, preseptal, and pretarsal (Fig. 19.3) (14). The orbital orbicularis oculi muscle extends from the eyebrow superiorly, temple

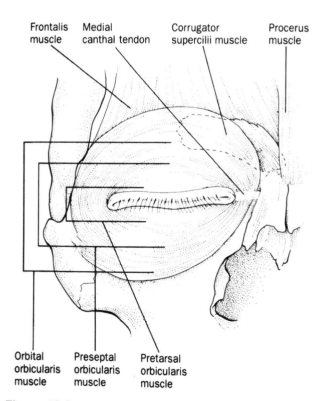

Figure 19.3 The orbicularis oculi muscles. [Reprinted with permission from Zide and Jelks (14).]

laterally, cheek inferiorly, and nose medially. The preseptal orbicularis oculi muscle covers the orbital septum. Medially, there is a deep head, Jones' muscle, which attaches to lacrimal sac fascia and a superficial head attached to the anterior medial canthal tendon. Laterally, the muscle covers the lateral canthal tendon and lateral orbital rim. The pretarsal orbicularis oculi muscle covers the tarsal plates. Medially, a deep head, Horner's muscle, helps form the posterior crus of the medial canthal tendon and attaches to the posterior lacrimal crest. The superficial head overlies the canaliculus and becomes part of the anterior crus of the medial canthal tendon (Fig. 19.4) (15).

4. Orbital Septum

A dense white connective tissue layer separates the eyelids from the orbit, called the orbital septum. In the upper eyelid, the orbital septum originates from the orbital rim at the arcus marginalis, a thickening of the periosteum, and then fuses with the levator aponeurosis near, but above the superior tarsal border (Fig. 19.5) (14). Medially, the septum attaches to the anterior and posterior lacrimal crests. Laterally, the septum travels anterior to the lacrimal gland and Whitnall's tubercle. In the lower eyelid, there is also the attachment at the orbital rim's arcus marginalis with extension to the inferior tarsal border (Fig. 19.6) (6).

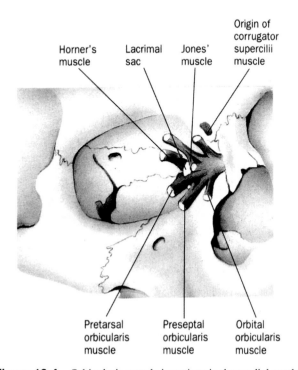

Figure 19.4 Orbicularis muscle insertions in the medial canthal area. [Reprinted with permission from Jordan and Anderson (15).]

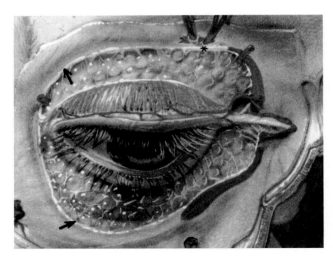

Figure 19.5 The orbital septum is a dense white connective tissue layer separating the eyelids from the orbit. Arrows: arcus marginalis. [Reprinted with permission from Zide and Jelks (14).]

Making a prominent eyelid crease is not an objective in Asians. Asian upper eyelids usually have a lower, more poorly formed eyelid crease. The orbital septum inserts lower down the levator aponeurosis preventing fibers from attaching to the subcutaneous tissue. A fuller upper eyelid is present since preaponeurotic fat is able to migrate further down the eyelid [Fig. 19.7(A–C)] (15).

5. Orbital or Preaponeurotic Fat

Posterior to the orbital septum is the orbital or preaponeurotic fat. In the upper lid, there are two preaponeurotic fat pads, a whiter medial pad and a more yellow central pad. The central fat pad often extends laterally and may be confused with the orbital lobe of the lacrimal gland. The lacrimal gland can be differentiated from fat by its pseudoencapsulated, firm white, cobblestone appearance (Fig. 19.8) (14). The lower lid has three fat pads including the whiter medial pad with the more yellow central and lateral pads. The medial and central fat pads are separated by the inferior oblique muscle (Fig. 19.9) (14).

6. Eyelid Retractors

The retractors of the upper and lower eyelids are found underneath the preaponeurotic fat and serve to open the eyelids. The elevators of the upper eyelid are the levator palpebrae superioris and Muller's muscles. The excursion of the upper lid from down gaze to up gaze is about 15–17 mm, mostly due to the levator muscle, with 2 mm coming from Muller's muscle (Fig. 19.10) (13). The levator muscle proceeds anteriorly from the orbital apex, inferior to the orbital roof, toward the superior

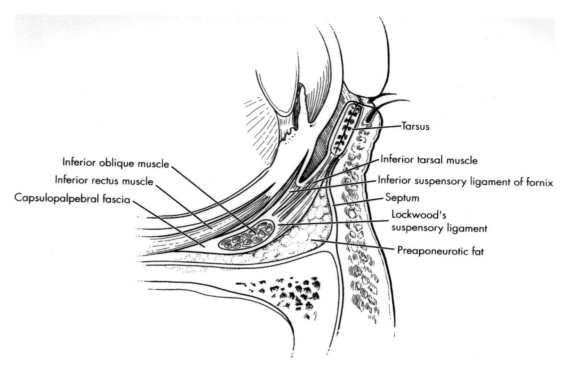

Figure 19.6 Lower eyelids orbital septum from orbital rim to the inferior tarsal border. [Reprinted with permission from Stern et al. (6).]

orbital rim. Whitnall's ligament or superior transverse ligament supports the levator muscle at the orbital aperture. This ligament is a glistening white fascial condensation that runs horizontally just below the rim. It extends from the trochlea medially to the lacrimal gland fascia temporally. The levator becomes a fibrous aponeurosis as it travels anterior to Whitnall's ligament and then inferiorly to insert on the anterior lower 7–8 mm of the tarsal plate. Whitnall's ligament acts as a pulley or fulcrum that helps change the levator muscle's direction from anterioposterior to superoinferior (Fig. 19.11) (14). Innervated by sympathetic nerves, Muller's muscle lies between the conjunctiva posteriorly and levator aponeurosis anteriorly. Muller's muscle travels from the level of Whitnall's ligament to insert on the superior margin of the upper tarsus (Fig. 19.12) (14).

Comparable to the upper eyelid, the lower eyelid also has two retractors, although much less mobile. This is because the lower lid equivalent to the levator muscle does not have a muscular component, but is only a fibrous band called the capsulopalpebral fascia. The fascia begins from the inferior rectus, splitting to surround the inferior oblique. The fascia reunites anterior to the inferior oblique forming Lockwood's suspensory ligament. Lockwood's ligament is equivalent to Whitnall's ligament of the upper lid. It helps to support the globe

and orbital structures (Fig. 19.13) (14). The capsulopalpebral fascia continues superiorly to insert at or near the inferior border of the tarsus (Fig. 19.14) (16). The lower eyelid equivalent to Muller's muscle is the inferior tarsal muscle. This poorly formed sympathetic muscle extends from Lockwood's ligament to the inferior tarsus between capsulopalpebral fascia anteriorly and conjunctiva posteriorly (14).

B. Special Considerations in Eyelid Burn Management

Dividing the eyelid into an anterior lamella (skin, orbicularis muscle), middle lamella (orbital septum), and posterior lamella (tarsus, conjunctiva) is helpful for reconstructive purposes (Fig. 19.15) (13). Anterior lamella may be replaced with myocutaneous flaps or full-thickness skin grafts to alleviate lid retraction and lagophthalmos. When reconstructing burned surfaces, attention must be made to support vascular graft and substitutes with a sufficient blood supply. Contraction and necrosis of reconstructed tissue is amplified in the eyelid area due to its importance for eye protection.

If a large area of upper eyelid skin is burned both above and below the eyelid crease, then two separate skin grafts may be placed to re-form the crease. The inferior edge of

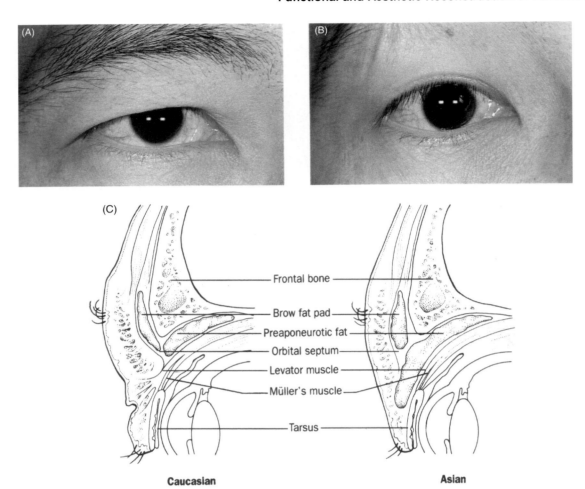

Figure 19.7 (A) Asian full upper eyelid. (B) Asian poorly formed eyelid crease. (C) In Asians, the preaponeurotic migrates further down the upper eyelid leading to a fuller upper eyelid and poorly formed eyelid crease. [Reprinted with permission from Jordan and Anderson (15).]

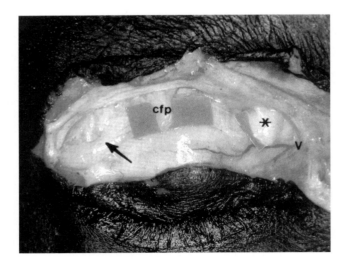

Figure 19.8 Upper-eyelid orbital fat. * indicates Whitish medial fat pad; cfp: central fat pad; arrow: extension of central fat pad to lateral upper lid. [Reprinted with permission from Zide and Jelks (14).]

the upper graft and the superior edge of the lower graft should meet at the eyelid crease. To re-create a prominent eyelid crease, the suture that attaches the skin graft to the recipient site should be placed at the superior margin of the tarsus. If a softer crease is wanted, then suturing the skin graft edges to more superficial subcutaneous tissue is needed.

A burn which penetrates deeper than the orbicularis oculi muscle to the orbital septum will further tether the eyelid open and prevent complete closure of the upper eyelid. This occurs because of the connection of orbital septum from the arcus marginalis at the superior orbital rim to the levator aponeurosis just above the superior tarsal border. Therefore, sharp dissection of this tissue plane will also be required to release the upper eyelid retraction.

To differentiate between involvement of just the skin/orbicularis complex vs. a deeper burn also scarring the orbital septum, a forced upward traction test should be performed. For lower lid reconstruction, the patient looks

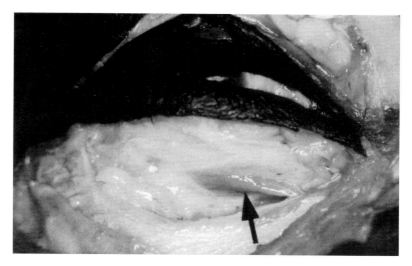

Figure 19.9   The inferior oblique muscle (arrow) separates the medial and central lower lid fat pads. [Reprinted with permission from Zide and Jelks (14).]

up while the examiner pushes the cheek and lower lid up to determine if the lower lid can be raised. For upper lid retraction, the patient looks down while the brow is depressed watching for upper lid closure. If the surgeon is able to elevate the lower lid or depress the upper lid, then only the anterior lamella is shortened. If the surgeon is unsuccessful, the middle lamella has also been involved and release of this tissue plane is required to alleviate the lid retraction.

If a burn injury extends down to tarsus or through orbital septum, blepharoptosis is possible from damage to the levator aponeurosis and muscle. Acutely, ptosis

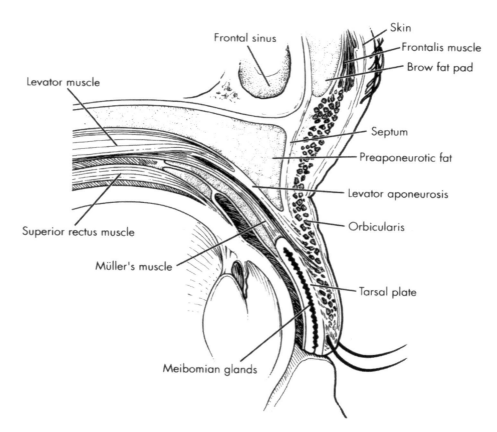

Figure 19.10   Upper-eyelid retractors: levator palpebrae superioris and Muller's muscles. [Reprinted with permission from Nerad (13).]

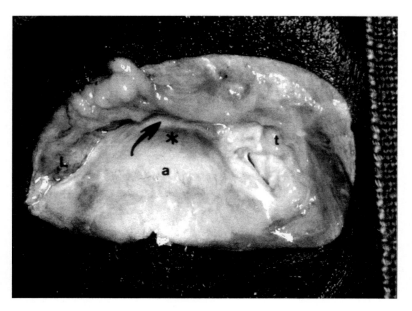

Figure 19.11   The orbital septum and preaponeurotic fat have been lifted to expose Whitnall's ligament (arrow) above the levator muscle (∗) and its aponeurosis (a). [Reprinted with permission from Zide and Jelks (14).]

is not a problem due to cicatricial lid retraction. After anterior lamella reconstruction is performed, ptosis may then present itself. Reattaching levator muscle to the tarsus will elevate the upper eyelid but care must be taken due to decreased orbicularis function. Under-correction of the ptosis repair may be necessary to prevent exposure keratopathy, due to decreased blink and lagophthalmos.

If the burn injury involves the full thickness of the eyelid, a tarsal and conjunctival graft, flap, or substitute will be needed to replace the lost posterior lamella. Without the firm support structure and nonkeratinized epithelial surface, the eyelids cannot function to protect the globe.

1.   Canthal Tendons

The lateral canthal tendon is a connective tissue band extending from the tarsal plate. Pretarsal orbicularis muscle from the upper and lower lid helps form the superior and inferior crus of the lateral canthal tendon.

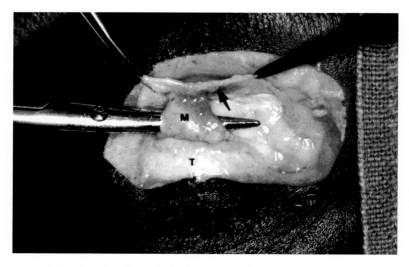

Figure 19.12   Muller's muscle (M) is found underneath the levator muscle (arrow) and inserts onto the superior border of the tarsus (T). [Reprinted with permission from Zide and Jelks (14).]

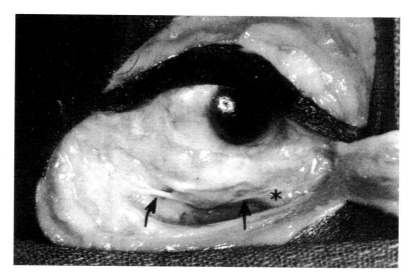

Figure 19.13 Arrows: Lockwood's suspensory ligament. (∗) Indicates inferior oblique muscle. [Reprinted with permission from Zide and Jelks (14).]

The tendon inserts onto Whitnall's or lateral orbital tubercle a few millimeters above the medial canthal tendon and 5 mm behind the orbital rim (Fig. 19.16) (13). A slight upward slant from the medial canthal tendon toward the lateral canthal tendon must be preserved to keep a normal "mongoloid slant" (Fig. 19.17) (13).

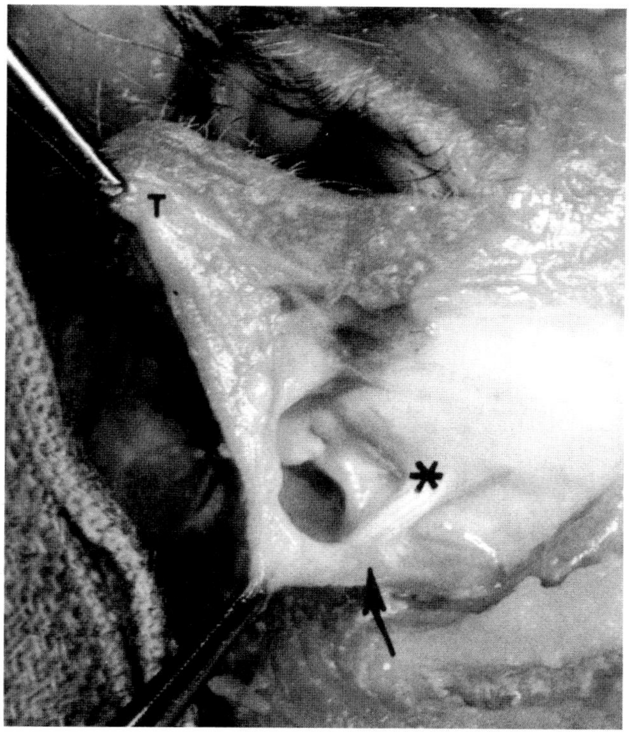

Pretarsal and preseptal orbicularis oculi muscles contribute to the medial canthal tendon, which has a superficial and deep head. The superficial head passes anterior to the lacrimal sac and attaches to the anterior lacrimal crest and frontal process of the maxilla. The deep head passes posterior to the lacrimal sac and inserts onto the posterior lacrimal crest of the lacrimal bone (Fig. 19.18) (13). Horner's muscle, a medial extension of

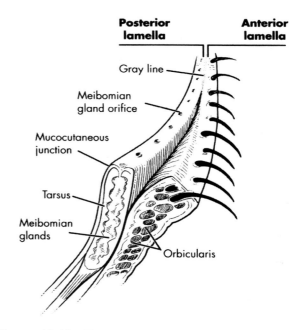

Figure 19.14 The capsulopalpebral fascia, grasped by the forceps, comes off the inferior rectus muscle (arrow) and inserts onto the inferior border of the lower lid tarsus (T). [Reprinted with permission from Victor and Hurwitz (16).]

Figure 19.15 The anterior and posterior lamellae of the eyelid. [Reprinted with permission from Nerad (13).]

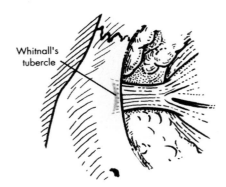

Figure 19.16 The lateral canthal tendon inserts onto Whitnall's tubercle. [Reprinted with permission from Nerad (13).]

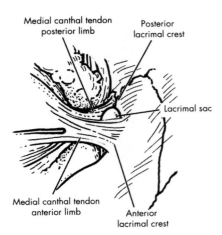

Figure 19.18 The medial canthal tendon. [Reprinted with permission from Nerad (13).]

the pretarsal orbicularis muscle, makes a significant contribution to the deep head. This posterior medial canthal tendon is the primary structure keeping the medial lower eyelid apposed to the globe.

Repairing the deep head of the medial canthal tendon is difficult due to the proximity of the canaliculi and lacrimal sac (Fig. 19.19) (13). However, because of the severity of the burn when the deep head of the medial canthal tendon is involved, irreversible damage to the canaliculi is also usually present. In that case, both a medial canthoplasty to the posterior lacrimal crest and a conjunctivodacryocystorhinostomy (C-DCR) are indicated.

2. Sensory Nerves

Sensory nerves of the eyelids originate from cranial nerve V, ophthalmic and maxillary divisions. The ophthalmic division has three branches lacrimal, frontal, and nasociliary, all of which to some extent innervate the upper eyelid. The lacrimal nerve supplies the lateral upper eyelid. The frontal branch splits into the supraorbital and supratrochlear nerves. The supraorbital branch leaves the orbit through the supraorbital notch of the frontal bone and supplies the skin of the forehead, scalp, and central upper eyelid. The supratrochlear branch exits the orbit above the trochlea and supplies the medial forehead and medial upper eyelid. The infratrochlear nerve, terminal branch of the nasociliary nerve, leaves the orbit below the trochlea and supplies the medial upper and lower eyelids, as well as the conjunctiva and nasolacrimal sac.

Two branches of the cranial nerve V, maxillary division, complete the innervation of the lower eyelid. The zygomaticofacial nerve through the zygomaticofacial foramen of the zygoma supplies the skin of the lateral lower eyelid. The infraorbital nerve exits from the orbit

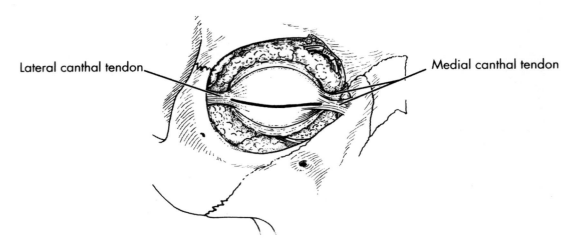

Figure 19.17 Slight upward slant from medial canthal tendon to lateral canthal tendon. [Reprinted with permission from Nerad (13).]

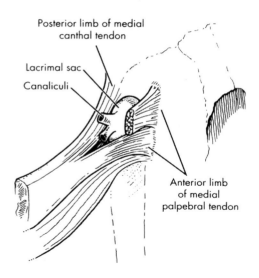

Figure 19.19 The medial canthal tendon surrounds the lacrimal sac. [Reprinted with permission from Nerad (13).]

via the infraorbital foramen of the maxilla supplying most of the lower lid skin, as well as the inferior conjunctiva.

Completing the sensation to the upper face, the zygomaticotemporal nerve innervates the skin of the anterior temple to the lateral orbital margin [Fig. 19.20(A–C)] (13).

3. Motor Nerves

In creating facial flaps for burn reconstruction, careful dissection in the area of cranial nerve VII or the facial nerve is extremely important to prevent paralytic brow ptosis, lagophthalmos, and lower lid ectropion. Emanating from the parotid gland, the upper temporofacial branch of the facial nerve further splits into the temporal and zygomatic branches supplying the upper face and eyelids (Fig. 19.21) (13).

The temporal branch travels over the proximal one-third of the zygomatic arch on its periosteal surface. The nerve at this point is usually 2.5 cm anterior to the external auditory meatus, with a range of 0.8–3.5 cm. The nerve continues in an oblique fashion on the undersurface of the superficial temporalis fascia 1.5 cm lateral to the lateral brow and enters the frontalis muscle <2 cm above the brow. The temporal branch supplies the frontalis, corrugator supercilii, procerus, and upper orbicularis muscles. The zygomatic branch travels across the zygomatic bone to innervate the lower orbicularis muscles (15).

All facial muscles, including the orbicularis oculi muscles, are innervated from their posterior surfaces. Therefore, dissection either superficial to the muscles or subgaleal beneath the course of the facial nerve will prevent damage to the muscle innervation (15).

4. Blood Vessels

The eyelids have a rich vascular network which is a combination of terminal branches from the internal and external carotid artery systems. The ophthalmic artery, the first branch off the internal carotid, travels from within the orbit to the eyelids giving rise to the dorsonasal, supratrochlear, supraorbital, and lacrimal arteries. Anastomoses with branches of the external carotid system, including the angular, facial, infraorbital, and superficial temporal arteries, complete the blood supply to the eyelids [Fig. 19.22(A–C)] (13).

The dorsonasal artery, which feeds the nasal bridge and medial forehead, exits the orbit between the medial canthal tendon and the trochlea and anastomoses with the angular artery. They proceed to form the medial superior and inferior palpebral arteries. On the lateral side of the eyelids, the lacrimal artery splits to form the lateral superior and inferior palpebral arteries. These palpebral arteries form the eyelid arcades, which may be identified during eyelid surgery. The superior palpebral arteries split to form the peripheral and marginal arcades of the upper eyelid. The peripheral arcade is found between the levator aponeurosis and Muller's muscle at the superior border of the tarsus. The marginal arcade travels atop the tarsus near the eyelid margin. In the lower eyelid, there is usually only a marginal arcade, which extends from the inferior palpebral arteries, also located near the eyelid margin anterior to the tarsus.

The supratrochlear artery exits the orbit above the trochlea and travels superiorly to supply the medial forehead and eyebrow. The supraorbital artery proceeds through the supraorbital notch superiorly providing the main blood supply to the forehead and eyebrow. The facial artery from the external carotid system travels around the mandible, proceeds superonasally running parallel to the nasojugal fold terminating into the angular artery. In an external dacryocystorhinostomy, careful blunt dissection is required to prevent laceration of the angular vessels. The infraorbital artery enters the orbit through the inferior orbital fissure, passes anteriorly within the infraorbital groove and canal, exiting out of the infraorbital foramen. The artery supplies the cheek and lower eyelid. The superficial temporal artery passes superonasally from just anterior to the external auditory canal toward the lateral orbit and temple which it supplies. Branches anastomose with the supraorbital artery, which may be identified during eyebrow surgery (13).

5. Lacrimal Pump

The pretarsal and preseptal orbicularis muscles are contiguous with the proximal lacrimal system and play an integral role in the lacrimal pump. Jones and Wobig (17) in 1976 proposed that eyelid closure and subsequent contraction of the deep head of the preseptal orbicularis muscle, Jones' muscle, attached to the lacrimal sac fascia, create negative pressure allowing tears to enter the opened lacrimal sac. The pretarsal muscles help by pushing tears through the canaliculi into the lacrimal sac. Upon relaxation, the sac collapses advancing tears into the nasolacrimal duct and nose. The canaliculi reopen allowing tears to re-enter and start the cycle again (Fig. 19.23) (14). If the function of the orbicularis muscle is hindered by a burn injury, epiphora occurs due to lacrimal pump failure. Although tears may be abundant which may lead you to believe the eye will keep moist, blink is reduced and lagophthalmos ensues. This will hinder exchange of tears over the entire surface

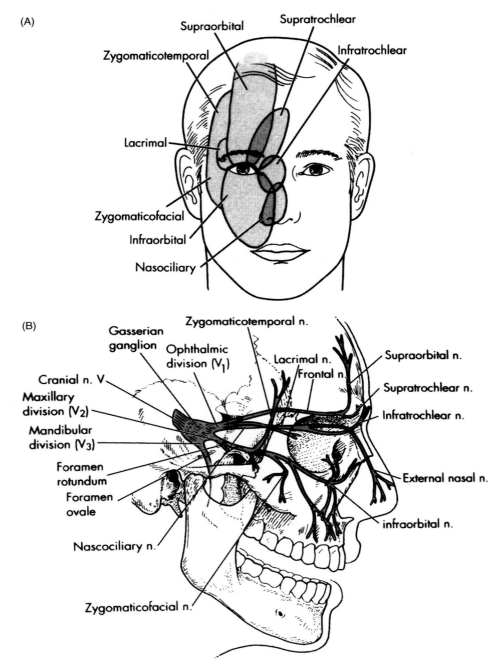

Figure 19.20 (A) Sensory distribution of the trigeminal nerve, CNV, ophthalmic and maxillary divisions. (B) The trigeminal nerve divisions: ophthalmic (CNV$_1$), maxillary (CNV$_2$), and mandibular (LNV$_3$). (C) The terminal branches of the ophthalmic (CNV$_1$) and maxillary (CNV$_2$) divisions of the trigeminal nerve. [Reprinted with permission from Nerad (13).]

(C)

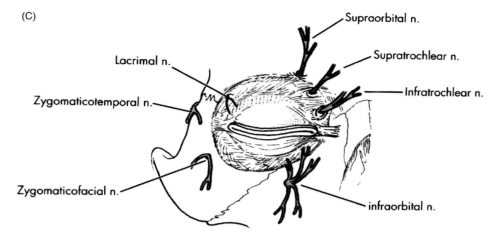

Figure 19.20 *Continued.*

of the cornea and, therefore, cause significant exposure keratopathy.

6. Lacrimal Anatomy

Complete evaluation of eyelid burns must include examination of the nasolacrimal system, in particular the puncta and canaliculi, to prevent persistent epiphora. The upper and lower puncta are located at the mucocutaneous junction, inverted toward the globe, so only with slight eversion may they be seen. They open 5–7 mm lateral to the medial canthus. The lower lid punctum is 1–2 mm lateral to the upper lid punctum. The puncta is 0.3 mm in diameter, enlarging into 1–2 mm diameter canaliculi.

The initial canaliculus travels 2 mm vertically then changes direction horizontally for 8 mm toward the

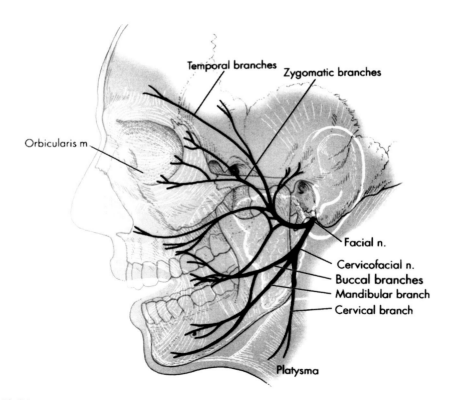

Figure 19.21 The branches of the facial nerve (CNV_{11}). [Reprinted with permission from Nerad (13).]

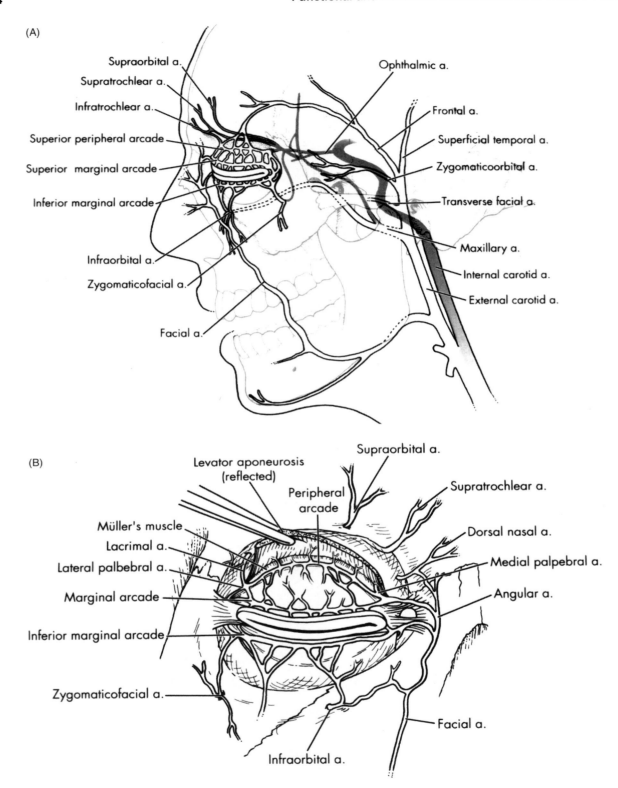

Figure 19.22   (A) The superficial arteries of the jaw. (B) The anastomoses of the anterior orbital and facial arteries. [Reprinted with permission from Nerad (13).]

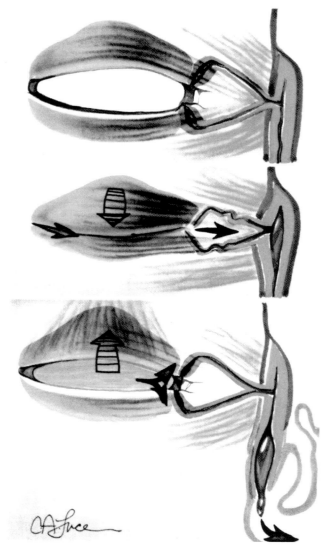

Figure 19.23 The lacrimal pump is dependent on the proper functioning of the orbicularis oculi muscles. [Reprinted with permission from Zide and Jelks (14).]

medial canthus. Usually, the upper and lower canaliculi come together to form a common canaliculus prior to entering the lacrimal sac. Infrequently, the canaliculi enter the lacrimal sac individually. The canaliculi are covered by pretarsal orbicularis muscle laterally and medial canthal tendon fibers medially (Fig. 19.24) (14).

At the end of the common canaliculus, as it enters the lacrimal sac, is the valve of Rosenmuller. This mucosal flap prevents reflux of tears back into the canaliculi. The common canaliculus enters the lacrimal sac, which lies in the lacrimal fossa formed by the frontal process of the maxilla and the lacrimal bone. The fundus of the sac located above the superior margin of the medial canthal

tendon is 3–5 mm. The body of the sac extends 10 mm inferiorly reaching the nasolacrimal canal of the maxillary bone. The nasolacrimal duct begins at this point for 12 mm within the canal until it enters the inferior meatus. The duct continues 5 mm along the lateral wall of the nose (Fig. 19.25) (14).

Medial eyelid burns must be examined carefully for proximal lacrimal drainage system damage and treated immediately (18). If punctal stenosis is identified, it should be dilated and probed to determine the amount of resistance. If the tissue injury and resistance are mild, then re-evaluation every 1–2 days with fluorescein dye disappearance testing and possible probing may defer surgical correction. If after 1 week, no signs of obstruction are present, then the lacrimal system should continue to function without epiphora.

However, if the puncta are not identifiable and/or the canaliculi cannot be easily probed, then punctoplasty and/or canaliculoplasty with silicone tube intubation is indicated. The tube should remain in place for 3–6 months. Later repair of punctal-canalicular burns by this method has poor outcomes. A C-DCR with glass, Jones' tube insertion is the most successful treatment after obliteration of the proximal lacrimal system.

7. Dacryocystorhinostomy

If a nasolacrimal duct obstruction is verified by punctal irrigation, then a dacryocystorhinostomy (DCR) is indicated. This procedure creates an anastomosis between the nasal cavity and the lacrimal sac at the level of the middle meatus bypassing the duct obstruction.

The procedure may be performed either under general or local monitored anesthesia care (MAC). If the patient can tolerate local anesthesia, intraoperative bleeding and recovery time is usually lessened. Whichever anesthetic method is used, a 1:1 solution of 2% lidocaine with epinephrine and 0.5% Marcaine with epinephrine is injected into the operative site. This includes subcutaneous infiltration at the incision site, an infratrochlear nerve block above the medial canthal tendon at the anterior and posterior lacrimal crests, and submucosal injection of the lateral nasal wall next to the anterior tip of the middle turbinate. The middle meatus is packed with two neurosurgical cottonoid pledgets soaked in a 4% solution of cocaine.

A 3 cm, oblique, straight line is marked on the skin just below the medial canthal tendon and 8 mm nasal to the medial commissure, extending over the inferior nasal rim of the orbit (Fig. 19.26) (19). The skin is incised with a no. 15 Bard-Parker blade. The subcutaneous tissue down to the periosteum is bluntly dissected with sharp iris scissors. Care should be taken not to lacerate the angular vessels (Fig. 19.27) (19).

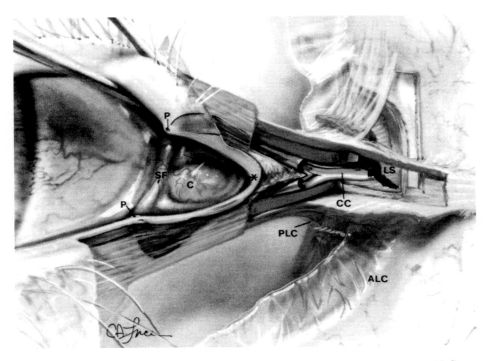

Figure 19.24   Proximal lacrimal drainage system. P: puncta; CS: common canaliculus; LS: lacrimal sac; PLC: posterior lacrimal crest; ALC: anterior lacrimal crest. [Reprinted with permission from Zide and Jelks (14).]

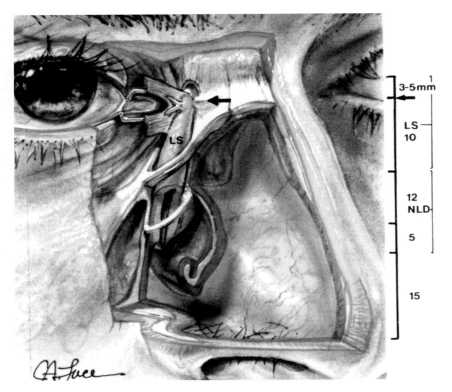

Figure 19.25   Distal lacrimal drainage system. Arrow: medial canthal tendon; LS: lacrimal sac; NLD: nasolacrimal duct. [Reprinted with permission from Zide and Jelks (14).]

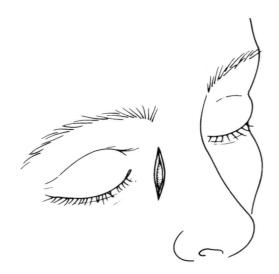

Figure 19.26 Skin incision for dacryocystorhinostomy. [Reprinted with permission from Stewart (19).]

The periosteum is incised with a no.15 Bard-Parker blade ~5 mm medial to the anterior lacrimal crest. Visualization for this step is improved by retracting with two small rakes. The lacrimal sac is reflected laterally by lifting the periosteum from the lacrimal fossa with a Freer elevator. The periosteum is also loosened anteriorly over the nasal bone to allow easier reapposition of the periosteum at the end of the procedure. Before removing the lacrimal fossa bone, the cottonoid strips should be removed from the nose to help prevent nasal mucosal trauma from the bur. The anterior lacrimal crest is then carefully removed using a medium-sized, olive-tip bur (Fig. 19.28) (19). Trauma to the nasal mucosa should be avoided by placing only light pressure on the bone by the bur. The lacrimal sac is protected by inserting the Freer elevator between the bone and sac. When inside the nose, the rest of the lacrimal fossa is extracted with rongeurs and Kerrison punches to form a 0.8 × 1.5 cm opening [Fig. 19.29(A) and (B)] (19). Bone wax and cautery may be used to acquire hemostasis.

The lacrimal sac is identified by placing a 00 naso-lacrimal probe into the canaliculus and tenting the sac (Fig. 19.30) (19). The periosteum and tear sac are cut with a no. 12 Bard-Parker blade that is wrapped with Steri-Strips so that only the tip remains clear. The anterior lacrimal sac flap is formed by making a semicircular incision, taking care not to go too deeply and thereby pierce the other side of the sac and enter the orbital fat. A posterior lacrimal sac flap is removed with Wescott scissors to widen the opening. The nasolacrimal probe should be seen coming through the sac. If not, the sac was not completely incised, or there is an obstruction at the common internal punctum. The blocked common internal punctum is opened by tenting it up with the naso-lacrimal probe and snipping it with Wescott scissors. Water is injected with a lacrimal cannula into the canaliculus.

The anterior lacrimal sac flap is isolated with one or two 4-0 vicryl sutures on a small half-circle needle. The suture is placed through once and left long. The two ends are held together with a serrefine. The suture is used later to appose the lacrimal sac and nasal mucosal flaps.

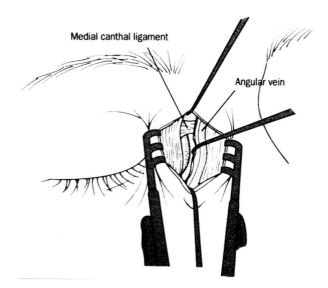

Figure 19.27 Deep blunt dissection revealing medial canthal tendon and the angular rein. [Reprinted with permission from Stewart (19).]

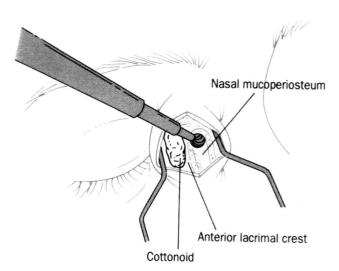

Figure 19.28 Olive-tip burr creates osteotomy. [Reprinted with permission from Stewart (19).]

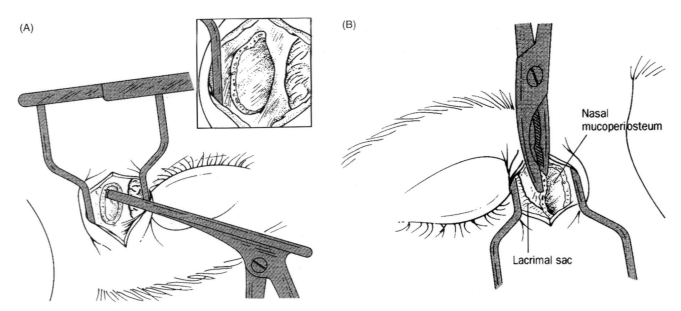

Figure 19.29 (A) Enlarging lacrimal fossa osteotomy with a Kerrison punch. (B) Further enlargement of the osteotomy with a rongeur. [Reprinted with permission from Stewart (19).]

Attention is then focused on creating an anterior nasal mucosal flap with a no. 12 Bard-Parker blade in a semi-circular fashion. A small hemostat inserted into the nose to tent the nasal mucosa laterally aids in making the flap. The posterior flap is excised with Wescott scissors. Hemorrhage is common at this point because the nasal mucosa is quite vascular. Packing the site with neurosurgical pledgets soaked in local anesthetic for a few minutes will aid in hemostasis. If necessary, gelfoam soaked in thrombin may be placed in the nose temporarily or allowed to remain there permanently.

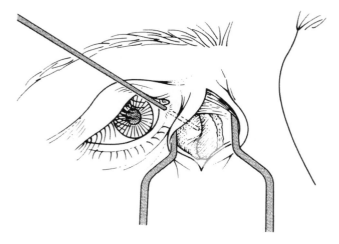

Figure 19.30 Tenting the lacrimal sac in preparation for its fenestration. [Reprinted with permission from Stewart (19).]

If the common internal punctum was occluded, a Crawford tube should be inserted. One of the Crawford probes is inserted through the superior punctum and into the nose. The probe is removed from the nose with a Crawford crochet-type hook. The other Crawford probe is inserted through the inferior punctum and removed from the nose.

Umbilical tape greased in antibiotic-steroid ointment is placed through the nostril in the surgical site for hemostasis. Approximately 20 cm is packed in the site and then cut at the nostril; it is removed on postoperative days 1–2. The Crawford tube metalends are pulled off, and the tubes are tied together in a 1 × 1 × 1 square knot (Fig. 19.31) (19). The serrefine is released from the 4-0 vicryl suture, and interrupted sutures are placed to appose the lacrimal sac and nasal mucosal flaps. Care is taken not to include the umbilical tape. The periosteum is reapposed with the 4-0 vicryl suture. Subcutaneous tissue is sutured with buried interrupted 5-0 vicryl sutures. The skin is closed with interrupted 6-0 mild chromic sutures. Antibiotic ointment is placed on the incision, and a folded eye pad is taped over the surgical site. The Crawford tube should be left in place for 2 months then removed through the nose (20).

The next procedure is referred to as C-DCR. Rather than nasolacrimal duct obstruction, epiphora in burn patients more commonly results from either punctal-canalicular occlusion or failure of the lacrimal pump. In these cases, a C-DCR is indicated. The primary difference between a DCR and a C-DCR is placement of a Jones tube.

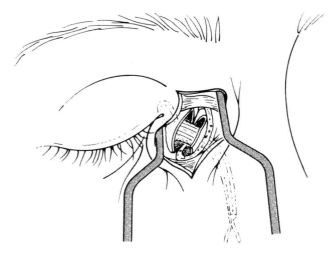

Figure 19.31 Silicone tube placement in the proximal lacrimal drainage system and tied inside the nose. [Reprinted with permission from Stewart (19).]

This Pyrex tube acts as a conduit for the passage of tears from the lacrimal lake into the nose bypassing proximal nasolacrimal obstructions or, in the case of lacrimal pump failure, allowing drainage due to the hydrophilic properties of glass.

A DCR is performed until the point of creating the anterior lacrimal sac and nasal mucosal flaps. The caruncle is excised with Westcott scissors. A 66 Beaver blade pointed in an inferior, posterior, nasal direction is advanced through the prior site of the caruncle. A fistula is created posterior to the lacrimal sac–nasal mucosal flaps and enters the nose near the anterior tip of the middle turbinate (Fig. 19.32) (19).

A no. 1 Bowman probe is placed through the opening until the nasal septum is felt. The probe is clamped with a mosquito hemostat at the level of the caruncle and removed to measure the length from tip to clamp. By subtracting 3 mm from this measurement, the correct length of the Jones tube is determined. The flange on the proximal end of the tube should be 3.5 or 4 mm depending on the size of the lacrimal lake. A double-armed 6-0 vicryl, which will later be used to prevent extrusion of the tube, should be knotted around the base of the flange.

The properly sized Jones tube is threaded onto the no. 1 Bowman probe. The probe is inserted back into the fistula and the tube advanced into the nose. If the anterior tip of the middle turbinate obstructs the end, then an anterior turbinectomy is performed with rongeurs. To verify drainage, a drop of balanced salt solution is placed into the lacrimal lake to observe for its disappearance. The position and/or size of the Jones tube should be adjusted as necessary. Each needle of the double-armed 6-0 vicryl should be driven through the full thickness of the medial lower lid and tied to the skin. The operation can then be completed as in a DCR (Fig. 19.33) (19).

Jones tubes can have a tendency to extrude and become obstructed. The patient should be reminded to close their eyes when nose blowing, sneezing, or coughing. The Jones tube must be immediately replaced if dislodged because the fistula may close within hours. To help clear the tube of mucus, artificial tears should be dropped into the lacrimal lake with the patient inhaling forcefully through the nose (21).

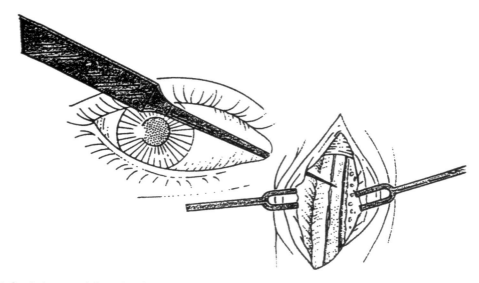

Figure 19.32 A fistula is created from the site of the caruncle into the middle meatus of the nose. [Reprinted with permission from Stewart (19).]

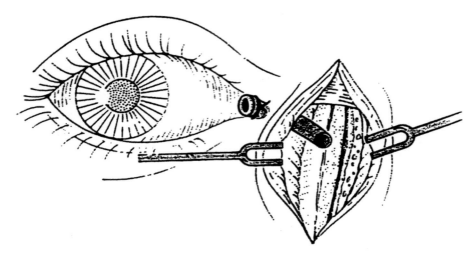

Figure 19.33   Jones tube sutured into place. [Reprinted with permission from Stewart (19).]

C. Acute Management and Early Reconstruction

Patients with acute facial burns involving the eyelids require careful ophthalmic evaluation. The use of fluorescin dye is crucial in the initial evaluation. Such an evaluation is crucial at the time of admission. Since eyelid swelling occurs early, this precludes an accurate

examination later. Although thermal injuries do not involve the cornea, when the cornea is involved 75% of corneal injuries heal with conservative management (22). It is well known that full-thickness injuries involving the orbicularis oculi can occur. However, involvement of the deep structures such as the levator muscle and tarsus is rare. Often such injuries occur in unconscious patients or in children unable to escape from fires. In 1875, Wolfe

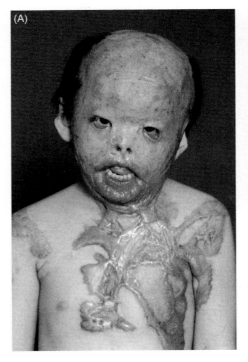
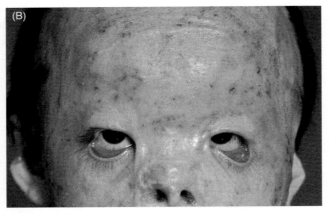

Figure 19.34   (A) Extrinsic lower-eyelid ectropion from a Grade IV neck contracture. (B) Close-up of lower-eyelid ectropions. (Courtesy of R. L. McCauley, MD.)

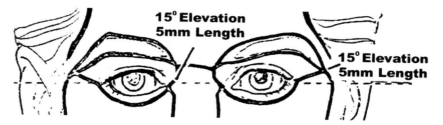

Figure 19.35 Approach to correction of eyelid ectropion. [Reprinted with permission from Huang et al. (7).]

was reportedly the first surgeon to describe the use of a full-thickness skin graft to correct a burn lid ectropion due to burn scar contracture (22). The acute management of thermal injuries to the eyelids includes the use of topical antibiotics, head elevation, and subsequent debribement of devitalized tissue if necessary and resurfacing with skin grafts. Although tarsorraphies have been used in the past, today, its general use is discouraged.Tarsorraphy does not prevent eyelid retraction, nor is it a substitute for appropriate repair of eyelids with skin grafts. Yet in rare cases, this may be the only option for protection of the globe (4,23–26).

Corneal exposure during the acute phase of treatment is accompanied by significant complications if not corrected (3). Nonsurgical approaches have been useful as a temporary method to prevent corneal perforation. Scleral contact lenses have been useful under these circumstances as well as the use of a thin polyethylene film (Saran wrap). Ophthalmic lubricating ointment is used to occlusively seal the film. Several surgical procedures have been useful during the acute phase of injury to prevent corneal ulcerations. The upper bulbar conjunctival flap, commonly referred to as the Gunderson procedures, is quite useful in preserving the integrity of the globe (22). Although initially described in 1958, this procedure continues to be utilized in current day management of the exposed cornea.

1. Reconstruction

Structural deformities to the eyelids in thermally injured patients do occur. The prevention of burn scar contractures

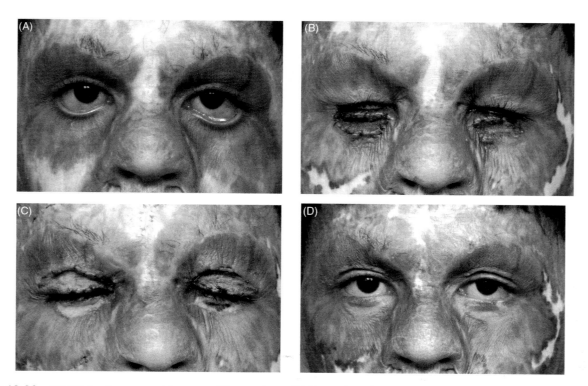

Figure 19.36 (A) Bilateral upper- and lower-eyelid ectropions. (B) Correction of lower-lid ectropions with full-thickness skin grafts. (C) Incomplete closure of eyes. (D) Correction of upper-eyelid ectropions with split-thickness skin grafts. (E) Final appearance. (Courtesy of R. L. McCauley, MD.)

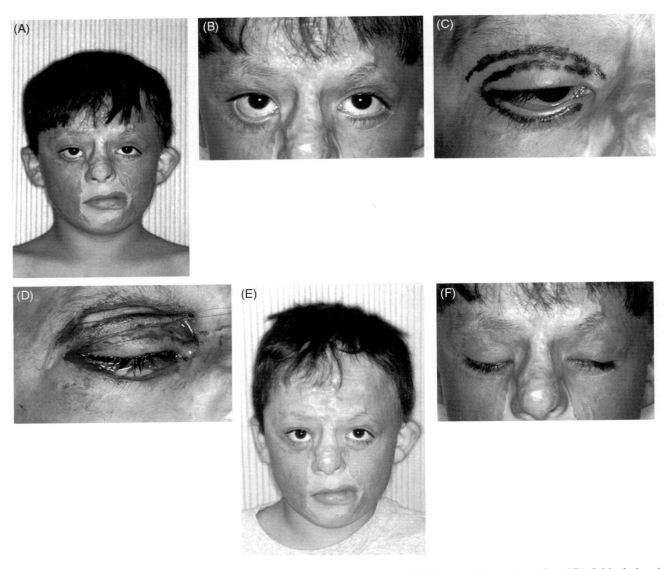

Figure 19.37   (A) Right lower-lid ectropion in a young boy with facial burns. (B) Close-up of ectropion. (C and D) Orbicularis oris myocutaneous flap designed from upper eyelid for correction of lower-lid ectropion. (E and F) Final appearance. (Courtesy of Dr. Ted T. Huang, Shriners Burn Hospital, Galveston, TX.)

of the eyelids is difficult. Pressure garments do not cover the areas and splinting, although described, is ineffective (27). Once corneal protection is achieved, it is still acceptable to wait until the scar matures before embarking on definitive reconstruction. These deformities may be classified as upper and lower lid ectropions, medial canthal hooding, palpebral fissure stenosis, and cannilicular obstruction (7). Full-thickness injuries may involve not only partial or complete loss of the lids, but also damage to the levator, the orbicularis oculi, and tarsal plate. Reconstruction of these defects is quite challenging.

2.   Eyelids

Burns involving the mobile upper eyelid or the static lower eyelid, if deep enough, can undergo wound contraction. The upper lid normally protects the cornea. Even with adequate early release, upper-lid ectropion may still occur (28).

3.   Ectropions

Ectropions continue to be a problem in burns to the eyelids. The early use of skin grafts and conformers does not eliminate this problem. One must alleviate problems associated with extrinsic ectropions before addressing the eyelid itself. Burn scar contractures of the cheek and neck can produce extrinsic lower-lid ectropions. In addition, contractures of the forehead may be implicated in extrinsic upper-eyelid ectropions. These problems should be addressed first. Intrinsic ectropions are only treated when extrinsic forces are not present or have been eliminated. In some patients with major thermal burns to the face and neck, eyelid ectropions may be a combination of both intrinsic and extrinsic factors (Fig. 19.34).

The classic approach to correction of eyelid ectropions has been described by Huang (6). (Fig. 19.35). Although early correction of eyelid ectropions may be indicated, recurrence is likely to occur (29). In the correction of lower-lid ectropions, it has been recommended that incisions be carried from the medial canthus to the lateral canthus and at least 15 mm beyond the canthus with a 15° angulation upward. This incisional release is believed to correct the majority of ectropions encountered, regardless of severity. Resurfacing of the defects with split-thickness skin grafts to the upper lid (0.018–0.020 in.) and full-thickness skin

grafts to the lower lid should provide adequate coverage. Due to the risk of recurrence, many surgeons feel that overcorrection of the defect is crucial. With this in mind, only one lid is recommended for surgical intervention at a time (Fig. 19.36). Usually, this is the eyelid with the most severe contracture. Correction of ectropions of the

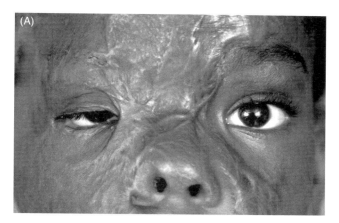

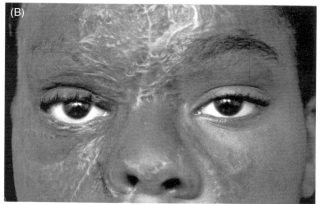

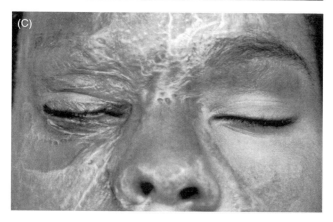

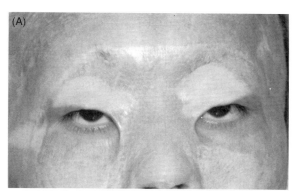

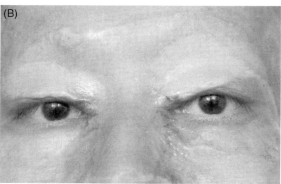

Figure 19.38 (A) Nine-year-old Asian with medial canthal hooding. (B) Six-years later; final correction with percent limb Z-plasties; 1 month since the last operation. (Courtesy of R. L. McCauley, MD.)

Figure 19.39 (A) Six-year-old patient with moderate medial canthal hooding impairing upper-lid movement (B) Five years after correction with local skin flaps. (Courtesy of R. L. McCauley, MD.)

upper and lower eyelids simultaneously does not allow for overcorrection.

4. Local Flaps

When eyelid burns involve only the upper or lower lid, other possibilities for reconstruction exist. Although skin grafts, harvested from the face, neck, or upper arm provide good color match, the use of local flaps may provide another dimension to this type of reconstruction. Unburned tissue from either the upper lid or the lower lid has been described as a method for correction of defects, a lateral eyelid transposition flap. This procedure was popularized by Gorney et al. (30) and Anderson and Edward (31). The width of the flap is determined with the eyelids closed to prevent secondary ectropions. The inclusion of the orbicularis oculi muscle may ensure flap survival. Kostakoğlo and Ożcan (32) reported successful use of the upper-lid orbicularis oculi myocutaneous flap for correction of lower-eyelid ectropin in seven patients with up to 40 months follow-up. The inclusion of muscle into this flap appears to be the key to its survival since the length to width ratio appears to be markedly increased (Fig. 19.37).

5. Tissue Expansion

The use of tissue expanders for eyelid reconstruction was reported by Victor and Hurwitz (16) who corrected a case of cicatricial ectropion following blepharoplasty.

In 1986, Garber and Lukash (33) reported the first case of tissue expansion in subtotal upper and lower eyelid reconstruction in a patient with severe eye burns. Upon completion of the expansion process, conchal cartilage was used for eyelid support prior to placement of the ocular prosthesis. The result was outstanding. Later in 1993, Tse and McCafferty (34) reported six cases of tissue expansion in the ocular region: one upper-eyelid expansion and five periocular expansions for correction of various periocular defects. Two complications were noted, one patient with a hematoma and another patient who developed partial flap necrosis. In 1998, Foster et al. (21) reported a series of 26 patients with eyelid defects who underwent rapid intraoperative tissue expansion (RITE) using a #14-French Foley catheter. The catheter was placed under the muscle skin flap and inflated twice for 5 min. The linear extent of the eyelid margin was decreased by 36% using this technique. More recently, Weislander and Weislander (35) in an experimental study with pigs, prefabricated advancement flaps for the reconstruction of lower-eyelid and cheek defects in pigs. It was felt that the expander capsule could serve as a conjunctival substitute providing a temporary physical shield and a template for mucosal regeneration.

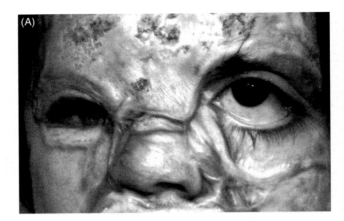

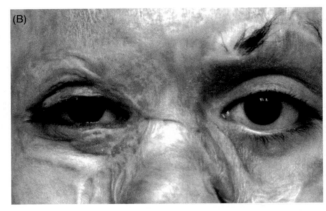

Figure 19.40 (A) Eight-year-old patient with significant facial scarring and severe right eye distortion with impaired lid function secondary to scarring. (B) Three-year follow-up after correction of upper and lower lids with skin grafts; local flaps were used to correct the medial canthal hooding. (Courtesy of R. L. McCauley, MD.)

6. Free-Tissue Transfer

The use of free-tissue transfers to reconstruct eyelid burns appears to be a last resort (36–40). Although the use of free-tissue transfers may be criticized in burn facial reconstructive because of bulkiness, the loss of facial expression, and poor color match, it often provides the only viable solution to a significant problem with eyelid burns. Both the patient and the surgeon recognize that in these circumstances, aesthetic will be compromised. Usually, these patients have severe upper and middle third facial deformities in which the use of local tissue is not feasible. The provision of soft tissue to correct severe deformities can only be achieved by free-tissue transfer. The radial artery forearm flap, the scapular flap, and the dorsalis pedis flap have all been used successfully for the reconstruction of full-thickness eyelid burns.

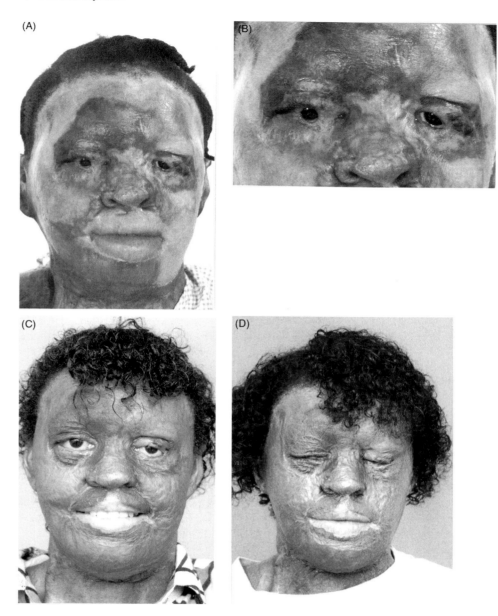

Figure 19.41 (A) Thriteen-year-old patient with palpebral fissure stenosis after severe facial burns and the use of tarsorrhaphy sutures for corneal protection. (B) Two-years after reconstruction of both the upper and lower eyelids with skin grafts. (C) Full closure of eyes noted. (Courtesy of R. L. McCauley, MD.)

7. Medial Canthal Hooding

Hooding around the medial epicanthus is a common problem seen in patients with burns involving the eyelids and nose. The early use of skin grafts with extensions medially may accentuate this deformity (7). The surgical correction of this problem is easily accomplished with the use of multiple Z-plasties and/or combined with skin resection. If the hooding obstructs the medial canthus, additional releases of the upper or lower lids may be warranted (Figs. 19.38–19.40).

8. Palpebral Fissure Stenosis

In patients with full-thickness burns to the eye, cicatricial adhesion along the tarsal margin may cause stenosis of the palpebral fissures. This condition, which has been described by Huang et al. (7), results in a characteristic spherical contracture of the eyelid margin producing the "port hole" deformity. This deformity is in contrast to a similar deformity created to protect the cornea in patients in whom the damage to the eyelids from full-thickness eyelid burns is compromised. The operative management of this problem includes correction of tissue deficits in the upper and lower lids prior to increasing the width of the palpebral fissure skin. The mucosal edges are usually reapproximated with 5-0 chromic catgut sutures. Presently, no clinical series addresses this unique problem (Fig. 19.41).

9. Canalicular Obstruction

Occasionally, patients present with lower-lid ectropion and epiphora. The majority of the time, correction of the ectropion with grafts or flaps repositions the lower lid to allow the drainage of tears. Under normal circumstances the lower lid accounts for the majority of the drainage system. On rare occasions, correction of the lower lid ectropion does not correct the epiphora. Canalicular obstruction is caused by scarring of the lid margins. Once canalicular obstruction is diagnosed, a C-DCR is indicated. This procedure creates a new fistulous tract when a medially based conjunctival mucosal flap is created through a bony window in the lateral nasal bones. The Jones tube is placed along the path of the flap and brought out through the nostril. Huang et al. (7) reported a series of four patients who successfully underwent correction of epiphora secondary to canalicular obstruction using C-DCRs. Their results were uniformly successful.

III. CONCLUSION

Burns to the eyelids and adnexa constitute major problems. Understanding of eyelid anatomy is imperative for determination of a surgical plan. Full-thickness injuries, or more commonly cicatricial lid retraction, require aggressive treatment to avoid problems of corneal exposure which can lead to blindness. Associated deformities are numerous and if improperly treated, can result in significant aesthetic and functional problems. Reconstructive efforts for major upper and lower-lid defects continue to evolve. Although coverage has been reported with the use of skin grafts, flaps, and free-tissue transfer, refinements in our techniques may allow the blending of function and aesthetics.

REFERENCES

1. Brou JA, Robson MC, McCauley RL, Herndon DN, Phillips LG, Ortega M, Evans EB, Alvarado MI. Inventory of potential reconstructive needs in the patient with burns. J Burn Care Rehabil 1989; 10(6):555–560.
2. Burns BF, McCauley RL, Murphy EL, Robson, MC. Reconstructive management of patients with >80% TBSA burns. Burns 1993; 19(5):429–433.
3. Barrow RE, Jeschke MG, Herndon DN. Early release of third degree eyelid burns prevents eye injury. Plast Reconstr Surg 2000; 105:860–863.
4. Guy R, Baldwin J, Kwedar S, Law EJ. A three year experience in a regional burn center with burns of the eyes and eyelids. Opthalmic Surg 1982; 13(5):383–386.
5. Frank DH, Wachtel Frank HA. The early treatment and reconstruction of eyelid burns. J Trauma 1983; 23:874–877.
6. Stern JD, Goldfarlo LW, Slater H. Ophthalmological complications as a manifestation of burn injury. Burns 1996; 22:135–136.
7. Huang TT, Blackwell SJ, Lewis SR. Burn injuries of the eyelids. Clin Plast Surg 1978; 5:571–581.
8. Pelletier CR, Jordan DR. An unusual and severe thermal burn to the eye and adnea. Can J Opthalmol 1996; 31: 319–323.
9. Kalish E, Steibel-Kalish H, Wolf Y, Robinpour M, Hauben DJ. Scorched eyelashes—do we treat them right? Burns 1998; 24:173–175.
10. Mannis MJ, Miller RB, Krachmer JH. Contact thermal burns of the cornea from electric curling irons. Am J Opthalmol 1984; 98:336–339.
11. Shokula PC. Ocular burns from microwaved eggs. Pediatr Emerg Care 1994; 10:229–231.
12. Vajpayee RB, Gupta NK, Angra et al. Contact thermal burns of the cornea. Can J Opthalmol 1991; 26:215–218.
13. Nerad JA. Oculoplastic Surgery, The Requisites in Ophthalmology. St. Louis: Mosby, 2001.
14. Zide BM, Jelks GW. Surgical Anatomy of the Orbit. New York: Raven Press, 1985.
15. Jordan DR, Anderson RL. Surgical Anatomy of the Ocular Adnexa: A Clinical Approach. San Francisco: American Academy of Ophthalmology, 1996.
16. Victor WH, Hurwitz JJ, Cicatricial ectropion following blepharoplasty: treatment by tissue expansion. Can L Ophthmol 1984; 19:317–319
17. Jones LT, Wobig JL. Newer concepts of tear tuct and eyelid anatomy and treatment. Trans Sect Ophthalmol Am Acad Opthalmol Otolaryngol 1977; 83:603–616.
18. Meyer DR, Kersten RC, Kulwin DR, Paskowski JR, Selkin RP. Management of canalicular injury associated with eyelid burns. Arch Ophthalmol 1995; 113:900–903.
19. Stewart BW. Surgery of the Eyelid, Orbit, and Lacrimal System. San Francisco: American Academy of Ophthalmology, 1995.
20. Bailey BJ, Calhoun KH. Atlas of Head and Neck Surgery—Otolaryngology. Philadelphia: Lippincott, Williams and Wilkins, 2001.
21. Foster JA, Scheiner, Wulc AE, Wallace IB, Greenbaum SS. Intraoperative tissue expansion in eyelid reconstruction. Ophthalmology 1998; 105:170–175.
22. Achauer BM, Adair SR. Acute and reconstructive management of the burned eyelid. Clin Plast Surg 2000; 27:87–96.
23. Astori IP, Muller MS, Pegg SP. Cicatrical post-burn ectropion and exposure keratitis. Burns 1998; 24:64–67.

24. Still Jr JM, Law EJ, Beclher KE, Mosses KC, Gleitsmann KY. Experience with burns of the eyes and lids in a regional burn unit. J Burn Care Rehabil 1995; 16:248–252.

25. Nose K, Isshiki N, Kusumoto K. Reconstruction of both eyelids following electrical burns. Plast Reconst Surg 1991; 88:878–881.

26. Gencosmanoglu R, Cuneyt, O, Alper M, Gundogan H, Cagdas A. Full thickness eyelid burn with intact levator function. Ann Plast Surg 2000; 44:234–235.

27. Feldman JJ. Facial burns. In: McCarthy J, ed. Plastic Surgery. Philadelphia: W.B. Saunders, 1990:2210–2218.

28. Warpeha RL. Resurfacing the burned face. Clin Plast Surg 1981; 8:255–267.

29. Sloan DF, Huang TT, Larson DL, Lewis SR. Reconstruction of eyelids and eyebrows in burn patients. Plast Reconstr Surg 1976; 58:340–346.

30. Gorney M, Falcea E, Jones W. One stage reconstruction of substantial lower eyelid margin defects. Plast Reconstr Surg 1969; 44:592–596.

31. Anderson RL, Edwards JJ. Reconstruction by myocutaneous eyelid flaps. Arch Ophthalmol 1979; 97:2358–2362.

32. Kostakoğlu N, Ożcan G. Orbicularis oculi myocutaneous flap in reconstruction of post-burn lower eyelid ectropion. Burns 1999; 25:553–557.

33. Garber PF, Lukash FN, Eyelid reconstruction using temporary tissue expanders and cartilage grafts. Ophthalmol Plast Reconstr Surg 1987; 3:253–257.

34. Tse DT, McCafferty P. Controlled tissue expansion in periocular reconstructive surgery. Ophthalmology 1993; 100:260–268.

35. Weislander JB, Weislander M. Prefabricated (expander) capsule-lined transposition and advancement flaps in reconstruction of lower eyelid and oral defects: an experimental study. Plast Reconstr Surg 2000; 105:1399–1407.

36. Yap LH, Earley MJ. The free "v"; a bipennate free flap for double eyelid resurfacing based on the second dorsal metacarpal artery. Br J Plast Surg 1997; 40:280–283.

37. Chat LA, Cort A, Braun J. Upper and lower eyelid reconstruction with a neuro vascular free flap from the first web space of the feet. Br J Plast Surg 1980; 33:132.

38. Thai KN, Billmire DA, Yakuboff KP. Total eyelid reconstruction with free dorsalis pedis flap after deep facial burns. Plast Reconst Surg 1999; 104:1048–1051.

39. Watanabe T, Furuta S, Hataya Y, Yuzuniha S, Otsuka Y. Reconstruction of the eyelids and nose after a burn injury using a radial forearm flap. Burns 1997; 25:360–365.

40. Rose EH. Aesthetic restorations of the severely disfigured face in burn victims: a comprehensive strategy. Plast Reconstr Surg 1995; 96:1573–1585.

20

Reconstruction of Cheek Deformities

ROBERT L. McCAULEY
University of Texas Medical Branch and Shriners Hospital for Children—Galveston Unit, Galveston, Texas, USA

MICHAEL K. OBENG
University of Texas Medical Branch, Galveston, Texas, USA

I. INTRODUCTION

Both the depth of injury and the subsequent acute management of facial burns have a tremendous impact on the reconstructive needs of the face. The issue of timing for the excision of facial burns is controversial. Initial investigators developed the time-honored practice of delayed excision of these wounds until deep partial-thickness or full-thickness injuries were clearly identified. Subsequent excision of eschar and resurfacing of aesthetic units with skin grafts was the standard of care (1–3). The recognition that delayed healing was associated with hypertrophic scars and wound contraction encouraged utilization of the face mask to control these problems. In many cases, this approach led to respectable outcomes. In recent years, the idea of early excision of facial burns has drawn attention (1–4). Proponents of this concept believe that early excision of deep second-degree or full-thickness wounds would not only lead to early wound closure, but also decrease hypertrophic scar formation and produce better aesthetic results. In addition, such an approach would also decrease the subsequent need for reconstructive procedures. Although all of these points can be easily embraced by both general surgeons and plastic surgeons involved in burn care, one problem continues to confound the issue. What is early excision? According to the literature, the definition of early excision can be within 24 h of burn injury to within 3 weeks of burn injury for facial burns. Without question, such a protracted time period prevents correlation and interpretation of data from other institutions. Since most facial burns are a combination of deep and superficial injuries with variable geographic patterns, these issues are apparently weighed prior to embarking upon early surgical excision. Yet, interinstitutional comparisons of early vs. late excision have been uniformly favorable for the early-excision group. Confounding the issue further is the fact that only a few studies used objective measurements to support their findings (3). Nevertheless, the idea of earlier excision of facial burn wounds and coverage with skin grafts may have significant benefits on facial aesthetics.

II. ANATOMY

Reconstruction of the burned cheek requires a thorough understanding of the concept of the facial aesthetic units as well as the regional anatomy of the cheek and surrounding structures. As classically described, the cheek subunit extends superiorly from the skin of the lower eyelid to the lower border of the mandible (5–7) (Fig. 20.1). Its medial border is defined by a line drawn from the medial canthus through the nasolabial line and around the oral commissure down to the lower border of the mandible. The lateral extent of the cheek unit is noted by a horizontal plane from the lateral canthus to the temporal hairline, extending inferiorly through the pretragal line to the inferior border of the mandibular angle.

Several authors have further divided the cheek aesthetic unit into three overlapping zones: the suborbital region, the preauricular section, and the buccomandibular region. The

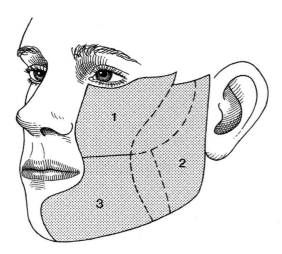

Figure 20.2 The three overlapping zones of the cheek aesthetic unit. [Reprinted with permission from Cabrera and Zide (8).]

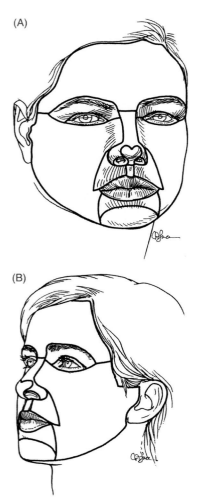

(A)

(B)

Figure 20.1 Aesthetic units of the face: (A) frontal view and (B) lateral view. [Reprinted with permission from Feldman (7).]

buccomandibular subunit encompasses the oral lining (8) (Fig. 20.2). The suborbital zone has been further subdivided into three subunits; A, B, and C (Fig. 20.3). Subunit C encompasses the lower-lid skin and extends from the lash line to the inferior orbital rim. Subunit A extends from the most caudal part of C and ends at the midpoint of the upper lip-nasal unit. Subunit B extends from the midpoint between the lateral canthus and tragus, then sweeps caudally in a curvilinear fashion anterior to the pretragal line, and ends at the most inferior border of A.

Chandawarker and Cervino (9) felt that the three-zone subunit of cheek aesthetic units did not account for the "anatomical contours and function" of the cheek. Nor did the three-zone concept account for the distribution of the neurovascular supply to the cheek. They, subsequently,

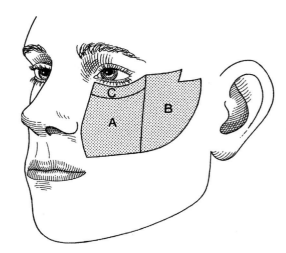

Figure 20.3 The subunits of Zone 1. [Reprinted with permission from Cabrera and Zide (8).]

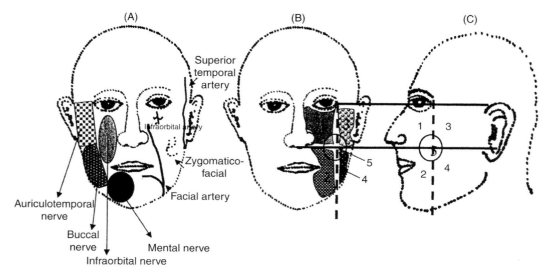

Figure 20.4   The five zone subunit classification of the cheek based on neurovascular anatomy. [Reprinted with permission from Chandawarker and Cervino (9).]

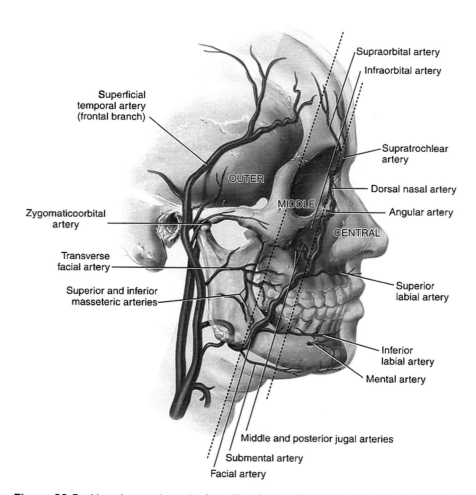

Figure 20.5   Vascular supply to the face. [Reprinted with permission from LaTrenta (10).]

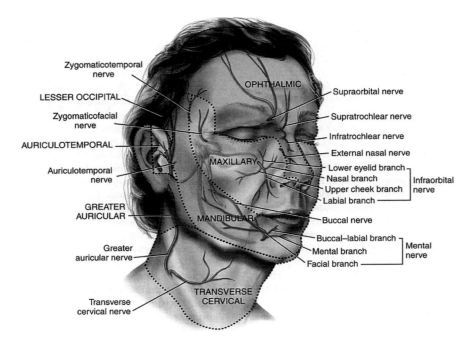

Figure 20.6   Sensory innervation of the cheek. [Reprinted with permission from LaTrenta (10).]

proposed a five-zone system (Fig. 20.4). Three horizontal and three vertical lines aid in this newly designed classification system. The horizontal line passes through the zygometric arch, and abuts the inferior border of the nasal sill and moves to the lower border of the mandible.

The vertical margin passes through the lateral margin of the nose, the lateral canthal line, and the preauricular region.

The importance of the aesthetic unit of the cheek, whether one uses the three or five-zone classification, is

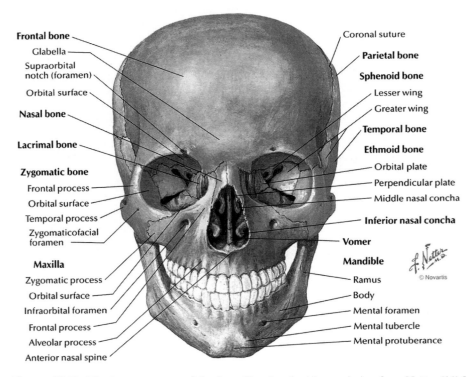

Figure 20.7   The bony structure of the face. [Reprinted with permission from Netter (11).]

to predict the effect of secondary problems on facial aesthetics after traumatic injury and to plan the correction of traumatic defects with skin flaps. The repair of these defects may be camouflaged based on the zone of injury. Because burn-related injuries to the cheeks characteristically pose unique problems, these subunits may be important in predicting contractures in burn patients. The classically described single unit of the cheek is too broad, and as such holds less promise when describing defects of the cheek. The development of the cheek subunit principle was not intended for burn patients. However, application of the three-subunit classification may be useful in the prediction of burn deformities.

The blood supply to the cheek is derived from the facial artery, the zygomatico-facial artery, the infraorbital artery, the transverse facial artery, and the superficial temporal artery, making this aesthetic unit of the face highly vascularized (9,10) (Fig. 20.5). The venous drainage is via the facial vein (10). Sensation to the cheek aesthetic unit is via the maxillary (V_2) and mandibular (V_3) branches of the trigeminal nerve (CNV) (9,10) (Fig. 20.6). V_2 arborizes

and terminates in three cutaneous branches: infraorbital, zygomatico-facial, and zygomatico-temporal nerves. The infraorbital nerve exits the intraorbital foramen and provides sensation to the upper part of this unit. V_3 also terminates and arborizes into three units: the auriculotemporal, the mental, and the buccal nerves. All three aid in providing sensation to this region. The auriculotemporal nerve innervates the skin in the preauricular region. The underlying bony structure of this aesthetic unit includes the maxilla, the zygomatic body and arch, and the mandibular body, angle, and ramus (10) (Fig. 20.7). These bones provide the bony framework to support the cheek aesthetic unit of the face. The muscles in this unit work in synchrony. The enormous amount of fibrils in each muscle and the ability of each fibril to contract independently make the cheek one of the most animated units in the face (9). These muscles are well layered and intertwine with both the superficial and deep fascial layers. The muscles of the face can be grouped into four main categories based on function and topology: epicranial; circumorbital and palpebral; nasal; and buccolabial group of muscles

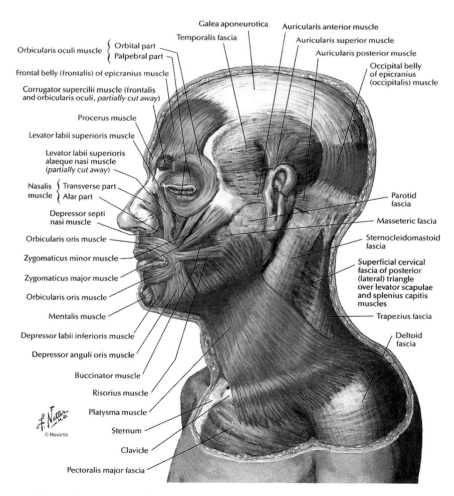

Figure 20.8 The muscles of facial expression. [Reprinted with permission from Netter (10).]

(Fig. 20.8). None of the epicranial or the nasalis group of muscles spans the cheek aesthetic unit. The inferior orbital portion of the orbicularis oculi muscle of the circumorbital and palpebral groups forms the upper part of Zone 1. This muscle arises from the nasal aspect of the frontal bone, the frontal process of the maxilla, and the medial palpebral ligament. Many of its fibers insert onto the skin and the subcutaneous tissue of the brow forming the depressor supercilii. The orbicularis oculi overlaps with some of the fibers of the levator labii superioris alaeque nasi, the levator labii superioris, and the zygomaticus minor. The action of the orbital portion of this muscle aids in eye closure by elevating the lower lid. It also helps with the transport of tears, especially the lacrimal part, by exerting tractional forces on the lacrimal fascia, which in turn dilates the lacrimal sac. It is clear that skin retraction may affect the position of the orbicularis oculi in burn patients with ectropions. In addition, the epiphora seen in these patients, in part, is due to the inability of the orbital portion of the orbicularis to provide adequate tractual forces for the transport of tears to the lacrimal sac (11,12).

The bulk of the muscles in the cheek aesthetic unit are part of the buccolabial group of muscles. These muscles shape and control the buccal orifice and the lips. The muscles of the buccolabial group that spans the cheek include levator labii superioris alaeque nasi, levator labii superioris, zyomaticus minor and major, depressor labii inferioris, depressor anguli oris, buccinator, orbicularis orbis, and the platysma (11,12).

The levator labii superioris alaeque nasi muscle originates from the upper part of the frontal process of the maxilla, and runs inferolaterally. It then splits into medial and lateral slips. The lateral slip inserts into the lateral part of the upper lip connecting with the orbicularis oris and the levator labii superioris. The lateral slip of this muscle aids in upper lip eversion and pulling of the nasolabial fold. Severe burn deformities of the upper lip and upper lip-nasal unit may be caused by skin contraction, which may also cause secondary pulling of the lateral slip of the levator labii superioris alaeque nasi muscle or the levator labii superioris (11,12).

The levator labii superioris originates from both the maxilla and the zygomatic bones above the infraorbital foramen. It inserts between the zygomaticus minor and the levator labii superioris alaeque nasi in the substance of the orbicularis oris. Like the levator labii superioris alaeque nasi, it helps with upper lip eversion and traction on the nasolabial fold.

The zygomatic minor originates from the lateral aspect of the zygomatic bone, passes inferomedially, and inserts onto the upper lip musculature. It connects to the levator labii superioris at its insertion. It elevates the upper lip and in so doing exposes the upper teeth. The zygomaticus major arises from the zygomatic bone, lateral to the

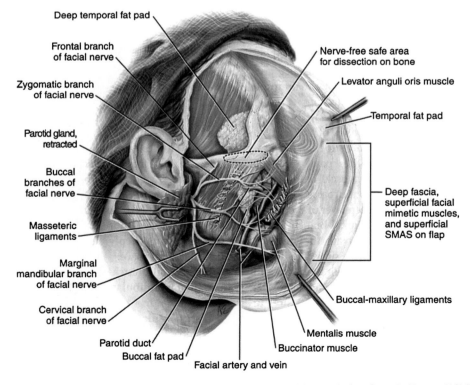

Figure 20.9   Anatomic layers of the cheek. [Reprinted with permission from LaTrenta (10).]

orbicularis oculi muscle. It inserts at the modiolus where it blends with some of the fibers of the upper lip musculature. It elevates the commissures, and also pulls the commissures laterally as one grins or smiles. In burn patients with microstomia it is possible that the zygomaticus minor muscle may be put on stretch as the orbicularis is pulled medially with scar contraction. The buccal branch of the facial nerve innervates both muscles. The depressor group of muscles consists of the depressor labii inferioris and the depressor anguli oris. They act to depress and evert the lower lip. The depressor anguli oris also acts on the commissures.

The buccinator occupies most of the space between the mandible and the maxilla. It attaches to the pterygomandibular raphe, the modiolus, the orbicularis oris, the maxilla, and the mandible. Most of its fibers attach deep to the submucosa in the cheek. Its actions include compressing the cheek against the gum and the teeth during mastication. It also aids the tongue in the direction of food to the molars. It also functions by expelling air from the oral cavity.

The platysma muscle originates from the neck and spans the lower aspect of Zone 3. It aids in lower lip eversion. The ansa cervicalis innervates the platysma. A "multilinked fibrous" system extending from the periosteum through the superficial musculoaponeurotic system (SMAS) to the dermis allows countless variations in facial expression through muscle contraction (10,12). The anatomic layers of this unit, beginning from skin,

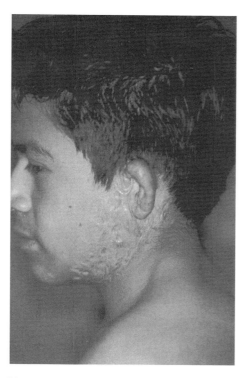

Figure 20.11 Fourteen-year-old patient with injury to Zone 2 with anterior displacement of the ear.

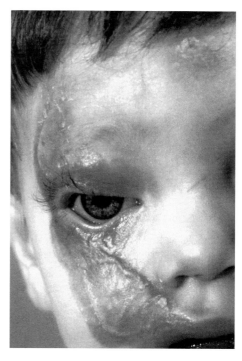

Figure 20.10 Five-year-old child with facial burns in Zone I producing a right lower eyelid ectropion.

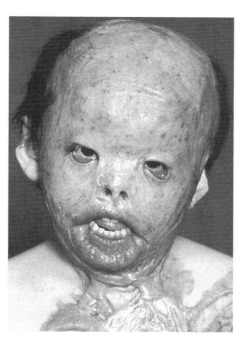

Figure 20.12 Nine-year-old female with grade IV neck contracture with lower eyelid ectropion and severe lower lip ectropion.

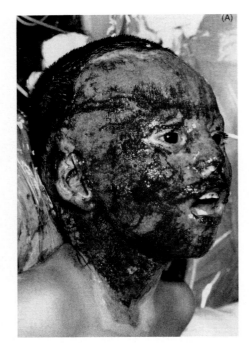
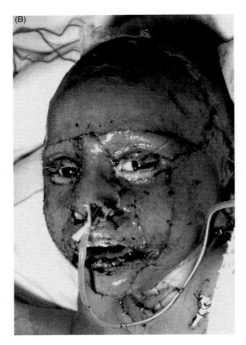
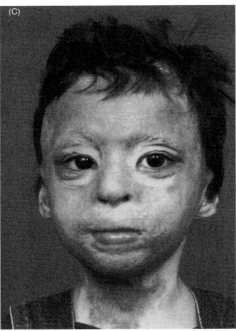

Figure 20.13   (A) Five-year-old patient with deep partial-thickness and full-thickness facial burns after early excision. (B) Resurfacing of face with scalp split-thickness skin grafts. (C) One-year follow-up. (Courtesy of Dr. S. E. Wolf and Dr. D. N. Herndon.)

are the superficial fat, the superficial SMAS, the mimetic muscles, and the deep layer of the SMAS. Underneath the deep layer of the SMAS is the plane containing the facial nerve, parotid gland and duct, facial artery and vein, and buccal fat pad (10,12) (Fig. 20.9).

The underlying bony framework with its overlying soft tissues gives the cheek the characteristic contour that typifies and helps to define the midface. In the superolateral to

the inferomedial trajectory, the nice smooth convexity of the malar eminence gradually transitions into the concavity of the nasolabial sulcus. The lateral aspects of the cheek flares into the defining mandibular angles that characterize the lower face. As the largest facial aesthetic unit, the cheek serves as a centerpiece for midface structures supporting the lower eyelids, nose, lips, and ears. Reconstruction of this unit not only restores aesthetic harmony, but also provides functional support (Figs. 20.10 and 20.11).

III. DEFORMITIES OF THE CHEEK

Deformities of the cheek can be produced by intrinsic factors or extrinsic forces. Since the cheek serves as the main buttress of the rest of the facial aesthetic unit, deformities of the cheek secondary to burns can distort the lower eyelids, the tragus, the nasal alae, and the commissures.

Intrinsic deformities are bound within the cheek subunits and can distort this aesthetic unit. These deformities can be produced by either hypertropic scars or burn scar contractures. Burn scar contractures can obliterate the smooth contours of the mid and lower face. The nasolabial fold can be effaced or accentuated as a result. Burn scar contractures in subunits C and A of the suborbital region (Zone 1) can produce ectropions of the lower eyelid (Fig. 20.12). Scars in the preauricular region (Zone 2) pose problems with auricular distortion producing anterior displacement (Fig. 20.13). Hypertrophic scars or contractures in this zone can also produce distortion in the lateral canthus of the eyes. Scars in the buccomandibular region (Zone 3) can produce microstomia. This not only interferes with the integrity of the oral cavity, but also may affect mandibular growth (1,2). In children, several studies have implicated retrognathia as a result of scarring and/or the use of pressure garments (13,14). Alae distortion and alteration of the nasolabial fold can also be witnessed with scars in Zone 2 and Zone 3.

Extrinsic deformities such as scar contraction in the surrounding aesthetic units can produce problems with cheek deformities. Most notably, cervical burn scar contractures, particularly Grade III and Grade IV contractures, can produce lower-eyelid and lower-lip ectropions (Fig. 20.14). Cervical contractures can also produce significant inferior pull on the buccomandibular region causing constriction of mandibular movement. Even in less severe contractures of the neck, the contour of the cheek is affected by the pull on the lower border of the cheek in a line parallel to the mandible (3). Other areas of concern include nasal burns and subsequent scarring that can affect the nasolabial fold. Also, auricular injuries can affect the preauricular region of the cheek subunit. Burn scars on the forehead subunit can cause distortion of the upper border of Zone 2. Deformities of this unit can be challenging to both the patient and even the most astute reconstructive surgeon.

IV. RECONSTRUCTION

A. Skin Grafts

The use of skin grafts for reconstruction of the chin units or subunits is well accepted. In the acute phase of injury, the

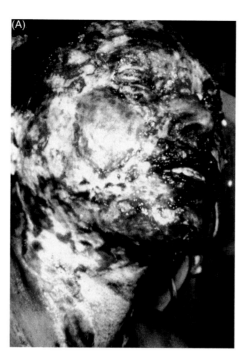

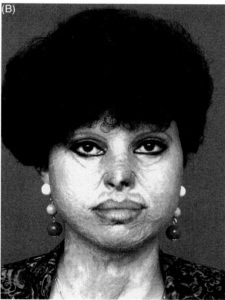

Figure 20.14 (A) Sixteen-year-old female with deep partial-thickness and full-thickness facial burns. (B) Final appearance after facial resurfacing, reconstruction of eyes, nose, and neck with skin grafts. Even after extensive reconstruction, cheek contour and facial features approach that of normal parameters.

use of skin grafts in the facial aesthetic units may decrease the need for subsequent reconstruction (Fig. 20.15). Unfortunately, in reconstruction, outside of the correction of lower-eyelid ectropions, the resultant reconstruction in Zones 2 or 3 using this technique may result in a patchwork appearance unless the entire cheek unit is grafted.

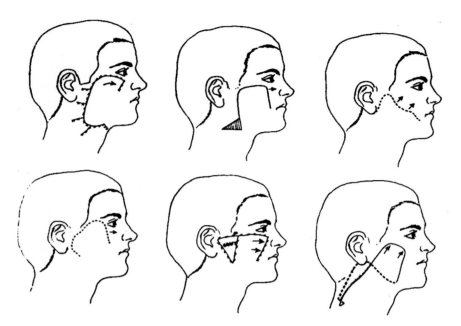

Figure 20.15 Various methods of cheek reconstruction. Variations in the rotation cheek flaps (above left). Esser (above center), Blascowcz (above right), Ferris Smith (below left), Mustarde (below center), Converse (below right), Stark, and Kaplan. [Reprinted with permission from Juri and Juri (15).]

It is well known that skin above the blush lines, above the supraclavicular region or from the inner aspect of the forearm provides the best appearance for skin grafts to the face. Yet this approach may not always be possible. In resurfacing the cheek unit with grafts because of contour irregularity and hyperpigmentation changes, if the majority of the cheek unit is involved, then resurfacing the entire cheek unit may be the best option (Fig. 20.16). However, obtaining a large sheet graft to resurface this region may only be possible in areas below the blush line such as the abdomen or flank. One method to obtain large grafts for resurfacing of burn defects is the use of expanded full-thickness grafts. Skin expansion is now a recognized surgical option in providing additional tissue for the resurfacing of soft tissue defects. In 1993, Bauer et al. (16) reported a series of 15 patients in whom expanded full-thickness skin grafts were used for reconstruction of defects either secondary to burn injury or due to the excision of congenital nevi. The burn patients underwent reconstruction of the aesthetic units of the face after burn injury using this technique. Uniformity of color and texture were reportedly excellent in comparison to nonexpanded full-thickness skin grafts. Expanded full-thickness skin grafts were felt to maintain all of the

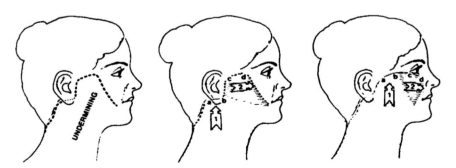

Figure 20.16 Method for advancement of cervicofacial flaps for cheek reconstruction. Our cervicofacial flap for cheek repairs (left). The incision line (dotted) and the area undermined (center). The cervical portion of the flap (vertically striped) is advanced upward and the horizontal portion (horizontally striped) is rotated forward. The arrows show the direction of movement (right). By comparing the location of points a, b, c, d, in this drawing with their location in the preceding drawing, the extent and direction of the movement become apparent. [Reprinted with permission from Juri and Juri (15).]

same characteristics with excellent aesthetic results and minimal graft size limitations. Without question, the use of buttock skin should be avoided at all costs. Its color mismatch in patients is striking, even from a distance.

B. Flaps

In 1918, Esser described the cheek rotation flap for the resurfacing of cheek defects (16). The disadvantage here was the visible scars left on the medial aspect of the face. Since that time, several variations in this technique have been published in an attempt to increase the surface area of the rotated cheek flap and to camouflage subsequent scarring (Fig. 20.17) (17–19). In 1979, Juri and Juri (15) combined advancement and rotation of large cervical cheek flaps for the reconstruction of cheek defects in which scars could be camouflaged (Fig. 20.18). Here, there is extensive undermining of the flap, which includes the cheek, the neck, the retroauricular and chin regions down to the clavicular line to enable complete mobilization. The cheek cervical flap is then advanced cephalad from the cervical area and rotated medially to resurface the cheek defect (16). Although their results were uniformly encouraging, the maximal size of the cervical defect that this flap corrects was not discussed. Later, Feldman employed this principle for resurfacing of large burn defects in patients with cheek burns but normal cervical skin (3,20).

C. Tissue Expansion

The use of tissue expansion in head and neck reconstruction of burn patients is well documented (21–25). However, these initial studies concentrated on the correction of burn alopecia. More recently, however, the use of tissue expansion in the neck to resurface cheek deformities has been addressed. In 1991, Weislander (26) documented his experience with tissue expansion in the head and neck in 28 patients. Similar to other investigators, the replacement of defects with local tissue of similar color match and texture was novel. Several general remarks were noted about the technical aspects of tissue expansion. The length and width of the expander should be as large as the defect. Avoidance of incisions bordering the defect is desirable. Dissection just below the subcutaneous flat is also recommended with the expander valve placed 7 cm or more away from the pocket. The gain in length of the expanded flap distance is measured by subtracting the base of the expander from the dome measurements. However, in reconstruction of cheek deformities using expanded cervicofacial flaps, it is difficult to always follow such guidelines. Incisions, although small, are usually placed at the junction of the defect and normal tissue. Secondly, because of the concavity of the

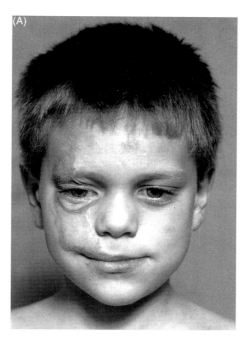

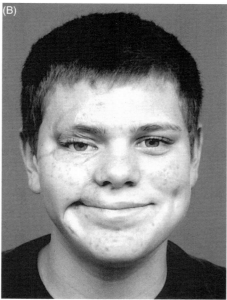

Figure 20.17 (A) Seven-year-old patient with right cheek scars with redundant full-thickness skin grafts after correction of right lower lid ectropion. (B) Six-year follow-up after revision of lower eyelid graft and cheek expansion to remove burn scars.

neck and the rotation advancement of these flaps, it is difficult to always estimate the amount of expanded flap movement. However, in the authors' experience 800–1200 cm^3 within an expander is necessary to resurface an entire cheek unit depending on the age of the patient. Although Weislander expanded tissue for reconstruction of the scalp, lips, ears, neck, and chin, cheek deformities were not addressed. Yet he did note that in expansion of the chin/neck angle, one case produced a neck contracture secondary to fibrosis in the subplatysma region. Later studies by Neale et al. (27) cautioned against the use of neck tissue expansion to resurface defects above the mandible. In a series of 37 patients, 52 expanders were placed for resurfacing of the neck and anterior face. However, long-term effects of gravity, growth, and scarring had a

significant impact on facial features. Neale et al. (27) cautioned that the use of expanded neck skin beyond the border of the mandible may be fraught with complications. In addition, the authors warned against linear scar formation and to only use expanded skin to correct facial defects in aesthetic units. In addition, it was felt that staged serial excisions, full-thickness grafts, local interdigitating flaps, or large neck flaps were preferable to expansion. The reported incidence of incomplete correction of

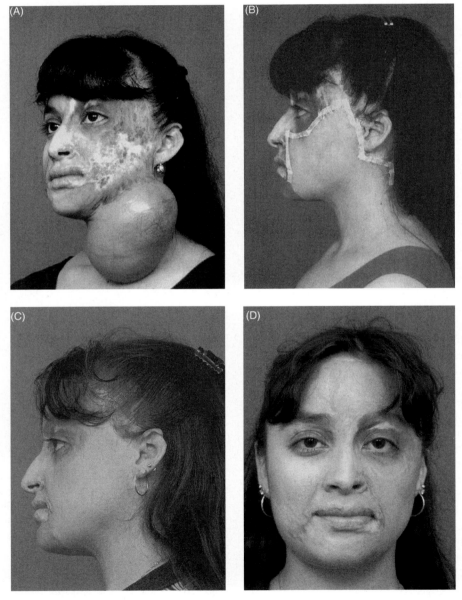

Figure 20.18   (A) Fourteen-year-old patient with left-sided facial scars, which included the cheek and (L) hemiforehead unit. A 680 cc tissue expander inflated to 800 cc. (B and C) Postoperative appearance after excision of cheek scars and rotation advancement of expanded cervicofacial flap; neck and chin contours are normal. (D) One-year follow-up after resurfacing of forehead with a full-thickness skin graft. Note normal cheek contour with an expanded cervicofacial flap.

the deformity and secondary deformities of the eyelids and lips leads to increased skepticism in the use of this technique for facial resurfacing (27). Because of the concerns voiced by Neale et al. (27) Hoekstra et al. (28) reported their experience using the pedicled expanded flap to resurface four patients with facial burns. Here, overexpanded flaps from the lower neck and chest were used to surface cheek defects. Division of the pedicle was performed 2 weeks later. Although this transfer did not fully correct the facial problems, a marked improvement was noted. It is important to note that in order to maximize the aesthetic results of tissue expansions, all contractures may require correction prior to resurfacing with expanded flaps. However, McCauley and Owiesy (29) reported excellent results in the use of expanded neck skin to resurface burn scars of the cheek without the use of a pedicled division later. Similar to the technique of advancement and rotation of nonexpanded cervical flaps described by Juri, the expanded cervicofacial flaps followed the same principles of rotation advancement with coverage of the entire cheek unit and minimal distortion of the normal facial features (Figs. 20.18–20.20). In a series of 28

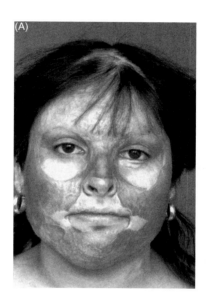 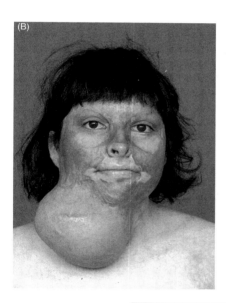 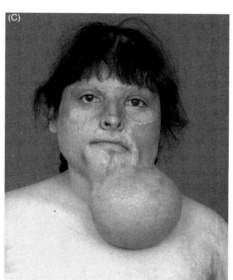

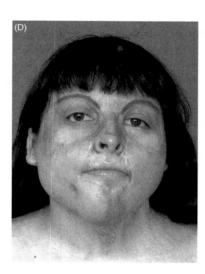 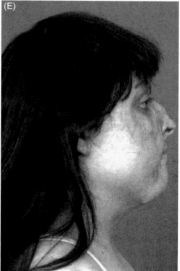

Figure 20.19 (A) Fifteen-year-old patient with hyperpigmentation of the chin and both cheeks. (B) Expansion of right side of neck for resurfacing of the right cheek. (C) Appearance 6 months later with expanded cervical skin on the left side. Patient previously sustained partial flap loss, necessary re-expansion. (D and E) Final appearance after resurfacing of both cheeks.

patients undergoing neck expansion for resurfacing of facial defects only, he noted that re-expansions were frequent but significant complications detected due to facial distractions were minimal. Although a major complication rate of 16.3% was noted (8/49 expanders removed for exposure or infection), the final results showed dramatic improvement in facial aesthetics. In 2000, Teot et al. (30) reported a series of seven patients who underwent prefabricated vascularized supraclavicular flaps for the resurfacing of burn scars of the face with excellent aesthetic improvement. Apparently, this flap can be made large enough to cover the entire facial unit, including the forehead, by simple advancement rotation of this flap with created openings for the eyes, nose, and mouth. Long-term follow-up, however, is not fully reported. Teot et al. (30) documented a 5-year follow-up of the first patient, indicating that the patient's facial movements have "progressively improved." Although details of insetting of the flap are omitted, it is extremely important not to produce an upper lip entropion and a lower lip ectropion using this technique.

The cheek is the largest aesthetic unit of the face. In spite of its elaborate contours, it is second only to the forehead in maintaining effective pressure using compressive garment therapy. Although recent studies have subdivided the cheek aesthetic unit into an additional three to five subunits, visualization of the face identifies the cheek as a single unit, which gradually blends the upper one-third and lower one-third of the entire lateral portions of the face.

The angular relationship between the lateral alar base and the cheek is difficult to reproduce after injury. The delicate contours of the cheek are important not only for facial shape, but also for facial harmony (31).

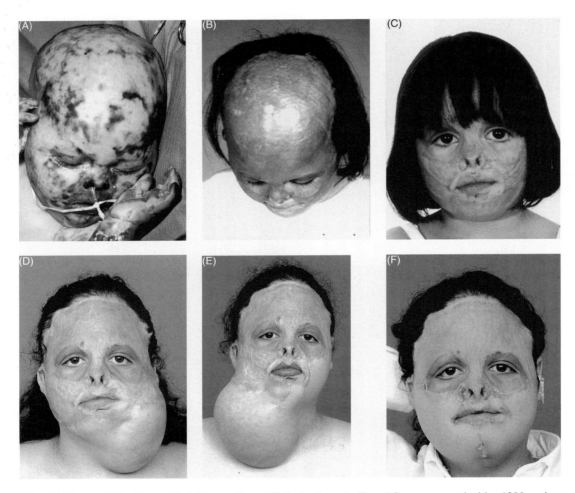

Figure 20.20 (A) Young child with total facial burns. (B and C) Scalp alopecia, Type 1C reconstructed with a 1200 cc tissue expander. (D) Age 14 with cheek and chin facial scarring and left-sided expanders in place for resurfacing the left cheek. (E) Right-sided neck expansion performed to resurface the right cheek. (F) Although the lower two-thirds of the face resurfaced, results were felt to be suboptimal. (G and H) Six months later, both cervical facial flaps elevated down to clavicle and advanced superiorly and medially for complete cheek resurfacing. (H) Six months' follow-up.

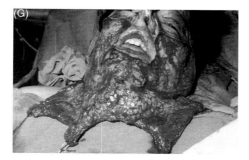
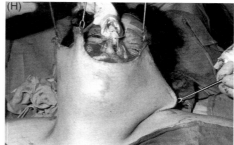

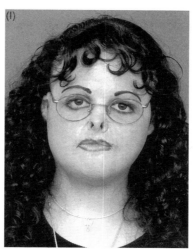

Figure 20.20 *Continued.*

D. Free-Tissue Transfer

The use of free-tissue transfer in the reconstruction of facial injuries is well documented (32–37). Even the groin flap has found a place in head and neck reconstruction, particularly for the treatment of hemifacial microsomia. However, it has given way to the scapular and parascapular flap for facial reconstruction, especially in the cheek region. In 1992, Upton et al. (33) reported their series of cheek reconstruction using the scapular and parascapular flap. Although none of these patients sustained thermal injuries, eight patients were treated for the sequela of irradiation burns. Aside from variations in the vascular anatomy, several points were made that influence the aesthetic outcome of these flaps. First, simultaneous dissection of the ipsilateral face and back is performed. In patients with postirradiation atrophy, extensions were needed to augment subcutaneous atrophy of the upper and lower lips. Secondly, Upton et al. (33) noted that the precise placement of the de-epithelialized flap to correct facial contours was the real challenge in this procedure. Unsatisfactory correction of facial contour was due to either overcorrection in the buccal region or underresection of fat and fascia in the proximal portion of the flap (38). In 1994, Pribaz et al. (38) described the use of a three-dimensional free flap for reconstruction of facial defects. Later, in 1995, Khouri et al. (36) reported his experience with the prefabricated induced expanded supraclavicular skin flaps. Later that year, Rose (35) addressed the issue of free-tissue transfer in patients with severe burn deformities. Although his results were successful, the approach was not met with uniform enthusiasm (39). Criticisms included poor texture, poor color match, bulk, and expense. However, the use of free-tissue transfer in facial burn injuries continues to be a part of the reconstructive options offered to burn victims.

The retroauricular temporal flap was described by Washio (40) as a pedicled flap for reconstruction of facial defects. Park et al. and others, reported the use of this flap as a free-tissue transfer (36,41,42). The vascular anatomy for this flap is based on the multiple anastomoses, which exist between the posterior auricular artery and the parietal branch of the superficial temporal artery. The thinness of this flap and its color match are touted as advantages for facial reconstruction. Thus, its use as a free flap in facial reconstruction seems to be advantageous.

However, one should bear in mind that resurfacing the entire cheek unit is not possible with this flap. In 1998, Milomir et al. (34) reported the use of the retroauricular temporal free flap for reconstruction of an electrical burn of the cheek nearly 3 months after injury. Debridement resulted in a defect measuring 12×7 cm that included partial removal of the zygomatic arch. Although a successful transfer was accomplished with excellent color match and with excellent patient satisfaction, facial deformities around the eyes and lips persisted.

There is little doubt that free-tissue transfer in the reconstruction of burn patients is not only possible, but in select cases, desirable. However, rarely do they represent the first line of reconstruction for burn patients. The indications for these procedures should be guided by the lack of availability of other techniques to provide adequate resurfacing of facial burns, and the need for composite tissue transfers (43). As we progress in search of ideal reconstructive procedures for the reconstruction of facial burns, free-tissue transfers will undoubtedly find its rightful place.

REFERENCES

1. Hunt JL, Purdue GF, Spicer T, Gennett G, Range S. Face burn reconstruction—does early excision and auto grafting improve results. Burns 1987; 13:39–44.
2. Jonsson CE, Dalsgaard CJ. Early excision and skin grafting of selected burns of the face and neck. Plast Reconstr Surg 1991; 88:83–94.
3. Fraulin FOG, Lllmayer SJ, Tredget EE. Assessment of cosmetic and functional results of conservative versus surgical management of facial burns. J Burn Care Rehab 1996; 17:19–29.
4. Voinchet V, Bardot J, Echinard C, Aubert JP, Magalon G. Advantages of early burn excision and grafting in the treatment of burn injuries to the anterior cervical region. Burns 1995; 21:143–146.
5. Gonzalez-Ulloa M, Castillo A, Stevns E et al. Preliminary study of the total restoration of the facial skin. Plast Reconstr Surg 1954; 13:151–161.
6. Gonzalez-Ulloa M. Reconstruction of the face covering by means of selective skin in regional aesthetic units. Br J Plast Surg 1956; 9:212–221.
7. Feldman JJ. Facial burns. In: McCarthy JG, ed. Plastic Surgery. Philadelphia: W.B. Saunders, 1990:2153–2236.
8. Cabrera RC, Zide BM. Cheek reconstruction. In: Aston SJ, Beasley RW, Thorne CHM, eds. Grabb and Smith's Plastic Surgery. Philadelphia: Lippincott-Raven, 1997:501–512.
9. Chandawarker RY, Cervino AL. Subunits of the cheek: an algorithm for the reconstruction of partial thickness defects. Br J Plast Surg 2003; 56:135–139.
10. LaTrenta GS. Atlas of Aesthetic Face and Neck Surgery. Philadelphia: W.B. Saunders, 2004.
11. Netter FH. Atlas of Human Anatomy. 9th ed. Teterboro: Icon Learning Systems, 2003.
12. Gray H. Gray's Anatomy: The Anatomical Basis of Medicine and Research. 38th ed. New York: Churchill Livingstone, 1999:791–800.
13. Fricke NB, Omnell L, Dutcher KD, Hollender LG, Engrav LH. Skeletal and dental disturbances after facial Burns and pressure garments use: a four-year follow-up. J burn Care Rehabil 1999; 20:239–249.
14. Fricke NB, Omnell L, Dutcher KD, Hollender LG, Engrav LH. Skeletal and dental disturbances after facial burns and pressure garments. J Burn Care Rehabil 1996; 17:338–345.
15. Juri J, Juri C. Advancement and rotation of a large cervico-facial flap for cheek repairs. Plast Reconstr Surg 1979; 64:692–696.
16. Bauer BS, Vicari FA, Richard ME, Schwed R. Expanded full thickness skin grafts in children. Plast Reconstr Surg 1993; 92:59–69.
17. Giles H, Millard DR. The Principles and Art of Plastic Surgery. Boston: Little, Brown & Co, 1957.
18. Start RB, Kaplan JM. Rotation flaps, neck to cheek. Plast Reconstr Surg 1972; 50:230.
19. McGregor IA. Eyelid reconstruction following total resection of upper or lower lid. Br J Plast Surg 1973; 26:346.
20. Feldman JJ. Reconstruction of the Burned Face in Children. In: Serafin D, Georglade NG, eds. Pediatric Plastic Surgery. St. Louis: Mosby Co., 1984.
21. Antonyshyn O, Gruss JS, Zucker R, MacKinnon SE. Tissue expansion in head and neck reconstruction. Plast Reconstr Surg 1988; 82:58–68.
22. Manders GK, Schenden MJ, Furrey JA, Hetzler PT, Davis TS, Graham WP. Soft tissue expansion: concepts and complications. Plast Reconstr Surg 1984; 74:493–507.
23. Manders GK, Graham WP, Schenden MJ, Davis TS. Skin expansion to eliminate large scalp defects. Ann Plast Surg 1984; 12:305–312.
24. Sasaki GH. In: Brent B, ed. The Artistry of Reconstructive Surgery: Scalp Repair by Tissue Expansion. St. Louis: Mosby Co., 1987.
25. McCauley RL, Oliphant JR, Robson MC. Tissue expansion in the correction of burn alopecia: classification and methods of correction. Ann Plast Surg 1990; 25(2):103–115.
26. Weislander JB. Tissue expansion in the head and neck. Scand J Plast Reconstr Hand Surg 1991; 25:47–56.
27. Neale HW, Kurtzman LC, Goh KB, Billmire DA, Yakuboff KP, Warden G. Tissue expanders in the lower face and anterior neck in pediatric burn patients: limitations and pitfalls. Plast Reconstr Surg 1993; 91:624–631.
28. Hoekstra K, Hudson DA, Smith AW. The use of pedicled expanded flaps for aesthetic resurfacing of the burned face. Ann Plast Surg 2000; 45:1–6.
29. McCauley RL, Owiesy F. Aesthetic reconstruction of facial burns in expanded cervicofacial flaps. Proc Am Burn Assoc 2001; 22:91.
30. Teot L, Cherenfant E, Otman S, Giovannini UM. Prefabricated vascularized supraclavicular flaps for face resurfacing after postburns scarring. Lancet 2000; 355:1695–1696.

31. Warpeha RL. Resurfacing the burned face. Clin Plast Surg 1981; 8:255–267

32. Goldsmith D, Sharzer L, Berkman MD. Microvascular groin flaps in the treatment of hemifacial microsomia. Cleft Palate-Craniofac J 1992; 29:44–71.

33. Upton J, Albin RE, Mulliken JB, Murray JE. The use of scapular and parascapular flaps for cheek reconstruction. Plast Reconstr Surg 1992; 90:959–971.

34. Milomir N, Hubli E, Anderl H. Facial reconstruction using a retroauricular-temporal free flap. Plast Reconstr Surg 1998; 102:1147–1150.

35. Ross HE. Aesthetic restoration of the severely disfigured face in burn victims: a comprehensive strategy. Plast Reconstr Surg 1995; 96:1573.

36. Khouri RK, Ozbek RM, Hruza GJ, Young VL. Facial reconstruction with prefabricated induced expanded (pig) supraclavicular skin flaps. Plast Reconstr Surg 1995; 95:1007–1015.

37. Fujino T, Harashina T, Nakajima T. Free skin flap from retroauricular to nose. Plast Reconstr Surg 1976; 57:338–341.

38. Pribaz JJ, Morris DJ, Milliken JB. 3-Dimensional folded free flap reconstruction of complex facial defects using intraoperative modeling. Plast Reconstr Surg 1994; 93:285–293.

39. Donelan MB. Invited commentary: aesthetic restoration of the severely disfigured face in burn victims: a comprehensive strategy. Plast Reconstr Surg 1995; 96:1578–1579.

40. Washio H. Retroauricular temporal flap. Plast Reconstr Surg 1969; 43:162.

41. Park C. The chondrocutaneous postauricular free flap. Plast Reconstr Surg 1989; 84:761–771.

42. Kolhe PS, Leonard AG. The posterior auricular flap: anatomic studies. Br J Plast Surg 1987; 40:562–569.

43. Park C, Shin KS, Kang HS, Lee YH, Lew JD. A new arterial flap from the postauricular surface: its anatomic basis and clinical application. Plast Reconstr Surg 1988; 82:498–504.

21

Reconstruction of the Burned Nose

MALACHY E. ASUKU
Ahmadu Bello University Teaching Hospital, Kaduna, Nigeria

ROBERT L. McCAULEY
University of Texas Medical Branch and Shriners Hospital for Children—Galveston Unit, Galveston, Texas, USA

I. INTRODUCTION

A. Historical Perspective

The history of nasal reconstruction is one that is richly recorded and is invariably synonymous to the history of the development of plastic surgery. Millard et al. (1) noted that the origins of plastic surgery are rooted in the correction of facial deformity and, specifically, in the restoration of the lost nose. The earliest account of a plastic surgical procedure is a description of an operation performed to reconstruct an amputated nose contained in the Indian *Sushruta Samhita* dated as far back as 600 BC (2–4). It is believed that at that time nasal reconstruction was performed by members of a caste of potters known as Koomas who utilized the forehead flap for their reconstructions. Their knowledge was said to have filtered through Persian, Greek, Arab, and Jewish scholars to the old Roman Empire (2–4). The excellence of the Indian

forehead flap is borne out by the fact that it is still being undertaken to this day with only minor modifications (2). Ben-Hur and Converse (3) noted that each human face is different and cannot be entirely reduplicated. They identified the nose as one of the main features responsible for the uniqueness of the individual face. Consequently, it comes as no surprise that ancient civilizations were concerned with the reconstruction of the nose in order to restore personality and identity (3).

The 16th century marked a major milestone in the history of nasal reconstruction and the development of plastic surgery. The Branca brothers of Sicily (1546–1599) introduced the concept of flap transplantation using pedicles from more distant points by successive migration. Yet it was Gaspare Tagliacozzi of Bologna who in his 1597 treatise titled "De Curtorum Chirurgia per Insitionem" described the use of the medial arm flap for the reconstruction of the nose. He discussed the concept of flap delay and emphasized the psychological benefits of a satisfactory outcome to the patient (3,4). In Tagliacozzi's own words, "we reconstruct and complete parts which nature had given but which were destroyed by fate, and we do so, not so much for the enjoyment of an eye, as for psychic comfort to the afflicted" (3). In the same century, Ambroise Pare wrote about a French man who following the loss of his nose in a fight went to Italy to have a new one reconstructed. He mentioned that the color match was not ideal and the nostrils differed from the original but that it was clearly better than an artificial silver nose, and more importantly, that the owner was happy with the new nose (3).

In 1816, Constantine Carpue, an English surgeon visited India to witness nasal reconstruction. He later published a book titled "an account of two successful operations for restoring a lost nose from the integuments of the forehead." He noted that the reconstructed nose was almost as good as the natural one and that the scar on the forehead was almost unnoticeable (2,4). This generated some enthusiasm among English surgeons. Keegan and Smith were among the first to adopt the technique and by 1823 they reported their successes with the technique. In 1836, Philibert Joseph Roux popularized the transplantation of pedunculated tissue into facial surgery. By 1857, T. P. Teale, a surgeon from Leeds General Infirmary, published an account of six cases of severe facial burns repaired by pedunculated flaps with impressive results (4). Though Baronio of Italy had performed experimental skin grafts on sheep in 1804, Bugner was the first to use the concept clinically. In 1823, he applied a skin graft from the thigh to the nose. In 1840, J. Warren Mason of Boston transplanted a full-thickness skin graft to the ala of the nose (3). It is rather interesting that by the turn of the 19th century, the two fundamental architectural principles which form the bedrock of plastic surgery, namely, the transplantation and manipulation of pedicled tissue and the grafting of tissue from one part of the body to another had both been introduced through reconstruction of no other organ than the nose (4). Today, following the experience that accrued from the reconstructions of extensive facial injuries during the two World Wars and the appreciation of the importance of form, color, contour, and harmony, the technique of nasal reconstruction has undergone infinite refinements in the search for perfection. Thus, nasal reconstruction has continued to constitute a daunting challenge to successive generations of reconstructive surge.

II. ANATOMY

The nose is a complexly contoured, multilayered three-dimensional structure occupying a central position on the face. It is composed of three distinct anatomical layers,

each of which serves a specialized function and contributes to the uniqueness of the nose. The outer covering of thin subcutaneous tissue and skin is protective and conforms to the contours of the underlying skeletal framework giving the nose its shape. The framework consists of thin and delicate scaffold of bone and cartilage providing projection at the root of the nose and support for the nasal sidewalls and alae. Millard (5) emphasized that the major function of the skeletal framework is in the maintenance of the nasal profile and patency of the airways. The innermost layer is a highly specialized and vascular hair-bearing mucous membrane. This layer nourishes the overlying cartilaginous structure and also contributes to the filtration and humidification of inhaled air. Burget and Menick (6) described the normal natural nose as being made up of thin vascular lining, sculptured alar tip cartilages, bone and cartilage braces that buttress the dorsum and the side walls, and a conforming canopy of thin skin that matches the face in color, texture, and hair distribution. The nose consists of two mirror image parts separated by the columella anteriorly and the nasal septum posteriorly. Spatially, the nose projects beyond the plane of the face and head, and is noticeable in the frontal and profile views making it rather prone to ridicule and assault. Despite its array of shapes and sizes, the nose has been aptly described as adding beauty to the face. Beyond that, however, it serves as the external route through which the respiratory function of gaseous exchange is made possible. Bernard (7) observed that the three-dimensional shape of the nose causes bright highlights and deep shadows, making any defects in form immediately noticeable even from a distance. They also noted that the nose, therefore, has a profound effect on an individual's perception of self-esteem and outlook to life.

III. CURRENT CONCEPTS IN THE ACUTE CARE OF THE BURNED NOSE

Fortunately, full-thickness burns of the nose occur less frequently when compared to partial-thickness burns, which are seen in about 70% of patients that suffer burns to the head and neck regions (8). Sir Archibald McIndoe (4) noted that following facial burns, the nose is partially or completely lost next in frequency to the eyelids; however, the loss may be limited to the covering skin with mild marginal loss of the nostril tip and columella. Treatment of the burn wound in the region of the face and neck differs from that in other parts of the body. Here, the concern over burn wound infection and subsequent sepsis in this region is minimal due to its excellent vascularity (8). Attention to minimizing edema by elevating the head of the bed and preventing infection by covering the affected areas with moist topical antimicrobials are, however, necessary to prevent conversion of partial-thickness burns to deeper burns. The rich vascularity and the high density of skin appendages allows for rapid re-epithelialization and early healing (8–10). Consequently, all but the most obvious full-thickness burns should be observed and treated conservatively prior to any consideration of skin grafting.

Deep partial-thickness burns of the nose may require no more than physiologic saline dressing with frequent changes if cartilage is not exposed. Alternatively, topical antimicrobial agents capable of eschar penetration and protecting the cartilage may be used (8). Debridement, if at all necessary, should be minimal and delayed until non-viable tissue is adequately demarcated. Boswick (8) observed that early surgical excision of full-thickness burns of the nose might damage the underlying cartilage, with a subsequent deformity that is a significant aesthetic problem. Pressure necrosis of the nasal soft triangles from placement of nasogastric and nasotracheal tubes may result in unwarranted tissue loss. The placement and fixation of such tubes should be undertaken with caution. Pressure points from these tubes should be relieved when found to produce further ischemia and subsequent necrosis (9,10). When skin graft is required, the supraclavicular area, posterior auricular region, and the inner upper arm are favored to provide grafts of satisfactory texture and color match (9). Lyle et al. (10) noted that meticulous technique and planning of the initial resurfacing with skin grafts could reduce the need for a secondary reconstructive procedure in the future. However, following healing of the acute burn wound, significant disfiguring problems may still occur as a result of scar hypertrophy and contractures (Fig. 21.1). The appropriate use of splints and appliances such as custom-made pressure garment, facial moulage, and the Uvex clear facemask may lessen this problem and result in earlier maturation of the burn scar, but secondary reconstruction is best undertaken when there is complete maturation of the scars. On occasion, however, severe cicatricial contraction of the nares may occur requiring the immediate use of custom-made nasal splints in mild cases and early reconstruction in severe cases with significant soft tissue loss.

IV. GENERAL CONCEPTS OF NASAL RECONSTRUCTION

According to Burget and Menick (11,12), the goal of nasal reconstruction must be the viewer's perception. They observed that tissues must be manipulated to achieve the desired visual result since success is not measured by the restoration of anatomy only, but also by the restoration of a naturally and aesthetically correct contour. They noted that the nose is not defined by its epithelial cover

or lining, or by the rigidity of its framework. The nose is defined by the specific shape that makes it look natural and attractive. They believed, therefore, that nasal reconstruction starts with visualizing an end result and then formulating a plan of action to achieve this goal. The reconstructive surgeon should analyze the defect and determine what is missing and what can be used to restore the defect. Like tissue must be used to replace like tissue as much as possible and in three dimensions. Successful reconstruction, therefore, depends on the judicious choice of donor materials, the precise use of nasal support, and the anticipation of the uncontrollable contractile forces of healing (11,12). However, one must realize that it is not always possible to re-create the perfect human nose, particularly in burn patients. This information may curb any unrealistic expectations by the patient. Appreciation of the detailed three-dimensional anatomy of the nose is key to any measure of success in nasal reconstruction. The principles proposed by Gonzalez-Ulloa in 1954 recognized that the nose is an aesthetic unit of the face. The later definition of its regional or topographic subunits by Burget and Menick in 1985 has been monumental in setting the standards for what should constitute nasal reconstruction today. Burget and Menick identified nine topographic subunits of the nose comprising the dorsum, nasal tip and columella, and the paired sidewalls, ala-nostril sills, and soft triangles (Figs. 21.1–21.3).

They observed that the dorsum, nasal tip, columella, and the ala-nostril sills are convex, while the sidewalls and soft triangles are concave in outline. They further noted that the outline of the subunits are derived by direct observation of surface contour and must be known and visualized during the planning and execution of nasal reconstruction. This subunit approach demands that nasal defects be analyzed on the basis of the aesthetic unit and its topographic subunits. Burget and Menick emphasized the need for the judicious choice and modification of recipient and donor tissue to provide for the exact replacement of nasal defects as subunits. These principles allow reproduction of the expected contours and landmarks that create the perception of the normal. They substantiated this concept by observing that when a large part of a subunit has been lost, replacing the entire subunit rather than simply patching the defect often gives a superior result. They also noted that when defects and reconstructions are made to fit topographic subunits, border scars of flaps tend to mimic the normal shadowed valleys and lighted ridges of the nasal surface. This allows the reconstructed part to blend into the residual nose and match the contralateral normal side. Although these general principles of nasal reconstruction remain valid, irrespective of the etiology of the nasal defect, one must admit the fact that when dealing with the burned nose, the difficulties are multiplied and

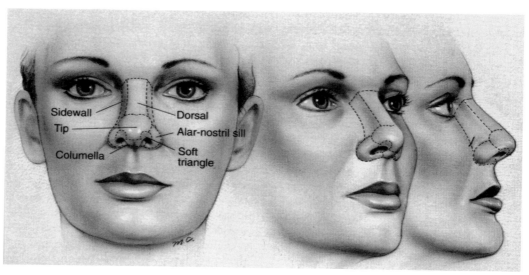

Figure 21.1   Aesthetic units of the nose. [Reprinted with permission from Burget and Menick (12).]

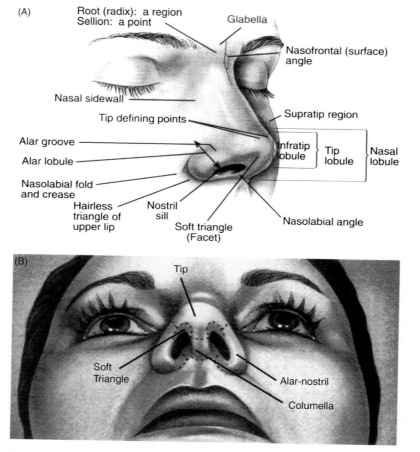

Figure 21.2   Surface anatomy of the nose. [Reprinted with permission from Burget and Menick (12).]

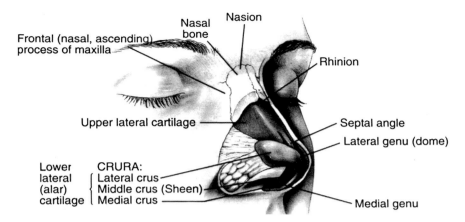

Figure 21.3 Bony and cartilaginous anatomy of the nose. [Reprinted with permission from Burget and Menick (12).]

additional considerations must be entertained. Most importantly, isolated nasal burns are rather unusual. When the nose is involved in burn injury, it is usually a part of more extensive facial burns. Lyle et al. (10) believed that in the reconstruction of postburn deformities of the face, the restoration of structures associated with active function should precede that for structures associated with passive function. They suggested that restoration of the burned nose should take highest priority considering its focal position both on the face and in the patient's perception and concerns. In practical terms, this means that only local tissues that survived the initial burn injury and were not used for reconstructions as the eyelids and lips would be available for nasal reconstruction. Another major issue is the choice of local tissue for postburn nasal reconstruction. In the presence of surrounding facial burns, nasal reconstruction with equally burned tissue is likely to produce a more harmonious appearance. Utilization of unburned tissue for nasal reconstruction in patients with total facial burns which required skin grafts may not only make the deformity more apparent but may also draw unnecessary attention to the rest of the face. Although the accurate and aesthetic reconstruction of the burned nose is critical, it may be unrealistic to have the same expectations that we have for patients undergoing isolated defects resulting from excision of congenital lesions and tumors. However, we should not underscore the zeal with which nasal reconstruction must be approached in the rehabilitation of the patient who has suffered the devastation of facial burns.

V. CLASSIFICATION OF POSTBURN NASAL DEFORMITY

Brou et al. (13) in a survey of 25 patients who suffered mean total body surface area (TBSA) burns of 71%

(65% full thickness) noted that 46% (235/512) of the reconstructive needs were in the head and neck region. Of these, the need for nasal reconstruction was third in frequency to reconstructive needs around the mouth and eyebrow/lid complex.

The need to reconstruct the burned nose is largely determined by the depth of the initial injury and the quality of acute care given to the burn wound. Fortunately, the nasal bones are rarely involved in burn injuries. However, the cartilaginous structures along with the overlying skin are frequently destroyed or severely distorted. The importance of making an accurate diagnosis before embarking on nasal reconstruction cannot be overemphasized. Classifying postburn nasal deformity in a manner that identifies the specific anatomical structures involved should serve as a template for developing a reconstructive plan. Postburn nasal deformities can be broadly classified into two groups: isolated soft tissue deformities and composite tissue deformities. While the composite tissue deformities may be partial or total, the soft tissue deformities which may affect the alae and/or the columella are frequently due to contraction of adjacent burned tissue (Table 21.1).

Table 21.1 Classification of Postburn Nasal Deformities

A. Soft-tissue defects
   I. Alar retraction/contractures
   II. Nostril stenosis
   III. Columella contractures
B. Composite defects
   I. Nasal alar loss—partial/total
   II. Columella and septal loss
   III. Total nasal loss
   IV. Total loss of cartilaginous vault
   V. Absence of nasal bones and cartilaginous vault

VI. RECONSTRUCTIVE OPTIONS

The first challenge in nasal reconstruction is to accurately define which structures are distorted or destroyed. Traditionally, nasal reconstruction is undertaken with emphasis on the replacement of lost tissue by anatomic layers (cover, lining, and support) and on methods of tissue transfers (grafts and flaps) (12). A broad knowledge of the reconstructive options using both local and distant tissues is of paramount importance. These options, as well as their advantages and disadvantages, should be fully discussed with the patient in order to ensure adequate cooperation through the often multiple stages of surgery (7,10). As opposed to defects following tumor excision, the burned nose usually has its upper half and bones intact while the skin is commonly compromised. The major deficit is the external covering of the nose, but scar contractures can severely deform the remaining tissues even when little is actually missing (7). Deformities of the alae and columella are often due to contractures of adjacent burned tissues and may be corrected by appropriate releases of the offending scar bands (10). Local transposition flaps such as the Z-plasty or any of its modifications and the V–Y advancement flap may be found suitable in this regard.

For most other deformities more extensive reconstructive efforts are often required. A common deformity that results from spontaneous healing of severe burns of the nose with loss of rim substance is the thin shiny nose with alar retraction and eversion of the nares. The lower lateral cartilages are rotated externally and are frequently seen as the leading edge of the nostril exposing the vestibule of the nose. According to Stephen and Brody (14) the goals in the correction of this deformity include restoration of the normal skeletal relationships, obtaining skin of normal thickness at the margin of the nose, and obtaining smooth and stable dorsal coverage with a minimum number of seams.

One surgical option involves the release of the nostril border by means of an incision on the cranial aspect of the lobule and turning down the resulting tissue in a caudal direction as a hinge flap to provide lining. This lengthens the nose; the margin and dorsum are then resurfaced with thick split-thickness or full-thickness skin grafts (7,10,14). Bernard (7) observed that the key to a good result with resurfacing is to use good quality skin grafts of sufficient size to cover an entire topographic subunit. They suggested the use of skin grafts obtained from above the level of the clavicle for better color and texture match. The supraclavicular and posterior auricular regions have long been recognized as suitable donor sites of full-thickness skin grafts. However, dermabrasion and overgrafting with a thick-split-thickness skin graft has also been suggested where the residual skin on the nasal dorsum is thin, irregular, or unstable (14).

The grafts are secured with tie-over bolsters at the alar bases while the vestibules are loosely packed with lubricated gauze. In order to add bulk to the alar skin and eliminate scar lines along the graft margins, the entire nasal unit can be dermabraded and overgrafted as the final stage of the reconstruction. Contracted nostrils can usually be opened by Z-plasties at the base or apex. However, the more severe stenosis often requires the use of skin grafts or flaps after the opening has been enlarged. The patient must then wear custom-made splints continuously for several months (4,15). Columellar contractures are often amenable to local tissue rearrangement. The V–Y advancement has been used in minor degrees of contractures. The use of forked skin flaps has also been useful in columellar lengthening. More severe contractures may require release and resurfacing with either thick split-thickness skin graft or full-thickness skin graft. In some cases reconstruction of the entire upper lip-nasal unit may be necessary (Fig. 21.4).

For composite loss of the ala, the reconstructive options will depend on the extent of the loss. When >50% of the ala is lost, two choices exist. The nasal ala may be converted to a total defect and corrected with the forehead flap for coverage. Alternatively, it may be corrected with a composite graft from the ear (Fig. 21.5). When the loss is less than 50%, the selected option must at least provide lining and coverage. The inclusion of cartilage though desirable may not be critical in reconstructing small defects. The nasolabial flap has been described as an ideal choice in these situations. The flap can be used even if scarred provided it is delayed and designed to include adequate subcutaneous tissue (7,16). Spear et al. (17) described the use of the folded nasolabial flap to provide both lining and cover. Flaps from the cheek and mouth based on various branches of the facial artery have also been described for correcting minor degrees of composite ala losses (18–20). Hataya et al. (19) described the reconstruction of the burned nasal alae with vascular island skin flaps pedicled on the infraorbital artery. They observed that while the technique obviates the need for secondary repair of a "dog ear," the donor site requires closure with a skin graft. The auricular composite graft obtained from the auricular helix has also been used extensively for the correction of composite ala losses (Fig. 21.6). This has previously been limited to correction of only small-sized defects due to the precarious survival of the composite graft in a scarred recipient tissue. Recently, however, various modifications have been introduced to improve survival of larger composite grafts. Soeda and Nakayama (21) described a modification with cartilage protruding from the inner edge of the graft to increase the contact surface of the graft and also contribute to fixation and support (Fig. 21.6). They also described the use of a composite graft from the helix in continuity with a

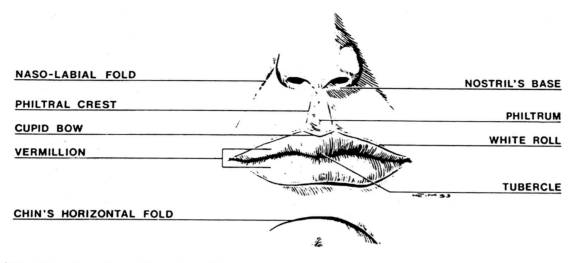

Figure 21.4 Dimensions of upper lip-nasal unit. [Reprinted with permission from Maillard GF, Montandon D. Reconstructive surgery of deep burns to the lips. Clin Plast Surg 1984; 11:655–668.]

retroauricular skin graft for the simultaneous correction of ala defect and replacement of scarred dorsal skin.

With extensive structural damage to the nose, options for subtotal and total nasal reconstruction become appropriate. These are often complex and may involve multiple stages. In the rare event of loss of nasal bones, auricular cartilage, rib, or cranial bone grafts have been used as struts for projection and support. Bernard (7) observed that critical to the success of this technique is the provision of adequate lining tissue and well-crafted septal and ala framework. Furthermore, Burget and Menick (6,12) observed that nasal support is best supplied at the time of soft tissue lining and cover construction. They also observed that loss of lining is the chief enemy of nasal reconstruction. Converse (22,23) observed that the forehead and scalp provide the best tissue for nasal reconstruction in terms of color match, texture, availability, and ease of reconstruction. This is evident in the multitude of techniques that have evolved over the years utilizing the forehead and scalp tissues in nasal reconstruction. These

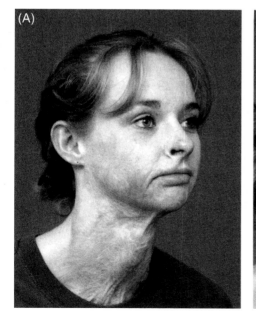 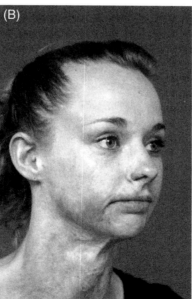 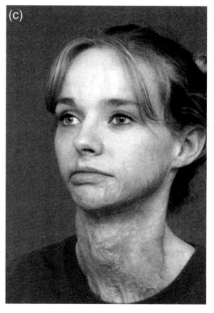

Figure 21.5 (A) Seventeen-year-old female with facial burns. (B) Composite graft from ear used for reconstruction with 6-month follow-up. (C) Contralateral preoperative appearance.

include the medial forehead flap based on the supratro-chlear vessels, the fronto-temporal flap, the Converse scalping flap, and the retroauricular-temporal flap described by Washio (24). The medial forehead flap is often favored and can be used even when scarred so long as the frontalis muscle is spared (7,25). The flap is harvested based on the supratrochlear artery, which can be identified by means of Doppler velocimetry. The base of the flap is narrowed to allow for unconstrained rotation while the distal end of the flap can extend into the hairline. The forehead flap may be augmented by preexpansion, which also allows the use of the flap with different orien-tations such as the superiorly based forehead flap

(7,10,26–29) (Figs. 21.7 and 21.8). The donor defect is reduced by direct closure while the residual defect is either skin grafted or allowed to heal secondarily. Bernard (7) observed that the latter heals surprisingly well and may become unnoticeable with time. This approach is now favored over closure of the donor defect with skin grafts.

In those patients whose forehead tissue is considered too extensively burned and in those who do not want additional scars on their forehead, distant flaps must be considered (7). Historically, such distant flaps were tubed and transferred in multiple stages. The classic medial arm flap described by Tagliacozzi three centuries

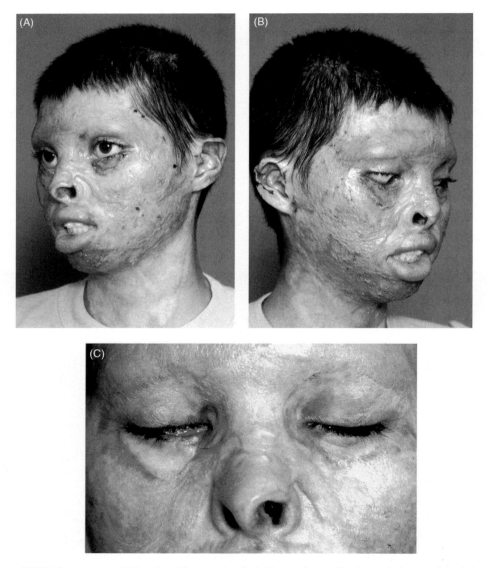

Figure 21.6   (A and B) Eighteen-year-old female with extensive facial burns. Loss of both nasal ala from burn injury; right-sided alar defect grather than left. (C) Close-up of both alar defects. (D) Extended composite grafts from ears for reconstruction. (E) One year after extended composite grafts. (F and G) Right and left nasal views at 2 years.

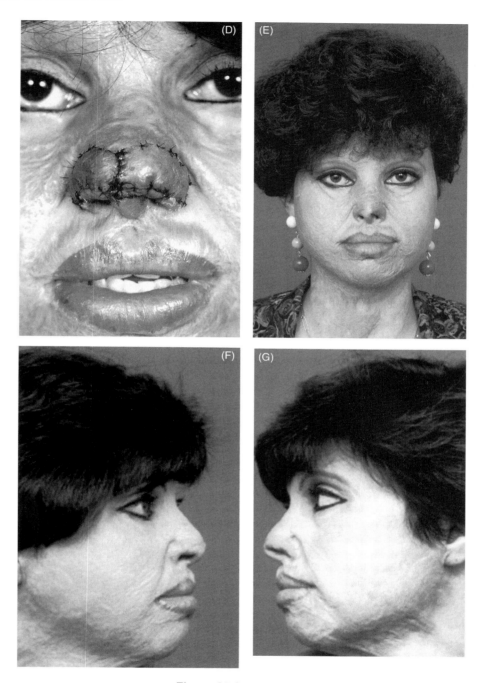

Figure 21.6 *Continued.*

ago was most popular for the reconstruction of the nose. Other tubed flaps used in nasal reconstruction include the deltopectoral flap and the transverse cervical flap (7,10,30,31). These flaps are cumbersome and can be fraught with complications. They have since been abandoned with the advent of microsurgical techniques.

Microsurgical techniques have allowed the one-stage use of well-tailored, high-quality tissues from remote

sites. Perhaps the first report on the use of free flaps in nasal reconstruction was that by Zhou and Cao (32) in 1989. They reported the use of a free flap based on the cutaneous branch of the acromiothoracic artery in correcting nasal deformities in nine patients, two of which were postburn. Subsequently, Benmeir et al. (33) in a case report described the use of the dorsalis pedis free flap for nasal reconstruction in a patient who had survived a

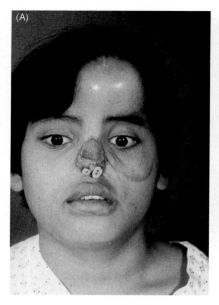 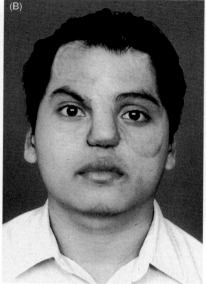 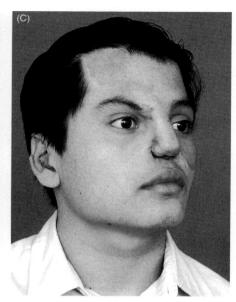

Figure 21.7 (A) Ten-year-old male referred after attempted nasal reconstruction using a scalping flap. Note: Expander inflated for second operation. (B and C) PA, lateral view after resurfacing with forehead flap and nasal tip augmentation.

75% full-thickness burn involving all other conventional flap donor areas. They used the superior labial artery and jugular vein as recipient vessels in a two-staged procedure. They recognized the larger vessels, the good texture match, and the large size of the flap, which enabled them to sculpture and refine the reconstructed nose at the second stage. However, it was noted that a significant donor site morbidity develops with the use of this flap. The thinness and adaptability of the radial forearm flap has made it a widely used free flap in reconstruction of the nose (34–36). Recent modifications of the flap have included pretransfer thinning of the flap and the inclusion of a portion of radial bone to provide structural support. The same concept has been extended to the dorsalis pedis flap with the inclusion of part of the metatarsal bone (37).

It would appear as though with microvascular capabilities, the options for nasal reconstruction are endless. Shenaq et al. (38) described the use of the composite auricular flap as free vascularized tissue to fill a large alar defect by harvesting the root of the helix with its feeding branch from the superficial temporal artery. Similarly, Pribaz and Falco (39) in 1993 reported the use of the auricular microvascular transplant for nasal reconstruction. A more recent innovation in the use of free flaps is the technique of prelamination and prefabrication of flaps (40). Khouri et al. (41,42) described the transfer of the radial forearm fascia to a subcutaneous pocket made from expanded supraclavicular skin. After 3 months, the tissue consisting of lining and coverage is then transferred on a vascular pedicle to the face for reconstruction of

complex contour deformities. Costa et al. (43) also reported the use of the radial forearm flap for prefabricated nasal reconstruction. Though the case presented in their report followed tumor excision, the concept can be applied to the reconstruction of the burned nose. One of the largest series in the literature on flap prelamination and prefabrication in the reconstruction of the burned nose is perhaps that reported by Pribaz et al. (44). They noted that tissue neovascularized by implanting a vascular pedicle can be transferred as a prefabricated flap based on the blood flow through the implanted pedicle. This technique potentially allows any defined tissue volume to be transferred to any specified recipient site, greatly expanding the armamentarium of reconstructive options. Pribaz et al. (44,45) and Pribaz and Fine (46) noted that this technique is particularly useful in patients who have survived large surface burns with marked facial disfigurement in whom thin donor sites are limited. It suffices to say that both of these techniques are relatively new and experience with them is limited. They also require multiple stages at prolonged intervals. Pribaz et al. (44) observed that in order to overcome venous congestion, prefabrication time might have to be extended to several months.

A. Nasal Prosthesis

The difficulties associated with the autologous reconstruction of contoured structures such as the nose and the ear have continued to allow the use of prosthesis in burn rehabilitation. Advancements in the techniques and materials used for prosthetic replacements have led some to

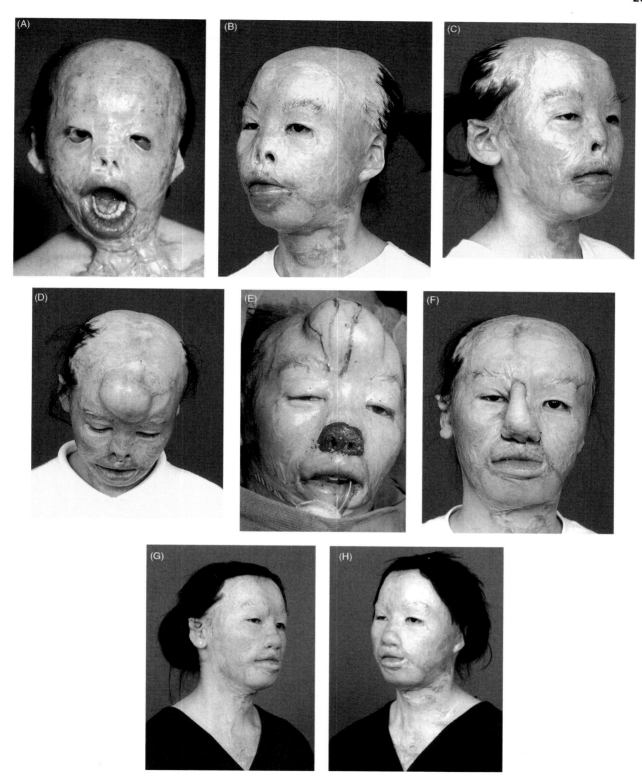

Figure 21.8 (A) Nine-year-old female with multiple facial deformities including eyelid ectropions, lower lip ectropion, and a Grade IV cervical contracture. (B and C) After correction of facial deformities, patient presents for correction of nasal tip deformity; 3 years have passed since the initial presentation. (D) Expanded forehead flap with expander placed under frontalis muscle and scar tissue. (E) Intraoperative photographs of turndown flaps for nasal lining and conchal cartilage grafts for support. (F) Turndown scar flaps were used for lining and cartilage grafts for support prior to resurfacing the nasal tip with the forehead flap. (G and H) Final appearance at 1 year with hairpiece.

believe that this option may be an acceptable alternative to reconstruction. Additionally, the increasing number of patients now surviving large surface area burns has led to increase in the number of patients who may be unsuitable for multistage reconstructive procedures. While some of these patients are unable to tolerate general anesthesia, others may have no pliable tissue to enable the required reconstructions (7). However, prostheses are usually not incorporated into the overall image of the patient. Its removal for cleansing further reminds patients of the anatomic loss of the nose and subsequent facial identity. The development of osseo-integration, techniques as a means of prosthetic anchorage has contributed to the renewed interest in the use of prostheses. This technique involves the placement of implants into the adjacent facial bone in the first instance. The overlying soft tissue is subsequently prepared by means of pegs and magnets to enable firm attachment of the fabricated prostheses. This has been largely successful though a number of complications and inadequacies continue to accompany the use of prostheses. Prostheses are not very suitable for very young patients who may be unable to adequately protect and maintain them. Furthermore, there is the constant need to review and replace the prosthesis as the child grows. Complications encountered even in the adult population include infections, minor skin reactions, and problems with anchorage. Despite these problems, however, prostheses may continue to play a role in the rehabilitation of the severely burned patient.

VII. POSTBURN NASAL RECONSTRUCTION IN THE PEDIATRIC PATIENT

Nasal reconstruction in the pediatric age group requires special considerations. Burget and Menick (12) observed that irrespective of the indication, nasal reconstruction in these diminutive patients imposes restraints. They noted that the immaturity of tissues coupled with normal growth and development have raised a number of questions, many of which are as yet unanswered. The principal issues are whether the rebuilt portion of the nose will grow in proportion to the developing face and the effects of surgical manipulation on residual nasal development. Other concerns are related to the appropriate time to initiate reconstruction. Here, quantity and quality of tissue is of concern. Furthermore, the technique and stages of reconstruction must be given due consideration in a bid to minimize the need for subsequent revisions. Generally speaking, it appears that several investigations in this field have agreed upon some principles. According to Burget and Menick (12), there is sufficient evidence to show that interference with the existing intranasal structures (the septum, naso-ethmoid complex, and nasal

vestibules) may arrest the growth of the nose. Consequently, they feel that surgery on the residual internal parts of the normal nose should be avoided until facial growth is complete. They also noted that there are few data to indicate the degree or rate of growth of skin flaps used as nasal cover. The experience in children has been that significant growth occurs in the skin and fat of the forehead flap at least in the first 4 years. The growth potential of the lining and the support is more unpredictable. They therefore, suggested that nasal reconstruction in the pediatric patient should be planned as a conservative and staged procedure. Adjacent normal tissue should be preserved in violation of the subunit principle. Donor tissues such as auricular cartilage are better preserved for the definitive procedure.

Postburn nasal reconstruction in the pediatric age group may constitute an even bigger challenge. Neale et al. (9) observed that an appropriate distinction must be made between the treatments of the burned face of the child and adolescent, and that of the adult. They observed that the burn wound of the child, in addition to being deeper, is complicated by relentless scar contractures and scar hypertrophy leading to significant secondary disfigurement. They further noted that the reconstructive efforts are not only directed at these complications, but are also subject to their effects. Consequently, satisfactory outcome takes longer to develop as the scars mature and remodel. Furnas et al. (31) espoused the principle of staged reconstruction of the burned nose in the pediatric patient. They suggested the use of distant pedicled tissue, initially, so that the best local donor sites are reserved for use in the final reconstruction after facial maturity. Although most authors believe in the delay of nasal reconstruction in children, we must keep in mind that the surgery comes at a time when the patient is expected to be overcoming the psychological effects of his injury. Some authors have also suggested reconstructing a relatively oversized or large nose in the pediatric patient so that as the face matures it catches up with the nose. This approach, however, must seek to define an oversized nose in practical and measurable terms. Finally, despite the poor suitability of the use of prostheses in children, this may offer an acceptable respite while awaiting facial maturity. The main advantage will be the fact that no surgery is undertaken at a time when growth potential of tissues may be jeopardized and final reconstruction will be spared of the scarring of earlier surgeries. However, recently, Giugliano et al. (47) reported their experience with nasal reconstruction using the forehead flap in 10 patients under 10 years of age. Although only one patient sustained burn injuries, this group made some interesting observations. It was felt that the subunit principal as noted by Burget and Menick required modifications (Fig. 21.9). Secondly, although the results are quite

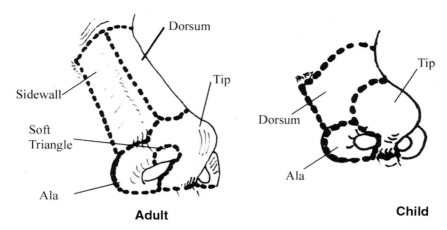

Figure 21.9 Comparison of adult and child nasal aesthetic units. [Reprinted with permission from Giugliano (47).]

acceptable, the mean follow-up of 5 years still leaves unanswered questions relative to the final aesthetic and functional evaluation of these patients. Yet, in spite of the success of this group with pediatric nasal reconstruction using the forehead flap, the issues of comparative aesthetic units and the timing of nasal reconstruction in the pediatric population continue to be debated (48).

VIII. CONCLUSION

Patients who have survived thermal injuries to the face suffer severe disfigurement. When the nose is involved, the deformities become immediately obvious with negative consequences on the patient's perception of self-image and self-esteem. The emotional and psychological effects can be crippling. The reconstruction of these defects requires a careful analysis of the missing segments as well as a detailed inventory of potential donor sites. Analysis of soft tissue defects vs. composite tissue loss is crucial to the selection of reconstructive options to provide the best aesthetic results. It is, therefore, important that all options available for improving the patient's appearance are brought to bear. The reconstruction should provide a sense of well-being associated with normal nasal breathing and a normal appearing nose. Through this long and often multistage process the patient needs continued reassurance and support in order to maintain their self-esteem and confidence. The ultimate reconstructive success of nasal restoration allows a better transition back into society.

REFERENCES

1. Millard DR. Total reconstructive rhinoplasty and a missing link. Plast Reconstr Surg 1966; 37:167.

2. Daver BM, Antia NH, Furnas DW. Handbook of Plastic Surgery for the General Surgeon. 2nd ed. Oxford University Press, 2000.

3. Ben-Hur N, Converse JM. The impact of plastic surgery on transplantation: from skin graft to microsurgery. Transplant Proc 1980; XII(4):616–620.

4. McIndoe AH. Total reconstruction of the burned face: the Bradshaw Lecture 1958. Br J Plast Surg 1983; 36:410–420.

5. Millard RD. Reconstructive rhinoplasty for the lower half of the nose. Plast Reconstr Surg 1974; 53:133.

6. Burget GC, Menick FJ. Nasal support and lining: the marriage of beauty and blood supply. Plast Reconstr Surg 1989; 84(2):189–203.

7. Bernard SL. Reconstruction of the burned nose and ear. Clin Plast Surg 2000; 27(1):97–112.

8. Boswick JA. Burns of the head and neck. Surg Clin North Am 1973; 53(1):97–104.

9. Neale HW, Billmire DA, Carey JP. Reconstruction following head and neck burns. Clin Plast Surg 1986; 13(1):119–136.

10. Lyle G, Robson MC, McCauley RL. Reconstruction of the head and neck. In: Herndon DN, ed. Total Burn Care. Philadelphia: W.B. Saunders, 1996:492–498.

11. Burget GC, Menick FJ. The subunit principle in nasal reconstruction. Plast Reconstr Surg 1985; 76(2):239–247.

12. Burget GC, Menick FJ. Aesthetic Reconstruction of the Nose. St. Louis: Mosby, 1994.

13. Brou JA, Robson MC, McCauley RL et al. Inventory of potential reconstructive needs in the patient with burns. J Burn Care Rehabil 1989; 10:555–560.

14. Stephen GG, Brody GS. Surgical correction of burn deformities of the nose. Plast Reconstr Surg 1978; 62(6):848–852.

15. Achauer BM. Nose reconstruction. In: Achauer BM, ed. Burn Reconstruction. New York: Thieme, 1991:52–63.

16. Feldman JJ. Facial burns. In: McCarthy JG, ed. Plastic Surgery. Philadelphia: W.B. Saunders, 1990:2153–2236.

17. Spear SL, Kroll SS, Romm S. A new twist to the nasolabial flap for reconstruction of lateral alar defects. Plast Reconstr Surg 1987; 79:915–920.

18. Fabrizio T, Savani A, Sanna M et al. The retro angular flap for nasal reconstruction. Plast Reconstr Surg 1996; 97:431–435.

19. Hataya Y, Kosaka K, Yamazaki M et al. Reconstruction of burned nasal alar with vascular island skin flaps pedicled on the infra orbital vessels. Burns 1995; 21:313–315.

20. Juri J, Juri C, Belmont JA et al. Neighboring flaps and cartilage grafts for correction of serious secondary nasal deformities. Plast Reconstr Surg 1985; 76:876–881.

21. Soeda S, Nakayama Y. Nasal deformities due to burns: their surgical treatment. Burns 1980; 6:266–270.

22. Converse JM. Clinical applications of the scalping flap in the reconstruction of the nose. Plast Reconstr Surg 1969; 43(3):249–259.

23. Converse JM. Burn deformities of the face and neck: reconstructive surgery and rehabilitation. Surg Clin North Am 1967; 47:323.

24. Washio H. Retro auricular-temporal flap. Plast Reconstr Surg 1969; 43(2):162–166.

25. Warpeha RL. Resurfacing the burned face. Clin Plast Surg 1981; 8(20):255–267.

26. Adamson JE. Nasal reconstruction with the expanded forehead flap. Plast Reconstr Surg 1988; 81:12.

27. Apesos J, Perofsky HJ. The expanded forehead flap for nasal reconstruction. Ann Plast Surg 1993; 30(5):411–416.

28. Zuker RM, Capek L, de Haas W. The expanded forehead scalping flap: a new method of total nasal reconstruction. Plast Reconstr Surg 1996; 98(1):155–159.

29. Furuta S, Hayashi M, Shinohara H. Nasal reconstruction with an expanded dual forehead flap. Br J Plast Surg 2000; 53(3):261–264.

30. Kobus K. Late repair of facial burns. Ann Plast Surg 1980; 5:191.

31. Furnas D, Achauer BM, Barlett RH et al. Reconstruction of the burned nose. J Trauma 1980; 20:25.

32. Zhou LY, Cao YL. Clinical application of the free flap based on the cutaneous branch of the acromio-thoracic artery. Ann Plast Surg 1989; 23:11.

33. Benmeir P, Neuman A, Weinberg et al. Reconstruction of the completely burned nose by a free dorsalis pedis flap. Br J Plast Surg 1991; 44:570–571.

34. Evans DM. Facial reconstruction after a burn injury using two circumferential radial forearm flaps, and a dorsalis pedis flap for the nose. Br J Plast Surg 1995; 48:471–476.

35. Frey M. The radial forearm flap as a pedicled flap for resurfacing a scarred nose. Ann Plast Surg 1994; 32:200–204.

36. Watanabe T, Furuta S, Hataya S et al. Reconstruction of the eyelids and nose after a burn injury using a radial forearm flap. Burns 1997; 23(4):360–365.

37. Ohmori K, Sekiguchi J, Ohmori S. Total rhinoplasty with a free osteocutaneous flap. Plast Reconstr Surg 1979; 63(3):387–394.

38. Shenaq SM, Dinh TA, Spira M. Nasal alar reconstruction with an ear helix free flap. J Reconstr Microsurg 1989; 5:63–67.

39. Pribaz JJ, Falco N. Nasal reconstruction with auricular microvascular transplant. Ann Plast Surg 1993; 31:289.

40. Pribaz JJ, Fine NA. Prelamination: defining the prefabricated flap. A case report and review. Microsurgery 1994; 15:618.

41. Khouri RK, Upton J, Shaw WW. Prefabrication of composite free flap through staged microvascular transfer: an experimental and clinical study. Plast Reconstr Surg 1991; 87(1):108–115.

42. Khouri RK, Upton J, Shaw WW. Principles of flap prefabrication. Clin Plast Surg 1992; 19(4):763–771.

43. Costa H, Cunha C, Guimaraes I et al. Prefabricated flaps for the head and neck: a preliminary report. Br J Plast Surg 1993; 46(3):223–227.

44. Pribaz JJ, Fine NA, Orgill DP. Flap prefabrication in the head and neck: a 10-year experience. Plast Reconstr Surg 1999; 103:808.

45. Pribaz JJ, Weiss DD, Mulliken JB et al. Prelaminated free flap reconstruction of complex central facial defects. Plast Reconstr Surg 1999; 104:357.

46. Pribaz JJ, Fine NA. Prefabricated and prelaminated flaps for head and neck reconstruction. Clin Plast Surg 2001; 28(2):261–272.

47. Giugliano C, Andrades PR, Benitez S. Nasal reconstruction with a forehead flap in children younger than 10 years of age. Plast Reconstr Surg 2004; 114:316–325.

48. Menick FJ. Discussion: nasal reconstruction with a forehead flap in children younger than 10 years of age. Plast Reconstr Surg 2004; 114:326–328.

22

Reconstruction of the Burned Ear

EVAN PICKUS
Shriners Hospital for Children—Galveston Unit, Galveston, Texas, USA

ROBERT L. McCAULEY
University of Texas Medical Branch and Shriners Hospital for Children—Galveston Unit, Galveston, Texas, USA

I. INTRODUCTION

The external ear is a highly visible, outwardly projecting appendage with a symmetrical twin. In light of this position of prominence, deformities of the ear as well as ear asymmetry can have profound psychological effects on one's self-image (1,2). The literature on ear reconstruction is extensive. Most of this is applicable to reconstruction of the auricle in the burned patient. However, there are two significant differences in the burned patient that deserve attention. In addition to the frequent loss of available surrounding cutaneous tissue for repair, these patients often suffer many additional injuries from their burns. Frequently, these major wounds are more life threatening than the ear wounds. Therefore, reconstruction of the ear is generally performed after more critical life-threatening needs are addressed.

Reconstruction of the external ear has been documented by Sushruta in Sanskrit as early as 900 BC in India (2–4).

Initial efforts consisted of the repair of severed earlobes with the use of pedicled flaps from the cheek (2,3,5). However, it was not until 1890 that Kuhnt and Schanz described total auricular reconstruction by using an ipsilateral auricular cartilage rudiment (6,7). In 1893, Randall constructed an auricular framework from rabbit cartilage (8). In 1905, Korte et al. (9) reported partial ear reconstruction when he harvested a composite graft from the contralateral healthy ear (9). In the past 100 years, over 40 types of materials for reconstruction of the auricular framework have been described (7). However, the majority of these have fallen into disfavor because of high complication rates and poor results (7). In addition, occasional reports have been made on attempts to create an auricle without the use of a supporting framework (10–12). Efforts made without a framework have all resulted in suboptimal results secondary to contractile forces on the reconstructed ear (7). Schmieden (13), in Germany in 1908, became the first surgeon credited with using autogenous costal cartilage in the reconstruction of an auricle. The construct was then buried in the abdomen and later transferred to the head using a "plastic migrating pedicle flap" (14). In 1959, Tanzer described his technique for microtia reconstruction using autogenous costal cartilage (15). Rapid acceptance of the use of costal cartilage for reconstruction of the ear occurred after Tanzer popularized this method (Figs. 22.1 and 22.2). The use of costal cartilage remains the predominant foundation for autologous ear reconstruction used today for total auricular reconstruction.

The primary concerns that surgeons have faced since initial attempts were made to reconstruct an auricle are the formation of a durable framework and stable skin coverage (7,16). Although these obstacles have been resolved, they can be problematic in patients with extensive facial burns. In addition to the above, problems such as bilateral ear loss and significant pigmentation changes continue to complicate ear reconstruction. In 1944, Suraci described seven conditions that must be considered when reconstructing an auricle. They are as follows: (1) correct size, (2) identical appearance to the contralateral ear, (3) identical auriculocephalic angles, (4) identical ear levels, (5) durability of the construct to withhold its size and shape, (6) the adequate selection of supporting and soft tissue for precise molding, and (7) an appropriate color match as compared with that of the contralateral ear (17). These principles still hold true today. Yet, attaining these standards in the burned patient is challenging. Although many reconstructive surgeons have made valiant efforts to fashion a duplicate ear, very few have been able to achieve superior results.

A. Ears

1. Anatomy

Anatomical relationships of the external ear are significant because of its unique shape and contour. Embryologically,

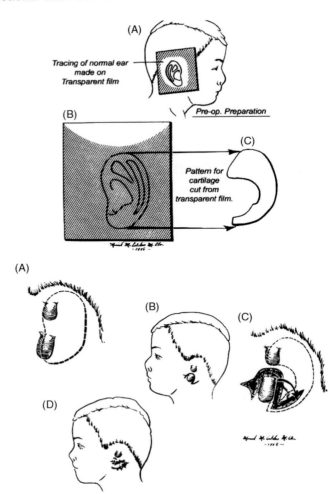

Figure 22.1 Tanzer's method of pattern preparation for auricular reconstruction. The use of an ear pattern to determine the relationship of existent tissue to the proposed site for total ear reconstruction (bottom A). Method of lowering and rotating existing auricular tissue to proper location (bottom B, C, and D). [Reprinted with permission from Tanzer (15).]

the ear is derived from the first (mandibular) and second (hyoid) branchial arches. Three hillocks are formed from the first branchial arch, which eventually give rise to the tragus, the root of the helix, and the superior rim of the helix (18). The hyoid arch also creates three hillocks which give rise to the antihelix, antitragus, and lobule. The external auditory meatus and the concha are formed by the first branchial groove. The length of the ear is ∼60 mm in adults and projects laterally between 20 and 30 mm from the skin covering the temporal bone (19). It lies in a plane equal to the superior rim of the orbit and the nasal spine (20). By age 3, the ear has achieved ∼90% of its adult size (18). The auricle is the external portion of the ear (Fig. 22.3). It is covered in its entirety with skin, which serves as the interface between deeper

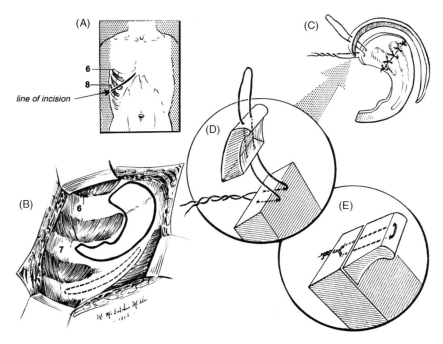

Figure 22.2 (A) Surgical approach to costal cartilage. (B) Pattern laid out on the sixth and seventh costal cartilages, overlying the synchondrosis and extending almost to the seventh costochondral junction. The eighth rib is removed for construction of helix. (C) Method of attaching helix to antihelixscapha unit with wire suture. (D, E) diagrammatic detail of the same. End of wire is bent flush with cartilage after completion of suture. [Reprinted with permission from Tanzer (15).]

structures and the environment. As with other areas of the body, auricular skin functions in a protective role to prevent deeper tissues from suffering insults secondary to trauma, thermal injury, or infection. Additionally, the skin contributes to thermoregulation, immunologic surveillance, sensory perception, and control of insensible fluid loss (21). Dermal appendages are deep intradermal

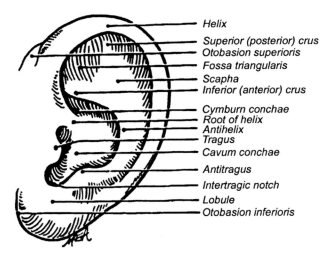

Figure 22.3 Structure of the external ear. [Reprinted with permission from Jones and Wellisz (2).]

structures lined with epithelial cells that have the potential for division and differentiation. These serve as a source for the regeneration of epithelial cells necessary for wound healing. In the ear, these include hair follicles, sebaceous glands, and sweat glands. Unlike most other organs, the ear has no appreciable soft tissue separating the skin from its underlying connective tissue. Deep to the skin is a single piece of elastic cartilage which gives the ear its distinctive shape. Medially, this cartilage is directly connected to the external acoustic meatus.

The anatomy of the lobule (earlobe) differs significantly from that of the auricle in that it has no underlying cartilage. Instead, it consists entirely of skin, fibroareolar tissue, and fat (17).

The ear contains six intrinsic and three extrinsic vestigial muscles. The anterior, superior, and posterior auricularis muscles comprise the extrinsic group. The anterior and superior muscles are connected to the epicranial aponeurosis and often there is a branch of the superficial temporal artery that separates the two (18). These are both innervated by branches of the temporal branch of the facial nerve. The posterior auricularis, the largest of the three extrinsic muscles, originates at the base of the mastoid process and is innervated by the posterior auricular branch of the facial nerve (18). Arnold's nerve, an auricular branch of the vagus, supplies the conchal skin as well as that of the posterior canal. The ear gets its vascular supply primarily from the posterior auricular and superficial temporal arteries and a complex collateralization of branches is present between them (22). The external carotid artery gives rise to the posterior auricular artery, which then travels alongside the posterior auricular branch of the facial nerve before sending branches to the parotid gland, a stylomastoid branch to mastoid cells and the tympanic cavity, a postauricular branch, and an occipital branch to the postauricular skin (20) (Fig. 22.4). Occasionally, the posterior auricular artery comes off of the occipital artery. Venous drainage is directed toward the external jugular vein via the posterior auricular vein (18). The anterior and superoposterior portion of the auricle drains into veins which are relieved into the superficial temporal and retromandibular veins. The latter structure runs deep to the great auricular nerve. Sensation to the superior and lateral surfaces inferior to the external acoustic meatus is provided by the greater auricular nerve with contributions from C2. The auriculotemporal nerve provides sensation to the skin superior to the meatus (21).

Lymphatic drainage from the lateral surface of the superior half of the auricle is directed anterior to the tragus in the superficial parotid lymph nodes. The retroauricular and deep cervical lymph nodes receive drainage from the superior surface of the upper portion of the auricle. The inferior portion of the auricle, as well as the lobule, drain into the superficial cervical lymph nodes.

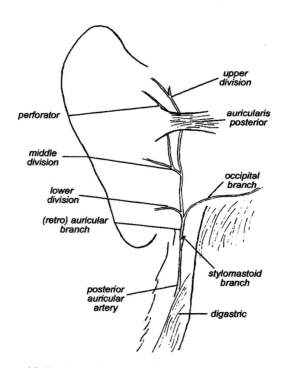

Figure 22.4 Arterial anatomy of the posterior auricular artery. [Reprinted with permission from Allison (20).]

2. Aesthetic/Functional Importance

The aesthetic significance of the ear is especially important in females who require them for purposes of adornment. However, both sexes are affected with regard to limitations on hairstyles. Furthermore, in certain cultures, the ear has spiritual and holistic importance (2). Some Asian cultures view large pendulous lobes to be aesthetically pleasing and to denote wisdom and longevity (2). If the face is to look normal, the appearance of the ears is vital. Additional functional ramifications of the external ear are limited to those who must wear eyeglasses.

B. Facial Burns

The face gives each person a distinct identity. Because of its exposure, the face is frequently involved in burn injury. Any disfigurement to the face is certain to cause the patient to suffer significant emotional injury in addition to their obvious physical involvement. The face has a rich vascular supply as well as numerous dermal appendages, both of which contribute significantly to re-epithelialization and rapid healing. In children, where the facial skin is generally thinner than what is seen in an adult, the face is substantially more vulnerable to both the initial burn injury as well as the ensuing scars that ultimately will result (23). Furthermore, in children, the disfigurement of the face caused by contractures and hypertrophic scarring frequently may exceed that from the initial burn injury. However, scarring is also a function of burn depth, infection, time from initial burn to wound closure, and type of closure.

In 1956, Gonzalez-Ulloa described the concept of facial reconstruction using anatomic subunits (24). By the utilization of this method, it is frequently possible to limit the scars that would be created by a patchwork of facial grafts and flaps. The use of similar tissue in its reconstruction by harvesting skin grafts from above the clavicle will further assist to minimize the disparity from uninvolved skin. Ultimately, no amount of medical care can restore the face to its normal appearance. However, by following the principles of judicious wound care and appropriate surgical intervention, reconstruction can be satisfactorily accomplished (23).

1. Involvement of the Ears

Auricular deformities may occur from the initial burn as well as from chondritis. Chondritis may result from the initial injury or from positional changes due to increased pressure on the ears and subsequent ischemia. The literature quotes between 42% and 60% of facial burns having ear involvement (25,26). Most auricular burns show partial ear involvement. The incidence of bilateral ear involvement differs by series but has been cited as high as 66% (27). The management of burns to the ear should proceed in a systematic fashion. During the acute phase of injury, the goals are to maximize tissue preservation and to prevent infection. Consequently, acute management of the burned ear is usually conservative (28). Initial efforts generally include the use of topical antibiotics and the avoidance of pressure.

Many different types of topical antibiotics have been used therapeutically in the management of burns to the ear. The list includes mafenide acetate, silver sulfadiazine, bacitracin, silver nitrate, and a host of other antibacterials. Mafenide acetate is a folate antagonist whose mechanism of action is the inhibition of folate synthesis. It has been the preferred topical antimicrobial for burns of the ear since its advent in the 1960s because of its ability to penetrate eschar and its broad antimicrobial spectrum (29). However, as with all medications, it has side effects which include pain on application and metabolic acidosis which results from carbonic anhydrase inhibition. The pain which patients often experience has been effectively reduced with the use of a 5% concentration compared to the standard 11.2% concentration (30). In a double-blind triple-crossover study, Harrison et al. (30) found that by using the 5% concentration, a two- to threefold decrease in pain could be achieved. Furthermore, they also determined that it was the hypertonicity of the concentration which led to the pain and not the decrease in cutaneous pH which had previously been suspected. Kucan and Smoot (31) used this solution as their primary topical antimicrobial in 276 burn patients without evidence of acid–base disturbances.

Pressure on the burned ear is to be avoided at all costs. Because of the avascular nature of the underlying cartilage and its reliance on the skin for providing its nutrition, any further insult to overlying burned skin can result in a full-thickness skin loss and exposure of the underlying cartilage. Pillows are generally avoided except when they have a central hole (foam donuts). A number of devices have been designed to alleviate pressure on the ears. Jordan et al. (32) described a "headgear" to alleviate pressure on the ears for those who are intubated. In their study, pressure necrosis was avoided in all survivors in whom this treatment was instituted. Harries and Pegg (33) described a foam ear protector which allowed for unimpeded visualization of the ear and enabled patients to sleep on their sides without any pressure on their ears.

Because of its avascular nature, auricular cartilage derives its nutrition from the surrounding skin and perichondrium (34,35). Unlike other burned areas where pressure is often used to minimize scarring and further disfigurement, pressure on the ears can cause significant tissue loss. Early excision of the eschar is not desirable as it functions as a biologic dressing and assists in preventing dessication of the delicate cartilaginous structures (35).

In summary, initial therapy for the thermally injured ear consists of gentle cleansing with soap and water, the liberal use of topical antibiotics, and avoidance of pressure (27). Mafenide acetate is the topical antibiotic of choice because of its unique ability to penetrate the burn eschar. The overwhelming majority of patients with burns to the ear go on to heal these injuries without long-term sequelae (27).

II. ACUTE CARE OF EAR BURNS

A. Partial-Thickness Injuries

Partial-thickness burns to the ear generally heal without complications (27). The determinant factor for auricular wound healing is the viability of the perichondrium except in the case of infection. If the perichondrium is intact, these injuries can re-epithelialize. Skin grafts cannot be placed directly on bare cartilage. However, if the perichondrium is present, skin grafts can close the defect. Skin grafts may be used in conjunction with local advancement flaps (35). In the case of deep partial-thickness injuries, concomitant edema and tissue loss both contribute to an environment where permanent injury is more likely to occur. In deep partial-thickness burns, debridement and the placement of skin grafts are vital in the prevention of further auricular embarrassment. However, the timing of operative intervention has varied depending on the surgeon (35).

B. Full-Thickness Burns

In full-thickness burns, there is total destruction of all layers of the epidermis and dermis. In the ear, full-thickness injuries may result in exposure or damage to the underlying cartilage. Surgical intervention is always required for both debridement and subsequent reconstruction (19). As with partial-thickness injuries, initial efforts consist of topical antibiotics and the avoidance of pressure. Once it is evident that a full-thickness injury is present, early operative intervention should be instituted to prevent further dessication and destruction of the ear cartilage. The options present in the surgical arsenal for coverage is dependant on the size of the defect, the presence of infection, and the condition of local tissue available. Frequently, full-thickness burns invade the auricular cartilage with subsequent tissue loss. The superficial temporoparietal fascial flap (STPF) for the salvage of denuded cartilage in burn patients was initially described by Tegtmeier and Gooding (36) in 1977 and further described by Cotlar (37) and Achauer et al. (38) (Fig. 22.5). The STPF flap receives its blood supply from the superficial temporal artery. Details of its elevation include the identification of the artery by Doppler exam. Incisions can be based on

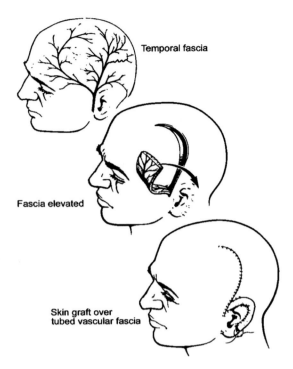

Temporal fascia

Fascia elevated

Skin graft over
tubed vascular fascia

Figure 22.5 The typical distribution of the superficial temporal artery is shown. A curved incision is designed after a dominant arterial pedicle has been mapped with the Doppler stethoscope. A relatively small flap is shown harvested to resurface damaged ear cartilage. The donor site is closed and a skin graft placed over the fascial flap and sutured into place. [Reprinted with permission from Achauer et al. (38).]

surgeon's preference. However, the curved and Y-incisions have been described. Once the incision has been made, the flap is elevated and either rotated or folded over the defect. As with any flap, care is taken not to disrupt the vascular pedicle. Following elevation and insetting of the flap, a split-thickness skin graft is used for coverage. If the flap is folded, a second procedure may be necessary for division of the pedicle. If required, this procedure can be done 7–10 days after the initial operation. However, full-thickness burns to the temporoparietal region may preclude the use of this flap (38).

C. Acute Problems with Ear Burns

1. Edema

As with any burn, thermal injuries to the ear are characterized by edema. This is especially troubling because of the avascularity of its underlying cartilage. Since the cartilage receives its chief means of nutrition via diffusion from the skin, edema of the skin with its concomitant constriction of the arterial supply can have disastrous complications down the line.

2. Chondritis

Chondritis is an infection that has invaded cartilage. Acute chondritis is a devastating late complication that may arise from burns to the external ear. Typically, it presents 3–5 weeks after the initial burn (25). The development of chondritis is irrelevant to the depth of the initial burn (i.e., second vs. third) (25). The final result is often severe disfigurement or total loss of the ear either by amputation or by autochondrectomy. Initially, it presents with dull pain but quickly manifests fever, erythema, edema, fluctuance, and exquisite tenderness. The auriculocephalic angle is increased with a pronounced protrusion of the ear. The helix and antihelix are the primary sites of occurrence. However, the tragus may be the only site of involvement. The inflammation may spread to the entire ear to encompass unburned areas of cartilage (26). Occasionally, the fluctuance may dissipate with spontaneous drainage of the purulent material. This is often accompanied by a decrease in pain and resolution of the fever. However, when this occurs, necrotic cartilage is usually present (26,28). Approximately 80–95% of these occurrences are due to *Pseudomonas aeruginosa* (25,39). However, *Staphylococcus aureus* is also found in ~50% of culture specimens (i.e., mixed flora) (25,26,39). *Providencia rettgeri*, *Proteus mirabilis*, *Enterobacter cloacae*, *Corynebacterium diphtheriae*, *Klebsiella pneumoniae*, *Escherichia coli*, and *Candida albicans* have also been cited (25,26,39). Chondritis has a very strong predilection for recurrence. However, its incidence has diminished significantly since the advent of mafenide acetate (Sulfamylon®) (25). Pressure on the ears must be meticulously avoided as ischemia is often the culprit for the initiation of chondritis. Nevertheless, chondritis is still seen occasionally and treatment options are lengthy. In addition to its role in the prevention of chondritis, mafenide acetate is often continued after the onset of chondritis. Systemic antibiotics are generally ineffective in the treatment of chondritis because of the avascularity of the auricular cartilage and the inability of the antimicrobial to reach therapeutic levels in the target tissue (40–42). Additionally, the use of systemic antibiotics allows for the development of resistance.

In 1908, LeDuc described iontophoresis (43). This was a novel method for the delivery of chemicals in solution across intact skin founded on the principle that an electric potential will cause ions in solution to migrate based on their respective charges (42). The use of iontophoresis held promise in the treatment of chondritis and was adequately reported in the burn literature (42,44–48). However, Desai et al. (42) in a dual clinical and animal study found that there were no differences in the incidence of chondritis in those patients who received iontophoresis vs. those who received routine care only (42).

Furthermore, 29% of the patients who received ionto-phoresis in their study developed gentamicin resistant organisms. The direct instillation of antibiotics without the use of iontophoresis, occasionally referred to as "dakinization," has also been reported for the treatment of auricular chondritis (44,49–51). However, both ionto-phoresis and the direct instillation of antibiotics into the ear have fallen into disfavor in most burn centers.

Surgical debridement also remains a treatment for chondritis. Operative debridement may be necessary. Bivalving of the ear involves making an anterior incision along the helical margin of the ear with subsequent debridement of the necrotic nonviable cartilage (Fig. 22.6). Once healthy white cartilage is reached, the debridement is concluded. Frequently, multiple episodes of operative intervention are required (39,52). The sequelae of this procedure often result in significant deformities of the ear.

Some burn surgeons advocate early debridement of third-degree burns to the ear with immediate autografting in order to prevent chondritis (25). However, this approach is not uniformly accepted (28). Furthermore, with early intervention, some healthy tissue is inevitably lost. Incision and drainage is generally inadequate in the treatment of chondritis as the abscess cavity is unable to contract because of the surrounding rigid cartilage (28). Once chondritis has been documented, operative debridement remains the most effective way of initiating a cure (28). Occasionally, an allergic reaction to mafenide acetate occurs in burned ears (52–54). However, this complication is not accompanied by fever, fluctuance, and pain. Care must be taken to diagnose this problem expeditiously in order to prevent unnecessary surgical intervention and subsequent tissue loss. However, in spite of our best efforts to maximize tissue preservation and control infection, deformities of the ear still occur.

3. Loss of Definition

Due to the intricate nature of its structures, any disruption of the ear anatomy is readily perceptible to the untrained eye. This is true both in the acute stage when edema distorts the normal configuration of the ear and produces an increased auriculocephalic angle as well as in the post-acute phase when the ear is often deformed.

III. RECONSTRUCTION

According to Salisbury and Bevin (55), the most common types of auricular burn deformities are the contracted ear, partial or complete loss of the helical rim, and total ear loss (55). Frequently, the ear burn is not an isolated injury and is secondary to more specific concerns on the face (55). In restoration of the ear, reconstructive efforts must be specifically tailored to achieve an optimal outcome.

The successful reconstruction of an ear is dependent on the integrity of the underlying framework (1). Initial reconstructive efforts can best be structured by viewing the ear in three distinct anatomic parts (19). These are the helix/lobule, the antihelix/antitragus, and the concha. Once the regions of the ear that will require reconstruction are determined, efforts should proceed systematically. In the contracted ear, Erikson and Vogt (19) advocate reconstruction in three steps: release of scar contractures, assessment of the framework defect and subsequent reconstruction, and finally cutaneous coverage. In contrast to the use of costal cartilage grafts in total ear loss, the majority of partial ear defects can be repaired with the use of local flaps and, if necessary, cartilage harvested from the contralateral ear (56). Auricular cartilage, in addition to its natural flexibility and resistance to trauma, is less likely to fall victim to the absorptive process that is often seen when using costal cartilage because of its minimal width (56). All efforts should be attempted to close these defects with similar tissues. Distant tissue, that is, rib cartilage, should only be used when all local options for tissue are exhausted or deemed inadequate (35,56). The location for placement of the ear in cases of total bilateral ear loss can be aided by the use of a parallelogram (Fig. 22.1). The axis of the ear is parallel to that of the profile of the nose. The vertical dimension can be determined by the glabella and subnasale.

A. Hypertrophic Scars and Keloids

In the burned patient, once closure of all wounds has occurred, either with autografts or healing by secondary intention, efforts are then directed toward the prevention

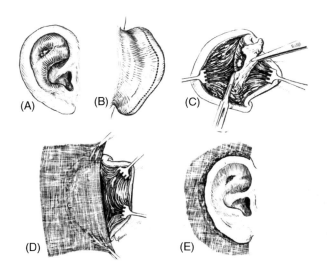

(A) (B) (C)

(D) (E)

Figure 22.6 Steps in chondrectomy using bivalving technique. [Reprinted with permission from Dowling et al. (25).]

and treatment of scarring and functional concerns. With respect to hypertrophic scars, three methods have received a significant amount of our attention. These are (1) the use of topical and injectable agents, (2) the use of pressure, and (3) surgery. Topical and injectable medicinal agents, usually steroids, have improved hypertrophic scars and keloids, but their results have not been uniform in the treatment of burned patients (57,58). Pressure is generally delivered via the use of fabricated plastic molds (24). In the ear, this method is controversial because of its propensity to lead to the development of chondritis. Surgery is always an option in the therapy for hypertrophic scars

and keloids of the ear. Frequently, these scars can be treated with excision and closure or skin grafts (Fig. 22.7). Depending on the size of the resultant defect, repair sometimes necessitates the use of a skin graft or local flap. The pitfall in the management of keloids is a high predilection for recurrence.

B.   The Constricted/Contracted Ear

Contractures of the ear most frequently center around the lobule and frequently the lobule becomes wedded to the

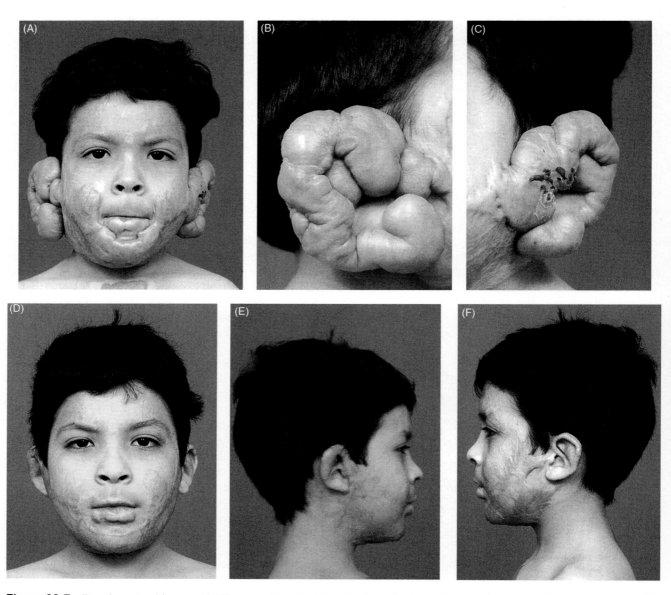

Figure 22.7   Burn hypertrophic scars (A) Six-year-old male status after burns to the head and neck regions with massive hypertrophic scars of the ears. (B) Close-up of right ear hypotrophic scars. (C) Close-up of left ear hypertrophic scars. (D) Frontal view $2\frac{1}{2}$ years after several excisions of bilateral ear hypertrophic scars using local flaps. (E) Close-up of right ear. (F) Close-up of left ear.

cheek (19,55). Often there is a downward pull on the lobule with concomitant loss of skin (55). However, the helical rim is also at risk. Deep partial-thickness injuries to the antihelix or the triangular fossa may heal secondarily, producing a contracted ear. In general, most of the cartilage framework is present and correction of the defect often requires anterior skin grafts and correction of the prominent ear with a pin back otoplasty. Contracture release followed by careful repair with V–Y advancement flaps or Z-plasties may also be required. In severe cases, cartilage grafts may be needed as well (Fig. 22.8). Skin grafts may be necessary. Care must be taken to ensure

that the flap will move superiorly and posteriorly as opposed to anteriorly or recontracture of the lobule is likely to occur (55). Burns to the helical rim if neglected can also lead to contractures. Surgical treatment is contingent upon the resulting defect after surgical release. Frequently, skin grafts or flaps are used to resurface the resulting cutaneous defects. Cartilaginous defects will also require correction.

C. Helical Rim Defects

The helical rim is the most prominent structure of the ear and is responsible for giving the ear its general outline and height. In the reconstruction of an auricle, it is the restoration of the helix which will ultimately determine the success of the procedure. Without integrity of the helical rim, any reconstruction would be suboptimal. Defects of the helical rim span the gamut from minimal to total loss of the helix. Direct closure of small defects is possible (Fig. 22.9). However, there may be some size discrepancy as compared to the unburned ear. Composite grafts will generally survive as long as they are small (usually 1 × 1 cm) (19,59). In cases where the retroauricular region has been spared, elevation of a postauricular flap may provide soft tissue cover for an entire ear framework. Occasionally, tissue expansion of the postauricular skin is utilized (19). However, the thick capsule may affect

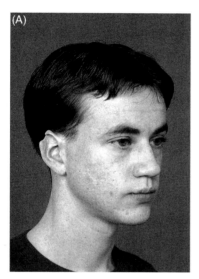

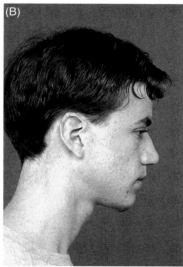

Figure 22.8 (A) seventeen-year-old male with small helical rim defect. (B) Appearance of right ear after reconstruction of the helical rim with ipsilateral cartilage graft and coverage with a postauricular flap: release and placement of a skin graft was performed after 1 month.

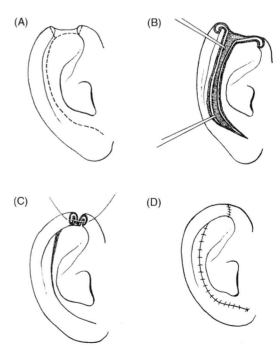

Figure 22.9 Operative plans for chondrocutaneous advancement flaps for marginal defects of the ear. [Reprinted with permission from Antia and Buch (60).]

definition of the ear. The superficial temporoparietal fascia with a split-thickness skin graft cover may also be utilized provided that the superficial temporal artery is intact (19). Because of the tenuous nature of the surrounding skin and the marginal blood supply, small areas of tissue loss are commonly seen following reconstruction (55).

D. Partial Ear Defects

Numerous procedures have been thoroughly detailed for the reconstruction of partial defects of the ear. The length of this list is prohibitive to describe all of them, but a number of them deserve further mention (1,36–38,59–68).

1. Small Defects

Small helical defects involving less than one-third of the rim can frequently be corrected with wedge excision and direct closure. Although some residual deformity may be apparent, the final result is often quite satisfactory (56). Depending on the size of the defect, local advancement flaps such as the chondrocutaneous flap described by Antia and Buch, can be employed (55,56,60) (Fig. 22.9). This is a chondrocutaneous flap which can be advanced from the inferior undamaged portion of the ear in a single-staged procedure. The principle utilized is advancement of the adjacent intact helical margin on a wide postauricular skin pedicle. The defect is then transferred to the more extensible lobule. If size discrepancy remains, a small wedge excision can be taken from the undamaged ear to allow for better size consistency. Although this technique was described initially in the repair of upper-third defects, Brent (1) states that it is even more effective in middle-third and lobule deformities. He noted that success with this flap requires that the helix be completely separated from the scapha by incising the helical sulcus through skin and cartilage until reaching but not violating the posterior auricular skin. Additional length can be obtained by advancing a V–Y flap of the helical crus (56). Tubed pedicle flaps from the postauricular sulcus may also provide the tissue necessary for small defects of the rim provided that the skin in this area is undamaged (69).

In reconstructions using retroauricular flaps, conchal cartilage can be used as the underlying support in order to avoid an additional donor site. Some authors feel that an antihelical strut is required to prevent collapse (56,70). However, this is not always necessary (Fig. 22.10). Distal tube flaps can also be harvested from the supraclavicular and neck regions although these should only be used in specific instances (56).

2. Medium-Sized Defects

Brent (1) described a procedure for repair when the helix as well as the entire scapha was lost in which he utilized the posterior border of the remaining ear as the new antihelix. In this technique, a retroauricular pocket is created in which a rib cartilage graft is then buried. It is elevated with a skin graft a few months later after healing has occurred, and will then serve as the helical rim. Frequently, in severe auricular burns, the peripheral structures including the helical rim and lobule are lost while the central portions remain intact and viable. The conchal transposition flap, originally described by Davis (70) for reconstruction of the superior helical rim, has been used for repair. The principle utilized in this flap is that a chondrocutaneous conchal flap can be elevated on an anterior pedicle to re-create the superior helix. Donelan (61) has modified and popularized this operation to allow for expanded procedures that may reconstruct the entire periphery of the ear (Fig. 22.11). In Donelan's modification, the superior transposition of the concha facilitates posterior and inferior rotation of the remaining scaphal and antihelical tissue, thereby expanding the entire ear. In his series of 24 ears in 18 patients, no major complications were seen and high patient satisfaction was attained. This procedure is also recommended for the contracted burned ear with cartilage loss. Unfurling of the ear contracture prior to transposition. Conchal donor sites were closed with split-thickness skin grafts. Lobule creation was based on a U-shaped incision made inferior to the lower pole. A caveat to this procedure is that maximum subcutaneous tissue as well as scar tissue must be included with the flap in order to substantiate the lobule (61). The posterior lobule as well as the resultant cheek defect may require closure with split-thickness skin grafts. Often the creation of a lobule will require composite grafts. These can be taken from the ipsilateral ear if the concha has been spared or from the contralateral ear if it has been burned (19,56,59,71). Alternatively, conchal cartilage grafts with coverage using a postauricular flap can produce excellent results (Fig. 22.8).

3. Large Defects

In situations where the overwhelming majority of the helical rim has been destroyed, the antihelix is often injured as well (35). Unlike traumatic defects where partial auricular loss can occur in any area of the ear, in the burned ear, the helical rim tends to bear the greatest insult. In such cases, helical rim reconstruction requires the use of rib cartilage grafts and coverage with a postauricular flap or the STPF flap. However, in significant thermal injuries, total ear loss has been noted. If central ear components are still present, it is possible to incorporate these structures into the final construct (Fig. 22.12).

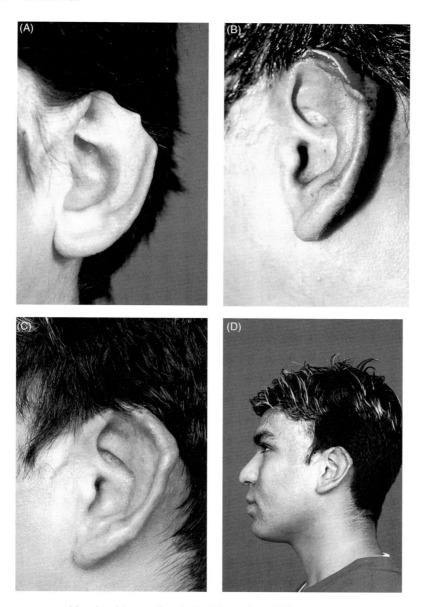

Figure 22.10 (A) Seventeen-year-old male with a medium helical rim defect. (B) Intraoperative photograph of conchal cartilage repair of defect prior to resurfacing with a postauricular flap. (C, D) Final result 6 months later.

4. Location of Helical Defects

Brent (56) believes that there are five primary ways to repair defects in the upper-third of the ear. In patients who have small defects of the rim, an advancement flap or preauricular flap can be utilized (56,60). More significant defects in the upper-third as defined here can be repaired by use of a Banner flap. Here, a small portion of cartilage must be grafted as well (72). This flap is based anterosuperiorly in the auriculocephalic sulcus. Adams (59) described a method for the reconstruction of larger defects in the upper portion of the auricle utilizing composite concha cartilage with perichondrium attached on both sides. The graft must be anchored to the helical remnant to prevent displacement of the graft. Defects in the middle-third of the auricle generally require cartilage grafts for repair (56). Converse (4) described a tunnel procedure for this type of repair. Additionally, local flaps such as the advancement flap of Antia-Buch may be required for coverage. Lower-third defects are especially challenging if the defect involves more than the lobe. In such cases, cartilage is often necessary to assist in restoring contour. Although Preaux has described a superiorly based flap by doubling it on itself (73), others advocate

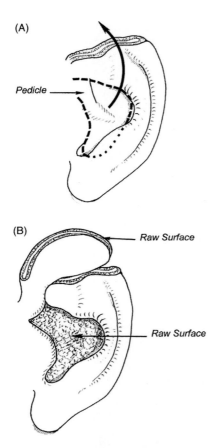

Figure 22.11 Operative technique for the conchal transposition flap. The concha is mobilized on an anterior pedicle and transposed superiorly to restore the upper third of the ear. The raw surface of the conchal donor site is closed with a split-thickness skin graft. [Reprinted with permission from Donelan (61).]

the addition of contralateral cartilage which is believed to improve the eventual restoration of contour as well as provide additional structural support. Further revision is then performed later by elevating a bipedicled chondrocutaneous flap described by Tanzer as a "valise handle" and skin grafting the posterior portion (15,56). Defects involving the lobe alone can frequently be repaired with rearrangement of local tissue. However, more elaborate methods of lobule repair have been described by Alanis (74), Kazanjian and Converse (75), and Brent (76).

5. Total Ear Loss

Total ear loss can occur in severe burns of the face. In a study by Goel et al. (27) of 100 patients with 166 burned ears, a total of 22 ears in 15 patients were completely lost. Seven of these were secondary to chondritis. Successful total ear reconstruction is dependent on both accurate framework fabrication and the availability of soft tissue coverage. The method currently in favor is based on that which was described by Tanzer in 1959 (15). The construct of the framework using costal cartilage grafts is the same in all patients (77). The determinant factor in selecting the type of reconstruction is the remaining skin and soft tissue (77). Bhandari (77) described a series of 76 total ear reconstructions following burn injury. He classified all burns resulting in total ear loss into five groups based on soft tissue availability and the type of coverage they would require. In group (1), the patients had healthy, viable periauricular skin suitable for a pocket. In group (2), the skin was either scarred or grafted but as in group (1), was supple enough for coverage. In group (3), local fascial flaps were required, and in group (4)

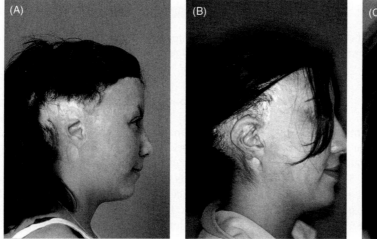

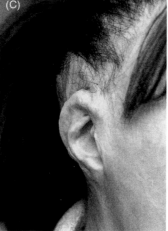

Figure 22.12 (A) Twelve-year-old female with total loss of the helical rim. (B) One year after reconstruction with a superficial temporal parietal fascial flap and STSG. (C) Oblique view of reconstructed ear.

where fascial flap options were nonexistent, free microvascular tissue transfer was necessary. In group (5), ear reconstruction was determined to be impossible and prostheses were recommended.

The undertaking of total ear reconstruction in a burned patient must begin with careful preoperative planning. Initial efforts should focus on the assessment of soft tissue availability and adequacy. A template of the contralateral unburned ear, if present, is used for determination of size and shape. Orientation of the ear is based on the unaffected ear, or 15–20° vertical to the nasal axis (77). Finally, the site is planned around the external auditory meatus with the superior limit level with the eyebrow (77).

Framework fabrication is initiated with a horizontal incision slightly superior to the costal margin. An extraperichondrial dissection is then carried out on the synchondrotic portion of the sixth and seventh ribs. The cartilage construct is then fashioned using the previously made template. Many authors (15,78) favor cartilage harvest from the contralateral side of the ear to be reconstructed. Alternatively, Bhandari (77) always harvests the cartilage from the right side so as to avoid the resultant defect that is created when harvesting full-thickness costal cartilage grafts using extraperichondrial dissection from being directly over the heart.

E. Implants

The use of prefabricated implants for ear reconstruction has a long history in plastic surgery. However, reported complication rates are high (79). Common complications of synthetic implants include extrusion, infection, and foreign body reaction of the host (79). Synthetic implants often give a superiorly pleasing cosmetic result. However, at present there remains no foreign substance that will behave as native tissue.

1. Medpor® Implants (Porous Polyethylene)

Medpor, porous polyethylene, is a relatively new option for framework reconstruction in burned patients and has been touted as an effective alternative to autologous rib cartilage grafts (80). It is composed of an inert material that entails both a flexible outer rim as well as a base for the central auricle (Fig. 22.13). Salient features include its strength, durability, and flexibility. The helical rim moves independently from the base and is compressible. The advantages of Medpor are similar to those which are seen with implants that were previously used in auricular reconstruction. Its use eliminates the necessity of harvesting autologous rib cartilage and eliminates the morbidity associated with this procedure. In addition, operative skill that is required for carving an auricular construct is eliminated. Disadvantages of

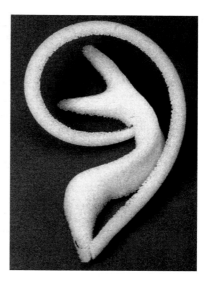

Figure 22.13 The pivoting helix ear framework is composed of two separate components. The helical rim is mobile and free to pivot around the base block. The framework can be modified by heating the Medpor in normal saline and molding it into its desired shape. Upon cooling, the implant maintains its new shape ans regains its previous mechanical characteristics. [Reprinted with permission from Wellisz (80).]

Medpor are a high rate of implant exposure, alopecia, poor skin graft healing, and the introduction of a foreign body (79). Additionally, a STPF flap is required for soft tissue coverage. Because of its porous nature, it encourages both vascular and soft tissue ingrowth as well as the deposition of cartilage (80). The framework construct is fashioned similarly as that which is done with autologous rib cartilage. Wellisz published a series of 26 ear reconstructions in 18 patients using Medpor. The results were reported to be durable over time. He stated that Medpor may be more effective for framework reconstruction in adults because of the calcification of rib cartilage that often is seen with aging. In his study, two cases of extrusion were seen, neither of which required extraction of the implant (80). However, the average follow-up in this series was only ten months and long-term data for outcomes were not available. Further data was presented by Wang (79) on 10 patients who underwent ear reconstruction using Medpor implant. However, these patients either had microtia or had suffered non-burn related trauma. In his study, there were two cases of extrusion and poor auricular detail in four patients. Thus, complication rates can be high. Reinish (81) reported a very low complication rate using Medpor. In a series of 103 patients with microtia, his exposure rate decreased from 44% to 7.3% over two separate time periods. However, this series did not contain ear reconstruction with Medpor in burn patients. Further evaluation of long-term outcomes of auricular reconstructions using Medpor must be investigated before a definitive assessment can be determined. It may be that Medpor® is an optimal choice for auricular reconstruction in select patients. Alternatively, it may follow a host of other one-time promising implants that have fallen into disfavor secondary to high complication rates and suboptimal results.

2. Osseointegration

Because of the intricate architecture of the ear, an accurate reconstruction is difficult at best. For this reason, many patients opt for a prosthetic ear. Consistent

attachment of the prosthesis to the skin has been problematic (19,82). Borrowing from the technique of dental implants, the introduction of osseointegration for ear reconstruction has allowed enhanced prosthetic attachment. The procedure involves the insertion of titanium implants into the temporal bone around the external acoustic meatus. A flap is elevated and then thinned over the implants. A 3–4 month window is then observed to allow for bony ingrowth into the titanium implants. Soft tissue invasion into the implants is prevented by a temporary plug. At the definitive procedure, the skin overlying the implants is punched out, and a metallic (titanium) bar is placed in the implant, which will allow for connection to the prosthesis (Fig. 22.14). The

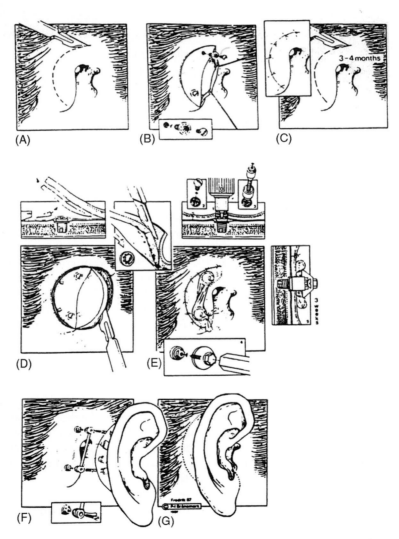

Figure 22.14 (A) Surgery for the bone-anchored auricular prosthesis skin incision. (B) Preparation and threading of holes in the mastoid area and insertion of the fixtures. (C) Incision is closed and the implants left unloaded for 3–4 months. (D) Exposure of the implants and a reduction in subcutaneous tissue. (E) Suturing of the thinned skin flap in place and punching of holes over the fixtures. Securing of cylinders and attachment of healing caps. (F) Construction of a bar for retention of the prosthesis. (G) The auricular silicone prosthesis in place.

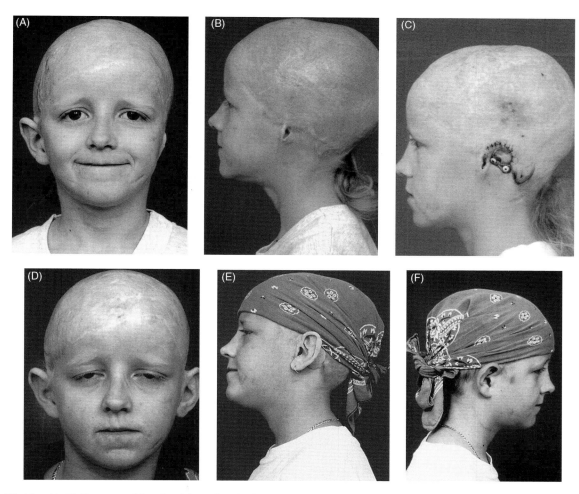

Figure 22.15 (A, B) Ten-year-old male with total auricular loss and skin grafts placed on to periosteum on the right side. (C) Appearance after placement of titanium implants in the mastoid region in preparation for the external bar for retention of the prosthesis. (D–F) Appearance, at one year after placement of osseointegrated ear on right side.

prosthetic is attached to the mastoid region via clips or magnets. Initially, this was performed as a multistaged procedure (Figs. 22.14 and 22.15). However, Tjellstrom and Granstrom (83) have performed the procedure in one stage. Problems and complications with implants include the following: (1) implants are temporary and must be replaced after a few years. In children, replacement may occur more frequently, (2) the anterior border where the prosthesis is attached to the skin can be observed, (3) there is often a skin/prosthesis color mismatch specifically when the patients facial color reddens from cold or when displaying emotion, (4) the tissue surrounding the implants may become infected, and (5) there can be a lack of bony ingrowth with the implant. Needless to say, long-term costs are higher secondary to the recurring need for implant replacement.

IV. CONCLUSION

Thermal injuries to the ear frequently result in permanent disfigurement. To minimize auricular deformity, therapy must begin promptly with meticulous cleansing and wound care. Initial objectives include the preservation of viable tissue and prevention of infection. Once the extent of the injury has been determined, initial planning for surgical intervention can proceed if necessary. Local flaps should be utilized whenever possible for closure of defects. Small to medium size defects may require local cartilage grafts. Large helical rim defects will require rib cartilage grafts. In either case, vascularized soft-tissue coverage is required. The type of vascularized coverage needed is a function of the size of the defect and status of the surrounding tissue. The external ear is an important part of the facial anatomy with specific aesthetic and functional correlations. Its loss can result in the compromise of overall facial aesthetics. Failure to correct or replace damaged ears in the thermally injured patient may also result in decreased self-esteem.

REFERENCES

1. Brent B. Reconstruction of ear, eyebrow, and sideburn in the burned patient. Plast Reconstr Surg 1975; 55:312–317.
2. Jones CE, Wellisz T. External ear reconstruction. Use of a pivoting helix, porous polyethylene implant. AORN J 1994; 59:411–415, 418–422.
3. Hauben DJ. Sushruta Samhita (Sushruta's Collection) (800–600 BC?). Pioneers of plastic surgery. Acta Chir Plast 1984; 26:65–68.
4. Converse JM. Reconstruction of the auricle. I. Plast Reconstr Surg 1958; 22:150–163.
5. Sushruta S. The classic reprint. Earlobe operations. Plast Reconstr Surg 1969; 43:515–522.
6. Schanz F. Wiedersatz einer verloren gegangenen Ohrmuschel: Korrespondenz-Blatter des allgem Arztl Vereins von Thuringen. 1890; 19:288–293.
7. Berghaus A, Toplak F. Surgical concepts for reconstruction of the auricle. History and current state of the art. Arch Otolaryngol Head Neck Surg 1986; 112:388–397.
8. Randall BA. An attempt to replace an auricle bitten off in childhood. Arch Otol 1893; 22:163–165.
9. Korte W. Fall von Ohrenplastik. Sitzung am Nov 13, 1905. Verh Fr Verein Chir Berlins 1905; 18:91–92.
10. Beck JC. The anatomy, psychology, diagnosis, and treatment of congenital malformation and absence of the ear. Laryngoscope 1925; 35:813–832.
11. De River PJ. Restoration of the auricle. Calif West Med 1927; 26:654–656.
12. Sarig A, Ben-Bassat H, Taube E et al. Reconstruction of the auricle in microtia by bipedicled postauricular tubed flap. Ann Plast Surg 1982; 8:221–223.
13. Schmieden V. Der plastische Ersatz von traumatischen Defekten der Ohrmuschel. Berl Klin Wochenschr 1908; 31:1433–1435.
14. Gillies HD, ed. Plastic Surgery of the Face. London: Oxford University Press, 1920:381–387.
15. Tanzer RC. Total reconstruction of the external ear. Plast Reconstr Surg 1959; 23:1–15.
16. Zeis E, ed. Handbuch der plastischen Chirurgie. Berlin: G Reimer, 1838:464–468.
17. Suraci AJ. Plastic reconstruction of acquired defects of the ear. Am J Surg 1944; 66:196–202.
18. Allison GR. Anatomy of the auricle. Clin Plast Surg 1990; 17:209–212.
19. Eriksson E, Vogt PM. Ear reconstruction. Clin Plast Surg 1992; 19:637–643.
20. Allison GR. Anatomy of the external ear. Clin Plast Surg 1978; 5:419–422.
21. Moore KL. Clinically Oriented Anatomy. 3rd ed. Baltimore: Williams and Wilkins, 1992:763.
22. Park C, Lineaweaver WC, Rumly TO, Buncke HJ. Arterial supply of the anterior ear. Plast Reconstr Surg 1992; 90:38–44.
23. Neale HW, Billmire DA, Carey J. Reconstruction following head and neck burns. Clin Plast Surg 1986; 13:119–136.
24. Gonzalez-Ulloa M. Restoration of the face covering by means of selected skin of regional aesthetic units. Br J Plast Surg 1956; 9:212–221.
25. Dowling JA, Foley FD, Moncrief JA. Chondritis in the burned ear. Plast Reconstr Surg 1968; 42(2):115–122.
26. Skedros DG, Goldfarb IW, Slater H, Rocco J. Chondritis of the burned ear: a review. Ear Nose Throat J 1992; 71:359–362.
27. Goel TK, Law EJ, MacMillan BG. Management of the acutely burned ear. Burns Incl Therm Inj 1983; 9:218–221.
28. Grant DA. Saving the burned ear. Texas Med 1967; 63:58–60.
29. Moncrief J, Lindberg R, Switzer W et al. Use of topical antibacterial therapy in the treatment of the burn wound. Arch Surg 1966; 92:558–565.
30. Harrison HN, Shuck JN, Caldwell E. Studies of the pain produced by mafenide acetate preparations in burns. Arch Surg 1975; 110:1446–1449.
31. Kucan JO, Smoot EC. Five percent mafenide acetate solution in the treatment of thermal injuries. J Burn Care Rehabil 1993; 14:158–163.
32. Jordan MH, Gallagher JM, Allely RR, Leman CJ. A pressure prevention device for burned ears. J Burn Care Rehabil 1992; 13:673–677.
33. Harries CA, Pegg SP. Foam ear protectors for burnt ears. J Burn Care Rehabil 1989; 10:183–184.
34. Caplan AI. Cartilage. Sci Am 1984; 251:84–87, 90–94.
35. Rosenthal JS. The thermally injured ear: a systematic approach to reconstruction. Clin Plast Surg 1992; 19:645–661.
36. Tegtmeier RE, Gooding RA. The use of fascial flap in ear reconstruction. Plast Reconstr Surg 1977; 60:406–411.
37. Cotlar S. Reconstruction of the burned ear using a temporalis fascial flap. Plast Reconstr Surg 1983; 71:45–48.
38. Achauer BM, Witt PD, Lamb R. Salvage of ear cartilage in patients with acute full-thickness burns. J Burn Care Rehabil 1991; 12:339–343.
39. Mills DC, Robers LW, Mason AD Jr, McManus WF, Pruitt BA Jr. Suppurative chondritis: its incidence, prevention, and treatment in burn patients. Plast Reconstr Surg 1988; 82(2):267–276.
40. Stroud MH. A simple treatment for suppurative perichondritis. Laryngoscope 1963; 73:556–563.
41. Stroud MH. Treatment of suppurative perichondritis. Laryngoscope 1978; 88:176–178.
42. Desai MH, Rutan RL, Heggers JP, Alvarado MI, McElroy K, Herndon DN. The role of gentamicin iontophoresis in the treatment of burned ears. J Burn Care Rehabil 1991; 12:521–524.
43. LeDuc S. Electronic ions and their use in medicine. London: Rebman Ltd, 1908.
44. Apfelberg DB, Waisbren BA, Masters FW et al. Treatment of chondritis in the burned ear by the local instillation of antibiotics. Plast Reconstr Surg 1974; 53:179–183.

45. Greminger RF, Elliott RA, Rapperport A. Antibiotic iontophoresis for the management of burned ear chondritis. Plast Reconstr Surg 1980; 66(3):356–360.

46. Macaluso RA, Kennedy TL. Antibiotic iontophoresis in the treatment of burn perichondritis of the rabbit ear. Otolaryngol Head Neck Surg 1989; 100(6):568–572.

47. Rigano W, Yanik M, Barone FA, Baibak G, Cislo C. Antibiotic iontophoresis in the management of burned ears. J Burn Care Rehabil 1992; 13(4):407–409.

48. Kaweski S, Baldwin RC, Wong RK, Manders EK. Diffusion versus iontophoresis in the transport of gentamicin in the burned rabbit ear model. Plast Reconstr Surg 1993; 92(7):1342–1349.

49. Stevenson EW. Bacillus pyocyaneus perichondritis of the ear. Laryngoscope 1964; 74:255–259.

50. Collentine G, Waisbren BA, Mellender J. Treatment of burns with intensive antibiotic therapy and exposure. J Am Med Assoc 1967; 200:939–942.

51. Wanamaker HH. Suppurative perichondritis of the auricle. Trans Am Acad Opathalmol Otolaryngol 1972; 76:1289–1291.

52. Pickus EJ, Lionelli GT, Woodall CE, Korentager RA. Mafenide acetate allergy presenting as recurrent chondritis. Ann Plast Surg 2002; 48:202–204.

53. Kroll SS, Gerow FJ: Sulfamylon allergy simulating chondritis. Plast Reconstr Surg 1987; 80(2):298–299.

54. Perry AW, Gottlieb LJ, Krizek TJ, Parsons RW, Goodwin CW, Finkelstein JL, Madden MR. Mafenide induced pseudochondritis. J Burn Care Rehabil 1988; 9(2):145–147.

55. Salisbury RE, Bevin AG. Atlas of reconstructive burn surgery. Philadelphia: W.B. Saunders, 1981:25–31.

56. Brent B. The acquired auricular deformity. Plast Reconstr Surg 1977; 59:475–485.

57. Lawrence WT. In search of the optimal treatment of keloids: report of a series and review of the literature. Ann Plast Surg 1991; 27:164–178.

58. Waymack JP, Pruitt BA. Burn wound care. Adv Surg 1990; 23:261–290.

59. Adams WM. Construction of the upper half of auricle utilizing composite concha cartilage graft with perichondrium attached on both sides. Plast Reconstr Surg 1955; 16:88–96.

60. Antia NH, Buch VI. Chondrocutaneous advancement flap for the marginal defect of the ear. Plast Reconstr Surg 1967; 39:472–477.

61. Donelan MB. Conchal Transposition flap for postburn ear deformities. Plast Reconstr Surg 1989; 83:641–652.

62. Costa H, Cunha C, Guimaraes I, Comba S, Malta A, Lopes A. Prefabricated flaps for the head and neck: a preliminary report. Br J Plast Surg 1993; 46:223–227.

63. Zhou G, Teng L, Chang HM, Jing WM, Xu J, Li SK, Zhuang HX. Free prepared composite forearm flap transfer for ear reconstruction: three case reports. Micosurgery 1994; 15:660–662.

64. Furuta S, Noguchi M, Takagi N. Reconstruction of stenotic external auditory canal with a postauricular chondrocutaneous flap. Plast Reconstr Surg 1994; 94:700–704.

65. Saraiya HA. A near closed book contracture of the ear: a case report. Burns 2000; 26:490–492.

66. Kumar P, Shah P. Preauricular flap for post burn ear lobe reconstruction—a case report. Burns 2000; 26:571–574.

67. Akin S. Burned ear reconstruction using a prefabricated free radial forearm flap. J Reconstr Microsurg 2001; 17:233–236.

68. Ellaban MG, Maamoun MI, Elsharkawi M. The bi-pedicle post-auricular tube flap for reconstruction of partial ear defects. Br J Plast Surg 2003; 56:593–598.

69. Stefanoff DN. Auriculo-mastoid tube pedicle for otoplasty. Plast Reconstr Surg 1948; 3:348.

70. Davis J. In: Symposium on Reconstruction of the Auricle. St. Louis: C. Mosby Co., 1974:247.

71. Gorney M, Murphy S, Falces E. Spliced autogenous conchal cartilage in secondary ear reconstruction. Plast Reconstr Surg 1971; 47:432–437.

72. Crikelair GF. A method of partial ear reconstruction for avulsion of the upper portion of the ear. Plast Reconstr Surg 1956; 17:438–443.

73. Preaux J. Un procede' simple de reconstruction de la partie inferieure du pavillon de l'oreille. Ann Chir Plast 1971; 16:60–62.

74. Alanis SZ. A new method for earlobe reconstruction. Plast Reconstr Surg 1970; 45:254–257.

75. Kazanjian VH, Converse JM. The surgical Treatment of Facial Injuries. 3rd ed. Baltimore: Williams and Wilkins Co., 1974:1334.

76. Brent B. Earlobe construction with an auriculo-mastoid flap. Plast Reconstr Surg 1976; 57:389–391.

77. Bhandari PS. Total ear reconstruction in post burn deformity. Burns 1998; 24:661–670.

78. Brent B. The correction of microtia with autogenous cartilage grafts: I. The classic deformity. Plast Reconstr Surg 1980; 66:1–12.

79. Wang PTH. Ear reconstruction using Medpor®. Proc Texas Soc of Plast Surg September, 2002.

80. Wellisz T. Reconstruction of the burned external ear using a Medpor® porous polyethylene pivoting helix framework. Plast Reconstr Surg 1993; 91:811–818.

81. Reinish. Proc Am Assoc Plast Surg 2004; 83:56.

82. Tjellstrom A. Osseointegrated systems and their applications in the head and neck. Adv Otolaryngol Head Neck Surg 1989; 3:39–70.

83. Tjellstrom A, Granstrom G. One-stage procedure to establish osseointegration: a zero to five years follow-up report. J Laryngol Otol 1995; 109:593–598.

23

Reconstruction of the Upper Lip and Commissure

ROBERT L. McCAULEY, GARRY W. KILLYON

University of Texas Medical Branch and Shriners Hospital for Children—Galveston Unit, Galveston, Texas, USA

I. UPPER LIP

A. Introduction

Burns to the face are common in large total body surface area injuries. The reconstructive needs can be numerous. Prioritization in the reconstruction of facial burns is a function of the depth of injury, the extent of the defect, and the severity of functional impairment. When these three issues are addressed, the eyes, nose, and mouth are the facial regions of most concern. Distortions in these areas can not only cause blindness, but also produce a loss of facial balance as well as impairment in our ability to speak, eat, and address issues related to dental hygiene. Burns to the upper lip nasal unit and the upper lip can have significant effects on facial aesthetics as well as impair our activities of daily living (ADLS). As we entertain the idea of aesthetic and functional reconstruction of the upper lip nasal unit and upper lip, we note that quantitative and qualitive assessments of normal function are often not known. Thus, in order to clearly define our reconstructive goals, an operative plan based on normal parameters needs to be devised. Mere attainment of a healed wound, today, is not satisfactory. Reconstruction with symmetry and balance of the lips and commissures is demanded.

B. Surface Anatomy

Although Gonzales-Ulloa (1) described the regional units of the face, Burget and Menick (2) defined the anatomic subunits of the upper lip to assist in the aesthetic reconstruction of this area. Gonzales-Ulloa concentrated on facial reconstruction using skin grafts, while Burget and Menick concentrated on the use of flaps to restore

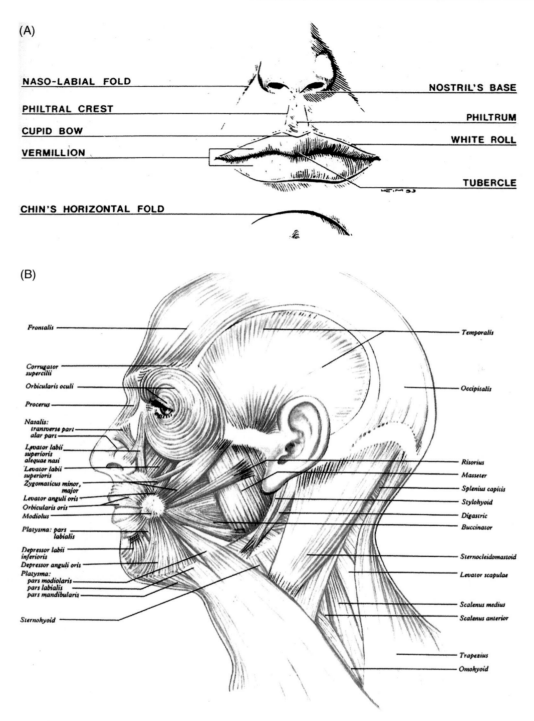

(A)

NASO-LABIAL FOLD

PHILTRAL CREST

CUPID BOW

VERMILLION

CHIN'S HORIZONTAL FOLD

NOSTRIL'S BASE

PHILTRUM

WHITE ROLL

TUBERCLE

(B)

Frontalis

Corrugator supercilii

Orbicularis oculi

Procerus

Nasalis:
transverse part
alar part

Levator labii
superioris
alequae nasi

Levator labii
superioris

Zygomaticus minor,
major

Levator anguli oris

Orbicularis oris

Modiolus

Platysma: pars
labialis

Depressor labii
inferioris

Depressor anguli oris

Platysma:
pars modiolaris
pars labialis
pars mandibularis

Sternohyoid

Temporalis

Occipitalis

Risorius

Masseter

Splenius capitis

Stylohyoid

Digastric

Buccinator

Sternocleidomastoid

Levator scapulae

Scalenus medius

Scalenus anterior

Trapezius

Omohyoid

Figure 23.1 (A) Soft tissue anatomy of the upper lip nasal unit and the lips and chin. [From Maillard and Montandon (3).] (B) Lateral view of perioral muscles. [From Gray's Anatomy (4).]

full-thickness defects in the upper lip nasal unit in an aesthetic manner. Both concepts are important landmarks in the spectrum of facial deformities seen today (Fig. 23.1). Burget and Menick divided the upper lip into smaller topographical subunits: two medial subunits and two lateral subunits. While viewing one half of the upper lip, the lateral subunit is bordered superiorly by the alar base and the nostril sill, medially by the philtrum, and laterally by the nasolabial crease (Fig. 23.2). The interlabial gap borders the upper lip-nasal unit inferiorly. It has two

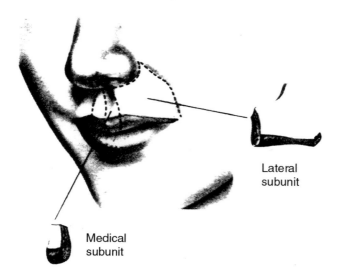

Figure 23.2 Subunit principle of the upper lip nasal unit. [From Burget and Menick (2).]

anatomic components of different color: the vermillion, which has lateral elements and a central tubercle, and the skin-covered lip, which consists of the lateral elements and a central philtrum. It is currently believed that when a large part of the subunit is destroyed, total replacement is warranted. Although these principles were not conceptualized with burn patients in mind, they serve as guiding points in our efforts to aesthetically reconstruct them.

C. Functional Anatomy

Understanding the functional anatomy of the blood supply, muscle, and nerves in the buccolabial is important for our understanding of what occurs in burn patients with subsequent deformities (Fig. 23.3). There are a number of muscle groups that interconnect with each other and have attachments to the skin and mucous membranes.

The orbicularis oris muscle in each lip originates in four quadrants from a modiolus at the corners of the oral fissure consisting of a pars peripheralis and a pars marginalis (4–8). The pars peripheralis is deeper and lies in the area under the lip skin whereas the pars marginalis is more superficial and is confined to the area under the vermillion (4,6,8). They meet at the mucocutaneous junction (4). The deeper layer of the orbicularis oris is continuous with the buccinator and the superficial layer is continuous with the facial muscles entering and leaving through the modiolus at the oral commissure (8). In the midline, the deeper layer of orbicularis oris is continuous with the muscle on the opposite side. The superficial layer of orbicularis interdigitates with its contralateral side and inserts into the dermis of the lateral aspect of the opposite philtral column (8). In burn patients with microstomia, especially those who have sustained electrical injuries, the orbicularis muscle may be partially destroyed during the injury or pulled medically as a result of contraction.

Tractors of the lip affect the action of the circumoral musculature. They are radially arranged as superficial and deep muscles and most have an attachment to the modiolus at the corners of the mouth (4,6). Direct tractors insert directly into the tissues of the lip without intervention of the modiolus (4). The force of contraction is at right angles to the oral fissure serving to elevate and/or evert the whole or part of the upper lip. These muscles also depress and/or evert the whole or part of the lower lip. In burn patients with ectropions, these muscles may be affected. The upper lip tractors from medial to lateral are the labial part of the levator labii superioris, alaeque nasi, levator superioris, and zygomaticus minor. They blend into a continuous sheet that inserts into the lip, anterior to the pars peripheralis. The lower lip tractors are the depressor labii inferioris medially and the platysma laterally (4). In patients with cervical contractures, the pull of the platysma muscle initially may accentuate lower lip ectropion. Again, they pass ventral to the pars peripheralis in coronal sheets.

The modiolar muscles are classified in terms of their general geometric relation to the modiolus as cruciate, or transverse (4). The cruciate muscles are the zygomaticus

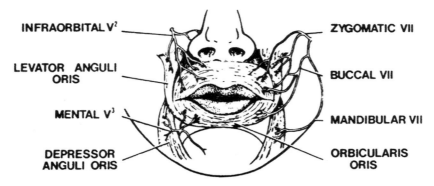

Figure 23.3 Muscular anatomy of the upper lip nasal unit. Lip and chin and innervation by V_2 and V_3. [From Maillard and Montandon (3).]

major, levator anguli oris, depressor anguli oris, and platysma. The transverse muscles are the buccinator, risorius, and incisivus superior and inferior.

The complex three-dimensional mobility of the modioli enables them to provide functional loci for integrated activities of the cheeks, lips and oral fissure, oral vestibule, and the jaws bearing teeth (4). These activities include biting, chewing, drinking, sucking, swallowing, changes in vestibular contents and pressure, variations in speech, modulations in music tone, harsher sounds in shouting and screaming, crying, and permutations of changes in facial expression. Some surgeons feel that severe electrical burns to oral commisures can affect the integrity of the modiolus and reconstruction may be indicated. The obicularis oris has a sphincter type mechanism. Its attachments are to the modioli laterally surrounding masculature and dermis. By itself, it has no bony attachment. This may explain why it is very susceptible to deformity forces from circumoral hypertrophic scarring. Also, with the attachment of the platysma to the modiolus, cervical contractures secondary to burn scarring may pull the modiolus and corners of the mouth in an inferior direction. In correcting microstomia, the freeing of these muscles may be necessary to return the modioli to its original position.

D. Function

Page and Stranc (9) recognized the need to quantitate the normal function of the lip. In any postoperative lip reconstruction, appearance and function are of paramount importance. However, in burn patients, little opportunity exists to assess how the severity of the acute injury affects function. In most cases, trying to determine the depth of injury and its subsequent management is of major concern. In patients referred for reconstruction, aesthetic concerns and functional impairments are evident. Decreased intraoral excursion is seen in patients with microstomia and oral incompetence with gum exposure is seen in patients with severe lower lip ectropions (Figs. 23.3 and 23.4).

Page (9) reviewed the parameters of normal lip function in adult patients. Four measurements were assessed. The intercommissural distance (ICD) was measured from one mucocutaneous junction of commissure to the other. Here, two sets of readings were made. One set of measurements occurred in repose; the second set was taken with the broadest possible smile. With maximum opening, soft-tissue gape (STG) was measured from the midpoint of the upper lip to a similar point on the lower lip. As an expression of the elasticity of the circumoral tissues, a lip index (LI) was devised (Fig. 23.5). The value obtained was equal to the size of the oral aperture plus its surrounding vermillion. Last, the depth of the intraoral sulcus (SD) was measured from a central midpoint. Maximal sphincter

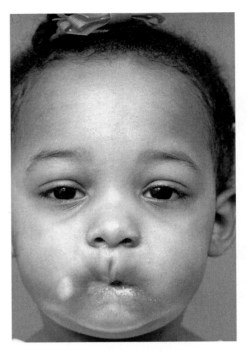

Figure 23.4 Three-year-old female with an electrical burn to the right oral commisure with severe microstomia.

power generated by the lip muscles was measured using a pommeter. Although these measurements were only made in white adults, it does form a basis by which future studies in children and nonwhite races can be centered. Later,

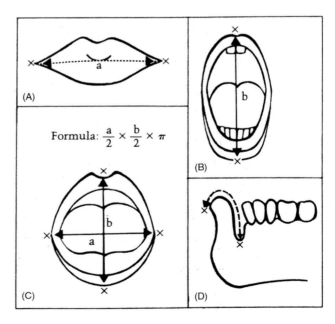

Figure 23.5 Measurements of lip function. (A) Intercommissural distance. (B) Soft tissue gap. (C) Lip index and formula. (D) Sulcus depth. [From Page and Stranc (9).].

Stranc et al. (10) reviewed the functional aspects of the reconstructed lip in a number of patients who had previously undergone lip reconstruction. Included in this study was a group of burn patients who sustained severe perioral burns which required excision of the burn wound and resurfacing with skin grafts. Each patient underwent measurements of ICD, STG, LI, SD, and pommeter readings. In addition, two-point discrimination, sensation, dribbling, oral access, dental status, and oral hygiene along with speech and EMG studies were documented. In Stranc et al. (10) assessment, dribbling was associated with a shallow sulcus, decreased sensation, limited intraoral access, and decreased muscle power. Patients with modest dribbling were noted to have at least two of these four parameters present. Of the various types of lip repair noted, only the Karapandzic flap, as expected, restored orbicularis alignment, but at the expense of partial denervation. In general, burn patients who underwent correction of deep perioral burn with skin grafts had less ICD at rest and smiling, a decreased LI, lower pommeter readings, and restricted intraoral access.

E. Acute Burn Care

In the past, facial burns have been generally treated conservatively. The use of topical ointments and allowing a superficial or deep partial thickening wound to heal secondary had been the mainstay of treatment. Later, the use of pressure garments and splinting controlled the hypertrophic scars and contracture until the scars matured. It has been shown that wounds that heal spontaneously within 14 days will heal without disfigurement. However, wounds that heal after 18–21 days, whether allowed to heal secondary or with skin grafts, show a greater tendency for scarring and secondary reconstruction. However, more recently, acute burns to the face have been treated more aggressively with early surgical excision and resurfacing of the defect with skin grafts (11–16). However, regardless of how early excision is defined when compared to later excisions, decreased hospital stay, decreased scarring, improved aesthetic results, and decrease in subsequent reconstructive procedures have been touted as advantageous. The lips are particularly vulnerable to a number of deformities for several reasons. First, compressive garments are ineffective in this region. Second, in men, healing in the mustache and bearded regions is protracted and particularly prone to folliculitis, leading to even more problems with delayed wound healing (17). The results of such delayed healing are hypertrophic scar formation and burn scar contractures. In children, the forces of contraction from burn scars and/or subsequent compression with pressure garments have been implicated in retarding the growth of

the mandible and being a factor in the development of malocclusion (18,19). In children with commissure injuries, the use of splints has been recommended. Yet, compliance issues can significantly compromise the ultimate outcome. In spite of these problems, the resurfacing of the upper lip-nasal unit from deep second-degree burns or third-degree burns is best accomplished with skin grafts that respect the anatomic units as outlined by Gonzales-Ulloa. Secondary reconstruction for burn scar contractures should also approximate these goals.

F. Reconstruction

Reconstruction of the upper lip-nasal unit is well described for nonburn injuries. The reconstruction of the resulting defects is a function of size, location, and the involvement of other surrounding structures such as the upper lip, columella, nasal vestibule, cheek, and nose (17).

1. Upper Lip Defects Without Involvement of the Vermillion

Assessment of burn scars to the upper lip includes not only a review of the soft tissue deficit, but also an assessment of involvement of the vermillion. Distortion beyond that of an upper lip ectropion and destruction of Cupid's bow are also important to note. In addition, determining the extent of the injury will determine if the philtrum, the nasal sill, or the nasolabial folds are involved. Outlining the deficits of the lateral and/or medial segments of the upper lip will allow us to determine the extent of the surface soft tissue defect (3). Functional assessment is also noted. Intraoral excursion is not only a function of the orbicularis muscle but also an indication of the pliability of the surrounding tissues. The contributions of surrounding aesthetic units to the contracture, in particular, must be assessed. The presence or absence of a philtrum is crucial in devising a surgical plan.

If the philtrum is present and the contractures are bilateral, excision of the lateral subunits of the upper lip and resurfacing with skin grafts are reasonable options. Tie-over bolster dressings are used and patients are given full liquids in the early postoperative period. Bolster takedown is carried out on postoperative days 5–7 to insure graft take. The use of a clear U-vex mask is desired to help prevent graft contraction. Nevertheless, in patients of color, hyperpigmentation of the grafts may compromise the aesthetic results (Fig. 23.6).

Reconstruction without the presence of a philtrum is more difficult. Unfortunately, most of our literature on reconstruction of the philtrum comes from correction of secondary cleft lip deformities (20–26). However, some of the techniques described are applicable to the reconstruction of the philtrum in burn patients. A number of

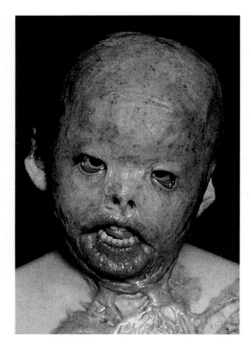

Figure 23.6 Nine-year-old female with severe lower lip ectropion after burn injury.

local subcutaneous flaps have been used to reconstruct the philtrum including the para-alar crescent subcutaneous pedicle flap and the local island pedicle flap (27,28). The use of local pedicle flaps is helpful when defects are small. However, major losses of the philtrum require more innovative techniques. In children with large facial burns, the use of local flaps may have a propensity for the development of a secondary deformity. In these patients, soft tissue laxity is usually not present. The use of composite grafts and fork flaps has also been noted.

Nevertheless, even with our best efforts, aesthetic reconstruction of the upper lip may be compromised and the results can be less than ideal. In adult male patients, there is an alternative solution. The use of hair-bearing flaps for reconstruction of the upper lip dates back to the mid-1900s (29,30). Hair-bearing scalp flaps based on the superficial temporal vessels were initially used as tubed flaps, which required multiple stages to complete (31,32). The subsequent development and use of the bitemporal artery visor scalp flap added some refinements and versatility to the reconstruction of the upper lip (33–35). Hafezi et al. (35) clearly demonstrated the aesthetic benefits that can be achieved with the use of this flap (Fig. 23.7). However,

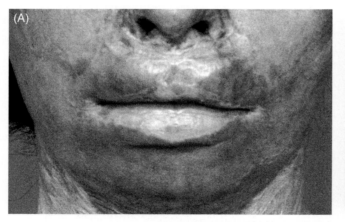

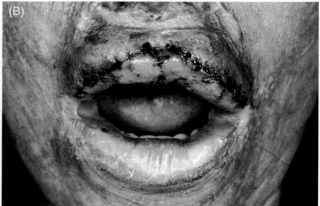

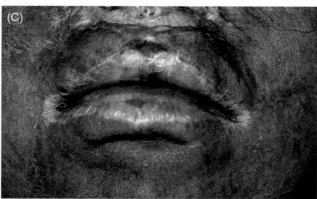

Figure 23.7 (A) Fifteen-year-old female with upper lip entropion. (B) Immediate appearance after correction. (C) Follow-up at 1 year.

a significant family history of baldness may preclude the use of this flap. In addition, it remains a multistage process, although some of the reported results are outstanding. With the advent of microvascular surgery, the use of hair-bearing tissue for reconstruction of the burned face evolved to a single-stage process (36,37). In spite of these advances, solutions to the aesthetic reconstruction of the upper lip in children and women remain elusive.

2. Reconstruction of the Upper Lip Defects with Involvement of the Vermillion

In many cases, once the vermillion of the upper lip is involved with burn injury, the healed wound shows loss of Cupid's bow with a rounding of the central features of the upper lip. This impacts negatively on facial balance (Fig. 23.8). Reconstruction of the upper lip-nasal unit requires careful recreation of Cupid's bow prior to addressing the medial and lateral segments. The low point on Cupid's bow is noted by the center of the columella. If soft tissue landmarks are distorted, the midpoint of the central incisors serves as a reliable landmark for reconstruction. All contractures of the upper lip-nasal unit must be relaxed prior to addressing Cupid's bow. Once these markings are assured, the peaks on Cupid's bow are created at an angle of 30°, usually 0.5–10 mm in height. Reconstruction of the philtrum can then proceed with the use of local skin flaps, composite grafts, or skin grafts. The lateral subunits are then addressed. Such an approach can provide reasonable reconstruction of the upper lip when the vermillion is distorted (Fig. 23.6).

3. Reconstruction of Major Upper Lip Defects

The reconstruction of major upper lip defects, those greater than one-third of the upper lip, is complicated. In such

situations, the need for functional reconstruction must include muscle replacement. In the central portion of the lip, the Abbe flap has been the work-horse for replacement of the central portion in the philtrum, with excellent results. However, its use in burn patients may be precluded if the lower lip is injured and cannot be utilized as a donor site for this flap.

Tobin et al. (38) discussed the need for reconstruction of major upper lip defects using motor and sensory innervated composite flaps. The innervated orbicularis oris flap was described by Karapandzic in 1974. This flap is mobilized to provide coverage to the upper lip in reconstructing major upper lip defects. This flap is composed of the orbicularis oris muscle with the overlying skin and mucosa attached to neurovascular pedicle, containing the fifth and seventh cranial nerves. The advantage of using this flap is the provision of a sensate and functional reconstruction. However, it can create microstomia (Fig. 23.9). Tobin suggests that the aesthetic frailties of this flap may be enhanced by use of the Abbe flap for columella reconstruction. The bilateral levator anguli oris flap has also been recommended for total upper lip reconstruction.

II. COMMISSURE INJURIES

A. Electrical Burns

Injuries to the commissures can occur as a result of both thermal and electrical trauma. Electrical burns to the mouth in children usually occur when they are <4 years of age. Although these injuries are never constituted, a large percentage of burn admissions, usually 1–3%, were quite devastating to the child and their parents (39,40). Fortunately, with new preventive measures, these injuries are even more infrequent. Electrical burns

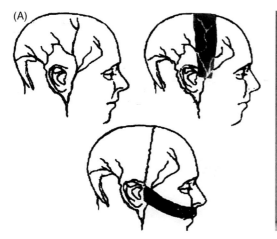
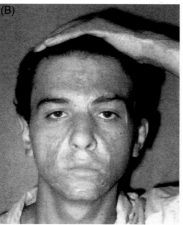
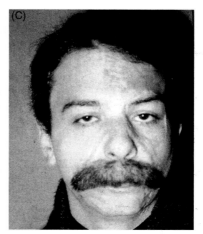

Figure 23.8 (A) Diagram of scalp visor flap for resonstruction of upper lip defect. (B) Twenty-two-year-old male with burns to the upper lip nasal unit. (C) Reconstruction with a scalp visor flap. [From Hafezi et al. (35).]

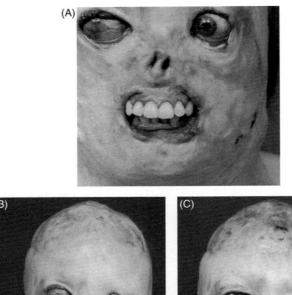

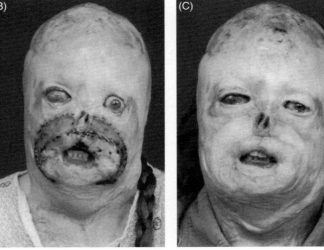

Figure 23.9 Twenty-year-old female referred with severe facial burns sustained as a child. Currently patient is blind. (A) Note severe upper and lower eyelid ectropions, total nasal loss, loss of the majority of the upper lip, and lower lip ectropion. (B) Reconstruction of the upper lip with a Karapandzic flap with a split thickness skin graft on the donor site. (C) Appearance 3 months after correction of upper and lower eyelid ectropions with skin grafts and lower lip ectropion with turnover scar flaps and skin grafts. Mild microstomia produced with Karapandzic flap. However, speech and the ability to feed were not impaired. Nasal reconstruction declined.

to the mouth can occur as a result of arc injuries or contact burns (41). Arc burns result from bridging of the polarity gap of the wires by saliva. As an arc or flash develops, temperatures are reported to rise as high as 3000 °C. Contact burns or thermoelectrical burns occur when the current follows a path of least resistance, that is, from the mouth to the ground. The duration of contact voltage, tissue resistance, current path, and current type determines the extent of injury (41,42). Although, the treatment of commissure injuries from electricity has evolved, controversy continues to exist over the initial management and subsequent reconstruction. A number of authors have advocated conservative management of patients with electrical burns to the oral commissures using mouth splints usually 10–14 days after injury before making any definitive surgical plans (43–46). Others have touted the use of splints to prevent the need for surgical intervention (Fig. 23.10). However, it should be noted that splinting alone will not replace the

full-thickness loss, including partial loss of the orbicularis oris; nor will it correct the subsequent deformities which result from the loss of bulk. Some authors questioned the use of splints indicating that scarring is increased (47). With the ultimate goal being that of aesthetics and functional uniformity, the management of these patients remains elusive. In addition, controversy over the timing of an operation in these patients remains variable. Yet several investigators believe that early surgical intervention offers fewer hospital stays and fewer operations with good aesthetic results (47,48). Without question, as we review the results of no surgical intervention vs. only surgical intervention as compared to early vs. late surgical therapy, with or without splints, the confusion is magnified. It is possible still that the timing and extent of injury influence the ultimate outcome. Orgell (49) in a retrospective study, evaluated the results of early surgical excision within 4 days of injury vs. conservative treatment with delayed eschar separation. The parameters measured

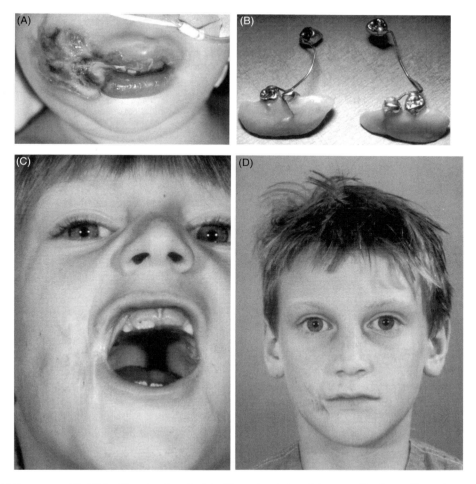

Figure 23.10 (A) Four-year-old child with extensive electrical burn involving right upper lip, lower lip, and commissure with extension into cheek. (B) Appearance of earlier splints attached to maxillary teeth. (C/D) Aesthetic and functional outcome 6 years later. [From McCauley and Barret (41).]

included lip roll, lip length, scar quality, and vermillion quality. He concluded that there was no difference between the two groups. Perhaps, controversy in the literature exists because the extent of the injuries was not delineated. Even Silverglade and Ruberg (50), staunch advocates of splinting only, admit to surgical intervention when most of the lip is involved with electrical injuries. In an attempt to correlate the ultimate aesthetic and functional outcome of electrical burns to the lips and commissures, Pitanquy et al. (51) developed a classification system for electrical burns of the commissure based on severity (Table 23.1). It is likely that such a classification scheme may allow us to compare apples to apples when we evaluate the many parameters involved with the type of early management, and nonsurgical vs. surgical intervention with the degree of injury and the ultimate functional and aesthetic outcomes. Zarem et al. (52) alluded to this management scheme when only patients deemed to have more extensive injuries underwent early surgical intervention.

Table 23.1 Classification of Commissure Injuries Secondary to Electrical Burns

Degree	Acute (0 to 4 days) and subacute (4 days to 2 months)	Sequela (more than 2 months)
Light	Up to one-third of upper or lower lip or up to one-sixth both lips without commissure involvement	Aesthetic impairment
Moderate	Over one-third of upper or lower lip or both without commissure involvement	Aesthetic and functional impairment
Severe	Over one-third of both lips with commissure; over two-thirds of upper or lower lip; local tissue involvement (tongue, gingivolabial, gutter, etc.)	Severe aesthetic and functional impairment

Source: Reprinted with permission from Pitanquy I, Vieira P, Muller P, Persichetti P, Piccolo N. Management of electrical injuries. Compend Cont Educ Dent 1986; 10:30–33.

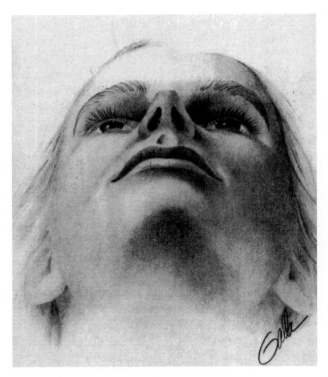

Figure 23.11   Natural position of oral commissures. [From Donelan (53).]

B.   Evaluation

Whether surgery is indicated during the acute phase or occurs after splinting and scar maturation, the type of operation selected attempts to recreate symmetry of the commissures and fill in any muscle bulk lost from the original injury (53). The selected procedure is usually chosen based on the degree of contracture, the functional deficit, and the extent of defect. One procedure does not fit all patients. Donelan (53) reviewed 135 cases of

commissure burns to assess various techniques of reconstruction. However, he noted that similar patterns of deformity follow soft tissue loss: first, there was lateral displacement of the central lip segments in the philtrum of the upper lip and the midline of the lower lip; second, there was the intermedial displacement of the commissure; and third, the scarred commissure was rounded, thick, and immobile (Fig. 23.11) (53).

Pensler et al. (54) felt that in order to minimize postoperative wound contraction after any type of repair, reconstruction of the modiolus labii by lateral advancement of the orbicularis oris was a significant part of the functional reconstruction. The new modiolus labii was sutured to the risorius, the platysma, and the triangulis muscles (Fig. 23.12) (54). It is clear that preoperative evaluation and the desire to taper procedures for aesthetic and functional reconstruction are the driving force behind a variety of techniques used for reconstruction of the oral commissure. The goals are to restore symmetry, match bulk, and re-establish normal function.

C.   Surgical Techniques

Although there are a plethora of techniques described for re-creation of a normal commissure, their use may be specific for the extent of the defect to be reconstructed (53–63). Using the classification scheme devised by Pitanquy (51), mild deficits that are noted to occur upto one-sixth of both lips may be managed in different fashions. If muscle loss is not an issue, mucosal advancement may be adequate to restore the normal contour of the upper and lower lips as well as the commissure. The technique of mucosal advancement was reported by Kazangian et al. (55) with variations in design reported by Gilles and Millard (56). Alternatively, if muscle loss has occurred, the rotation advancement flap with attached muscle as described by Barach (42) and popularized by

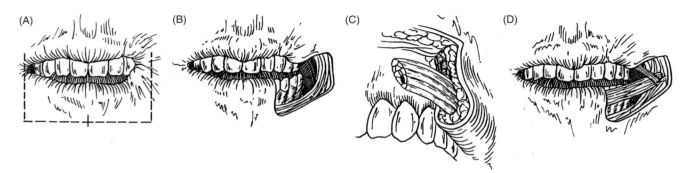

Figure 23.12   Restoration of the modiolus. (A) The position of the new modiolus is established with distance from the unburned commissure to the interdental space between the maxillary centra incisors as a guide. (B) Area of scar excision from lower lip to distance comparable to the unburned modiolus. (C) The orbicularis oris muscle is advanced laterally. (D) The orbicularis oris muscle from the upper and lower lip is advanced laterally to the location of the new modiolus. [From Pensler and Rosenthal (54).]

Canady (57) is useful. As a variation of mucosal advancement flap, the triangular pedicle intraoral flap as described by Johns (58) may be appropriate.

Although popularized in acute reconstruction of commissure burns, the tongue flap as modified by Donelan (53) has been used in smaller defects because of its versatility and reportedly superior aesthetic results (52).

Medium-sized defects, those which involve up to a third of the upper and lower lips and commissure, may require more extensive approaches for commissure and lip restoration. Although the tongue flap and the rotation advancement mucosal flaps may still be useful, other innovative techniques have been reported (59–61). If the commissure is not involved, the cross-lip pedicle flap is an alternative choice. In addition, Hagan (62) reported the use of the nasolabial musculocutaneous flap for correction of medium-sized defects.

More severe defects, those greater than one-third of the lip, are added challenges to the reconstruction of these defects. The availability of local tissue large enough for reconstruction will surely limit our choices. The use of distant tissues, although adequate, may compromise aesthetics. Again, the tongue flap appears to be able to provide adequate tissue for commissure reconstruction and may be the work-horse under these conditions. Other uses of regional tissue include the use of the island submental flap in combination with a nasolabial flap (63). Although function is maintained, the aesthetic results are less than optimal.

III. CONCLUSION

Our constant search for the ideal reconstruction of the upper lip and commissures continues to elude us. The question of whether to operate or not operate still resurfaces. The use or nonuse of splints, interestingly enough, may continue to be controversial. The selection of the type of operation to perform on these patients is based on a multitude of factors. However, issues related to the extent of the defects, the functional impairment, and the best operation for aesthetic reconstruction will always guide our decision as to which operation to choose. Realistic expectations on the part of our patients, their families, and ourselves can prepare us all for the sometimes less than ideal results seen in the reconstruction of very large defects. Nevertheless, as reconstructive surgeons, our goal is to continue to pursue these difficult reconstructions with refinements and new innovative techniques in order to obtain facial harmony and aesthetic balance.

REFERENCES

1. Gonzalez-Ulloa M, Castillo A, Stevens E, Alvarez-Fuertes G, Leonelli F, Ubaldo F. Preliminary study of total restoration of the facial skin. Plast Reconstr Surg 1954; 12:151–161.
2. Burget GC, Menick FJ, Aesthetic restoration of one half the upper lip. Plast Reconstr Surg 1986; 78:583–593.
3. Maillard GF, Montandon D. Reconstructive surgery of deep burn to the lips. Clin Plast Surg 1984; 11:655–668.
4. Williams P, Warwick R, Dyson M, Bannister L, eds. Gray's Anatomy. 37th ed. London: Churchill Livingstone, 1989:570–580.
5. Thorek P, ed. Anatomy in Surgery. 2nd ed. Philadelphia: Lippincott, 1962:110–154.
6. Millard DR, ed. Cleft Craft (The Evolution of Its Surgery). 1st ed. Little Brown & Co., 1976:19–40.
7. Fernandez-Villoria JM. A study of the development of the orbicularis oris muscle. Plast Reconstr Surg 1975; 55(2):205–213.
8. Briedis J, Jackson IT. The anatomy of the philtrum: observations made on dissections in the normal lip. Br J Plast Surg 1981; 34(2):128–132.
9. Page RE, Stranc MF. Normal lip function in adults. Ann Plast Surg 1982; 9:502–505.
10. Stranc MF, Page RE. Functional aspects of the reconstructed lip. Ann Plast Surg 1983; 10:103–111.
11. Hunt JL, Purdue GF, Spicer T, Bening HG, Range S. Facial burn reconstruction: does early excision and autografting improve results? Burns 1987; 13:39–44.
12. Jonsson CE, Dalsgaard CJ. Early excision and grafting of selected burns of the face and neck. Plast Reconstr Surg 1991; 88:83–94.
13. Fraulin FOG, Lilmayer SJ, Tredget EE. Assessment of cosmetic and functional results of conservative vs. surgical management of facial burns. J Burn Care Rehab 1996; 17:19–29.
14. Voinchet V, Bardot J, Echinard C, Aubert JP, Magalou E. Advantages of early burn excision and grafting of burns to the anterior cervical region. Burns 1995; 21:143–146.
15. Jougard JP, Echinard C, Carlin G, Manelli C, Palyret D. Severity and prognosis after early excision from one to twenty one percent of the body surface area. Scand J Plast Reconstr Surg 1972; 12:121–125.
16. Engrav LH, Heimbach DM, Walkinshaw MD, Marvin JA. Excision of burns of the face. Plast Reconstr Surg 1986; 77:744–749.
17. Weerda H, Siegert R. Reconstruction of the upper lip. Facial Plast Surg 1990; 7:72–83.
18. Rothman DL. Pediatric orofacial injuries. Pediatrics 1996; 4:37–42.
19. Fricke NB, Omnell ML, Dutcher KD, Hollender LG, Engrav LH. Skeletal and dental disturbances after facial burns and pressure garments. J Burn Care Rehab 1996; 17:338–345.
20. Onizuka T, Akagawa T, Tokunaga S. A new method to create a philtrum in secondary cleft lip repairs. Plast Reconstr Surg 1978; 62:842–847.
21. Onizuka T. Philtrum formation in the secondary cleft lip repair. Plast Reconst Surg 1975; 56:522–526.
22. Reichert H. Philtrum formation in cleft lip surgery. Ann Acad Med 1983; (suppl 2):337–340.

23. Namnoum JD, Hisley KC, Graepel S, Hutchins GN, Vander Kolk CA. Three-dimensional reconstruction of the human fetal philtrum. Ann Plast Surg 1997; 38:202–208.

24. Tange I. The lambda flap for secondary cleft lip repair. Cleft Palate Craniofac J 1997; 34:357–361.

25. Kinnebrew MC. Use of the Abbe flap in revision of the bilateral cleft lip-nose deformity. Oral Surg Oral Med Oral Pathol 1983; 56:12–19.

26. Sadove AM, Eppley BL. Correction of secondary cleft lip and nasal deformities. Clinics Plast Surg 1993; 20:793–801.

27. Suzuki S. Para-alar crescentric subcutaneous pedicle flap for repair of skin defects in the philtrum. Ann Plast Surg 1989; 23:442–446.

28. Velasco VS, Martinez SA, Diez ME, Pena DA. Hemi-philtrum rotated flap. Ann Plast Surg 2003; 50:480–483.

29. Jurkiewicz MJ, Krieck TJ, Mathes SJ, Ariyan. Plastic Surgery: Principles and Practice. St. Louis: Cv Mosby Co., 1990:419–439.

30. McCarthy JG, May JW, Little WJ. Plastic Surgery. London: W.B. Saunders, 1990:614–622.

31. New GB. Sickle flap for nasal reconstruction. Surg Gyncol Obstet 1945; 90:497.

32. Kazanjian VH, Converse JM. The Surgical Treatment of Facial Injuries. 3rd ed. Baltimore, MD: Williams and Wilkins Co., 1974.

33. Kim JC, Hadlock T, Varvares MA, Cheney ML. Hair-bearing temporoparietal facial flap reconstruction of upper lip and scalp defects. Arch Facial Plast Surg 2001; 3:170–177.

34. Datubo-Brown DD, Khalid KN, Levick PL. Tissue expanded visor flap in burn surgery. Ann Plast Surg 1994; 32:205–208.

35. Hafezi F, Naghibzadeh B, Nouhi A. Facial reconstruction using the visor scalp flap. Burns 2002; 28:679–683.

36. Walton RL, Bunkis J. A free occipital hair-bearing flap for reconstruction of the upper lip. Br J Plast Surg 1983; 36:168–170.

37. Lyons GB, Milroy BC, Lendvay PG, Toeston LM. Upper lip reconstruction: use of the free superficial temporal artery hair-bearing flap. Br J Plast Surg 1989; 42:333–336.

38. Tobin GR, O'Daniel. Lip reconstruction with motor and sensory innergrated composite flaps. Clin Plast Surg 1990; 17:623–632.

39. Richardson DS, Kittle PE. Extraoral management of a lip commissure burn. J Den Child 1981; 352–356.

40. Davies MR. Burns caused by electricity. Plast Reconstr Surg 1958; 11:288–292.

41. McCauley RL, Barret JP. Electrical injuries. In: Erickson E, ed. Plastic Surgery: Indications, Operations and Outcomes. St. Louis: Mosby, Inc., 2000:375–387.

42. Canady TW, Thompson SA, Barach J. Oral commissure burns in children. Plast Reconstr Surg 1996; 97:738–744.

43. Czerepak CS. Oral splint therapy to manage electrical burns of the mouth in children. Clin Plast Surg 1984; 11:685–692.

44. Port RM, Cooley RO. Treatment of electrical burns of the oral and perioral tissues in children. J Am Dent Assoc 1986; 112:352–354.

45. Sandove AM, Jones JE, Lynch TR, Sheets PW. Appliance therapy for personal electrical burns: a conservative approach. J Burn Care Rehab 1986; 9:391–395.

46. Neale HW, Billmire DA, Gregory RO. Management of perioral burn scarring in the child and adolescent. Ann Plast Surg 1985; 15:212–217.

47. De La Plaza R, Quetglas A, Rodriguez E. Treatment of electrical burns to the mouth. Burns 1983; 10:49–60.

48. Ortiz-Monesterio F, Factor R. Early definition treatment of electrical burns to the mouth. Plast Reconstr Surg 1982; 69:169–173.

49. Orgell MG, Brown HC, Woolhouse FM. Electrical burns of the mouth in children: a method for assessing results. J Trauma 1975; 15:285–289.

50. Silverglade D, Ruberg Rl. Non-surgical management of burns to the lips and commissures. Clin Plast Surg 1986; 13:87–94.

51. Pitanquy I, Vieira P, Muller P, Persichetti P, Piccolo N. Management of electrical injuries. Compend Cont Educ Dent 1986; 10:30–33.

52. Zarem HA, Green DM. Tongue flap for reconstruction of the lips after electrical burns. Plast Reconstr Surg 1979; 53:310–312.

53. Donelan MB. Reconstruction of electrical burns of the oral commissure with a ventral tongue flap. Plast Reconstr Surg 1995; 95:1155–1163.

54. Pensler JM, Rosenthal A. Reconstruction of the oral commissure after an electrical injury. J Burn Care Rehab 1990; 11:50–53.

55. Kazangian VH, Roopenian A. The treatment of lip deformities resulting from electrical burns. Am J Surg 1954; 88:882.

56. Gilles H, Millard DR. Lip trauma. In: Gilles H, Millard DR, eds. Principles and Art of Plastic Surgery. Vol. II. Boston: Little, Brown and Co., 1957:508–509.

57. Bardach J. Local flaps and free skin grafts. In: Head and Neck Reconstruction. St. Louis: Mosby, Inc., 1992.

58. Johns FR, Sandler NA, Ochs MW. The use of the triangular pedicle flap for oral commissure plasty: report of a case. J Oral Maxillofac Surg 1998; 56:228–231.

59. Low D, Clark R, Jimenez F, Deitch EA. The bipedicled lip flap for reconstruction of the vermillion border in the patient with severe perioral burn. Oral Surg 1987; 63:526–529.

60. Leake JE, Curtin JW. Electrical burns of the mouth in children. Clin Plast Surg 1984; 11:669–683.

61. Cosman B, Gong K, Crikelair GF. Horizontal cross lip flap with pedicle at commissure: a case report. Plast Reconstr Surg 1968; 41:273–275.

62. Hagan WE. Nasolabial musculocutaneous flap in reconstruction of oral defects. Laryngoscope 1986; 96:840–845.

63. Daya M, Mahomva O, Madaree A. A multiple reconstruction of the oral commissures and upper and lower lip with an island submanial flap and a nasolabial flap. Plast Reconstr Surg 2001; 108:968–971.

24

Reconstruction of the Lower Lip and Chin

ROBERT L. McCAULEY

University of Texas Medical Branch and Shriners Hospital for Children—Galveston Unit, Galveston, Texas, USA

I. INTRODUCTION

Lip reconstruction can be dated back to ancient India around 1000 BC (1). However, the first reports of lip reconstruction in the Western world were first cited by Celsius in AD 60 (1,2). Later in the 16th century Tagliocozzi popularized lip repair by using local flaps and distant forearm transfers (3). As cited by Maltz, Ambrose Pare further refined some of Tagliacozzi's techniques in 1627 (2). His surprise in achieving excellent outcomes is indicated by his quote "I took care of him but God cured him." In the late 1700s Louis described the "V" excision of a tumor and Chopart described an advancement flap from the anterior neck to close a lower lip defect (1). The nasolabial flap was introduced as a technique for lower lip reconstruction by Von Bruns and later popularized by Zymanowski in the 19th century (2). By 1830, Romand was able to classify the different procedures for lip reconstruction into three groups—the French method: the use of sliding or advancement flaps; the Indian method: the use of rotation flaps; and the Italian method: the use of distant flaps (1). In 1848, Stein recommended the use of upper lip flaps to repair defects of the lower lip, and Eastlander, in 1872, reported the use of rotation flaps from the oral commissures of the mouth for closure of lip defects (3). In 1957, Gilles and Millard (4) introduced the fan flap in which lateral full-thickness flaps were utilized for upper or lower lip reconstruction by rotating them around the corners of the mouth. Clearly, the modification of many of these techniques by Kazangian and Converse improved (5) the aesthetic quality of these techniques. In addition, the concept of reconstruction of lip defects by aesthetic units as advocated by Burget and Menick (6) clearly represents current state of the art thinking.

Although many of these historical developments are key to our understanding of the principles of lower lip reconstruction, significant loss of tissue in the lower lip–chin complex rarely occurs in burn patients. Here, soft tissue deformities result from scar contractures producing eversion of the lower lip or microstomia. In addition, cervical contractures may accentuate deformities of the lower lip and chin. Regardless of the initial acute therapy, deep partial-thickness burns or full-thickness burns to the lower lip chin region usually result in some type of deformity. The perioral tissues are not amenable to compression therapy and may be distorted by burn scar contractures and hypertrophic scars (7). Some authors feel that postburn deformities of the lower lip are more devastating than those of the upper lip (8). The restoration of contour to the lower lip and chin represents a challenge. As noted, problems associated with distortion include ectropions and lower lip incompetence secondary to the loss of the enterolabial sulcus. The presence of cervical burn scar contractures producing extrinsic ectropions of the lower lip can further complicate the reconstructive plan (Fig. 24.1). Yet, it is clear that the aesthetic and functional reconstruction of burn patients requires the blending of harmony between the lower one-third of the face and the upper two-thirds of the face.

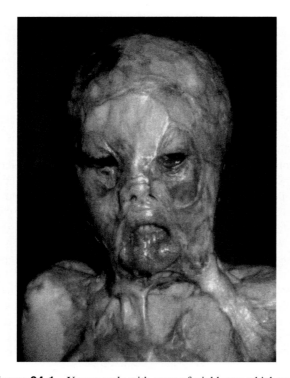

Figure 24.1 Young male with severe facial burns which were neglected. Now with severe ectropion which is both intrinsic and extrinsic. The extrinsic component is secondary to a Grade IV neck contracture.

II. ANATOMY

A. Muscular Anatomy of Lip and Chin

The orbicular oris muscle acts as a sphincter to support the lips. Its primary function is that of lip closure and its superficial fibers help protrude and purse the lips. Additional lip support is attributed to the buccinator and risorius muscles, which help approximate the lips to the alveolus for the clearing of food and saliva from the gingivobuccal sulcus (9). Lower lip function is controlled by the risorius muscle. This muscle lies horizontally and may be contiguous with the fibers of the platysma. Its fibers converge at the angle of the mouth and insert into the skin (10). This allows the risorius to retract the angle of the mouth playing a large part in producing our smile (Figs. 24.2 and 24.3). The depressor anguli oris, the depressor labii inferioris, and the platysma muscles all contribute to produce retraction and depression of the lower lip (9). It is possible that in patients with microstomia, the medial border of the orbicularis oris can be altered with displacement of the modiolus. Lower lip ectropions also can occur indirectly by the inferior pull of the plastysma muscle and skin as seen in cervical contractures. In addition, intrinsic ectropion of the lower lip secondary to burn injuries affects the function of the orbicularis oris, the depressor anguli oris, and the depressor labii inferioris.

The primary muscle of the chin is the mentalis. This muscle passes from the lower incisor downward to the skin over the chin. When it contracts, it raises the skin over this region and accentuates the transverse fold (10). In 1989, Zide and McCarthy (11) noted the importance of the mentalis muscle in chin and lower lip position. Although the role of the depressors in lower lip function is crucial, these muscles do not address the movement of the central portion of the lower lip. It is felt that in the absence of the mentalis muscle, the lower incisors may become visible at rest. This muscle arises from the anterior mandible at the level below the incisors but above the pogonion. As this muscle contracts, the skin of the chin is forced against the front of the mandible. Since the mentalis has no fibers which insert into the lower lip, an indirect effect is lower lip elevation. Zide and McCarthy (11) described three clinical problems which may affect the mentalis muscle: its origin, its displacement, and elongation and deficits. In patients with partial-thickness burns or full-thickness burns requiring skin grafts, the mentalis may be affected by scar formation. Feldman (12) noted that in the reconstruction of burn patients, the removal of fat and muscle is necessary at the labiomental crease to accentuate the natural folds in resurfacing of the chin region. However, the effect of this procedure on mentalis function is unclear. Although the muscle is deep to the plane of excavation, scarring still may alter its function.

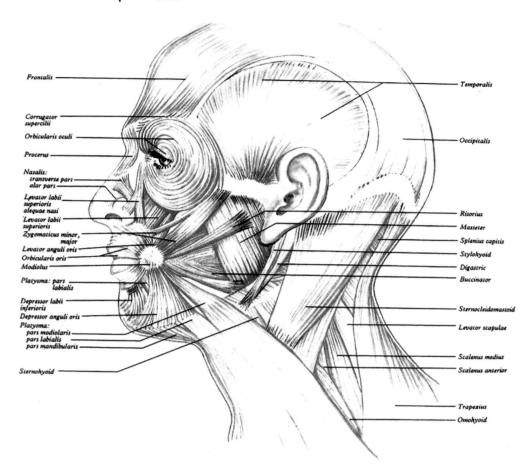

Figure 24.2 Muscles from the lateral aspect of the face. [Reprinted with permission from Williams PL, Warwick R, Dyson M, Bonnister LH. Myology. In: Williams PL, Warwick R, Dyson M, Bonnister LH, eds. Gray's Anatomy. New York: Churchill Livingston, 1989.]

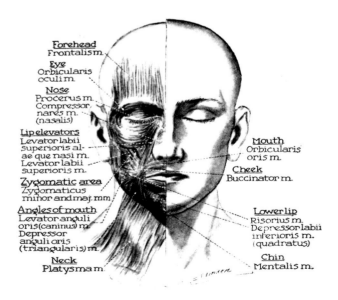

Figure 24.3 Muscles of the lower lip and chin. [Reprinted with permission from Thorak (10).]

B. Surface Anatomy of the Lip and Chin

As plastic surgeons, we usually view deformities of the lip and chin as problems seen in patients seeking cosmetic surgery. As reconstructive surgeons, we can apply these same principles to the aesthetic reconstruction of facial burns. Classically, facial height is measured in thirds. The upper one-third includes the distance between the hairline and the glabella. The middle one-third includes the region from the glabella to the base of the columella. Lastly, the lower one-third of the face encompasses the area between the columella and the lowest point in the mandible, the mentum (Fig. 24.4) (13).

If the height of the lower two-thirds of the face is measured, the middle one-third would constitute 43% of the distance known as the distal one-third of the face. The area between the subnasale and the mentum would constitute 57% of the distance (1) (Fig. 24.5). The height of the lower one-third of the face is further divided into two separate units. The upper one-third is the distance from the stoma to the subnasale and the lower two-thirds,

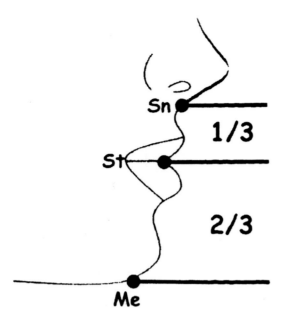

Figure 24.4 The lower one-third of the face. [Reprinted with permission from Frodel (13).]

is the distance from the stomion to the mentum (Fig. 24.4). The upper lip is slightly anterior to the lower lip and is one-third thinner (13). In evaluating the position of the chin, two vertical lines are passed from the nasion. The pogonion, or the most anterior portion of the chin, should be at this line or slightly behind it. Alternatively, chin projection can be determined by a vertical line from the subnasale (Fig. 24.6). The pogonion should be 4 mm behind

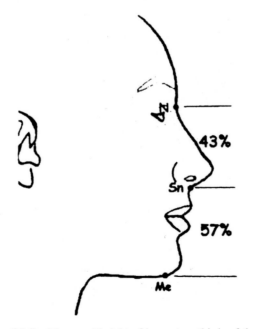

Figure 24.5 Measured height of lower two-thirds of the face. [Reprinted with permission from Frodel (13).]

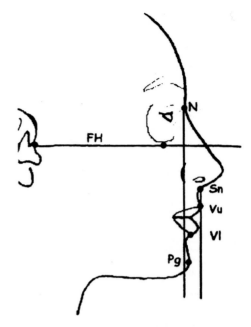

Figure 24.6 Chin projection. [Reprinted with permission from Frodel (13).]

the line. It is important to note that the dental occlusion plays an important role in the assessment of chin deformities. Patients with Angel's Class II occlusion suggest overprojection of the maxilla and/or underprojection of the mandible (13). Lower lip position is influenced by the inclination of both the maxillary and the mandibular incisions and the position of the maxilla and the mandible.

Anatomy of the lip can vary based on ethnicity. In many ways this has been altered with the increase in lip augmentation procedures. However, regardless of the thickness of the lips, the aesthetic balance between the upper and the lower lips is desirable. The length of the lips is defined as being the distance between either both lateral or both midpupillary lines. The lower lip is one-third wider than that of the upper lip.

III. ACUTE FACIAL BURNS

The management of acute facial burns is well described (14–17). Controversy exists as to the timing for early vs. delayed excision of partial-thickness injuries. However, the goal is to minimize the resection of viable tissue and decrease the need for subsequent reconstructive efforts. In patients with deep partial-thickness or full-thickness facial burns, the primary areas of concern are the eyes, the mouth, and the neck (7,8). These high-risk areas are prone to the development of contractures which can alter facial aesthetics and impact function. With respect to the mouth and the neck, the development of intrinsic or extrinsic lower lip ectropions can totally alter the aesthetic

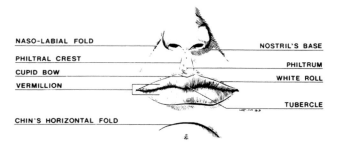

Figure 24.7 Diagram of normal proportions in lip and chin anatomy. [Reprinted with permission from Maillard and Montandon (18).]

integrity of the lower lip–chin unit (18) (Fig. 24.7). Even with minimal alterations in this area, the goal is to restore the balance of the lower one-third of the face with that of the upper two-thirds. Clearly, principles of aesthetic surgery are crucial in our decision making process. Once we incorporate these guidelines, we can now develop a template onto which our reconstructive efforts in burn patients may be addressed. Without question, differences in color match and texture may compromise our aesthetic results. However, notwithstanding these problems, we need to approach these areas of reconstruction with tempered enthusiasm.

IV. SURGICAL CONSIDERATION

A. Lower Lip

The lower lip and the mentolabial sulcus is a striking feature of the lower one-third of the face. Reconstruction of this region requires a detailed understanding of the complex contours noted in the lip–chin complex. Cardoso et al. (19) describe the contour of this unit as that of a dumbbell. The soft tissues in the region of the men- tolabial sulcus are condensed to form an isthmus between the lip and the chin (12). Cardoso et al. (19) also studied the histological nature of the mentolabial sulcus. It is felt that the muscles of the lower lip are responsible for the function and maintenance of the sulcus. In deep burns of the lower lip, the underlying tissue and the cutaneous inser- tion of the muscle are destroyed only to be replaced by scar. The inelastic scar now produces a fixed and altered contour (19,20). Lower lip ectropion is a sequela of this process as is loss or blunting of the mentolabial angle.

One of the major concerns with burns to the lower one- third of the face is the correction of lower lip ectropions. These problems can be secondary to intrinsic factors or extrinsic factors. Often in severe cases, the presence of the lower lip ectropion is a combination of both factors. Cervical contractures are the primary cause of extrinsic lower lip ectropions. The contracture of the platysma

muscle has a direct effect on lower lip eversion. The degree of lower lip ectropion which is intrinsic can only be determined after correction of the extrinsic problem. Only then is the lower lip contour re-evaluated and assessed for correction. In cases where intrinsic lower lip ectropion is severe, several abnormalities exist: displace- ment of the commissures inferiority, decrease in the intra- oral sulcus, increase of the horizontal length of the lower lip, and possibly an increase in the width of the lower lip (Fig. 24.8). In these long-standing defects, releasing the lower lip only will not always correct oral incompetence if the commissures are not addressed.

In addition, the nonuse of compression facemasks after the acute injury may accelerate the development of lower lip ectropions. Consequently, oral incompetence and exposure of the teeth can also become important issues.

B. Chin

The chin is an important component of the lower one-third of the face. Burns to this region can encompass other areas of the face as well as the neck. These problems are divided into two categories: soft tissue deformities only and deformities involving the mandible itself. Soft tissue deformities are those that result form deep partial- or

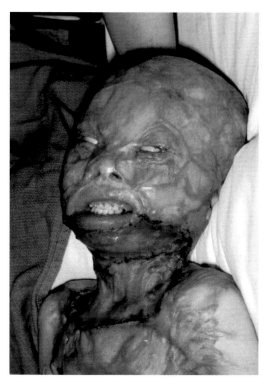

Figure 24.8 After neck release note the interior displacement of the lower lip, the increased horizontal length of the lip, and the increased width of the lower lip.

full-thickness injuries. The development of hypertrophic scars and keloids can become problematic. In addition, in men, this bearded region is prone to the development of folliculitis, which can delay healing. Such injuries can later have an effect on the contour of the lower lip and chin.

Clearly, associated neck contractures will not only alter the contour of the lower lip, but can also allow the chin to become encased in neck scar. Grade IV contractures of the neck usually involve significant scar contractures of the chin which subsequently can affect function (Fig. 24.9).

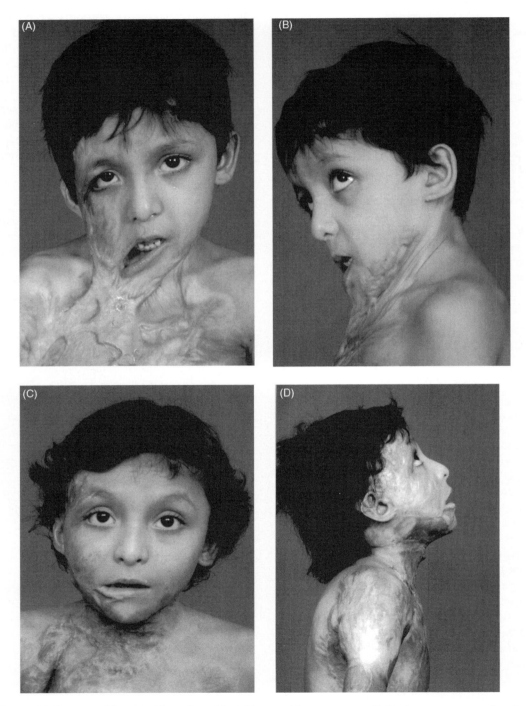

Figure 24.9 (A, B) Ten-year-old male with neglected facial burns with encasement of chin in scars connected to the anterior chest wall. (C, D) Normal chin contour after correction of the neck contracture with split-thickness skin grafts and a full-thickness skin graft to correct the lower lip ectropion.

Problems associated with bony deformities of the chin are divided into two categories: (1) chin deformities that occur with full-thickness burn injuries and directly involve the bone and (2) chin deformities which occur indirectly because of encasement in burn scars or from the treatment of these scars with compression garments. In either case, restriction of mandibular growth is believed to be affected (21,22).

V. RECONSTRUCTION

A. Lower Lip Reconstruction

1. Mentolabial Sulcus

Major soft tissue loss of the lower lip after thermal injury is rare. However, it is possible that electrical injuries can produce major soft tissue loss. But, more common are deformities associated with the development of microstomia or ectropions. Even with perfect facial resurfacing during the acute phase of care, loss of contour in the lower third of the face can occur. This will detract from the overall aesthetic results. Blunting of the mentolabial sulcus not only makes the chin appear smaller, but secondary lower lip ectropions, even though mild, can compromise the final appearance (23). Initial methods to correct this problem with excavation of fat and muscle do not have uniform success (23,24). Cardoso et al. believe that projection is lost at a later stage due to gravitational pull and subsequent sagging. They recommend reconstruction of the mentolabial sulcus by excision of scar tissue, lateral flap advancement of the underlying tissues and resurfacing with skin grafts (19). Feldman believes that excisional releases and re-contouring of the underlying tissues gives us the best chance in re-establishing the normal appearance of the mentolabial angle (24). All of these factors need to be addressed in order to achieve successful and aesthetically pleasing results.

2. Ectropions

The use of local flaps for reconstruction of the lower two-thirds of the face is well described. However, in facial burns, this problem is magnified because the surrounding tissue may also be involved in burn injury. Consequently, the use of these flaps is prohibited during the acute phase of injury or even in the early maturation phase of wound healing. Needless to say, local burn tissue can be safely moved once wounds have matured (Fig. 24.10). The use of local flaps is excellent for correction of small lower lip ectropions. However, in burn patients, the availability of local tissue for correction of these problems may be limited.

In patients with severe lower lip ectropions, simply correcting the upper segment of the chin unit by incisional or

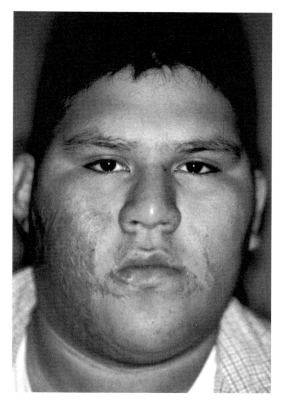

Figure 24.10 Correction of a lower lip ectropion with a local transposition flap.

excisional release and resurfacing the defect with skin grafts may not produce the desired results. The commissures, and the increased length and width of the lip may need to be addressed. A combination of procedures are often required to correct severe deformities. A complete release of the lower lip–chin unit is required as a first step. In long-standing lower lip ectropions, the orbicularis oris muscle may be attenuated. This problem along with the inferior displacement of the commissure is addressed with bilateral commissuroplasties, reconstruction of the modiolus, and partial vermillionectomy. Tightening of the orbicularis muscle by advancing the commissures superiorly and revising the modiolus provides the necessary suspension needed for lower lip function. The increased width of the lower lip may also be noted after the above procedures have been performed. The lower lip is usually one-third more of the width than the upper lip. Consequently, a partial vermilionectomy may be necessary in order to achieve lip balance. These procedures have been shown to achieve significant improvement in lower lip function and aesthetics in the most dramatic cases of lower lip ectropions (Fig. 24.11).

The use of pedicled flaps has been described for lower lip reconstruction (25–30). Although many of these techniques have found a place in oncologic reconstruction or

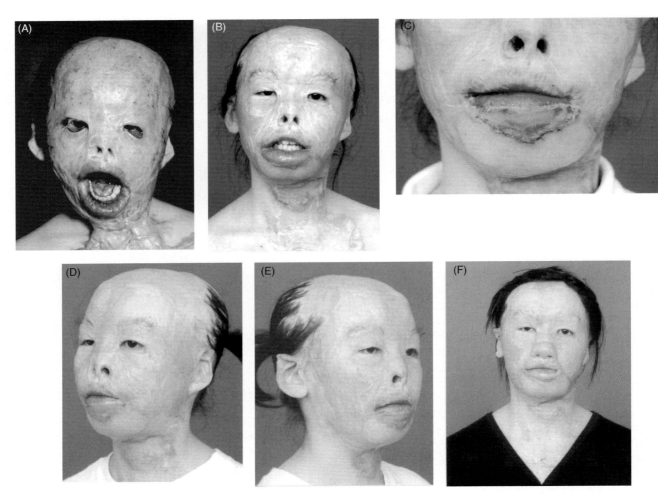

Figure 24.11 (A) Young boy with neglected facial burns. (B) Appearance of lower lip after the neck release with split-thickness skin grafts. Note commissure position after release with inferior displacement. (C) Note lower lip and chin region in the final stages of the reconstruction approach.

nonburn traumatic injuries, reports of their use in reconstruction of the burned lower lip is scarce. However, contour problems and the occasional destruction of the lip musculature may render these procedures as a secondary line of defense in burn reconstruction. Similarly, free-tissue transfers have also been used to reconstruct complex deformities of the lip and chin (31–34). But again, most of the reports do not include burn patients. However, it suffices to say that the sensate composite radial forearm flap seems to be popular for reconstruction in this region.

B. Chin Reconstruction

1. Skin Grafts

Most burn surgeons contend that facial burns that do not heal within 2 weeks should be excised and grafted (14,35). Studies have shown that the incidence of hypertrophic scars increases in areas of delayed wound

healing (36). Excision of scars and resurfacing of the defect as part of the chin subunit or the entire subunit of the chin can produce excellent results.

2. Flaps

In adult men, partial-thickness burns to the hair-bearing regions of the face can be complicated by folliculitis, thereby increasing the chances for the development of unsightly scars. In some instances, resection of these areas and resurfacing with skin grafts may be the only solution to this problem. However, the aesthetic results may be less than optimal. Several authors have suggested excision of these unsightly scars and reconstruction with a beard (14,36–39). Although several techniques have been advocated, recent studies by Hafezi et al. (39) using the bitemporal artery scalp flap has produced excellent results (Figs. 24.12 and 24.13). Although this group

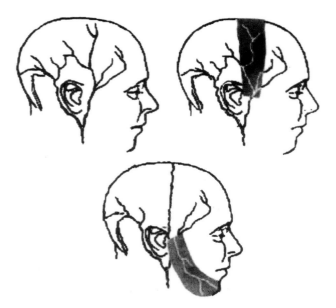

Figure 24.12 Diagram of the use of the visor scalp flap for reconstruction of the lower one-third of the face as a band. [Reprinted with permission from Hafezi et al. (39).]

used this flap as a bipedicle visor flap, it can also be used as a free-tissue transfer for reconstruction of the beard. The primary limitation of this technique is the orientation of the hair follicles. In addition, patients who have a strong family history of male patterned baldness may not be suitable candidates.

3. Tissue Expansion

Although visor flaps can produce excellent results in men, some patients opt for other alternatives. Also, in women and children alternative methods for the reconstruction of pronounced chin scars are crucial. Tissue expansion is a well-accepted method in the reconstruction of patients with head and neck burns (40–43). The use of expanders for the correction of cheek and chin defects is still in a state of infancy (42,44). Nevertheless, dramatic results can occur without the development of secondary lower lip ectropions. As noted in principle of tissue expansion, small incisions are used and the expander is placed in a subcutaneous pocket. Expansion is typically started 2–3 weeks after surgery and the stitches have been removed. Once expansion is complete, the expander is removed and the expanded flap is advanced cephalad with the neck in slight extension. Tension on the suture line should be avoided at all costs since the development of a secondary ectropion is of some concern. Patients are placed in a loose extended chinstrap to help the flap contour to the chin and upper neck for the first week (Fig. 24.14).

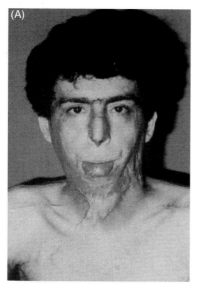

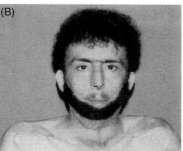

Figure 24.13 (A) Preoperative appearance of patient with chin scars after burn injury. (B) Postoperative appearance after reconstruction with the visor scalp flap. [Reprinted with permission from Hafezi et al. (39).]

4. Chin Augmentation

Thermal burn injuries involving the central portion of the mandible, or bony chin, is uncommon (Fig. 24.15). Although, it is conceivable that such injuries may occur more frequently in electrical burns, this is not well documented. Consequently, the effects of these injuries on growth and development of the chin is nonexistent. However, to date, several studies have implicated the use of compression therapy with subsequent underdevelopment of the chin after burn injury (21,22) (Fig. 24.16). For reconstructive surgeons, this now becomes another focus in facial reconstruction burn patients. The evaluation of chin deformities is only part of a comprehensive facial analysis. McCarthy et al. (45) developed a surgical system for the correction of bony chin deformities (Figs. 24.17 and 24.18). Although, it is clear that a number of authors have proposed various systems to evaluate chin size and shape, McCarthy et al. noted that none are perfect and surgical decisions should not be solely based on these

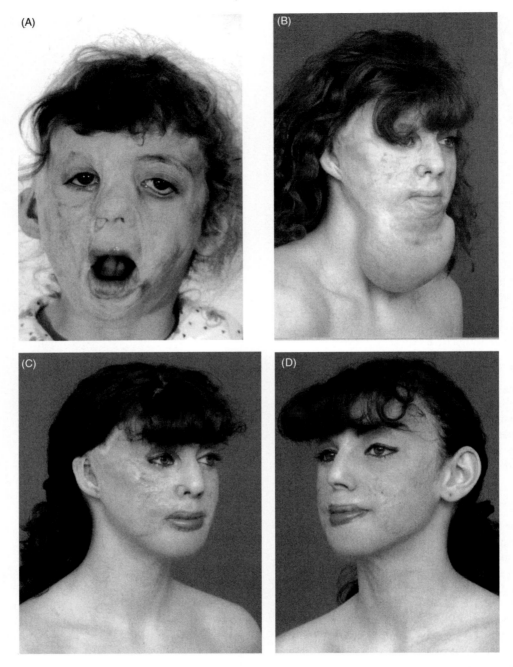

Figure 24.14   (A) Young girl with facial burn scars. (B) Improvement of burn scars on the cheek regions improved surgically, but patient unhappy with chin scars, particularly the graft in the upper part of the chin subunit. Tissue expander (100 cm^3) placed and over-inflated. (C, D) Appearance 6 months after removal of chin tissue expander and resurfacing with the expanded flap.

parameters. However, according to Frodel (13), microgenia is a term that describes a recessive or short chin in the sagittal and vertical dimensions. Retrogenia is essentially microgenia in the sagittal plane. In burn patients, the most commonly seen chin deformity is retrogenia. The etiology of this deformity has been attributed to burn injuries to the lower one-third of the face in combination with compression therapy. Although the exact incidence of this problem in burn patients is unknown, retrogenia is the most common chin abnormality noted in the overall population. Vertical microgenia is commonly a reflection of retrognathia with Class II malocclusion. Patients may have a deepened labiomental sulcus and a procumbent lower lip.

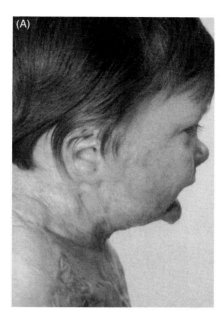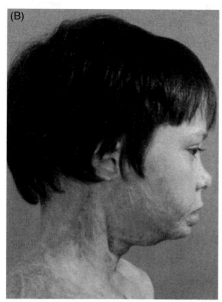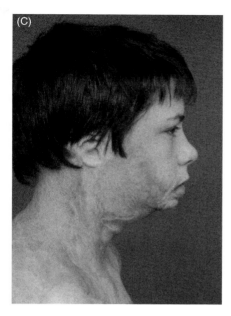

Figure 24.15 (A) Infant with facial burns with full-thickness burns to the chin with extensive debridement of tissue over the chin. (B) Early indications of a small chin in vertical and horizontal dimensions 5 years later. (C) As a teenager, the lack of chin projection is more pronounced.

Guyuron et al. (46) introduced a practical classification of chin dysmorphology in an analysis of 2879 patients over a 10-year period. The most common dysmorphism noted was microgenia (63.8%). It is clear that the acceptable methods of chin augmentation are the sliding genioplasty or augmentation with alloplastic implants. In 2001, Chang et al. (47) reviewed their experience with sliding genioplasty for correction of retrognathia. In the eight

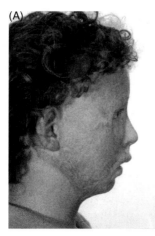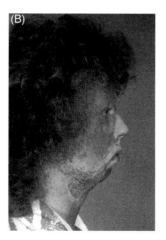

Figure 24.16 (A) Young boy with microgenia. (B) Four-year-old follow-up demonstrating pronounced chin deformity.

patients requiring chin reconstruction, the average advancement was 8 mm. Their follow-up of 6 months to 5 years (2.3 years mean) showed excellent aesthetic results with minimal complications. In 1985, Thomson (48) described the sagittal genioplasty which has been effectively shown to perform reduction, augmentation, pushback, and advancement genioplasties. A lower labial incision is made through the mucosa. The dissection is continued downward with division of the mentalis muscle and division of the periosteum to expose the chin. A horizontal subapical cut through the mandible is performed avoiding the apices of the teeth and both mental nerves. Rigid function is obtained with the use of lag screws. Thomson reported minimal complications as a result of this versatile approach for the correction of chin dysmorphology. Vuyk (49) reviewed his experience in the treatment of chin retrusion with silicone implants. In his review of 40 patients who underwent augmentation genioplasty, bone resorption was noted in 13 patients (61%) (49). However, the majority of these patients (8/13) experienced minimal resorption. Interestingly, Peled et al. (50) reported his experience in the use of silicone implants in children with Downs syndrome. In his series of 50 patients with a mean age of 9, all underwent augmentation of the nose, cheek, and/or chin with silicone implants. Of the 12 patients who underwent chin augmentation, 9 patients (75%) developed crater-like bone resorption. All implants were subsequently removed with bony regrowth back to its preoperative status. To

CHIN DEFORMITY
(WITHOUT OCCLUSAL PROBLEMS)

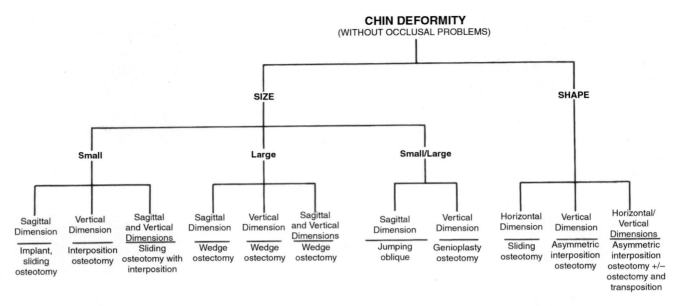

Figure 24.17 Classification of chin deformities without occlusion problems. [Reproduced with permission from McCarthy et al. (45).]

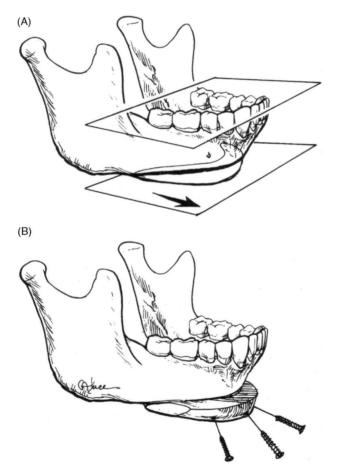

(A)

(B)

Figure 24.18 Sliding Genioplasty. (A) Osteotomy made in plane parallel to the occlusal surface. No significant change, in the vertical dimension. (B) Lag screws provide fixation. [Reproduced with permission from McCarthy et al. (45).]

date, a large series of burn patients undergoing genioplasty either by advancement or with alloplast implants does not exist. However, from these reports, several points are important to note. First, chin implants in children or even young adults appear to have an increased risk of bone resorption. The younger the patient, the greater the resorption. Second, although relapse occurs with advancement genioplasties, this seems to be a reliable alternative (Fig. 24.19). Needless to say, in burn patients any type of advancement genioplasty requires the presence of soft regions that are pliable in the upper neck and chin, to ensure the success of the procedure.

VI. CONCLUSION

Clearly, much is to be learned about reconstruction of the lower one-third of the face in burned patients. The correction of lower lip ectropions needs to be addressed only after correction of cervical contractures, which may contribute to the severity of the problem. In long-standing ectropions an increase in the horizontal and the vertical dimensions of the lower lip may be noted. Here, after correction of all extrinsic components, a complete release of the lower lip combined with bilateral commisuroplasties, reconstruction of the modiolus, and a partial vermilionectomy may be considered. Approximation of the normal aesthetic balance of the lips is possible with preservation of function. The correction of soft tissue defects of the chin is a function of the extent of the depth of the injury. Although resurfacing of these defects appears to be adequate with the use of skin grafts, sculpturing of the labiomental crease prior to placement ensures a more natural appearing result. Bony defects of the chin rarely occur in thermal injury. However, burns to the chin and the associated use of compression therapy have been implicated in the development of retrognathia. However, to date, no extensive epidemiologic studies have been performed to compare the incidence to that of the normal population.

Regardless of this issue of incidence, the correction of this problem with advancement genioplasty or alloplast implants will most likely require the placement of additional tissue in the chin–upper neck region. Reported long-term follow-up of these procedures in burn patients

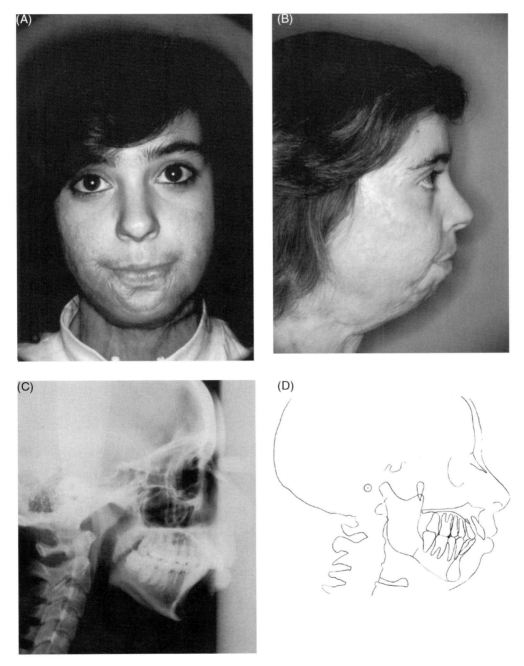

Figure 24.19 (A and B) Fifteen-year-old child with retrognathia; anterior and lateral views. (C) Preoperative lateral cephalogram. (D) Preoperative planning model. (see page 344 for E–I) (E) Preoperative planned movement of mandible by 8 mm and chin advancement by 10 mm. (F and G) Postoperative follow-up after surgery, anterior and posterior views. (H) Lateral postoperative cephalogram. (I) Postoperative panorex. (Courtesy of Elgene Manious, MD, Chief, Division of Maxilliafacial Surgery, University of Texas Medical Branch, Galveston, TX.)

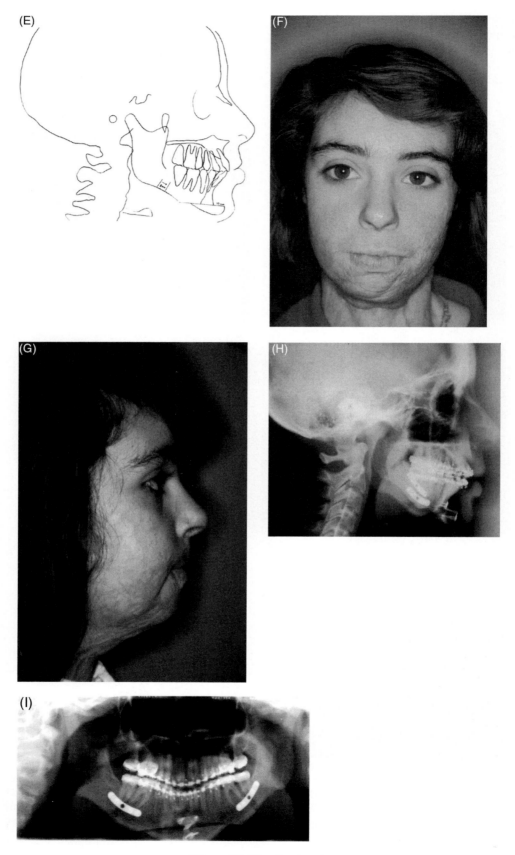

Figure 24.19 *Continued.*

appears to be currently lacking. Nevertheless, we should remain ever vigilant in our efforts to restore all aspects of facial burn injuries to their normal parameters.

REFERENCES

1. Mazzola RF, Lupo G. Evolving concepts in lip reconstruction, Clin Plast Surg 1984; 11:584–617.
2. Malte M. Evolution of Plastic Surgery. New York: Theo Gaus Sons Inc., 1946.
3. Gullane PJ, Maring GC. Minor and major lip reconstruction. J Otolanyngol 1983; 12:75–82.
4. Gilles HD, Millard DR Jr. Principles and Art of Plastic Surgery. Boston: Little Brown and Co., 1957.
5. Kazangian VH, Converse JM. In: The Surgical Treatment of Facial Injuries. 2nd ed. Baltimore: Williams and Wilkins, 1959.
6. Burget G, Menick FJ. Aesthetic restoration of one-half the upper lip. Plast Reconstr Surg 1986; 78:583–593.
7. Warpeha RL. Resurfacing the burned face. Clin Plast Surg 1981; 8:255–257.
8. Neale HW, Billmire DA, Carey JP. Reconstruction following head and neck burns. Clin Plast Surg 1986; 13:119–136.
9. Guillan PJ, Martin GC. Minor and major lip reconstruction. J Otolanyngol 1983; 12:75–82.
10. Thorak P. Anatomy in Surgery. 2nd ed. Philadelphia: J.B. Lippincott, 1962.
11. Zide BM, McCarthy J. The mentalis muscle: an essential component of chin and lower lip ectropion. Plast Reconstr Surg 1989; 83:413–420.
12. Feldman JJ. Reconstruction of the burned face in children. In: Serafin D, Georguade NG, eds. Pediatric Plastic Surgery. St. Louis: Mosby, 1984:522–632.
13. Frodel JL. Evaluation and treatment of deformities of the chin. Facial Plast Surg Clin N Am 2002; 10:221–232.
14. Hunt JL, Purdue GF, Spicer T, Gennett G, Range S. Face burn reconstruction—does early excision and autografting improve results. Burns 1987; 13:39–44.
15. Jonsson CE, Dalsgaard CJ. Early excision and skin grafting of selected burns of the face and neck. Plast Reconstr Surg 1991; 88:83–94.
16. Fraulin FOG, Lllmayer SJ, Tredget EE. Assessment of cosmetic and functional results of conservative versus surgical management of facial burns. J Burn Care Rehabil 1996; 17:19–29.
17. Voinchet V, Bardot J, Echinard C, Aubert JP, Magalon G. Advantages of early burn excision and grafting in the treatment of burn injuries to the anterior cervical region. Burns 1995; 21:143–146.
18. Maillard GF, Montandon D. Reconstructive surgery of deep burns of the lips. Clin Plast Surg 1984; 655–668.
19. Cardoso ERL, Amondo-Kuofi HS, Hawary MB. Postburn deformity of lip–chin complex: a method to restore the mentolabial sulcus. Int J Oral Maxillofac Surg 1995; 24:148–150.
20. Cardoso ERL, Amondo-Kuofi HS, Hawary MB. Mentolabial sulcus: a histologic study. Int J Oral Maxillofac Surg 1995; 24:145–147.
21. Fricke NB, Omnell L, Dutcher KD, Hollender LG, Engrav LH. Skeletal and dental disturbances after facial burns and pressure garments use: a four-year follow-up. J Burn Care Rehabil 1999; 20:239–249.
22. Fricke NB, Omnell L, Dutcher KD, Hollender LG, Engrav LH. Skeletal and dental disturbances after facial burns and pressure garments. J Burn Care Rehabil 1996; 17:338–345.
23. Mazzola RF, Lupo G. Evolving concepts in lip reconstruction. Clin Plast Surg 1984; 11:584–617.
24. Feldman JJ. Facial burns. In: McCarthy JG, ed. Plastic Surgery. Philadelphia: W.B. Saunders, 1990:2153–2236.
25. Yoshida T, Sugihara T, Ohura T, Minakawa H, Igawa H. Double cross lip flaps for reconstruction of the lower lip. J Dermatol 1993; 20:351–357.
26. Bayramicli M, Numanoglu A, Tezel E. The mental v-y island advancement flap in functional lower lip reconstruction. Plast Reconstr Surg 1997; 100(7):1682–1690.
27. Jemec B, Sanders R. A functional variant of lower lip reconstruction. Br J Plast Surg 1999; 52:232–235.
28. Yotsuyanagi T, Nehei Y, Yokoi K, Swada Y. Functional reconstruction using a depressor anguli oris musculocutaneous flap for large lower lip defects, especially for elderly patients. Plast Reconstr Surg 1999; 103(3):850–856.
29. Moschella F, Cordova A. Platysma muscle cutaneous flap for large defects of the lower lip and mental region. Plast Reconstr Surg 1998; 101(7):1803–1809.
30. Rudkin GH, Carlsen BT, Miller TA. Nasolabial flap reconstruction of large defects of the lower lip. Plast Reconstr Surg 2003; 810–817.
31. Ozdemir R, Ortak T, Kocer U, Celebioglu S, Sensoz O, Tiftikcioglu YO. Total lower lip reconstruction using sensate composite radial forearm flap. J Craniofac Surg 2003; 14:393–405.
32. Jeng S-F, Kuo Y-R, Wei F-C, Su C-Y, Chien C-Y. Reconstruction of concomitant lip and cheek through and through defects with combined free flap and an advancement flap from the remaining lip. Plast Reconstr Surg 2004; 113:491–498.
33. Serletti JM, Tavin E, Moran SL, Coniglio JU. Total lower lip reconstruction with a sensate composite radial forearm-palmaris longus free flap and a tongue flap. Plast Reconstr Surg 1997; 99:559–562.
34. Sandove RC, Luce EA, McGrath PC. Reconstruction of the lower lip and chin with the composite radial forearm-palmaris longus free flap. Plast Reconstr Surg 1991; 88:209–214.
35. Jonsson CE, Dalsgaard CJ. Early excision and skin grafting of selected burns of the face and neck. Plast Reconstr Surg 1991; 88:83–94.
36. Deitch EA, Wheelahan TM, Rose MP, Clothier J, Cotter J. Hypertrophic burn scars: analysis of variables. J Trauma 1983; 231:895–898.
37. Argrawal K, Panda KN. Moustache reconstruction using an extended midline forehead flap. Br J Plast Surg 2001; 54:159–161.

38. Datubo-Brown P, Khalid NK, Paul LL. Tissue expanded visor flap in burn reconstruction. Ann Plast Surg 1994; 32:205–208.

39. Hafezi F, Naghibzzdeh B, Nouhi AH. Facial reconstruction using the visor flap. Burns 2002; 28:679–683.

40. McCauley RL, Oliphant JR, Robson MC. Tissue expansion in the correction of burn alopecia: classification and methods of correction. Ann Plast Surg 1990; 25(2):103–115.

41. Weislander JB. Tissue expansion in the head and neck. Scand J Plast Reconstr Hand Surg 1991; 25:47–56.

42. Neale HW, Kurtzman LC, Goh KB, Billmire DA, Yakuboff KP, Warden G. Tissue expanders in the lower face and anterior neck in pediatric burn patients: limitations and pitfalls. Plast Reconstr Surg 1993; 91:624–631.

43. Antonyshyn O, Gruss JS, Zucker R, MacKinnon SE. Tissue expansion in head and neck reconstruction. Plast Reconstr Surg 1988; 82:58–68.

44. McCauley RL, Owiesy F. Aesthetic reconstruction of facial burns in expanded cervicofacial flaps. Proc Am Burn Assoc 2001; 22:91.

45. McCarthy JG, Ruff GL, Zide BM. A surgical system for the correction of bony chin deformity. Clin Plast Surg 1991; 18(1):139–152.

46. Guyuron B, Michelow BJ, Willis L. Practical classification of chin deformities. Aesth Plast Surg 1995; 19:257–264.

47. Chang EW, Lam SW, Karen M, Donlevy JL. Sliding genioplasty for correction of chin abnormalities. Arch Fac Plast Surg 2001; 3:8–15.

48. Thomson ERE. Sagittal genioplasty: a new technique of genioplasty. Br J Plast Surg 1985; 38:70–74.

49. Vuyk HD. Augmentation mentoplasty with solid silicone. Clin Otolaryngol 1996; 21(2):106–118.

50. Peled IJ, Wexler MR, Ticher S, Lax E. Mandibular resorption from silicone chin implants in children. J Oral Maxillofac Surg 1986; 44:346–348.

25

Correction of Cervical Burn Scar Contractures

ROBERT L. McCAULEY

University of Texas Medical Branch and Shriners Hospital for Children—Galveston Unit, Galveston, Texas, USA

I. INTRODUCTION

Facial and neck burns present quite a challenge for reconstructive surgeons. Whereas the incidence of neck burns vary, they remain an integral part of acute burn care. Under most circumstances, deep partial-thickness burn injuries and full-thickness burn injuries are tangentially excised and resurfaced with split-thickness skin grafts. Superficial partial-thickness wounds are allowed to heal secondarily. In either case, early wound closure and the prevention of neck contracture is crucial. The use of neck splints and physical therapy are part of the postoperative regimen to prevent subsequent contractures. However, even under the best circumstances, burn scar contractures of the neck can occur. The degree and severity of the contractures have been classified according to their effects on the range of motion in the neck (Table 25.1). Neck motion is classified into these areas: flexion, extension, rotation, and lateral flexion (Table 25.2). All of these movements are crucial to performing our activities of daily living (ADLs). Of these four movements, extension seems to inhibit function the most in burn patients and certainly is the focus of our efforts in defining burn scar contractures of the neck. Grade II contractures or greater not only affect neck extension and lateral rotation, but may also distort facial features. The combination of these forces often produces significant facial distortion complicated by limitations in performing ADLs. The reasons for development of significant neck contractures are easily dissected. The concavity of the neck, the thinness of the skin, and its increased mobility all contribute to the propensity for the development of neck contractures. However, treatment of these problems is complex. Long-term follow-up is scarce.

II. ACUTE CARE

Early excision and grafting of burn wounds is a well-accepted concept in the management of patients with

Table 25.1 Burn Scar Contractures of the Neck—Classification

Grade I	Symptomatic; no limitations in range of motion; no facial distortion
Grade II	Symptomatic; may have mild limitations in neck extension and/or rotation; distortion of lower one-third of face may be noted on extension
Grade III	Symptomatic; cannot extended head past neutral position; limited extension; distortion of lower one-third of face
Grade IV	Symptomatic; loss of cervicomental angle; severe facial distortion; possible fusion of chin to anterior chest wall

major thermal burns. However, relative to the head and neck, even the most aggressive of acute burn surgeons may temper their approach. Although the concept of early excision offers the advantages of early wound closure, the prospect of decreased hypertrophic scarring, and improved aesthetics, one main problem exists. What is considered early excision? A review of the literature indicates that early excision can occur within 24 h of burn injury to nearly 3 weeks after burn injury (1–3). In each of these studies, however, early excision of burn wounds was touted to be effective in decreasing hypertrophic scarring and improving aesthetics. Yet, the concept of timing for early excision remains elusive. As we look closer at the acute management of cervical burns, yet another dimension is brought to light. In 1995, Voinchet et al. (4) reported their series of early excision and grafts of anterior neck burns (within 24 h) as compared to patients who underwent delayed excision (after 5 days, but within 3 weeks) (4). These authors noted that the incidence of hypertrophic scars and subsequent scar contractures of the neck were lower in the early-excision group. In addition, subsequent revisions were more common in the early-excision group. Similar to previous studies, Voinchet et al. (4) supported the concept of early excision of acute neck burns noting its impact on subsequent reconstructive procedures. However, it should be noted in this study that the extent of neck burns and the frequency in which meshed skin grafts were utilized within each group were not addressed. The use of meshed split-thickness skin grafts or thin-sheet grafts may affect the subsequent development of

Table 25.2 Degrees of Normal Cervical Spine Range of Motion According to American Association of Orthopedic Surgeons (AAOS)

Flexion	0–45	0–30
Extension	0–45	0–30
Lateral flexion	0–45	0–40
Rotation	0–60	0–30

cervical contractures. In addition, postoperative compliance is also a factor in the prevention of these problems. However, even with these issues factored in, early excision in facial and neck burns seems to be favored.

When acute cervical burns require coverage of the soft tissues with split-thickness skin grafts (STSG), insuring graft survival is crucial. The intraoperative techniques of obtaining hemostasis and insuring contact of the graft to the concave recipient bed are crucial for graft survival. Postoperatively, the prevention of graft shearing may be accomplished by placement of a tie-over bolster. Ideally, patients are positioned supine on a short mattress so that the neck is in extension. The head of the bed is put on shock blocks to simulate the reverse Trendelenberg position to facilitate oral intake. A full liquid diet is instituted for a few days in cases where large grafts are used to resurface the neck. Prism glasses are important to improve visualization of the surroundings while in this position. If bolsters are used, grafts are exposed in 5–7 days. Once graft take is deemed acceptable, patients are placed in hard neck collars to maintain neck extension between 90° and 105°. This collar is worn during the day. At night, the short mattress supine position is encouraged. Alternatively, the neck collars can be worn at night but they tend to be less comfortable. Physical therapy is instituted during this time to maintain and improve range of motion. Yet, in spite of these measures, cervical burn scars continue to be problematic.

III. NORMAL NECK CONTOUR

The recreation of the youthful neck has been a topic in plastic surgery for years (5–9). Over time, various techniques have been devised to improve the aging neck and return it to its youthful appearance. Today, most approaches to this operation have utilized variations of transection or plicatiar of the platysma muscle to achieve this goal. In addition, submental fat resection or liposuction has become a standard adjunct to rejuvenate the neck. Ellenbogen and Karlin (8) produced five visual criteria for the youthful neck. These criteria include: (1) a distinct mandibular border from mention to angle; (2) a subhyoid depression which gives the neck the appearance of being long and thin; (3) a visible thyroid cartilage bulge; (4) a visible, anterior border of the sternocleidomastoid muscle; and (5) a cervicomental angle between 105° and 120° (Fig. 25.1). These criteria are important parameters to keep in mind when reconstructing patients with severe cervical burn scar contractures. In burned children, the type of operation performed will affect neck contour later. In order to achieve as normal a contour as possible, aside from prominence of the thyroid cartilage, these measurements approximate what we would like to achieve in the correction of severe cervical contractures.

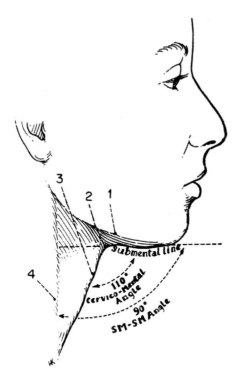

Figure 25.1 Criteria for the youthful neck: (1) distinct inferior mandibular border, (2) subhyoid depression, (3) visible thyroid cartilage bulge, (4) visible anterior sternoclesidomastoid border, and (5) SM–SM angle of 90° (cervico-mental angle between 105° and 120°). [Reprinted with permission from Ellenbogen and Karlin (8).]

In Grade II cervical contractures or greater, scar excision is necessary to obtain a complete release of the neck. Transection of the platysma muscle here is routine. Protection of the overlying fascia adjacent to the submandibular gland is often overlooked in this type of surgery. However, it is crucial that the fascial layer here remains intact. Violation of this fascia will produce glandular ptosis and compromise the final aesthetic results. Currently, a number of procedures are described to correct severe cervical burn scar contractures. They range from the use of skin graft to free-tissue transfers (9). The decision as to how one should proceed to correct these difficult problems should be guided by tissue availability, patient circumstances, and our visualization of the resultant neck aesthetics.

A. Reconstruction

The surgical management of cervical contractures is dependent on the severity of the contracture, the availability of acceptable donor sites, and the compliance of the patient. The support of the family to encourage the patient to follow through with the postoperative plan is also crucial. In addition, the availability of local resources to assist with physical therapy may have an impact on the choice of tissue used for reconstruction. For the surgeon, the goal is to provide stable soft tissue coverage which corrects facial deformities, returns range of motion to normal, reconstructs the cervicomental angle, and blends in well with patient's color and skin texture. Needless to say, the reconstructive choice should provide normal contour to the neck. To date, these ideals are not uniformly accomplished in the reconstruction of cervical deformities. Current methods used to address cervical contractures range from the use of skin grafts and local skin flaps to complex reconstruction with expanded pedicled myocutaneous flaps and free-tissue transfers. Needless to say, the experience of the surgeon plays a large role in determining the choice of procedure. The choice as to which reconstruction to proceed with is influenced by all of the above factors.

IV. CLASSIFICATION OF NECK CONTRACTURES

All cervical burn scar contractures are not equal. Consequently, their management differs. It may be useful to classify these contractures based on their effects on range of motion as well as their effects on the production of secondary facial distortion. Although it is clear from the literature that a multitude of procedures exist for the correction of these problems, analysis as to which procedure is appropriate is lost since the degree of contracture is either omitted or presented as a case report or in a limited series. In addition, long-term follow-up is often missing.

A. Grade I Contractures

Grade I cervical contractures are mild contractures. Usually, the patient has full extension, but complains of tightness in the neck. Facial distortion on full extension is not present. However, on physical examination, neckbands of varying widths are present. Narrow neckbands can be corrected with multiple Z-plasties, which lengthens the neck tissue and reorients the scar. Rarely are skin grafts necessary to correct this problem (Fig. 25.2).

B. Grade II Contractures

Grade II cervical contractures are moderate contractures in which patients are able to extend the neck, but facial distortion is noted. The range of motion is past 90°, but may fall short of full extension. This indicates that there is a significant soft tissue deficit. Occasionally, the neck extension will also cause cephalad migration of the nipple–areola complex in female patients. Correction of the contractures may require large transportation flaps.

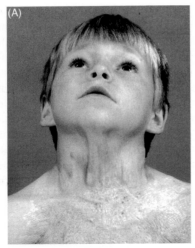

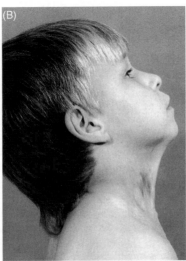

Figure 25.2 (A) Grade 1 neck contracture: full extension: no facial distortion but a central band is present making patient symptomatic. (B) Blunting of cervicomental angle is noted. [Reprinted with permission from Ellenbogen and Karlin (8).]

Large cervical flaps, either alone or in combination with other cervical flaps, may be used for closure (Fig. 25.2). Alternatively, the use of full-thickness skin grafts (FTSG) provides adequate correction, if available. If FTSG are unavailable, thick STSG may be used. However, when skin grafts are used, splinting is crucial in the postoperative phase to prevent recurrence.

C. Grade III Contractures

Grade III cervical contractures are diagnosed when neck extension past the neutral plan of 90° cannot be achieved. Facial distortion is usually present (Fig. 25.3). These patients require extensive neck releases, not only of the skin, but also of the underlying platysma muscle. Soft

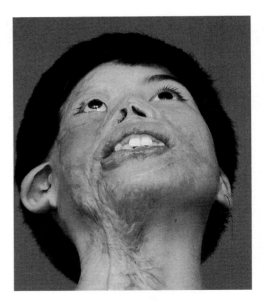

Figure 25.3 Grade II neck contracture. Near complete extension is noted; however, lower lip ectropion with inferior displacement is noted on the right side.

tissue coverage of defects in Grade III contractures has sparked utilization of a variety of surgical procedures, all with purported superiority over the standard technique of resurfacing with skin grafts (Fig. 25.4) (10–14).

D. Grade IV Contractures

Grade IV contractures are described as those in which patients are unable to reach the neutral position.

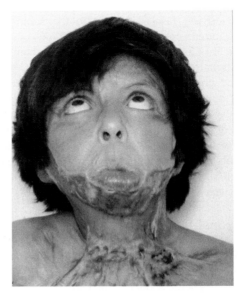

Figure 25.4 Grade III neck contracture; limited range of motion; patient unable to extend beyond neutral position.

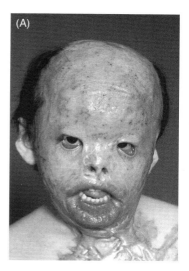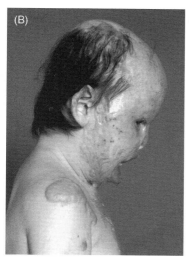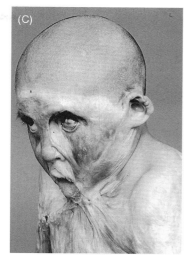

Figure 25.5 (A and B) Grade IV neck contracture with patient unable to extend neck to neutral position. (C) Grade IV neck contracture with fusion of chin to the anterior chest wall.

Occasionally, such patients can present with fusion of the neck to the anterior chest wall (Fig. 25.5). These patients have fixed neck contractures with severe impairment in ADLs. Needless to say, facial distortion is always present. Although airway obstruction does not appear to be present, the quality of life for these patients is dismal. Similar to patients with Grade III neck contractures, various methods for correction have ranged from the use of skin grafts to free-tissue transfer. Yet, regardless of which techniques are utilized, functional and aesthetic considerations must be taken into account.

V. SKIN GRAFTS

To many investigators, the time-honored use of skin grafts remains the standard method of treatment for severe mentosternal contractures. The advantage of this procedure is the ability to resurface large areas of the neck, the ease of the procedure, and the ability to restore aesthetics of the neck. However, recurrent contractures are a common concern unless a protracted course of splinting is followed. McCauley et al. (15) retrospectively evaluated the use of STSG vs. FTSG in the management of Grade IV cervical burn scar contractures in 18 children referred to his institution. Ten patients with a mean age of 7.6 years underwent STSG with a mean thickness of 17/1000 in. These patients were compared to eight children with a mean age of 9 years who underwent an FTSG placement for correction of Grade IV cervical contractures. The mean time from injury to reconstruction was ∼18 months for all patients. Although 7 out of 10 patients with STSG required additional revisions with STSG at ∼17 months, only 3 out of 8 patients with FTSG required additional releases at

$2\frac{1}{2}$-years. Although splinting was required from 3 to 6 months, all patients ultimately had successful outcomes (Figs. 25.6–25.8). It is important to recognize that the use of STSG in these patients were not failures. This study does emphasize the fact that STSG are not always able to keep up with the growth of children. However, FTSG appear to be better suited.

VI. FLAPS

Grade III and IV burn scar contractures of the neck usually involve the anterior neck, lateral neck, and submental region. The earliest use of flaps to address this problem was reported by Mutter in 1842 (10). This flap is a cutaneous skin flap oriented over the lateral shoulder and is believed to have been limited, since neither fascia nor muscle was included in the pedicle (11). Arufe referred to this cervicoacromial flap as the epaulette flap and successfully used it to resurface defects after the release of burn scar contractures of the neck (16). In a series of 286 cases, the procedure was performed in stages, one of which included a delay procedure. Several investigators recognized the value of this flap in the correction of cervical burn scar contractures (17,18). They also recognized from Arufe's experience that there were limitations in width and length. Consequently, the use of the expanded version of this flap has been reported on several occasions (17,18). In a series of 12 patients, Almeida et al. (18) reported the use of the expanded cervicoacromial flap in an attempt to minimize limitations of length and width. The complication rate from exposure of the expanders was only 8.3% (one patient). However, the correction of dog-ears at the base of the flap was frequent (67% of

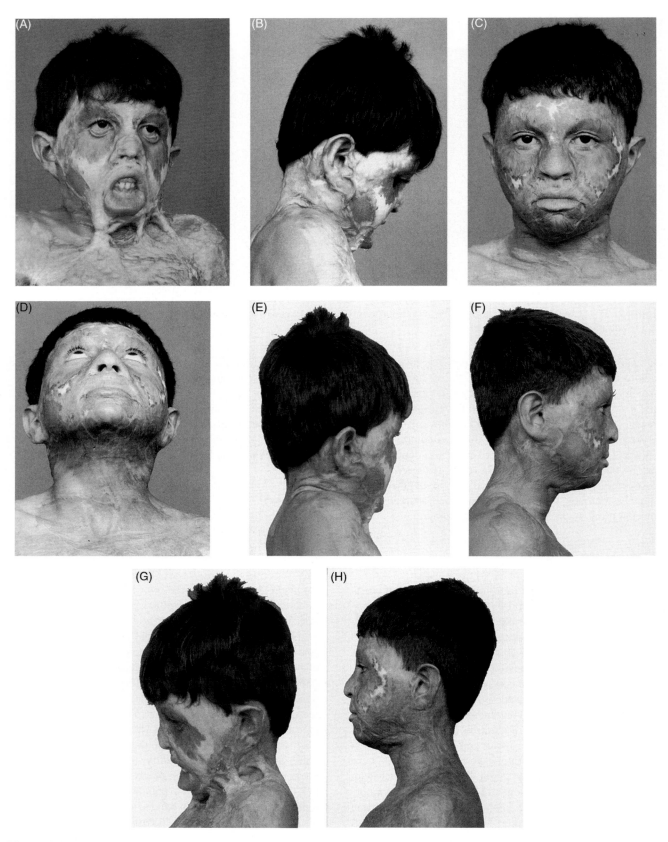

Figure 25.6 (A, B) Seven-year-old male with Grade IV neck contracture; severe facial distortions noted. (C, D) Five years later after two operations to the neck using split-thickness skin grafts and one operation using a large Z-plasty to correct contour problems: no operative intervention in $2\frac{1}{2}$ years; note full neck extension. (E, F) Pre- and postoperative right lateral view: note normal neck contour. (G, H) Pre- and postoperative left lateral view: note normal neck contour.

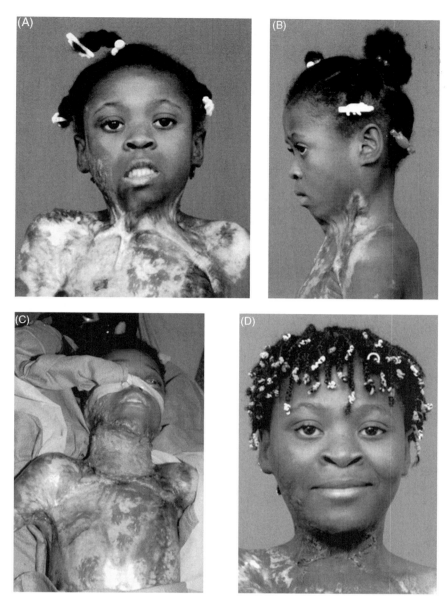

Figure 25.7 (A, B) A 6-year-old female with Grade IV neck contracture. (C) Patient underwent excision of burn scars with allograft placement. Four days later, patient returned to the operating room for allograft removal and resurfacing with FTSG taken from the abdomen. (D) Two-year follow-up with contour of the neck maintained. Patient 1 week earlier, underwent Z-plasties within the FTSG to correct lateral bands.

patients). The author noted that expansion not only allowed for an increase in flap width, but also provided a thinner flap with better contouring of the neck.

Aranmolate utilized the bilobed skin flap to correct Grades III, IV contractures of the neck. This procedure is offered as an alternative to the use of skin grafts (19). In nine patients, most of who were children, the prerequisite for use of this flap was a scar-free shoulder, including the lateral two-thirds of the clavicular region. The flap is designed and transposed in a fashion similar to multiple modified Z-plasties with excellent results initially. Early results show excellent neck contour, re-creation of the normal cervicomental angle, and a reasonable range of motion. However, long-term follow-up for this promising procedure is not available.

The use of myocutaneous flaps in correction of cervical burn scar contractures is controversial. Several pedicled myocutaneous flaps have been described, not all with ideal designs or outcomes (11–14,20). Isenberg et al. (11) described the use of the longitudinal trapezius

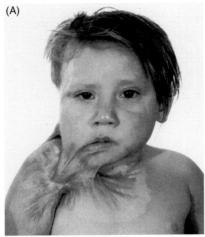

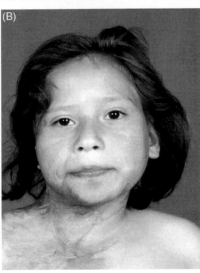

Figure 25.8 (A) A 6-year-old child with Grade IV lateral neck and shoulder contractures. (B) Three and a half years of follow-up, 2 years since the last release of contractures of neck and shoulder with STSG (two operations required).

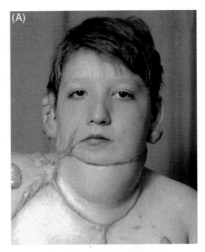

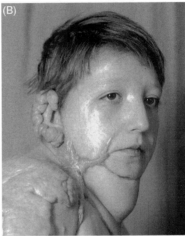

Figure 25.9 (A, B) A 15-year-old male referred to our institution after correction of cervical contracture using a parascapular flap. Obliteration of cervicomental angle is noted. Although the flap survived, aesthetics were severely compromised.

fasciocutaneous flap for correction of severe burn scar contractures of the neck. This flap is based on the transverse cervical artery. Although length may not be a problem, flap width is limited and may not fully correct the neck contracture. Long-term follow-up for this procedure is absent. The latissimus dorsi myocutaneous flap (LDMF) was originally described as a fasciocutaneous flap by Tolhurst and Haesecker in 1982 (12). At that time, it was advocated for correction of axillary contractures. The inclusion of the latissimus dorsi muscle into this flap has been used for the correction of anterior neck contractures (14). Wilson et al. (13) described the use of the LDMF in six patients with Grade IV neck contractures. Although this flap corrects the defect in a single stage, they admit that the dissection is difficult, the size of the skin

paddle is limited, and partial necrosis of the skin, although minor, is common. However, again, long-term follow-up is lacking. In addition, it is unclear as to whether complete correction of these contractures was obtained (14). Aesthetically, the cervicomental angle was not fully corrected with this technique. One of the major problems associated with the use of myocutaneous flaps for cervical reconstruction is its bulkiness and color mismatch. Ohba et al. (20) described the extended serratus anterior myocutaneous flap as a thin, reliable pedicled flap, which maintains the contour and aesthetics of the neck. However, some limitations exist. The width of the skin paddle should be < 10 cm in an adult. This makes reconstruction of the entire neck difficult. Consequently, only contractures in the upper half of the neck are recommended for correction with this flap.

VII. MICROVASCULAR FREE-TISSUE TRANSFER

The use of free flaps in the correction of cervical contractures has been extensively reported (21–26). Most commonly, the scapular or parascapular fasciocutaneous free flap has been used owing to its increased size to cover large skin defects (21–23). With free-tissue transfers having a >95% survival rate, safety is usually not an issue (24,27). What is of concern is aesthetics. These flaps may require multiple revisions to obtain definition of the cervicomental angle as well as improve lower neck contour (25) (Fig. 25.9). Yet, without the proper design of flap width, disasters can occur even with flap survival (Fig. 25.10). Recently, Yang et al. (26) also recognizing the problem of the neck contour with free-tissue transfer, described the use of the anterolateral thigh flap, combined with cervicoplasty, to correct cervical burn scar contractures. This group was the first to compare preoperative and postoperative range of

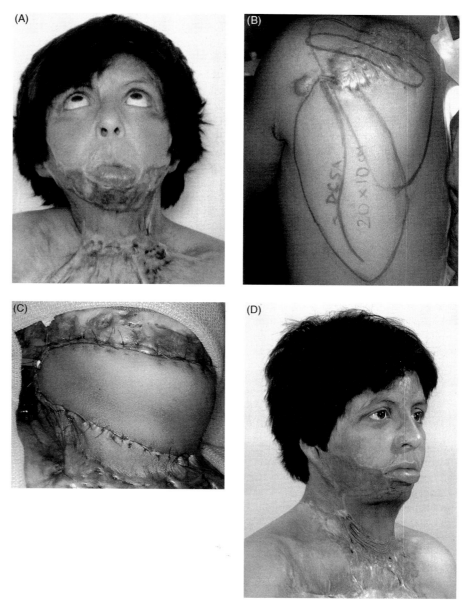

Figure 25.10 (A) A 12-year-old male referred for correction of Grade III cervical contracture. (B) Near complete scar excision necessitated a large (10 × 20 cm) parascapular free flap for coverage. (C) Insetting of parascapular flap: head is at the top. (D) Final result after three procedures to debulk the flap.

motion measurements. The mean extension in this group of patients preoperatively was 95° (almost Grade III neck contractures). Postoperative improvements in extension and lateral rotation were noted although follow-up was only 5 months. However, width limitations prevent the use of this flap for resurfacing of the entire neck.

Tissue expansion has found a permanent place among the reconstructive options available to surgeons. It is not surprising that it has found a place in the reconstruction of burn patients with head and neck deformities. Expanded free-flap transfers have been reported in the correction of cervical contractures (25,28,29). In an attempt to further provide thin vascularized tissue to the neck for correction of cervical contractures, Woo and Seul (28) reported the use of the expanded arterialized venous free flap. The pre-expansion of this flap in three patients, eliminated problems of flap necrosis and provided a large, thin segment of vascularized tissue for resurfacing of the neck. Celikoz et al. (29) utilized the expanded sensate radial artery free flap for resurfacing of cervical contractures. However, this flap is of limited size, although its thinness and pliability are ideal for the neck. With a variety of techniques reported for the reconstruction of cervical burns, very few comparative studies exist. Recently, Adant et al. (30) reported the long-term follow-up of a study which compared skin grafts, tissue expanded flaps, and free-tissue transfer in the correction of cervical contractures (30). Although the series is small, five patients within each group, with follow-up of at least 1 year, produced some interesting observations. Apparently, all patients had Grade III/IV neck contractures. In a comparison of morbidity, skin elasticity, skin sensation, color match, and scar recurrence, the use of full-thickness skin grafts appears to be preferred.

VIII. CONCLUSION

The management of cervical burns during the acute phase of injury, along with rehabilitation efforts, can avoid major burn scar contractures. However, most circumstances are not ideal and burn scar contractures still occur. Our approach to the reconstruction of these problems depends on both severity and tissue availability. Most contractures are mild or moderate (Grade I or II), and are easily corrected with local flaps or skin grafts. As contractures become more severe, the methods used for correction become more diverse. The use of split skin grafts continues to deliver excellent results. However, postoperative splinting is necessary. In addition, in children, frequent revisions using skin grafts are negative aspects of this procedure. FTSG may be of better benefit. Pedicled flaps, both

expanded and nonexpanded, have shown some promise (10–14,16–20). The use of free-tissue transfers, both expanded and unexpanded, has also been successful (21–23,25–31). However, with respect to achieving aesthetic contours of the neck and restoring the cervicomental angle, multiple revisions after free-tissue transfer including defatting and Z-plasties are required (25,26). The use of arterialized venous free flaps may help minimize these problems (28). The results from the use of tissue substitutes are early. Yet, some results have been less than optimal (32). Still, it appears that the standard for correction of cervical contractures by which all techniques are judged may be of use for skin grafts. Here, the extent of coverage is not limited to the anterior neck as noted with many other techniques. With FTSG, a two-stage approach may be required for the resurfacing of extensive neck defects. A complete incisional or excisional release is carried out in stage 1, followed by autografting at stage 2 (15). However, in spite of the report by Adant et al. (30), which indicates that the skin grafts may be preferred to tissue expansion or free-tissue transfers, these patients will require a protracted course of splinting. Yet, the results can be outstanding. As we continue to search for ideal methods for the reconstruction of cervical burn scar contractures, the restoration of the cervicomental angle and providing contour for the lower neck region should be the focus by which to direct our surgical intervention. Many of the described techniques were developed and utilized in the neck to address these issues. Although there may be a place for all of these techniques, the severity of the contracture, donor site availability, patient compliance, and expected aesthetic results will help in the selection of the most appropriate procedure.

REFERENCES

1. Hunt JL, Purdue GF, Spicer T, Bennett G, Range S. Face burn reconstruction—does early excision and autografting improve results. Burns 1987; 13:39–44.

2. Jonsson CE, Dalsgaard CJ. Early excision and skin grafting of selected burns of the face and neck. Plast Reconstr Surg 1991; 88:83–94.

3. Fraulin FOG, Lllmayer SJ, Tredget EE. Assessment of cosmetic and functional results of conservative vs. surgical management of facial burns. J Burn Care Rehab 1996; 17:19–29.

4. Voinchet V, Bardot J, Echinard C, Aubert JP, Magalon G. Advantages of early burn excision and grafting in the treatment of burn injuries to the anterior cervical region. Burns 1995; 21:143–146.

5. Webeter RC, Smith RC, Smith KF. Face lift, part 2: etiology of platysma cording and its relationship to treatment. Head Neck Surg 1983; 6:590–595.

6. Newman J, Lolsky RL, Mai ST. Submental liposuction extraction with hard chin augmentation. Arch Otolaryngol 1984; 110:454–457.
7. Connell BF. Neck contour deformities—the art, engineering, anatomic diagnosis, architectural planning, and aesthetics of surgical correction. Clin Plast Surg 1987; 14(4):683–692.
8. Ellenbogen R, Karlin JV. Visual criteria for success in restoring the youthful neck. Plast Reconstr Surg 1980; 66(6):826–837.
9. Stamatopoulos C, Panayotou P, Tsirigotou S, Ioannovich JD. Use of free flaps in the aesthetic reconstruction of face and neck deformities. Microsurgery 1992; 13:188–191.
10. Mutter TD. Cases of deformities from burns relieved by operation. Am J Med Sci 1842; 4:66–80.
11. Isenberg JS, Price G. Longitudinal trapezius fasciocutaneous flap for the treatment of mentosternal burn scar contractures. Burns 1996; 22:76–79.
12. Tolhurst DE, Haesecker B. Fasciocutaneous flaps in the axillary region. Br J Plast Surg 1982; 25:430–435.
13. Wilson IA, Lokesh A, Schubert A, Benjamin CJ. Latissimus dorsi myocutaneous flap reconstruction of neck and axillary burn contractures. Plast Reconstr Surg 2000; 105:27–33.
14. Argarwal R, Chandra R. Latissimus dorsi myocutaneous flap reconstruction of neck and axillary burn contractures; correspondence and brief communication. Plast Reconstr Surg 2000; 106:1216–1217.
15. McCauley RL, Owiesy F, Dhanraj P. Management of Grade IV neck contractures in children. Proc Am Burn Assoc 2001; 22:89.
16. Arufe HN, Cabrera VN, Sica IE. Use of the epaulette flap to relieve burn contractures of the neck. Plast Reconstr Surg 1978; 61:707–714.
17. Karacaoglan N, Uysal A. Reconstruction of post burn scar contractures of the neck by expanded skin flaps. Burns 1994; 20:547–550.
18. Almeida MF. Expanded shoulder flap in burn sequela. Act Chir Plast 2001; 43:86–90.
19. Aranmolate S, Attah AA. Bilobed flap in the release of postburn mentosternal contractures. Plast Reconstr Surg 1989; 83:356–361.
20. Ohba S, Inoue T, Ueda K, Takamatsu A. The pedicled, extended serratus anterior musculocutaneous flap for cervical contracture release. Ann Plast Surg 1995; 35:416–419.
21. Tseng WS, Cheng, Tung TL, Wei FC, Chen HC. Microsurgical combined scalpular/parascapular flap for reconstruction of severe neck contractures case report and literature review. J Trauma Inj Infect Crit Care 1999; 47:1142–1147.
22. Angrigiani C, Grilli D. Total face reconstruction with one free flap. Plast Reconstr Surg 1997; 99:1566–1575.
23. Xu J, Li SK, Li YQ, Ma XB, Li SY. Superior extension of the parascapular free-flap for cervical burn scar contracture. Plast Reconstr Surg 1995; 96:58–62.
24. Wei FC. Overview of microvascular surgery. In: McCauley RL, ed. Aesthetic and Functional Reconstruction of Burns. New York: Marcel Dekker, 2005.
25. Fan JC. Post-transferred tissue expansion of a musculocutaneous free-flap for debulking and further reconstructure. Ann Plast Surg 1997; 38:523–526.
26. Yang JY, Tsai FC, Chana JS, Chuang SS, Chang SY, Huang WC. Use of free thin anterolateral thigh flaps combined with cervicoplasty for reconstruction of post burn anterior neck contractures. Plast Reconstr Surg 2002; 110:39–46.
27. Inigo F, Jimenez-Murat Y, Arroyo O, Martinez A, Ysunza A. Free flaps for head and neck reconstruction in non-oncological patients: experience in 200 cases. Microsurgery 2000; 20:186–192.
28. Woo SH, Seul JH. Pre-expanded arterialised venous free flaps for burn contracture of the cervicofacial region. Br J Plast Surg 2001; 54:390–395.
29. Celikoz B, Sengezer M, Guler MM, Selmanpakoglu N. Reconstruction of anterior neck contractures with sensate expanded radial forearm free flap. Burns 1996; 22:320–323.
30. Adant JT, Bluth F, Jacquemin D. Reconstruction of neck burns. A long-term comparative study between skin grafts, skin expansion and free flaps. Acta Chir Belg 1998; 98:5–9.
31. Angrigiani C. Aesthetic micosurgical reconstruction of anterior neck burn deformities. Plast Reconstr Surg 1994; 93:507–518.
32. Hunt JA, Moisidis E, Haertsch P. Initial experience of Integra® in the treatment of postburn anterior cervical neck contractures. Br J Plast Surg 2000; 53:652–658.

26

Correction of Soft Tissue Defects of the Back and Shoulders

NELSON SARTO PICCOLO

Instituto Nelson Picolo and Pronto Socorro para Queimaduras, Goiânia, Goiás, Brazil

I. INTRODUCTION

Burn wounds of the back and shoulders can be an isolated injury or part of a more complex, larger burn. In the pediatric population, younger children frequently have deep and extensive injuries, caused by scalding liquids, commonly involving the head, neck, shoulders, and back.

Flame burns are only responsible for about 8% of all our burns, but they are the most frequent cause of major burns in adults. Although rarer in Brazil, but very frequent in the United States and Europe, the wounds generated in these accidents are usually very deep, large burns, which require aggressive surgical treatment (Fig. 26.1).

The surgical management will be dictated not only by the depth of injury, but also by the extent of the injury. In addition, the experience or method with which the treating burn team is acquainted influences outcome. The choice and timing of treatment may influence both functional and aesthetic results in the immediate and in the long term since backs may be grafted later or with "lesser quality" meshed skin in major burns. Better quality skin grafts are typically used to cover more critical areas, such as face, hands, and major joints.

Since scald burns are not all treated the same way by the various services, particularly in children, the reconstructive surgeon may also be faced with patients who present with hypertrophic scars as a result of nonexcised, nongrafted areas. These sequelae are generally accompanied by various degrees of functional deficit, which may influence the surgeon to take a more immediate approach for the patient's reconstruction, even before complete maturation of the scar tissue has occurred.

More recently, the advent of bioengineered skin substitutes, has allowed earlier closure of burn wounds. Accordingly, this has led to earlier hospital discharge and rehabilitation procedures in most burn centers (1–3). In the vast majority of burn patients, the sequelae of major burn injuries involve the skin and scar contractures. In most cases, then, planning a reconstructive procedure rests on how to promote the substitution of scarred skin with healthy, normal looking skin. Obviously, injuries involving deeper tissues, such as electrical burns, will have to be reconstructed accordingly (4,5) (Fig. 26.2).

Whatever the method chosen for the surgical correction of these soft tissue defects, the operating surgeon should provide a timely procedure, which will yield a profitable

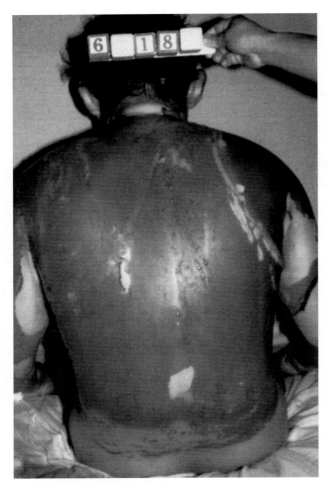

Figure 26.1 Patient with extensive flame burn, also involving the back and shoulders.

result for the patient. The results should not only be functional and aesthetic, but also reflect positively on the patient as a whole to improve self-esteem and his or her abilities to relate socially and to function better in his/her activities of daily living (ADLs). The ultimate goal for the reconstructive team then is to bring the patient back to his preinjury status, which, unfortunately, cannot always be achieved.

II. PREOPERATIVE EVALUATION

Although preoperative assessment must be performed to not only identify functional deficits, but also address patient's complaints. Planning for an operative procedure for a specific patient will obviously be influenced by the injury as a whole. But, for the purpose of this chapter, we will present considerations on the treatment of burn sequelae of the back and shoulders only. Although one may have significant functional deficits as a result of back burns, impairment may be more important as a result of shoulder burns. Hypertrophic scarring and contractures are the main cause of poor functional results. However, patient compliance with occupational therapy and physical therapy (OT and PT) can influence the outcome. This aspect of care must always be closely followed.

Continuity of the treatment offered to the patient may require an even larger commitment of all involved. As the burn team and the patient initially pursued survival during the acute phase of injury, all who were engaged in this process must now pursue the same direction with a broader view. Here, the goals are restoration of function,

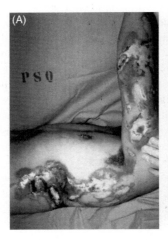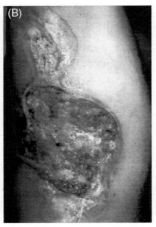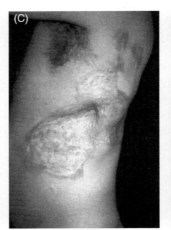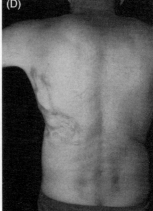

Figure 26.2 (A) Electrical injury to the left trunk and back. (B) Same patient, postexcision. (C) Same patient, after skin grafting. (D) Same patient, after skin grafting, posterior view.

improvement in the cosmetic aspect of the burn scar, and adaptation of the patient to a new image and a new life (6). Compliance with the use of pressure garments and frequent visits to the PT/OT department all influence the outcome of the surgical procedure. The patient must be aware that a similar or even better performance at the PT/OT suite will be requested of him in the immediate postoperative period to insure the success of the operative procedure. Important considerations are the continuation of the rehabilitative program initiated early, during the acute phase of treatment, with continuous and progressive active range of motion in all joints and proper positioning at rest. In addition, avoiding techniques that unnecessarily immobilize the patient or body parts is essential (7).

The burn injury may have left a severe, disfiguring as well as functionally crippling scar. The patient may be depressed or undergoing psychological counseling, which will require continuous support toward the planning, execution, and result of the proposed surgical treatment. In our institution, the patient is evaluated by the surgeon, the physiotherapist, the occupational therapist, and the psychologist. As a result of this evaluation, his or her complaints are noted and his or her needs are prioritized in accordance with the degree of disability or severity of the disfigurement. The entire team involved in the treatment of the patient must be aware of the patient's case as well as acquainted with him or her personally. A thorough evaluation of the patient's psychological status may be the single most important step of the preoperative evaluation. Although the adult, male patient is more frequently concerned with functional aspects, cosmesis may be the stronger issue in the cases of children and female patients. The patient must deal with realistic expectations for an already difficult situation. The injuries or disfigurements may be severe and he may be experiencing difficulty in coping with his everyday life. This issue may be even more complex when the patient is a child. Here, parents may feel guilty about the initial event, and may be obtrusive relative to following the usual sequential treatment in rehabilitation, willing to "burn steps" and go immediately into surgery. The other end of this complex spectrum is rejection of the patient by one or both parents. Forced seclusion, not allowing the child to go to school, play, or participate in social activities with his or her peers is a difficult challenge (8). The surgeon may also have to enforce proper timing of the procedures when regional habits and custom influence the requests for reconstruction. This is frequently the case in Brazil, where the weather is always hot, and female patients will very often ask for immediate reconstruction of the burn sequelae concerning the back, so they can soon go back to sun tanning and wearing light or minimal clothing.

III. SURGICAL OPTIONS

When considering how to correct back and/or shoulder soft tissue defects, the surgeon will soon realize that in most cases, wound closure was attained with skin grafts acutely. The exception usually happens in electrical burns, or deep friction burns, when deeper tissue injury is the rule and skin or muscle flaps may have to be used (9) (Fig. 26.3). The method of acute treatment will, of course, influence the method of reconstruction. Local tissue may have already been spent for the initial injury problem, and there may be different types of tissue covering the posterior trunk. Local tissue may have been utilized as pedicled flaps to reconstruct more mobile, extensile parts like the neck or the axilla. In cases where the back and/or shoulder injury has been an isolated injury, with normal skin in the periphery of the sequela, the treatment of choice will be tissue expansion (Fig. 26.4). Tissue expansion has been widely used all over the world, in all age brackets, for removal of burn scars. It is a very versatile technique, with an infinity of implant shapes and sizes. Better results are generally obtained when the scar tissue is already mature and the patient comprehends the sequence of treatment required in this technique. The learning curve is relatively short and swift, for both the surgical team and the patients. The later benefits are that these patients can be taught to expand the implants themselves, at home (10,11).

In cases where tissue contraction has resulted in functional impairment in an area within a larger scar, it may be necessary to surgically correct the lack of local tissue, usually with incision and grafting, and/or with Z-plasties, when there are contracture bands. Other options may include the rotation of skin or composite flaps, and, more rarely, even the transfer of distant tissue by microsurgical techniques (12) (Fig. 26.5).

In the rarer cases where skin grafting was placed onto deeper structures like periosteum or deep muscle layers, peripheral soft tissue can be expanded compositely,

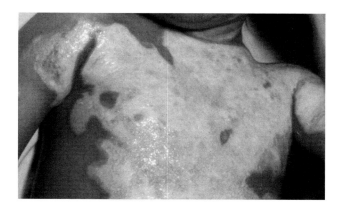

Figure 26.3 Scald burn.

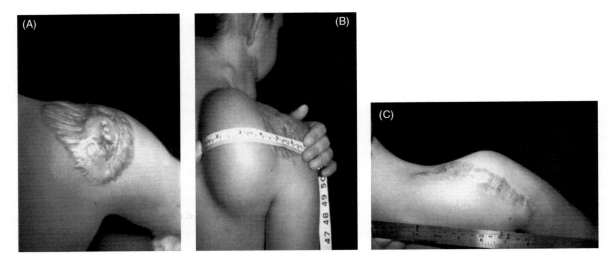

Figure 26.4   (A) Patient with postburn shoulder scar. (B) Tissue expander inflated. (C) Postoperative appearance after removal of burn scar and resurfacing with expanded flap.

advancing skin, subcutaneous layer, fascia, and/or muscle. The surgeon must not forget that all soft tissue above the expander is expanded, including vessels and nerves, and he should take advantage of these facts when planning an adequate reconstruction for a particularly difficult problem.

IV.   INTRAOPERATIVE CONSIDERATIONS

Most procedures in these areas are done under general anesthesia in an intubated patient. Complete control of the airway is imperative in back and shoulder

reconstructive procedures due to the fact that awkward positioning may result in respiratory obstruction if an airway is not properly secured.

Skin markings for the placement of implants or expanders, indicating the shape and rotation of a flap, should be performed immediately before surgery, with the patient awake and standing. Whenever possible, the natural skin lines and creases should be respected. Failure to do so may result in uneven anatomical placement of incisions and, subsequently, unsightly scar lines.

Special care should also be taken when considering using the normal skin of the axilla for the posterior shoulder flap, particularly in the prepubertal patient,

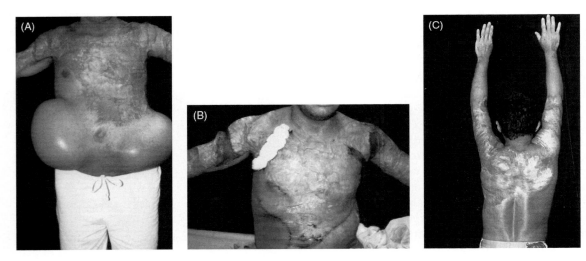

Figure 26.5   (A) Patient with severe restriction of shoulder movement, being expanded for full-thickness expanded skin graft, to be placed on both axillas for bilateral shoulder release. (B) Patient 8 days postremoval of tissue expanders, partial scar removal and full-thickness expanded skin grafting to both axillas. (C) Same patient with full functional recovery of shoulder movement.

when this area is hairless. These flaps can rarely be advanced further than a few centimeters, because of the risk of transferring hair-bearing tissue to a non-hair-bearing area, such as the posterior inferior shoulder. Although tissue expansion is probably the most widely used technique for reconstruction in burn care today, there are several issues to be considered and the seasoned surgeon will take several precautions to minimize the incidence of complications. A common misjudgment in planning, at the time of ordering or choosing the tissue expander, is that although the expander is presented as a tri-dimensional implant with height, width, and length in the catalog, when it is placed in the dissected surgical pocket, it is placed flat or with minimal volume within. Thus, its base now has an increased dimension on each side. The implant now is much larger than the measures described on its label. Consequently, it is most important when creating the pocket for the tissue expander that one considers the size of the base of the implant (width and length) plus the folded sides, which will also be a part of the flat cookie shape of the expander (Fig. 26.6). Implants with a thick base should be reserved for areas with thicker overlying tissues like the paramedian back area. Thinner prosthesis should be the choice, to be placed on the shoulders, and on or around the base of the neck. Beware of the placement of an expander with a stiff base over a curved surface like an upper arm or leg in a child. The stiff base may project up into the skin as the base straightens out increasing the risk of expander exposure. We often inject a small amount of volume into the expander, through the skin, into the expander port, after it is in its place, under healthy or scar tissue. This will insure that the connection is working properly. In addition, this provides a certain massaging/buffer effect to the underlying tissue as the patient moves or is moved in the immediate postoperative period. Failure to consider the issues mentioned earlier may cause folds or edges of the still flat expander to project into healthy tissue or suture lines, which may result in local discomfort, tissue necrosis, contamination of the surgical pocket, and premature extrusion. If the surgeon chooses to place continuous vacuum drainage for the first 24–48 h, as we usually do, the drain should be placed before the expander to avoid its displacement or folding, which may occur if the drain is forced within the surgical cavity after the expander is already in place. The drain should never be brought out through healthy, scarless tissue, but via a stab wound in a neighboring scar. When considering shoulder expanders, dissection should be limited to the size and shape of the compressed expander. Wider pockets in this area may facilitate "to and fro" movements of the continuously growing implant, and it may dislocate with gravity, into the lateral arm. This will result in less tissue being expanded in the desired area, where the tissues are firmer and thicker (Fig. 26.7).

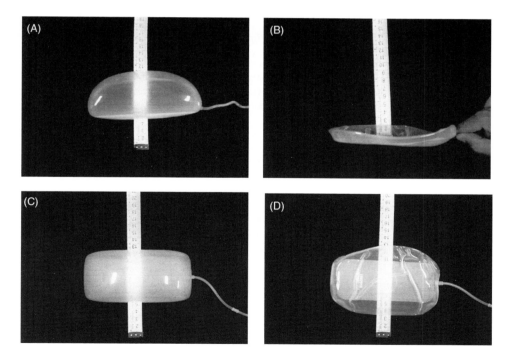

Figure 26.6 (A) Rectangular expander with "full" volume, seen from the side. (B) Same expander without any volume, "flat," as it is usually placed into the surgical cavity. Note the height of the empty prosthesis. (C) Rectangular expander with "full" volume, seen from the top. (D) Same expander, "flat." Note the larger area taken by the folded sides.

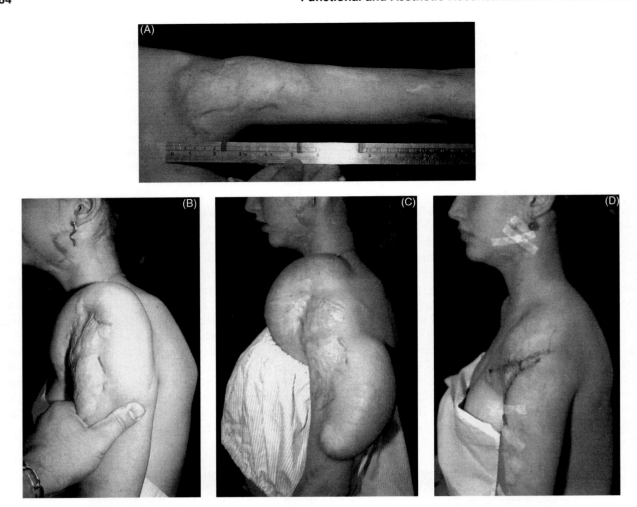

Figure 26.7   (A) Patient with hypertrophic shoulder scar. (B) Same patient with expanders placed on left shoulder, being held up, on the original surgically placed position. (C) Same patient, when expander is not held up, demonstrating the effect of gravity on the filled prosthesis, on the looseness of the soft tissue in young patients. (D) Immediate postop result, demonstrating the lesser resection at shoulder level, from where the prosthesis has been "taken" by gravity.

V.   PITFALLS

Although most plastic surgeons involved in burn reconstruction have collected a vast experience with different techniques of reconstruction, one must be aware of the complications related to each technique and be prepared for the occasional poor result. The patient and/or his or her families must be made aware of these possible occurrences. A burn survivor may be under a varied load of stress, and dealing with frustration could be very difficult, when compared to other plastic surgery patients.

The surgeon must be honest with the patient and the patient's family, discussing the surgical plan, its expected outcome, and possible complications and pitfalls. Patients with a failed surgical procedure will rarely blame the surgical team if they were made aware of this possibility

beforehand. The surgeon must also assure the prospective patient that even though complications occur, the surgical team is prepared to deal with them accordingly, taking the appropriate measures in due time. It is widely accepted to show pictures of unidentifiable patients with previous similar cases, to give an idea of the expected results. The author is personally against the use of computer images that are modified on the screen to give an idea of the expected results. Such images may not be representative of the true results.

In our experience, the most frequent complication, when considering tissue expansion, is the formation of striae, followed by scar widening and implant dislocation. Other failures are usually due to unrealistic surgical expectations, as in the rare case where the surgeon may think that more tissue can be removed. The resulting tight suture line closure may result in dehiscence of the suture line. This can produce a long-lasting wound where previously only a scar existed. This may have happened to several of us, generally, in earlier years of surgical practice, when the eagerness to please the patient was greater than common sense and the geometric reality would dictate.

VI. NURSING ISSUES

The nursing staff as an integral part of the burn team must be intimately involved in the direct care and treatment of the burn patient or victim who is planning to undergo surgical reconstruction. Understanding the reconstructive plan will allow for a smoother postoperative period, when appropriate actions will be taken at the correct time. Positioning may be a major issue and the nursing staff will be working closely with the PT/OT group to ensure the success of the operative procedure. Also, the nursing staff may bring important input on how the patient behaved after previous acute or reconstructive procedures. This helps the surgeon to recommend a more realistic approach to certain patients who were considered problem patients or difficult patients. Compliance with positioning is absolutely necessary in the postoperative care of most procedures in the back and shoulders. The staff must be completely informed about each and every case, and the requirements relating to their care and expected outcome.

VII. REHABILITATION ISSUES

The physiotherapist and the occupational therapist work very closely in the recovery of the burn patient as a whole. Since admission for the care of an acute burn, these professionals control important issues which will influence the outcome and result for that particular patient. It is no different when reconstruction is considered. The patient who is a candidate for surgical treatment of burn sequelae must be cleared by the rehabilitation team in relationship to timing, necessity, and compliance for the planned operation. The presence of the PT or OT in the operating room is as routine nowadays as the presence of the circulating or scrub nurse, anesthesiologist, or surgeon. Most splints are made during or right after the procedure to insure proper positioning of the joints or extremities. This is frequently necessary when considering shoulder or back procedures. The patient as a whole is very important because most splints may engage several parts of the body. Consequently, the influence of support or motion to other body parts must be taken under consideration. Preoperative consultation with the rehabilitation team members will clear

any doubt as to where to reconstruct first, based on orthesis placement, pressure garment requirements, and physiotherapy progress.

VIII. LONG-TERM OUTCOME

Good results are undoubtedly the goal of any operative procedure. Planning for sequential procedures in a burn survivor is relatively standard procedure, since most patients have several problems that cannot all be dealt with simultaneously. In the usual case, the patient or the parents will be made aware of the planned procedures and how one previous procedure influences the next one. Shoulders are generally treated earlier than backs, as the patient may also have other areas that were prioritized in the sequence of reconstruction.

Complete scar removal may be obtained with one or more operations in the case of localized shoulder or back scars, but pressure garments may have to be worn for months or even more than 1 year after the procedure. If scar widening still occurs, a revision may be in order. Scar removal may not be the objective in some cases where functional restriction is the concern. The patient will be submitted to the technique that will fit the need. Usually, incisions of the retraction area and thick split-skin graft or full-thickness skin graft application may be necessary. Alternatively, rotation of a local pedicled flap may be the procedure of choice. The result here may be appreciated earlier, and the patient may be back to his usual function in a matter of weeks or months. Whatever is the case, long-term good results are more prevalent when the surgeon insures adequate, sequential procedures, and the patient is realistic in his or her expectations.

IX. CONCLUSION

As with any other part of the body which may have been injured during a burn accident, the shoulder and the back may have residual scarring and consequently functional and aesthetic disabilities may ensue. The patient must be prepared to face the challenges of reconstruction in order to return to normal life as possible. This may require psychological support as well as rehabilitative support. However, these support systems must be put in place as early as possible. There are a wide array of possibilities at hand for the reconstructive surgeon who will obviously choose the ones he or she is most acquainted with using. Although complications may occur, the patient must be assured that the burn team as a whole is prepared to deal with whatever problem or difficulty he or she may have.

REFERENCES

1. Heimbach D, Heimbach D, Luterman A, Burke J, Cram A, Herndon D, Hunt J, Jordan M, McManus W, Solem L, Warden G. Artificial dermis for major burns: a multicenter randomized clinical trial. Ann Surg 1988; 194:413–428.
2. Tompkins RG. Increased survival after massive thermal injuries in adults: preliminary report using artificial skin. Crit Care Med 1989; 17:734–740.
3. Fitton AR, Drew P, Dickson WA. The use of a bilaminate artificial skin substitute (Integra) in acute resurfacing of burns: an early experience. Br J Plast Surg 2001; 54:208–212.
4. MacKinnon C, Klaassen M, Widdowson P. Reconstruction of a severe chest and abdominal wall electrical burn injury in a pediatric patient. Plast Reconstr Surg 1999; 103(6):1775–1777.
5. Foyatier JL, Comparin JP, Masson CL. Skin flaps and extended full-thickness skin grafts. Indications in the repair of burn sequelae. Ann Chir Plast Esthet 1996; 41(5):511–532.
6. Petro JA, Salzberg CA. Ethical issues of burn management. Clin Plast Surg 1992; 19(3):615–621.
7. Boswick JA Jr. Comprehensive rehabilitation after burn injury. Surg Clin N Am 1987; 67(1):159–166.
8. Patridge J, Robinson E. Psychological and social aspects of burns. Burns 1995; 21:453–457.
9. Xu X, Zhu W, Wu Y. Experience of the treatment of severe electric burns on special parts of the body. Ann NY Acad Sci 1999; 888:121–130.
10. Manders EK. Soft tissue expansion. Concepts and complications. Plast Reconstr Surg 1984; 74:495–507.
11. Hudson DA, Grobbelaar AO. The use of tissue expansion in children with burns of the head and neck. Burns 1995; 21:209–211.
12. Ono I, Tateshita T. Reconstruction of a full-thickness defect of the chest wall caused by friction burn using a combined myocutaneous flap of teres major and latissimus dorsi muscles. Burns 2001; 27:283–288.

27

Reconstruction of Axillary Contracture

JUI-YUNG YANG

Chang Gung Memorial Hospital, Taipei, Taiwan

I. INTRODUCTION

Axillary burn scar contractures are common problems after deep thermal burns involving the upper trunk or extremities because they are neither easily positioned initially nor easily rehabilitated later. The contractures can produce both functional and anatomical deformities. A vicious cycle, caused by both repeated ulcers after exercise and scar contracture after wound healing, frequently develops during the rehabilitation stage. Surgical intervention is usually needed if contractures are established. However, surgical correction for axillary contractures is still a challenge because the axilla is a unique three-dimensional pyramid-shaped hollow formed by the junction of the upper extremity and trunk (1). Thus, a satisfactory reconstruction needs detailed preoperative evaluation of the anatomy of axilla involved by scar contracture and prioritizing available donor tissues.

II. PREOPERATIVE EVALUATION

Axilla contractures are characteristically divided into two groups: those involving the hairy dome and those that do not. Grishkevich classified the contractures into two types: edge contractures caused by a tight web and strip contractures caused by a wide scar (2). Achauer (3) classified them into four types, namely, type 1, anterior or posterior axillary fold only; type 2, both anterior and posterior fold with the apex spared; type 3, the entire axilla; and type 4, scars of the axilla and the adjacent areas. Hallock's (4) classification of axillary contractures is modified from Salisbury and Bevin (5) and also divided into four types: (1) solitary anterior or posterior web; (2) scar bands adjacent to axilla; (3) anterior and posterior webs with the cupola spared; and (4) total axillary obliteration. The key point of the classification of the axilla contracture is to differentiate whether the dome of the axilla is involved or not. If the dome is spared and most of the axillary hairs exist, the reconstructive procedure may be aimed at the release of contracture utilizing local cutaneous tissue such as Z-plasty, etc. If the dome was already destroyed, the reconstructive procedure may be aimed at the replacement of the entire scar tissue utilizing local or distant flaps or skin grafts.

Besides the local tissue condition, the abduction function of the upper limb should also be considered. Huang et al. (6) used the range of motion and defined the severity of the contracture as follows: mild, <25%; moderate, 25–50%; and severe, >50% (6). Usually a releasing procedure, using local tissue is enough for the mild cases and a tissue replacement procedure is needed for the severe cases. The surgical considerations for the moderate cases depends on the local tissue condition.

III. SURGICAL CONSIDERATIONS

The use of skin grafts is the basic technique to correct the contracture. A full-thickness skin graft (FTSG) is the first choice for replacement of the scar tissue if the graft donor site is available. Less secondary contraction will occur with FTSG than with split-thickness skin grafts (STSG). However, the donor site of the FTSG should be closed primarily or grafted with STSG. The shortage of graft donor site is the main limitation in using FTSG for burn scar axillary contractures. The use of STSG, although more donor sites may be available, will have more secondary contraction. Prolonged immobilization initially and splinting later is needed after application of STSG for the correction of these scar contractures. The advantage of the use of skin grafts in correcting burn scar contractures of the axilla is that the reconstruction is also suitable, from minor contractures to total obliteration of the axilla (Figs. 27.1–27.3). Recently, artificial dermis has been applied to the reconstruction of burn scar contractures of the axilla, especially when skin graft donor sites were not available or a greater underlying dermal tissue cushion is needed such as in the axilla or in the elbow (7,8). However, this new technique requires a two-stage operation and is cost-ineffective. The postoperative rehabilitation such as pressure therapy is still needed.

A. Local Flaps

In the mild cases of scar band deformity, local Z-plasties may be enough for the release of the contracture. Examples in Figs. 27.4 and 27.5 show how a simple Z-plasty can solve the problem of scar band deformity in the anterior axilla. Sometimes, multiple Z-plasties may be needed to correct a longer linear contracture band (Figs. 27.6–27.9). In this case, the scar bands extended from the elbow across the axilla to the upper chest and

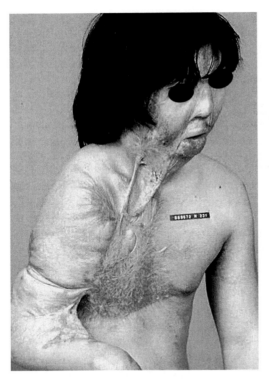

Figure 27.1 Severe scar contracture of the neck, axilla, and elbow after flame burn since childhood.

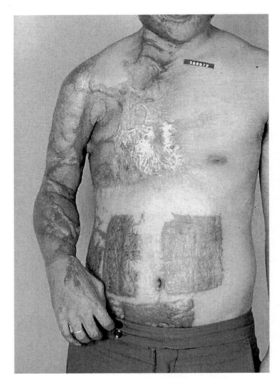

Figure 27.2 Release contracture with thick STSG taken from the abdomen. Two years' follow-up showed satisfactory results.

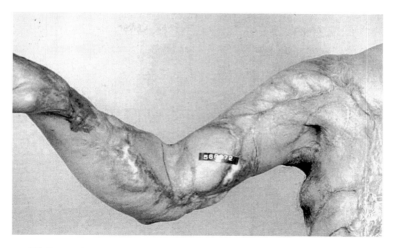

Figure 27.3 Follow-up for 5 years showed good function of the shoulder function.

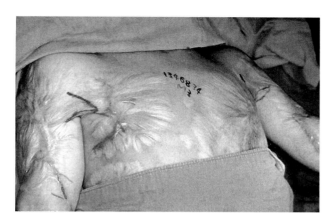

Figure 27.4 Multiple scar bands in anterior axilla and arm. Z-plasties were applied for release of contracture.

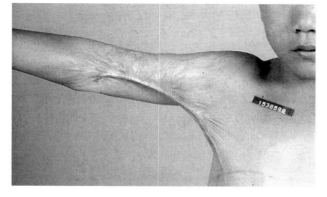

Figure 27.6 Long linear scar bands involving elbow, axilla, and upper chest.

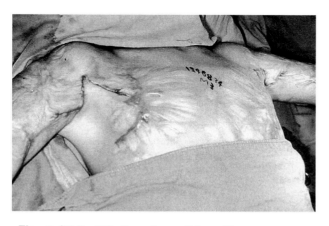

Figure 27.5 Effective release of the axillary contracture.

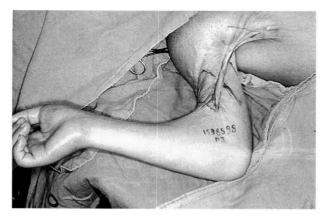

Figure 27.7 Multiple different directions of Z-plasties were applied.

caused limitations in extension of the upper limb. Various directions of the Z-plasties not only solve the problem but also provide the chance to excise some redundant scar tissue. The Hirshowitz's five-flap procedure is also very effective in the release of the scar band deformities (9,10). The triangular flaps of two opposite Z-plasties and a Y–V advancement flap constitute the five flaps (Figs. 27.10–27.13).

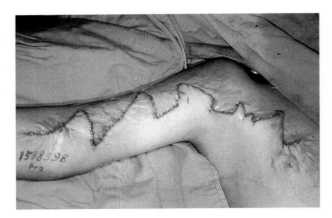

Figure 27.8 Immediate results of transposition of skin flaps of those Z-plasties and excision of some redundant scar tissues.

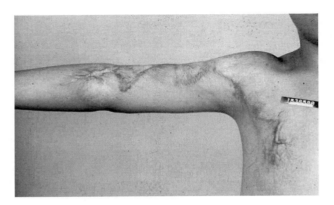

Figure 27.9 Follow-up for one more year revealed satisfactory results.

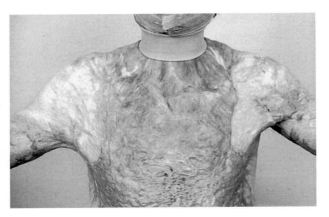

Figure 27.10 Interior scar fold deformities caused limitation of arm abduction and shoulder elevation.

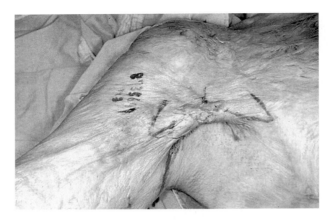

Figure 27.11 Design of a five-flap plasty for anterior scar fold in the axillary region.

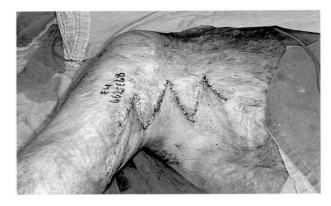

Figure 27.12 The result of five-flap plasty after interpolation of the flap.

The V–Y plasty may also be used for correction of burn scar contractures of axillary fold or adjacent areas (Figs. 27.14 and 27.15). The triangular flap was advanced and rotated to achieve a greater release and avoid a linear scar in the axillary fossa. Olbrisch's running Y–V plasty can be applied to longer scar band deformity like the multiple Z-plasties (11).

Karacaoglan's seven-flap plasty may be used in patients with linear postburn axillary contracture (12). The geometry of the seven-flap plasty consists of two half Z-plasties and one W–M plasty. Vaubel's V flap designed for correction of the axillary defect can also be used for reconstruction after scar excision and the release of contracture (13). The V-flap is a combination of V–Y advancement and two Limberg transposition flaps.

Whenever healthy local tissue is available, the scar shape should be taken into consideration to make a better design in the reconstructive procedure. A specially designed square flap applied to a patient with scar band deformity in the posterior axillary fold is useful

(Fig. 27.16). The square flap method basically consists of a square flap and 45° and 90° angled triangular flaps. After joining these flaps, an elongation rate of +180% is obtained (14). The effect of the release of contracture is

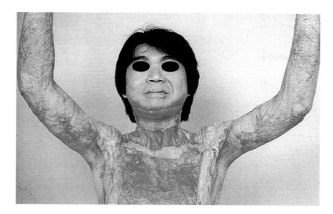

Figure 27.13 Follow-up 1 year later revealed satisfactory results.

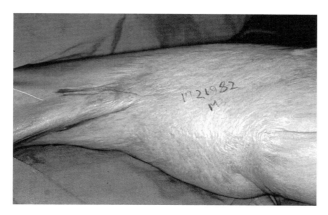

Figure 27.14 A big scar band in the anterior axillary fold that caused contracture.

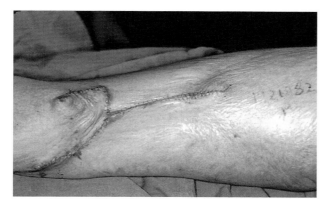

Figure 27.15 The scar tissue was nearly matured and could be used as an advancement and rotated flap in a modified V–Y plasty.

greater than with the Y–V advancement flap because the head of the flap is a square not a triangular shape. The advancement of the square flap also can provide more chances to excise more scar tissue (Fig. 27.17).

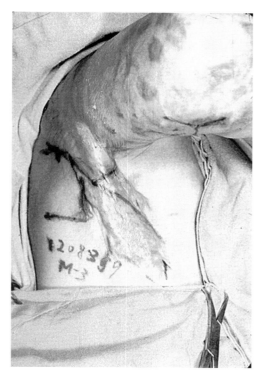

Figure 27.16 A square flap was designed for scar band deformity in a patient with posterior axillary fold contracture.

B. Fasciocutaneous Flaps

When extensive adjacent scar tissue or even dome obliteration is noted in axillary contractures, local cutaneous flaps such as the Z-plasty is usually not enough for a complete release. In this situation, larger local pedicle flap such as fasciocutaneous flap is a better choice. The most local random patterned transposition flap is elevated at a safe base–length ratio of 1:1. However, the raising of fasciocutaneous flaps with ratios of 1:3 or more can survive (10,15). The blood supply to the deep fascia is rich enough to support this flap so that the presence of burned skin or grafts on part of the flap is not a contraindication for use (16). Usually this flap is designed along the lines of the contracture. Wherever possible, the flap should be in an area where there is low tension in the tissue at right angles to the scar axis so that the secondary defect can be closed primarily (17). This flap may be elevated from the lateral chest, the lateral back, or the parascapular, cervicohumeral, or thoracoacromial regions. In addition, the posterior upper arm and inner arm can be used depending on the relationships between the scar tissue and the available donor site (17–22). A schema for a reasonable flap selection process has been devised based on the relative severity and anatomic location of the axillary burn scar contracture (5) (Figs. 27.18–27.21).

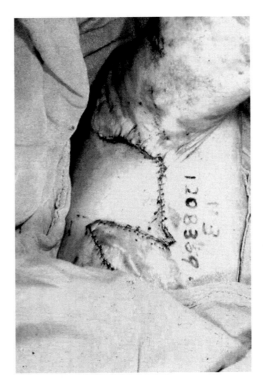

Figure 27.17 The postoperative results of advancement of the square flap after excision of the most severe scar tissue and release contracture.

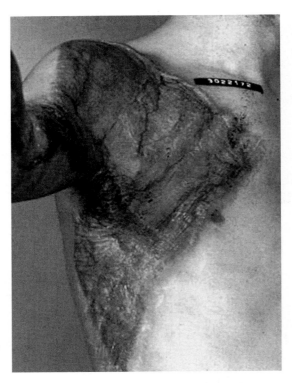

Figure 27.18 Scar contracture with total obliteration of axillary dome after flame burn.

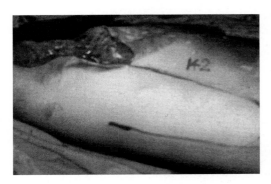

Figure 27.19 A big fasciocutaneous flap, 8 × 24 cm, was designed in the lateral back.

These photographs document a young man with a scar contracture involving the entire axilla including the dome being treated with a fasciocutaneous flap with good results. The range of motion of the shoulder improved from 70° to ~180°. Figures 27.22–27.24 document a scar contracture not only in the axillary dome but also in the anterior shoulder. A long fasciocutaneous flap, 5 cm × 18 cm, was elevated from the lateral back and transposed 90° to cover the defect in the axilla and anterior shoulder after releasing the contracture. The donor site can be easily closed primarily. The results showed that the flap is well suited for this situation.

Most of the fasciocutaneous flaps were designed as pedicled flaps. They may have dog-ears at the pedicle after transposition. The movement of the flap is limited due to the pedicle attachment. The island flaps may solve this problem. For example, the scapular island flap utilizing the circumflex scapular artery, a branch of the subscapular artery, as its vascular pedicle can be rotated 180° on this pedicle to insert into the axillary defect after contracture release (23–25).

Depending on the three cutaneous branches of the circumflex scapular artery, the scapular flap is designed horizontally in the middle scapular region, the parascapular flap obliquely in the lower scapular region, and the ascending scapular flap vertically in the upper scapular region. All can be used for axillary reconstruction (23,26,27).

Some modifications of the island flaps have been noted to minimize the residual contractures or to increase the width of the flap for coverage. A posterior arm fasciocutaneous flap with its feeding vessels from the brachial vessels can also be elevated as an island pedicle flap to increase the arc of rotation to cover the axillary defect (21). The parascapular flap may be folded on to itself in a "U" shape to double the width of the flap for greater coverage (26) (Figs. 27.25 and 27.26). An axial bilobed flap, based on the transverse and ascending branches of the circumflex scapular artery, is also successfully used to reconstruct severe burn scar contractures of the axilla (28). The primary flap may have greater width up to 12 cm and the

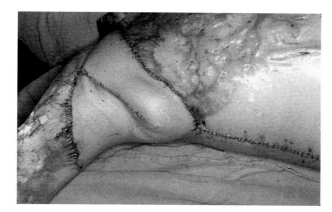

Figure 27.20 Complete release of the contracture and the defect was covered by transposition of that flap. The donor site was closed primarily.

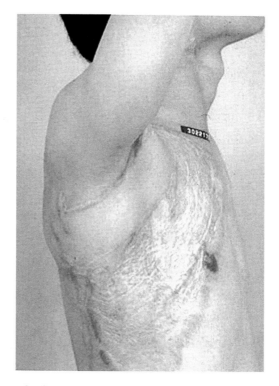

Figure 27.21 Follow-up for two more years revealed satisfactory results.

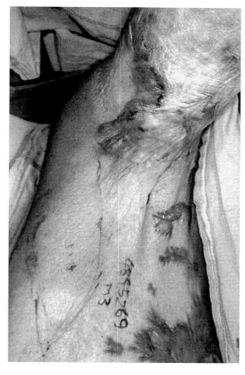

Figure 27.22 Patient sustained scar contracture in axillary dome and anterior shoulder. A long fasciocutaneous flap, 5 × 18 cm in size, was designed at the lateral back.

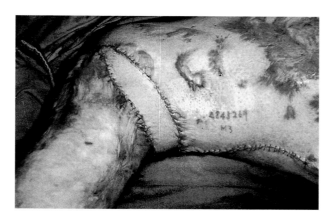

Figure 27.23 The flap was transposed 90° to cover the defect after complete release of contracture.

secondary defect can be closed primarily without tension. Recently, the thoracodorsal perforator-based cutaneous island flap was successfully used for extensive axillary burn scar contractures (29). This flap offers some advantages over other island flaps such as scapular or subscapular flaps. The exit points of the perforators are usually far from the burn injury and the length of the vascular pedicle permits the design of a large flap. In addition, the donor site is easy to close primarily.

C. Muscle and Myocutaneous Flaps

The muscle or myocutaneous flaps, sometimes, are an alternative choice for correction of extensive burn scar contractures of the axilla. After releasing of the contracture, the lateral portion of the latissimus dorsi (LD) muscle is chosen to transpose and fill the defect in axillary area. Skin grafts are placed over the muscle (30). In unusual circumstances, when simple options are

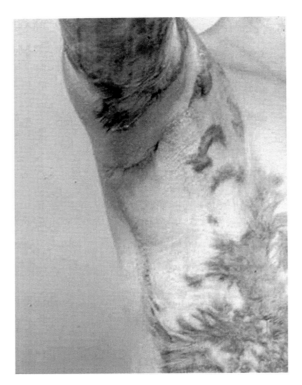

Figure 27.24 Follow-up for several months showed satisfactory results.

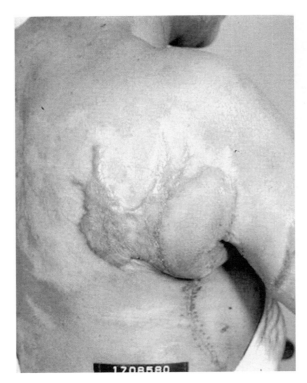

Figure 27.26 The flap totally survived and the shoulder function was restored.

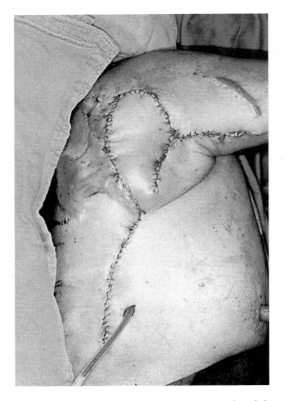

Figure 27.25 A patient with scar contracture involving the entire axilla was reconstructed with the folded parascapular flap.

unavailable, the skin-grafted long head of the triceps muscle flap may serve admirably as another vascularized flap alternative for releasing of either anterior or posterior axillary web contractures (31). The LD myocutaneous flap is part of the armamentarium to reconstruct the axillary region after wide releases of burn scar contractures (32). The main disadvantage of using the LD myocutaneous flap is its bulkiness. Dividing the thoracodorsal nerve will, over time, reduce the bulkiness of the flap secondary to muscle atrophy.

D. Microvascular Free-Tissue Transfer

Microvascular free-tissue transfers, especially the free perforator flaps, are now more popular. The ultrathin cutaneous flap based on either septal or intramuscular perforators, such as the anterior lateral thigh flap, is a good choice to reconstruct the deformities in concavity area such as the neck or axilla (33).

E. Tissue Expansion

Tissue expansion is a very useful technique for aesthetic replacement of postburn scar deformities. It provides skin flaps around the affected region with similar color, texture, and composition for reconstruction (34,35). This technique also provides minimal donor site morbidity. Figures 27.27 and 27.28 show a tissue expander being placed in the shoulder area. The scar tissue was excised and the contracture was corrected. The resultant defect was covered by advancement of the expanded skin flap.

IV. INTRAOPERATIVE CONSIDERATIONS

Usually, the scar in the axillary dome should be totally excised and then the residual underlying fibrotic bands should be cut to achieve complete release for the patients with total obliteration of the axillary dome. Care must be taken not to injure the brachial plexus and greater vessels during the procedure. The brachial plexus may also be injured by exerting too much stretch on the plexus when extending the upper arm during the release. In addition, it should be mentioned that every effort must be made not to disturb the axillary hairs during transposition of the local flaps for those patients with anterior or posterior axillary scar bands. Multiple Z-plasty or continuous VY-plasty with moderate-sized skin flaps may have less possibility to disturb the axillary hairs than a single large Z-plasty or VY-advancement flap. When fasciocutaneous flaps are used for reconstruction, care must be taken to include the deep fascia in the flap dissection or the

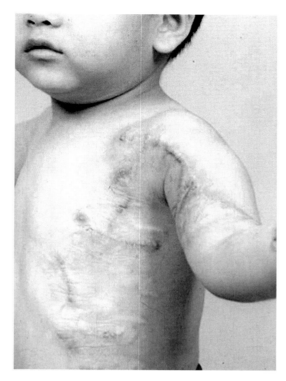

Figure 27.28 The scar was excised and contracture relieved after reconstruction with expanded skin flap. There was no donor site morbidity.

circulation might be compromised. Because of scar contractures, the skin and the subcutaneous tissues are thicker in the back and the adjacent tissues surrounding the axilla are usually thinner than normal tissue. Thinned flaps such as thinned musculocutaneous perforator-based flaps are recommended by some authors (36).

V. PITFALLS

Waiting for scars to mature before the correction of axillary contractures is not always necessary. Because these contractures will cause functional impairment, especially for the pediatric patients, early intervention is necessary (37). If the axillary dome is spared in the burn scar contracture, the axillary hairs are better preserved during the reconstruction. The male patient may complain more if the axillary hairs are displaced. Figures 27.29–27.32 show a patient who complained of malposition of his axillary hairs after local flap reconstruction for the axillary contracture was performed at another clinic. The original axillary hairs were located at the lower axilla but not at the dome. A large Z-plasty to elevate the entire hair-bearing skin flap to the middle axilla was performed during a secondary reconstruction. The final result showed correct position of axillary hairs and the patient felt satisfied.

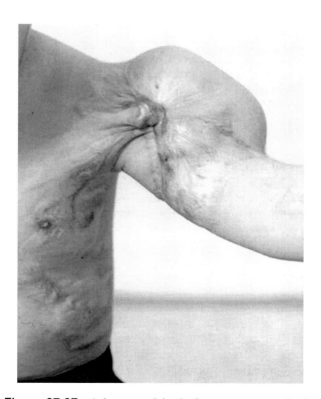

Figure 27.27 A boy complained of scar contracture in the anterior axilla. A tissue expander was placed at the shoulder near the scar tissue.

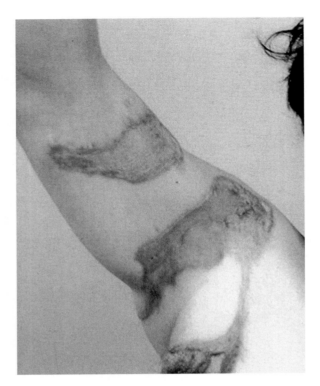

Figure 27.29   A patient with malposition of the axillary hairs after transposition of a fasciocutaneous flap.

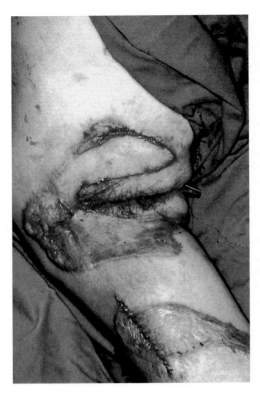

Figure 27.31   The axillary hairs were moved to the axillary dome after transposition of the hair-bearing flap.

In addition, one should mention that the burned or grafted skin over the fasciocutaneous flap usually causes no problems if the skin is mature or stable. In the early stages of the burn injury or with immature skin grafts, gentle manipulation of this tissue is required to avoid superficial necrosis of the overlying of the skin when raising fasciocutaneous flaps. Because the vascular pedicle in the flap is easily kinked or compressed after transposition to the axilla, proper position to avoid these conditions is very important to prevent partial flap necrosis.

VI.   NURSING ISSUES

Postoperative immobilization is very important. The tie-over dressings for graft skin should be kept clean and dry postoperatively. The splint if any should be kept in place. Frequent check-up of the dressings and change, if necessary, is needed to prevent maceration of the surrounding skin. Poor hygiene of the axillary area frequently causes wound infection and subsequent loss of skin grafts.

Sometimes tip necrosis of a Z-plasty can be prevented after releasing the tension by removing one or two stitches around the tip. In cases where flaps are used for correction of axillary contractures, one should watch out for impaired

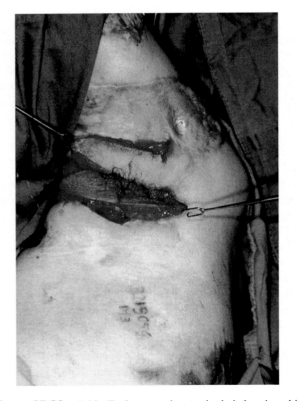

Figure 27.30   A big Z-plasty to elevate the hair-bearing skin flap was performed.

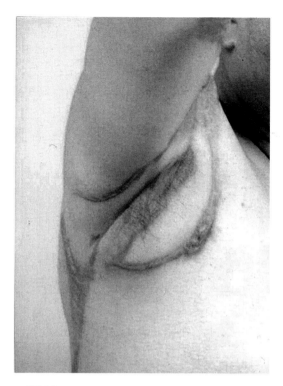

Figure 27.32 Two more years of follow-up showed satisfactory results.

circulation of the entire flap. Artery insufficiency causes the flap to look pale and venous congestion produces a dark-reddish appearance to the flap. Poor function of the drainage system may possibly cause hematoma formation beneath the flap. Postoperative follow-up at the outpatient service and the rehabilitation unit should be arranged for every patient who receives this type of reconstructive surgery.

VII. REHABILITATION ISSUES

It is very important to understand that postoperative rehabilitation after correction of the burned axillary contractures is crucial to achieve the best results. Traditionally, airplane splints have been used after reconstruction (37,38). The airplane splint is used from 5 days to 2 weeks for postoperative immobilization. Following immobilization, using the splint at night is routinely recommended for 3–6 months (39). The figure-of-eight soft brace applied for scapular positioning can also be used for the postgrafted pressure therapy in the axillary region (38,39). The combination of free abduction splinting, use of pressure garments, and adequate physiotherapy is advocated as a satisfactory method for postoperative care after treating axillary burn scar contractures (40).

Because the burn axilla in a child is a difficult area to immobilize during the postgrafted stage, a device, called the "papoose," was designed by Macdonald et al. (41) for this situation. The papoose, which is made of 4 in. thick foam, fixes the child with the arms in 20° horizontal abduction and 90–160° shoulder abduction, according to the patient's needs. This position is maintained by the use of foam axillary wedges and velfoam straps attached to the papoose and secured around the arm, waist, etc. However, the axillary splint is difficult to keep in place and may be uncomfortable for those patients who have some daily activities. A salute splint designed by Abhyankar (42) has the same results as other splints but may be more easy to use and more comfortable for patients. The splint is made of a narrow-width cotton fabric and consists of four straps to help stabilize the arm in abduction during surgery, to place the hand on the forehead while the patient is lying down, and to put the hand on the head while the patient is ambulatory. While splinting is emphasized after the use of skin grafts, exercise of the shoulders should not be neglected. Routine follow-up to receive evaluation and comments from the physical and occupational therapists is very important. When flaps are used, a shorter period of immobilization is required. The decreased incidence of secondary contractures and the greater extensibility of the flap is an advantage over the use of skin grafts.

VIII. LONG-TERM OUTCOMES

Complete release of the scar contracture with postoperative rehabilitation will result in good outcomes even after long-term follow-up in patients who underwent local flap reconstruction for severe axillary contractures (Figs. 27.6, 27.21, and 27.32). Local cutaneous flaps such as Z-plasties are useful for longitudinal scar bands, while fasciocutaneous transposition or island flaps are useful for more extensive scar contractures in the axillary region. From a review of the literature and the evidence-based results in this article, we know why Donelan (43) recommends that it is advantageous to correct axillary contractures by rearranging local tissues as flaps whenever possible (11–29).

REFERENCES

1. Woodburne RT. Essentials of human anatomy. 4th ed. New York: Oxford University Press, 1969:75–86.
2. Grishkevich V. The basic types of scar contractures after burns and methods of eliminating them with trazezplasty flaps. Plast Reconstr Surg 1991; 88:1044–1054.
3. Achauer BM. The axilla. In: Achauer BM, ed. Burn Reconstruction. New York: Thieme Medical Publishers, 1991:87–99.

4. Hallock GG. A systematic approach to flap selection for the axillary burn contracture. J Burn Care Rehabil 1993; 14(3):343–347.

5. Salisbury RE, Bevin AG. The axilla. In: Salisbury RE, Bevin AG, eds. Atlas of Reconstructive Burn Surgery. Philadelphia: W.B. Saunders, 1981:108–111.

6. Huang TT, Blackwell SJ, Lewis SR. Ten years of experience in managing patients with burn contractures of axilla, elbow, wrist, and knee joints. Plast Reconstr Surg 1978; 61:70–76.

7. Moiemen NS, Staiano JS, Ojeh NO, Thway Y, Frame JD. Reconstructive surgery with a dermal template: clinical and histologic study. Plast Reconstr Surg 2001; 108(1):93–103.

8. Chou TD, Chen SL, Lee TW, Chen SG, Cheng TY, Lee CH, Chen TM, Wang HJ. Reconstruction of burn scar of the upper extremities with artificial skin. Plast Reconstr Surg 2001; 108(2):378–385.

9. Hirshowwitz B, Karev A, Levy Y. A 5-flap procedure for axillary webs leaving the apex intact. Br J Plast Surg 1977; 30:48–51.

10. Kurtzman LC, Stern PJ. Upper extremity burn contractures. Hand Clin 1990; 6(2):261–279.

11. Olbrisch RR. Running Y–V plasty. Ann Plast Surg 1991; 26:52–56.

12. Karacaoglan N, Uysal A. Use of seven-flap plasty for the treatment of axillary and groin postburn contractures. Burns 1996; 22(1):69–72.

13. Vaubel E. The V flap. A combination of V–Y advancement and two Limberg transposition flaps. Ann of Plast Surg 1991; 26(1):64–69.

14. Hyakusoku H, Fumiiri M. The square flap method. Br J Plast Surg 1987; 40:40.

15. Tolhurst DE, Haeseker B. Fasciocutaneous flaps in the axillary region. Br J Plast Surg 1982; 35:430.

16. Achauer BM, Spenler CW, Gold ME. Reconstruction of axillary burn contractures with the latissimus dorsi fasciocutaneous flap. J Trauma 1988; 28:211–213.

17. Roberts AHN, Dickson WA. Fasciocutaneous flaps for burn reconstruction: a report of 57 flaps. Br J Plast Surg 1988; 41(2):150–153.

18. Tiwari P, Kalra GS, Bhatnagar SK. Fasciocutaneous flaps for burn contractures of the axilla. Burns 1990; 16(2):150–152.

19. Hallock GG. Regional fasciocutaneous flaps for the burned axilla. J Burn Care Rehabil 1991; 12(3):237–242.

20. Hallock GG, Okunski WJ. The parascapular fasciocutaneous flap for release of the axillary burn contracture. J Burn Care Rehabil 1987; 8:387–390.

21. Elliot D, Kangesu L, Bainbridge C, Venkataramakrishnan V. Reconstruction of the axilla with a posterior arm fasciocutaneous flap. Br J Plast Surg 1992; 45(2):101–104.

22. Budo J, Finucan T, Clarke J. The inner arm fasciocutaneous flap. Plast Reconstr Surg 1984; 73:629–632.

23. Diamond M, Barwick W. Treatment of axillary burn scar contracture using an arterialized scapular island flap. Plast Reconstr Surg 1983; 72:388–390.

24. Teot L, Bosse JP. The use of scapular skin island flaps in the treatment of axillary postburn scar contractures. Br J Plast Surg 1994; 47(2):108–111.

25. Nisanci M, Er E, Isik S, Sengezer M. Treatment modalities for postburn axillary contracures and the versatility of the scapular flap. Burns 2002; 28(2):177–180.

26. Yanai A, Nagata S, Hirabayashi S, Nakamura N. Inverted-U parascapular flap for the treatment of axillary burn scar contracture. Plast Reconstr Surg 1985; 76:126–129.

27. Maruyama Y. Ascending scapular flap and its use for the treatment of axillary burn scar contracture. Br J Plast Surg 1991; 44(2):97–101.

28. Karacalar A, Guner H. The axial bilobed flap for burn contractures of the axiilla. Burns 2000; 26(7):628–633.

29. Kim DY, Cho SY, Kim KS, Lee SY, Cho BH. Correction of axillary burn scar contracture with the thoracodorsal perforator-based cutaneous island flap. Ann Plast Surg 2000; 44(2):181–187.

30. Knowlton EW. Release of axillary scar contracture with a latissimus dorsi flap. Plast Reconstr Surg 1984; 74:124–126.

31. Hallock GG. The triceps muscle flap for axillary contracture release. Ann Plast Surg 1993; 30(4):359–362.

32. Wilson IF, Lokeh A, Schubert W, Benjamin CI. Latissimus dorsi myocutaneous flap reconstruction of neck and axillary burn contractures. Plast Reconstr Surg 2000; 105(1):27–33.

33. Yang JY, Tsai FC, Chana JD. Use of free thin anterolateral thigh flaps combined with cervicoplasty for reconstruction of postburn anterior cervical contractures. Plast Reconstr Surg 2002; 110(1):39–46.

34. Marks MW, Argenta LC, Thornton JW. Burn management: the role of tissue expansion. Clin Plast Surg 1987; 14(3):543–548.

35. Yamamoto Y, Yokoyama T, Minakawa H, Sugihara T. Use of the expanded skin flap in esthetic reconstruction of postburn deformity. J Burn Care Rehabil 1996; 17(5):397–401.

36. Kim DY, Jeong EC, Kim KS, Lee SY, Cho BH. Thinning of the thoracodorsal perforator-based cutaneous flap for axillary burn scar contracture. Plast Reconstr Surg 2002; 109(4):1372–1377.

37. Greenhalgh DG, Gaboury T, Warden GD. The early release of axillary contractures in pediatric patients with burns. J Burn Care Rehabil 1993; 14(1):39–42.

38. Jordan RB, Daher J, Wasil K. Splints and scar management for acute and reconstructive burn care. Clin Plast Surg 2000; 27(1):71–85.

39. Leman CJ. Splints and accessories following burn reconstruction. Clin Plast Surg 1992; 19(3):721–731.

40. Whitaker J, Lamberty Ma BGH. Pressure garments in the treatment of axillary burns contracture. Physiotherapy 1981; 67(1):5–7.

41. Macdonald LB, Covey MH, Marvin JA et al. The papoose: device for positioning the burn child's axilla. J Burn Care Rehabil 1985; 6(1):62–63.

42. Abhyankar SV. The salute splint for axillary contractures. Br J Plast Surg 2001; 54(3):213–215.

43. Donelan NB. Reconstruction of the burned hand and upper extremity. In: McCarthy JG, ed. Plastic Surgery. Philadelphia: W.B. Saunders, 1990:5452.

28

Reconstruction of the Burned Breast and Nipple–Areolar Complex

ROBERT L. McCAULEY, GARRY W. KILLYON
University of Texas Medical Branch and Shriners Hospital for Children—Galveston Unit, Galveston, Texas, USA

KANIKA BOWEN
University of Texas Medical Branch School of Medicine, Galveston, Texas, USA

I. INTRODUCTION

Thermal injuries to the anterior chest wall can have severe psychological impact because of scarring and contractures. In adult female patients, such injuries, which can be severe in nature, can lead to severe distortion of the involved breasts. In children, breast development becomes an important issue. Thus, deformities related to scar contractures in the developing breast can be significant and surgical intervention may be necessary. In the prepubescent female, the management of the burn injury during the acute phase of treatment is of paramount importance. Previous studies have documented development of breasts in female adolescent patients even in the absence of the nipple–areola complex (NAC) (1). Needless to say, these patients underwent conservative management of their initial injuries after demarcation of eschar with tangential excision of burns on the anterior chest wall or blunt eschar separation (eplúchage) with subsequent coverage with a split-thickness skin graft. In both types of treatment, preservation of the underlying breast bud was of primary concern. In a review of 28 patients treated in such a fashion, McCauley et al. (1) showed that all patients subsequently developed breasts. To date, numerous studies have documented the psychological impact of thermal injuries and their subsequent deformities in burn patients (2–5). These problems very well may be accentuated in female patients with such injuries who develop significant breast deformities. As reconstructive surgeons, our goal is to transform, as much as possible, significant breast deformities to the ideal breast shape that is desired within our society.

II. INCIDENCE

In recent years, patients have continued to survive increasingly large total body surface area burns. In general, this increased survival has been attributed to better resuscitation, control of burn wound sepsis, improved support of the hypermetabolic response and early closure of the burn wound. Burvin et al. (3) evaluated 421 female patients admitted to their institution over a 3-year period, focusing on female patients with breast burns. Of the 138 female burn patients identified, only 9% had nonisolated breast burns. Although the overall total body surface area burn was not identified, 66% of the breast burns were secondary to scald injuries (6). In 1989, Brou et al. (7) evaluated 25 patients with a mean total body surface area burn of 71%. In this series of patients, 512 reconstructive problems were identified. In the trunk and perineal regions, 70 problems were identified. In 1993, Burns et al. (8) analyzed reconstruction issues associated with 28 patients who survived burns of at least 80% of the total body surface area. In this series, 564 reconstructive problems were noted. In each series, ∼20 reconstructive problems identified per patient. In the series by Burns et al. (8), the trunk was the most frequently injured area in the torso/lower extremity section. Interestingly enough, the trunk

was only second to the hand with respect to the most frequently injured anatomic section. In addition, the breasts were the most frequently injured region within the truncal/perineal region. McCauley et al. (1) noted that subsequent analysis of the donor sites usually revealed that the tissue available for reconstruction was usually less than optimal. Without question, these issues are of significant concern since it has been recognized that 71% of female patients with burns to the anterior chest wall with involvement of the NAC will require surgical intervention to assist with breast development (1) (Figs. 28.1 and 28.2).

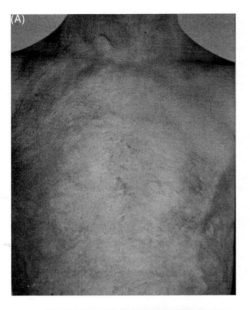

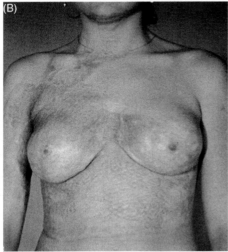

Figure 28.2 (A) An 8-year-old girl, 1-year after a 30% total body surface area burn involving both nipple–areolar complex after constructive debridement and coverage with split-thickness skin grafts. (B) Ten-year follow-up, breast development after additional release using split thickness skin grafts. [Reprinted with permission from McCauley et al. (1).]

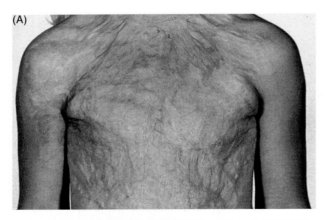

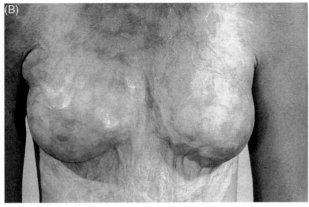

Figure 28.1 (A) A 5-year-old girl after conservative debridement of burns to the anterior chest wall involving both nipple–areolar complex: subsequent split-thickness skin grafts placed over the chest wall. (B) Breast development noted in teenage years.

III. ACUTE MANAGEMENT OF BURNS TO THE ANTERIOR CHEST WALL

Early tangential excision of burns to the anterior chest wall is currently the standard of care in the management of burn patients. Numerous studies have documented both a significant decreases in morbidity and length of hospital stay when compared to the more conservative approach of delayed eschar separation (9,10). However, this approach is modified at many burn centers when dealing with anterior chest wall burns in young female patients (1,6,11,12). In such cases, the eschar may be allowed to demarcate and separate prior to tangential excision. MacLennon et al. (11) even suggested marking the areas of the breast bud prior to surgical intervention in order to avoid destruction during debridement. Several investigations have previously shown that even with the destruction of the NAC, the breast bud may be uninjured (1,11). In prepubescent females, since the majority of burns to the anterior chest wall are scald injuries, it is believed that the subcutaneous tissue is still quite viable (6,13). This is significant since the mammary gland in children is believed to be 4–8 mm located in the subcutis. It is believed to be attached to the overlying nipple by the epithelium of the parsinfundibularis of the milk ducts (13).

Clearly, when deep thermal injures to the anterior chest wall occur, removal of the nonviable issues is important. Flame or electrical injuries may necessitate excision deep into the subcutaneous tissues or even to fascia. Burn wound sepsis may also necessitate deep excision of subcutaneous tissues. In such instances, fascial excision may be the minimal operation necessary to either remove all nonviable issue or to treat burn wound sepsis. Unfortunately, if the underlying breast bud is involved in the excised specimen, these patients will not develop breasts. Should this occur, a difficult problem now exists with respect to breast reconstruction.

IV. RECONSTRUCTION OF THE BURNED BREASTS

Reconstruction of the burned breasts encompasses a variety of techniques (14–21,43). Most reconstructive surgeons view this issue in two parts: reconstruction of the breast mound and reconstruction of the NAC. Choosing the best option available is dependent upon the age at which the patient sustained injury, the type of injury and the extent of surgical management during the acute phase of treatment. Obvious restriction in the breast development as a result of scar contracture has been the classic indicator for surgical intervention. However, the timing for such intervention varies with each patient. McCauley et al. (1) in a review of 28 patients with burns to the anterior chest wall with involvement of the NAC, 71% of these patients required surgical intervention to assist with breast development.

Traditional methods of breast reconstruction after mastectomy for breast cancer may not be an option in these young girls during their developmental years. Often, areas of significant burn injury and lack of tissue bulk may preclude the use of the transverse rectus abdominus myocutaneous (TRAM) flap as a method for reconstruction. The need for bilateral breast reconstruction in many of these patients further complicates the issue. The use of the latissimus dorsi myocutaneous flap, is an option and has been utilized by a number of surgeons (11,12,17). Some success has been achieved with the use of tissue expansion and subsequent placement of submuscular breast implants. Because of significant scarring in the inframammary region in many of these patients, the transaxillary approach may be the best operative approach.

The burned male breast represents a challenge due to a decrease in subcutaneous tissue and lack of desirable outcomes for those who undergo reconstruction of the NAC. Most male patients opt not to undergo aesthetic breast and NAC construction, thus making the opportunity to reconstruct the male breast rare (23). Literature on the subject of male breast and NAC reconstruction is limited and significant data are not available. The initial surgical reconstruction of the burned male breast centers on scar excision and contracture release by multiple W-plasty and Z-plasties (24). The male NAC can either be reconstructed using a full-thickness graft from non-hair-bearing scrotal skin or from full-thickness skin grafts from the thigh. Tattooing of the areola should be adequate to define the areola (23). If attempting to raise the nipple, stacked cartilage grafts can be placed beneath the areolar graft (11). Although many men opt to forego aesthetic treatment for breast and NAC reconstruction, the option should be made available.

A. Reconstruction of the Burned Breast Mound

In patients with anterior chest wall burns, the goal is to allow breast development to proceed in an unimpeded fashion. In patients with unilateral breast burns, scar contractures can be detected quite early as the uninjured breast clearly serves as a landmark for distortions in shape or displacement of the NAC. A number of factors are assessed preoperatively to best determine the type of reconstruction required in these patients. The extent of the deformity, the location of the deformity and status of the surrounding soft tissue are all assessed prior to embarking on any surgical plan. Extensive deformities over the breast mound itself is approached quite differently than deformities in the inframammary region alone. The incision or excision of

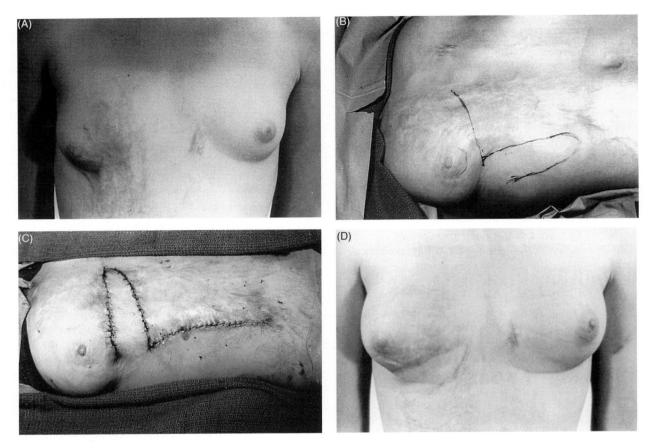

Figure 28.3   (A) A 13-year-old girl with early breast development and entrapment of right breast in burn scar with inferior displacement. (B) Proposed outline of a fasciocutaneous flap along with proposed incised release. (C) Transposition flap with place. (D) One-year follow-up.

scars over the breast mound itself is carried out to improve breast contour. If the deformity is minimal and located in the inframammary region the use of local fasciocutaneous flaps are an option (Fig. 28.3). However, extensive burns over the breast mound may require excisional release and resurfacing with thick (15–20 times one-thousandths of an inch) split-thickness skin grafts (Fig. 28.4). In some cases of bilateral breast entrapment, an inverted

T incision is required to separate the developing breasts and relax the scar tissue over the breast mound.

1.   Bilateral Breast Burns: Amastia

As previously stated, patients who have sustained injuries to the underlying breast bud will not develop breasts. During the adolescent years, this becomes a significant

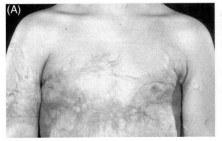
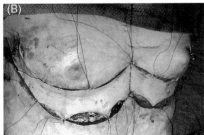
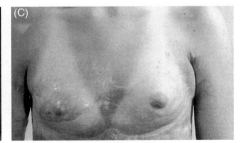

Figure 28.4   (A) 6-year-old girl after recovery of anterior chest wall burns treated with conservative debridement and coverage with skin grafts. (B) Six years later with breast development, patient required bilateral inframammary releases and coverage with skin grafts. (C) Symmetric breast development noted 2 years later.

issue to young girls. The use of the TRAM flap for reconstruction may not be an option because of the lack of tissue bulk. The latissimus dorsi myocutaneous flap is an option with implant placement. The author's approach has been to release the scar contractures using thick split-thickness skin grafts with an inverted T incision. Once the new grafts have matured, a transaxillary approach is then used for placement of submuscular tissue expanders. Once expansion is completed, the expanders are removed and breast implants are then inserted using the transaxillary approach. The use of the transaxillary incision avoids problems which may develop with wound healing if the inframammary approach is undertaken (Figs. 28.5 and 28.6).

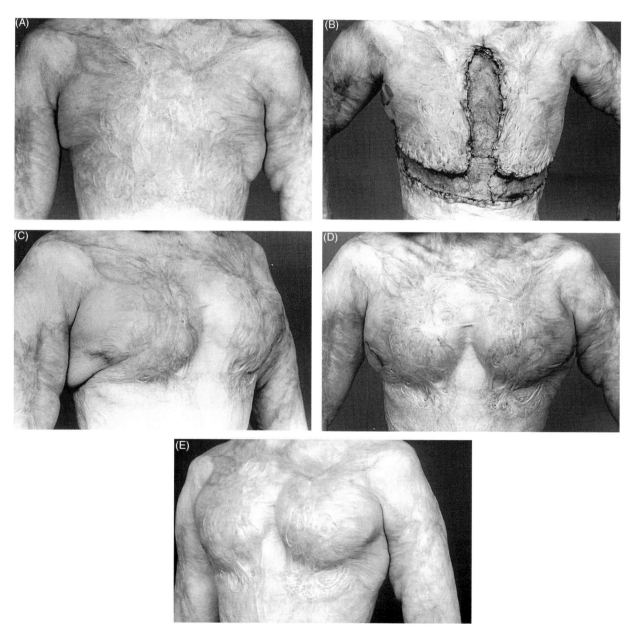

Figure 28.5 (A) A 15-year old patient who survived a 60% total body surface area burn but necessitated fascial excision of deep burns over anterior chest wall. Note lack of breast development. (B) Inverted "T" incision performed to release chest contractures. (C) Trans axillary approach used for insertion of tissue expanders (200 cc expanders). Expanders placed under poctoral muscle and over inflated six months after inverted "T" release of anterior chest wall tightness. (D) Final appearance after removal of expanders, insertion of saline implants and bilateral revision of lateral redundant tissue over the breasts. (E) Right oblique view.

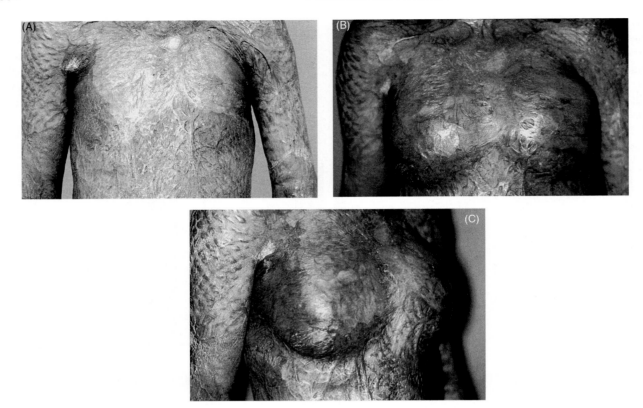

Figure 28.6   (A) A 14-year-old girl with fascial excision over anterior chest wall and resurfacing of the defect with meshed skin grafts. (B) Final appearance after placement of tissue expanders using the trans axillary approach and replacement with saline implants. (C) Left lateral view showing projection of implants for breast enhancement.

The use of tissue expansion and placement of an implant is employed in reconstruction of the burned breast when it is believed that there is adequate skin to result in primary coverage of the prosthesis after placement. Becker (25) introduced the permanent breast expander implant in 1984. Tissue expanders are placed in the subglandular or submuscular plane and are expanded incrementally until the desired growth is obtained (16).

In burned patients, who have undergone fascial excisions, placement in the submuscular plane is the only option. Some authors have recommended that reconstruction be delayed several months to allow for scar softening to take place (15). Afterwards, the expander can be temporarily deflated to assess tissue laxity (18,26). At this point, insertion with a subpectoral breast implant proportional in volume to the tissue expander provides a

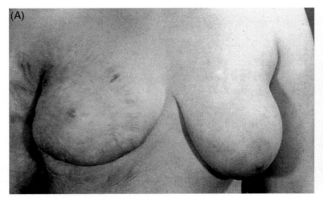

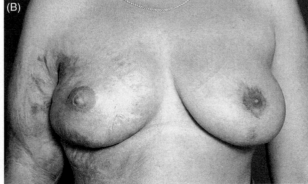

Figure 28.7   (A) A 17-year-old female with burns to the right breast. Previously, skin grafts were used to assist breast development. Now patient complains of breast asymmetry because of the larger more ptotic left breast. (B) Six months postoperative appearance after reconstruction of the right areola with a full-thickness skin graft from the inner thigh and a left-sided mastopexy.

breast mound that is not under tension. Some common complications that are seen with the use of tissue expander and implants include exposure of the injection port, infections, spontaneous deflation, and capsule formation (26).

2. Bilateral Breast Burns: Mammary Hyperplasia

Although uncommon, mammary hyperplasia can occur in the postburn breast (27). This condition may occur unilaterally in which a reduction mammoplasty may be required

for breast symmetry (Figs. 28.7 and 28.8). Alternately, bilateral reduction mammoplasties may be required if both breasts are hyperplastic. Thai et al. (27) have established certain principles in the management of such patients. First, the release of all contractures prior to embarking upon a procedure which reduces breast volume is recommended. Second, reduction mammoplasty using the inferior pedicle technique is quite safe in these patients. In their series, six patients (10 breasts) underwent removal of 454 g of tissue per breast without major

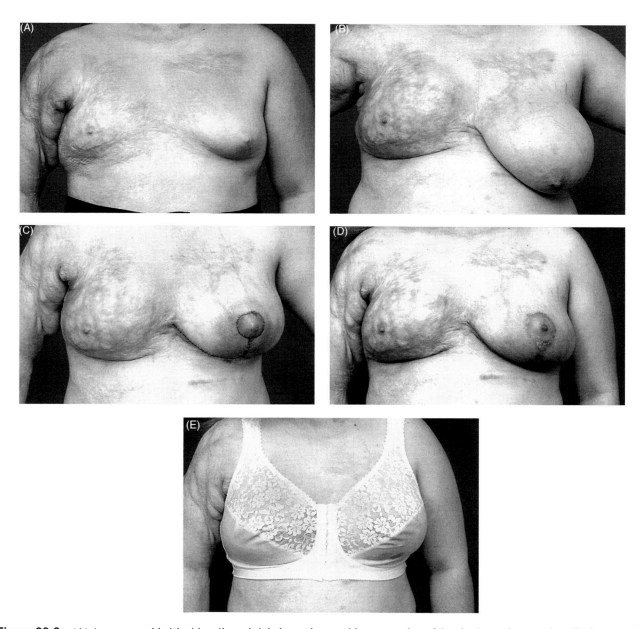

Figure 28.8   (A) A ten-year-old girl with unilateral right breast burns with preservation of the nipple areolar complex. (B) Same patient at age 17 with unilateral macromastia on the left. Note normal breast shape without ptosis on the right side. (C) Postoperative appearance after left unilateral reduction mammaplasty. (D) Four-month follow-up. (E) Patient is satisfied with results being able to wear a brassiere for adequate support for both breasts.

complications noted. It is important to note that only patients with split-thickness skin grafts over the breasts were included in this series. El-Khatib (28) also confirmed the safety and reliability of the inferior pedicle technique in postburn breast reduction (28).

3. Unilateral Breast Burn

The Hypoplastic Burned Breast

Correction of the hypoplastic breast is challenging. When burn injury is involved, reconstruction becomes increasingly difficult. In burn patients, it is unclear as to whether the event would have occurred without injury or if it happened because of partial loss of the breast bud. Reconstruction of the hypoplastic breast, ideally, is undertaken at the time of complete breast development. Tissue expanders, implants, and myocutaneous flaps have been used to augment the hypoplastic breast (Fig. 28.9). Correction of this defect is important in maintaining a symmetrical appearance of the reconstructed breast mound. The TRAM flap and the latissimus dorsi flap has been used in the reconstruction of the hypoplastic breast. When

tissue expansion with subsequent placement of an implant is the treatment plan, a period of over expansion is advised not only to achieve a more naturally appearing breast, but to also possibly reduce capsular contracture (29–32). Subsequent reduction mammoplasty of the uninvolved breast may be required to achieve symmetry.

Mastopexy/Reduction Mammoplasty

Symmetry of the burned breast is desired and should be the driving force behind breast reconstruction. Correction of asymmetry is complicated and must address skin contractures, nipple dystopia and volume asymmetry (33). The most difficult technical problem has been that of achieving volumetric and geometric equality (34). Assessment of proper volume status between the two breasts can be closely approximated perioperatively, but geometric equality will change over time.

In patients with unilateral breast burns, the uninjured breast serves as a guide for shape and symmetry. Unfortunately, in some patients achieving breast symmetry may be challenging. Occasionally, even as breast development proceeds with the injured breast, its subsequent development

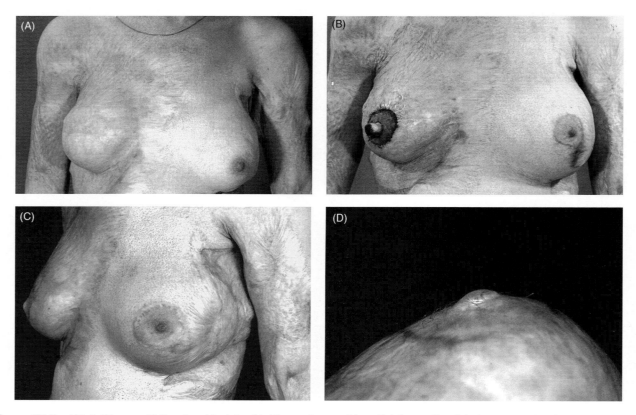

Figure 28.9 (A) A 17-year-old female with right-sided breast burns with a slightly smaller right breast noted. Skin grafts were used in the past to assist right-sided breast development. (B) Left pericresant mastopexy performed to lift the nipple–areolar complex with right-sided augmentation. The right nipple areolar complex reconstructed with a skate flap and inner thigh full-thickness skin graft. (C) Two-year follow-up. (D) Note projection still of the skate flap.

may still pose a problem with respect to shape and size when compared to the normal breast. The choices of reduction mammoplasty or a mastopexy on the uninjured breast vs. augmentation of the injured breast depends on the extent of the asymmetry and the patient's desires (Fig. 28.10). Sometimes different procedures may be required on each breast to achieve symmetry.

4. Unilateral Breast Burn: Breast Ptosis

Burns to the breast even after extensive releases with skin grafts maintain a very strong outer envelop for breast support. Thai et al. (27) noted that the thick inelasticity of skin grafts creates a sling that does not become ptotic with age. In patients with unilateral breast burns, over time, the contralateral uninjured breast may become ptotic when compared to the reconstructed burned breast (Fig. 28.10). In cases where at least a grade II ptosis is present, a mastopexy of the uninjured breast may be necessary. This procedure not only improves breast symmetry but also improves superior pole fullness.

B. Reconstruction of the Nipple – Areola Complex

Reconstruction of the NAC constitutes the second stage of breast reconstruction. The literature has numerous articles to address this issue (35–39). The NAC reconstruction is often delayed until the reconstructed breast mound has had time for scars to mature. This may be 9–12 months after breast mound reconstruction. In general, reconstruction of the NAC is undertaken when the breasts have fully developed. In the reconstructed breast, several problems may exist: malpositioning of the NAC and partial or total absence of the NAC. In cases of malpositioning of the NAC in the burned breast, Mohmand and Nassan (35) suggested the use of two double U-plasty for correction. This technique is quite similar to a Z-plasty in which the NAC is transposed inferiorly or superiorly to match the contralateral unburned breast (Fig. 28.11). Of course, the technique can only be performed in patients with no evidence of breast contraction and in patients in which there is minimal displacement of the NAC.

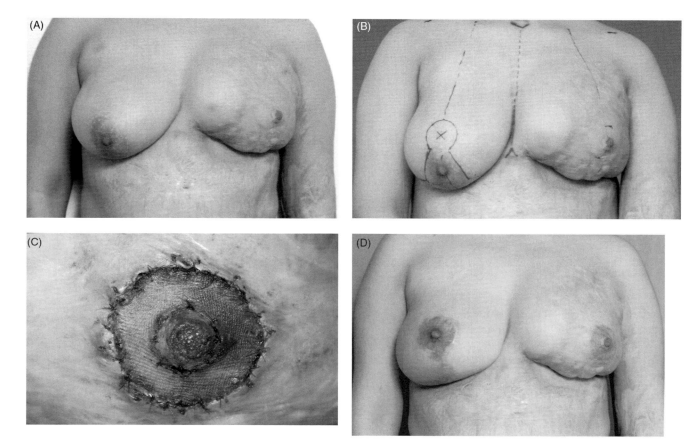

Figure 28.10 (A) A 19-year-old woman complaining of breast asymmetry. Note left-sided breast burn with preservation of the nipple but loss of the areola. Grade III ptosis noted on right side. (B) Outline for proposed right-sided mastopexy and reconstruction of the left areola. (C) Inner thigh full-thickness skin graft used for the left areolar at time of right-sided mastopexy. (D)Final results at 6 months.

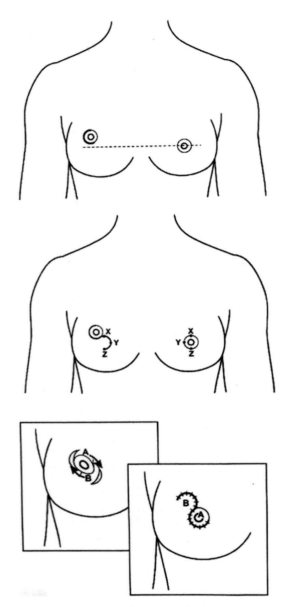

Figure 28.11   Diagram of the double V plasty. [Reprinted with permission from, Mohmand and Nassan A. (35).]

Reportedly, there is minimal interference with the sensation of the NAC with this technique.

In situations where the nipple is present but the areola is partially or totally lost treatment alternatives differ. Partial loss of the areola can be addressed with tattooing of the region to blend in with the color of the remaining areola. In situations where the entire areola is lost, tattooing of the areola or resurfacing with full-thickness skin grafts are useful. The upper inner thigh as a donor site produces excellent contrast with the surrounding tissues in this situation (38). In unilateral breast burns, the technique utilized may be guided by the color match of the unaffected side.

However, in bilateral breast burns with areola loss, either technique provides acceptable results.

Total loss of the NAC presents a difficult problem in the burned patient. Although numerous techniques are available, their role in the reconstruction of the burned breast has yet to be fully evaluated (35–37). In the absence of the native NAC, a nipple can be constructed from numerous composite graft donors, including toe pulp, postauricular cartilage and skin, or the opposite nipple (11). The use of labial skin to reconstruct the NAC has been replaced with more current procedures. Reconstruction of the NAC using auricular skin and cartilage can be used in patients where nipple sharing is not an option and yields fair to good results (40). The conchal cartilage is used to simulate Montgomery glands. Free toe pulp grafts as well as composite grafts taken from the second to fourth toe has been utilized in NAC reconstruction. Pensler et al. (36) reviewed different results of various techniques in reconstructing the burned NAD. They recommended the use of full-thickness skin grafts from the superomedial thigh for reconstruction of the areola. This group also

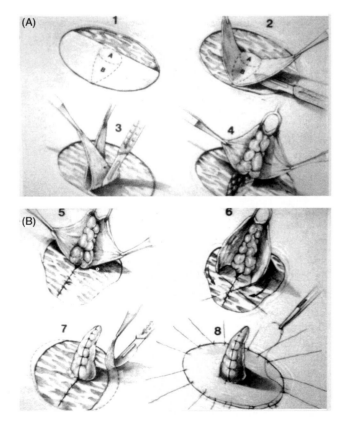

Figure 28.12   (A) Design of the skate flap as described by Little with elevation of the pedide. (B)Design of the skate flap as described by Little with reconstruction of the areolar and coverage with a full thickness skin graft. [(Reprinted with permission from, Little (41).]

recommended the use of the quadrapod flap for nipple reconstruction if there is adequate surrounding dermis (36). This technique appeared to be superior to the composite grafts and the "double-bubble" technique over a 1-year period. Several authors have been skeptical with respect to the use of skin flaps in reconstruction of the NAC (11). Since these flaps require normal dermal elements and subcutaneous tissue to maintain viability to the skin, it was felt that the role of skin flaps in the reconstruction of the NAC in the burned patient was limited. In 1984, Little described

the "skate" flap for NAC reconstruction (Fig. 28.12) (41). Its use in reconstruction of burn patients has received little attention. However, McCauley and Robson (42) reported the successful use of the "skate" flap in reconstruction of the nipple in the burned breast (Fig. 28.13). This finding clearly demonstrates the re-establishment of an adequate subdermal plexus in burned patients after resurfacing with skin grafts. Virtually all techniques that involve the projection of a nipple will succumb to some degree of flattening. Several factors have been cited for this

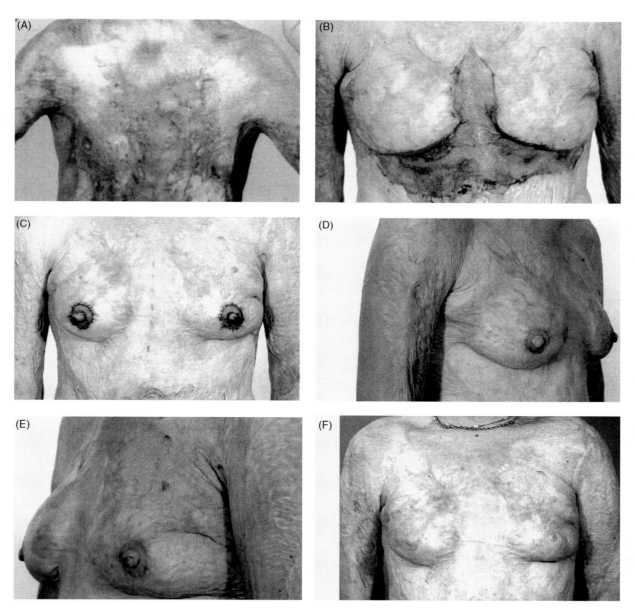

Figure 28.13 (A) A 20-year-old girl with immature scars with open drainage over the anterior chest wall: patient was treated conservatively. The nipple–areolar complex was absent bilaterally. (B) After wound maturation of an inverted "T" incision was performed to assist breast development. (C) Three years later, bilateral "skate" flaps were utilized to create the nipple. (D and E) Excellent projection noted at 4 months. (F) Seven-month follow-up: patient still has projection of the nipples, but loss of contrast around the areola.

phenomenon including surface tension of skin, lack of normal infrastructure, and centrifugal forces (26,29,30).

V. CONCLUSION

Reconstruction of the burned breast encompasses a number of complex issues. Management of such burns in prepubescent females during the acute phase of injury is extremely important in determining the need and ultimate outcome of subsequent reconstructive procedures. The use of skin grafts and/or fasciocutaneous flaps to assist breast development and prevent deformities is crucial. The use of tissue expansion and breast implants play an important role in the reconstruction of patients with significant breast asymmetry or in patients who do not develop breasts because of fascial excision. Problems associated with breast asymmetry may require augmentation or even a reduction mammaplasty depending on the extent of the deformity and patient's desires. Clearly, the literature demonstrates the reliability and safety of these procedures in the burned breast. Macromastia of the burned breasts is also safely addressed with reduction mammoplasties. The NAC requires multiple procedures to complete the reconstructive efforts. Intradermal tattooing of the areola or the use of full-thickness skin grafts provide acceptable results. The successful use of the "skate" flap in reconstruction of the nipple is the authors' preferred method. It is reliable and safe.

Regardless of the type of reconstructive procedure utilized in the burned breast, the goal of the reconstructive surgeon is to provide symmetric breasts which should be as aesthetically pleasing as possible. Such efforts are rewarded as we come closer to the reintegration of burned patients into our society with positive self-images.

REFERENCES

1. McCauley RL, Beraja V, Rutan RL, Huang TT, Abston S, Rutan TC, Robson MC. Longitudinal assessment of breast development in adolescent female patients with burns involving the nipple–areolar complex. Plast Reconstr Surg 1989; 83(4):676–680.
2. Cahners SS. Young women with breast burns: a self-help "Group by Mail". J Burn Care Rehabil 1992; 13:44–47.
3. Burvin R, Robinpour M, Milo Y, Tamir G, Wolf Y, Hauben DJ. Female breast burns: conservative treatment with a reconstructive aim. Israel J Med Sci 1996; 12:1207–1301.
4. Bernstein N. Emotional Care of the Facially Burned and Disfigured. Boston, MA: Little, Brown and Co., 1976.
5. Stoddard FJ. Body image development in burned children. J Am Acad Child Adolesc Psychiatry 1982; 21:502.
6. Watson EJ, Johnson AM. The emotional significance of acquired physical disfiguration in children. Am J Orthopsychiatry 1958; 28:85.
7. Brou JA, Robson MC, McCauley RL, Herndon DN, Phillips LG, Ortega M, Evans EB, Alvardo MI. Inventory of potential reconstructive needs in the patient with burns. J Burn Care Rehabil 1989; 10(6):555–560.
8. Burns BF, McCauley RL, Murphy FL, Robson, MC. Reconstructive management of patients with greater than 80 per cent TBSA burns. Burns 1993; 19(5):429–433.
9. Herndon DN, Barrow RE, Retan RL, Rutan TC, Desai, MH, Abston, S. A comparison of conservative versus early excisional therapies in severely burned patients. Ann Surg 1989; 209(5):547–553.
10. Herndon DN, Parks DH. Comparison of serial debridement and autografting and early massive excision with cadaveric overlay in the treatment of large burns in children. J Trauma 1986; 26:149–152.
11. MacLennon SE, Wells MD, Neale HW. Reconstruction of the burned breast. Clin Plast Surg 2000; 27(1):113–119.
12. Al-Qattan MM, Zuker RM. Management of acute burns of the female pediatric breast: delayed tangential excision versus spontaneous eschar separation. Ann Plast Surg 1994; 33:66–67.
13. Kunert P, Schneider W, Flory J. Principles and procedures in female breast reconstruction in the young child's burn injury. Aesth Plast Surg 1988; 12:101–106.
14. Guan W, Jin Y, Cao H. Reconstruction of post-burn female breast deformity. Ann Plast Surg 1988; 21(1):65–69.
15. Pakhomov SM, Dmitriev GI. Scar deformities of the mammary glands—surgical treatment. Acta Chir Plast 1984; 26(3):150–157.
16. Versaci AD, Balkovich ME, Goldstein SA. Breast reconstruction by tissue expansion for congenital and burn deformities. Ann Plast Surg 1986; 16(1):20–30.
17. Kalender V, Aydim H, Karabulut AB, Özcan M, Amiraslanov A. Breast reconstruction with the internal mammary artery pedicle fasciocutaneous island flap: description of a new flap. Plast Reconstr Surg 2000; 106(7):1494–1498
18. McCauley R. Reconstruction of the trunk and genitalia. In: Herndon DN, ed. Total Burn Care. Philadelphia, PA: Elsevier Ltd., 2001:707–709.
19. Ozgur F, Gokalan I, Mavili E, Erk Y, Kecik A. Reconstruction of post-burn breast deformities. Burns 1992; 18(6):504–509.
20. Psillakis JM, Woisky R. Burned breasts: treatment with a transverse rectus abdominis island musculocutaneous flap. Ann Plast Surg 1985; 14(5):437–442.
21. Slator RC, Phil D, Wilson GR, Sharpe DT. Post-burn breast reconstruction: tissue expansion prior to contracture release. Plast Reconstr Surg 1992; 90(4):668–674.
22. Bishop JB, Fisher J, Bostwick J. III The burned female breast. Ann Plast Surg 1980; 4(1):25–30.
23. Spence RJ. Bilateral reconstruction of the male nipple. Ann Plast Curg 1992; 28:288–291.
24. Lewis JR. Reconstruction of the breasts. Surg Clin of North Am 1971; 51:429–440.

25. Becker H. Breast reconstruction using an inflatable breast implant with detectable reservoir. Plast Reconstr Surg 1984; 73:678–683.

26. Loss M, Infanger M, Kunzi W. The burned female breast: a report of 4 cases. Burns 2002; 28:601–605.

27. Thai KN, Mertens D, Warden G, Neale HW. Reduction mammaplasty in postburn breasts. Plast Reconstr Surg 1999; 103(7):1882–1886.

28. El-Khatib HA. Reliability of inferior pedicle reduction mammaplasty in burned oversized breasts. Plast Reconstr Surg 1999; 103(3):869–873.

29. Kneafsey B, Crawford DS, Khoo CTK, Saad NM. Correction of developmental breast abnormalities with a permanent expander/implant. Br J Plast Surg 1996; 49:302–306.

30. Becker H. The permanent tissue expander. Clin Plast Surg 1987; 14:519–527.

31. Becker H. Expansion augmentation. Clin Plast Surg 1988; 15:587–593.

32. Persoff MM. Expansion-augmentation of the breast. Plast Reconstr Surg 1993; 91:393–403.

33. Payne CE, Malata CM. Correction of post-burn deformity using the Lejour mammoplasty technique. Plast Reconstr Surg 2003; 111:805–809.

34. Corso PF. Plastic surgery for the unilateral hypoplastic breast. Plast Reconstr Surg 1972; 50:134–141.

35. Mohmand H, Nassan A. Double U-plasty for correction of geometric malposition of the nipple–areola complex. Plast Reconstr Surg 2002; 109(6):2019–2022.

36. Pensler JM, Haab RL, Perry SW. Reconstruction of the burned nipple–areola complex. Plast Reconstr Surg 1986; 78(4):480–485.

37. Adams WM. Labial transplant for correction of loss of the nipple. Plast Reconstr Surg 1979; 4: 295–298

38. Broadbent PR, Woolf RH, Metz PS. Restoring the mammary areola by a skin graft from the upper inner thigh. Br J Plast Surg 1977; 30:220–222.

39. Becker H. Nipple–areola tattooing using intradermal tattooing. Plast Reconstr Surg 1988; 81:450.

40. Brent B, Bostwick J. Nipple–areolar reconstruction with auricular tissues. Plast Reconstr Surg 1977; 60: 353–361.

41. Little JW. Nipple–areolar reconstruction. Clin Plast Surg 1984; 11:351–364.

42. McCauley RL, Robson MC. Reconstruction of the nipple–areola complex in the burned breast using the 'skate' flap. Proc Am Burn Assoc 1994; 26:14.

43. Neale HW, Smith GL, Gregory RO, MacMillan BG. Breast reconstruction in the burned adolescent female (an 11-year, 157-patient experience). Plast Reconstr Surg 1982; 70(6):718–724.

29

Reconstruction of Chest Contractures

JUI-YUNG YANG

Chang Gung Memorial Hospital, Taipei, Taiwan

I. INTRODUCTION

Burn injuries of the chest are not uncommon. Flame burns with ignition of clothes, scald burn due to pouring hot water over upper trunk, chemical burns with direct or indirect involvement of the chest; friction burns or electrical injuries to the chest can frequently produce deformities of the chest. Sometimes, the electrical burn involves deeper tissue injuries than others (1,2). However, no matter what kind of injury is involved, the most serious complications may occur in the female chest (3).

The significance of breast development to women is not only for nursing but also a symbol of sexuality. It could be a disaster when the breast is destroyed in any accident including burns. Thus both functional restoration and aesthetic reconstruction should be taken into consideration during correction of burn breast deformities. In this chapter, the literature about burn breast reconstruction is reviewed. The principles of conservative debridement in the acute stage and complete scar release in late stage along with nipple areolar complex (NAC) reconstruction and proper choice of replacement tissue are still valid for burn breast reconstruction. Free flaps including trimmed perforator flap reconstruction is also discussed.

II. PREOPERATIVE EVALUATION

In the acute stage, the depth of the injury should be carefully evaluated. Possible involvement of the ribs should be kept in mind in deep burns especially in electrical burns. The choice of reconstruction procedure is related to the extent and depth of injures. Involvement of NAC in burn injury should also be assessed.

In the delay reconstructive stage, any possibility of developmental limitation is usually a high priority. Extensive chest scar contractures may result in kyphosis. The scars in the pediatric female breast can possibly cause hypoplasia or even aplasia of the breasts. The status of NAC should be cited in the chart. The breast deformities may be classified into several groups including: 1—caudal contracture, which might results in marked asymmetry and restriction of breast contour; 2—lateral contracture, which causes displacement of the breast; 3—loss of breast volume and destruction of the NAC, which usually is due to direct burn injury to the breast; and 4—NAC deformities, either distorted or completely destroyed (4). The classification may be simplified as: (1) adjacent scar contracture, which causes a disfigured breast; (2) volume decrease with or without NAC destruction; and (3) isolated

393

NAC destruction. The preoperative evaluation of the relationship between breast deformities and surrounding available healthy tissues is very important for decision-making about the reconstructive timing and procedure.

III. SURGICAL OPTIONS

In the acute stage every effort should be made to preserve the breast tissues. Skin grafts after spontaneous eschar separation or after delayed tangential excision when wound demarcation is clear for the burns of the female pediatric breast makes no difference in later breast development (5). In spite of the significant thermal injury to the anterior chest wall with involvement of the NAC, no patient failed to develop breasts. This is a finding of McCauley et al. (6) in 28 patients with long-term follow-up of 15 patients. Initial conservative treatment with preservation of breast buds for burned female children is recommended. By recognizing that the breasts are specialized structures and that burns to the breast, especially if lactating, delayed tangential excision and cessation of lactation by using bromocriptine were suggested to achieve successful reconstruction (7). Thus, conservative management of the acutely burn breast in children, especially girls, to preserve breast buds is the first choice of surgical options (8,9).

Deep thermal burns involving chest and/or breasts may be reconstructed with conservative debridement and skin grafts. However, a full-thickness chest wall defect following high-voltage electrical injury requires prompt, secure, and stable repair. Immediate reconstruction with flaps such as latissimus dorsi myocutaneous flap is better than skin graft after granulations appeared (10). If the defect is located at the upper chest accompanied by costal bone exposure, the cervicohumeral flap has been described for reconstruction. It can be raised undelayed with a length-to-width ratio of 2:1 or 3:1 and transposed to cover the anterosuperior chest wall (11). Sometimes costal bones or cartilages involved in deep burns should be aggressively excised to ensure subsequent reconstruction successful (12). Reconstruction of a full-thickness defect of the chest wall caused by friction burn using a combined myocutaneous flap of teres major and latissimus dorsi muscle has been reported (13).

In the late stages the goals of reconstruction are aimed at complete release of contractures to prevent or to correct the deformities especially the female chest. Complete release of the scar contracture by means of scar revisions with Z- or VY-plasty, proper replacement of tissue defects utilizing skin grafts, local flaps (i.e., square flaps and slide-swing plasty, fasciocutaneous flaps, myocutaneous flaps), tissue expansion, free flaps, or combined utilization of these methods are advocated by some authors

(3,8,9,14–29). Some methods of NAC reconstruction are also proposed (30–35). All the aforementioned methods are reasonable to achieve the goals of both functional and aesthetic reconstruction for burn breast deformities (36–39). The surgical options and clinical examples are noted in the following text.

Case 1: This case involves a young girl with multiple burn scars in her chest and abdomen with caudal contracture of the left breast (Fig. 29.1). Excision of scars and reconstruction with a Limberg flap from the abdomen and V-Y plasty for the left breast were performed to correct all contractures (Fig. 29.2). Seven years later the breast started to develop without any contracture (Figs. 29.3 and 29.4).

Case 2: This deals with a lateral burn scar contracture of the breast, which resulted in lateral deviation of the NAC (Fig. 29.5). The deformity was corrected by scar excision and a V-Y advancement flap (Fig. 29.6).

Case 3: This case relates to a 5-year-old girl who sustained a third degree flame burn over the entire chest–abdomen with destruction of the NAC (Fig. 29.7). In the acute stage, every effort was made to preserve the breast buds. The breast areas were the first priority for sheet skin graft (Fig. 29.8). Seven years later at adolescent age, the development of the breasts was restricted by scar contracture around the chest (Fig. 29.9). Complete release of scar contracture was achieved by means of multiple Z-plasties and scar revisions (Fig. 29.10). A 4-year follow-up of the patient showed good development of both breasts with acceptable symmetry. A comparison can be made between pre- and postoperative appearances as shown in Figs. 29.11 and 29.12, respectively. The patient did not desire NAC reconstruction.

Case 4: Upper and lateral scar contracture with distortion of the left breast occurred in a woman who sustained a flame burn in her childhood (Fig. 29.13). Excision of the scars, complete release of contracture by means of cutting the underlying fibrotic bands, and resurfacing with a thick split-thickness skin graft (STSG) were performed (Fig. 29.14). Postoperative pressure therapy was done to prevent secondary graft skin contraction using custom-made garments (Fig. 29.15). The breasts were restored to their natural contour and symmetry (Fig. 29.16).

Case 5: This case relates to a 22-year-old female, who sustained a flame burn since childhood. A severe caudal scar contracture with underdevelopment of both breasts especially the left side, which was retracted down to the abdomen, was noted (Fig. 29.17). Complete scar release with preservation of the breast mounds was achieved by means of wide incisions and cutting of fibrotic bands. The resultant extensive defect was covered by thick STSG with tie-over suture (Fig. 29.18). Postoperative compression garment was applied to prevent secondary

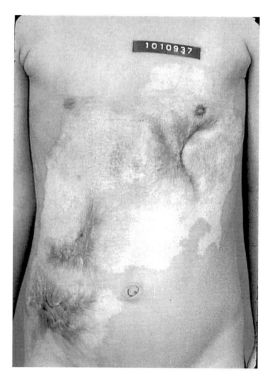

Figure 29.1 Scar contracture of the chest and abdomen with caudal retraction of the left breast.

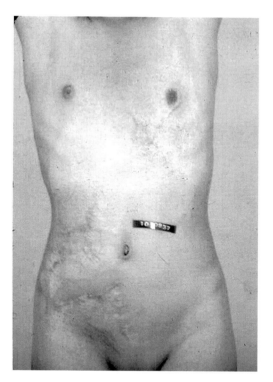

Figure 29.3 Follow-up for 3 years showed satisfactory results.

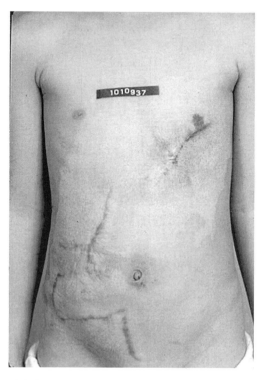

Figure 29.2 Scar excision and V-Y advancement flap for the left breast.

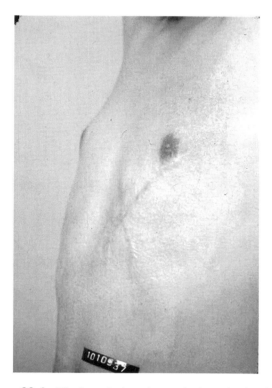

Figure 29.4 The lateral view shows nipple projection being started without limitation.

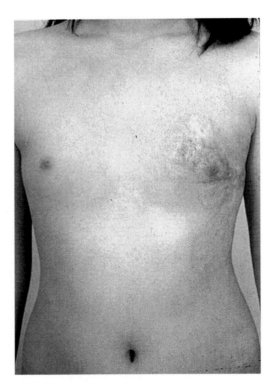

Figure 29.5 A patch of scar tissue over the left chest with lateral retraction of the breast.

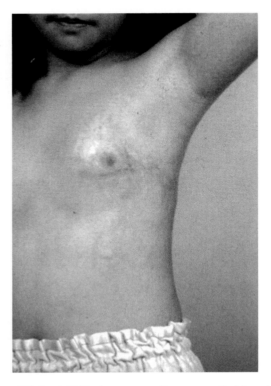

Figure 29.6 A V-Y advancement flap was applied for release of contracture to allow unlimited development of the breast.

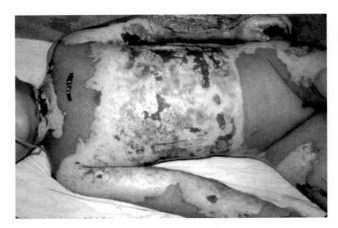

Figure 29.7 A 5-year-old girl suffering from third degree flame burn over the entire chest–abdomen with destruction of the nipples.

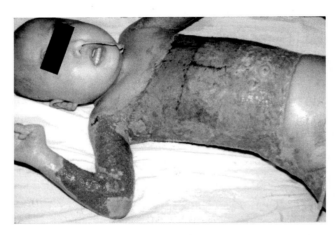

Figure 29.8 Conservative debridement with preservation of breast buds and proper sheet STSG.

contracture of the skin graft (Fig. 29.19). Follow-up of the patient at 1 year showed a satisfactory result. For comparison, the pre- and postoperative appearances are shown in (Figs. 29.20–29.23). Augmentation mammoplasty was suggested but not accepted.

Case 6: This involves a 14-year-old girl with a deformity of her right breast due to burn scar contracturea around the inframammary area. For reconstruction, design of an inferior-based fasciocutaneous flap from her flank was performed (Fig. 29.24). A relaxation incision was placed along the inframammary fold. The contracture was released as much as possible and the breast mound was well preserved but not undermined (Fig. 29.25). Immediate postoperative result of transposition of the fasciocutaneous flap showed good release of the contracture (Fig. 29.26). A 2-year follow-up showed good projection of the right breast from lateral view (Fig. 29.27).

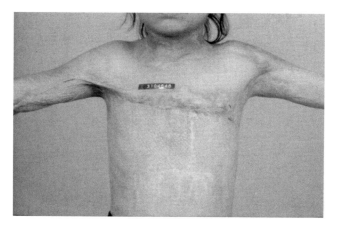

Figure 29.9 Seven years later at adolescent age, development of the breasts was restricted by scar contracture around the chest.

Preoperative appearance of her chest at puberty showed marked distortion and hypoplasia of the right breast (Fig. 29.28). However, after reconstruction with a local flap, the development of both breasts seemed rather symmetric and the contour of right breast was satisfactory (Fig. 29.29).

Case 7: This case presented a 10-year-old girl, who developed a burn scar contracture over the entire chest with restricted development of both breasts. The nipples were destroyed but could still be identified (Fig. 29.30). Combined use of local fasciocutaneous transposition flaps from the flanks to the inframammary fold and a full-thickness skin graft (FTSG) for the intermammary area was done before puberty. Three years later, development of both the breasts is noted (Fig. 29.31). The pre- and postoperative lateral views are shown in Figs. 29.32 and 29.33, respectively. The third degree burns sustained, severe scar contracture after wound healing, limitation of breast development, and the corrected deformities after

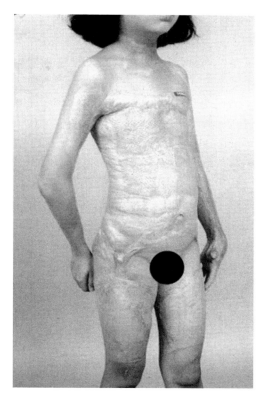

Figure 29.11 Preoperative oblique view before reconstruction for comparison.

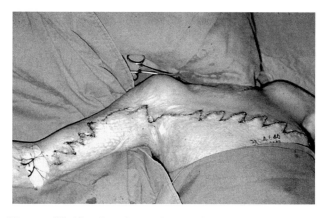

Figure 29.10 Complete release of scar contracture was achieved by means of multiple Z-plasties and scar revisions.

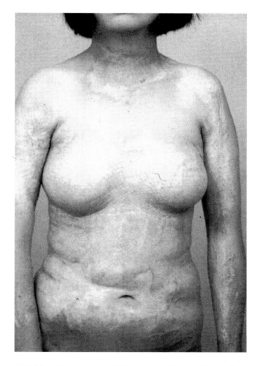

Figure 29.12 Four-year-follow-up of the patient showed well development of both breasts with acceptable symmetry. Patient had no desire to do NAC reconstruction.

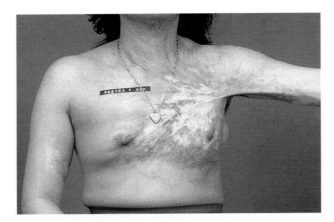

Figure 29.13   Upper and lateral scar contracture of the chest with distortion of left breast in a woman after flame burn.

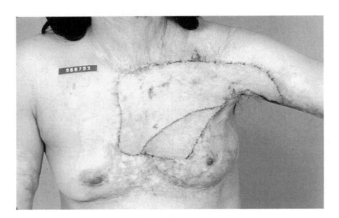

Figure 29.14   Thick STSG was used to cover the defects after scar excision and complete contracture release.

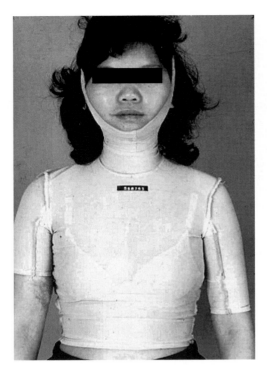

Figure 29.15   Postoperative pressure therapy with custom-made garment worn for 6 months.

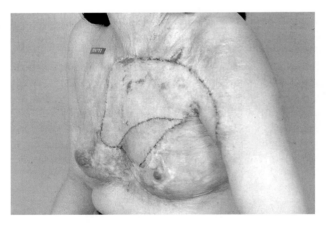

Figure 29.16   The oblique view shows symmetric breasts.

local fasciocutaneous flap reconstruction are shown in Figs. 29.34–29.37, respectively.

Case 8:   This is a case involving a 6-year-old boy, who sustained a scald burn over his chest and abdomen 1 year before reconstruction. Some kyphosis of the trunk and asymmetry of both nipples is noted (Fig. 29.38). Tissue expansion was used and most of the scar tissue was excised (Fig. 29.39). The location of the nipples was regulated during each time of reconstruction, which finally resulted in symmetry (Fig. 29.40).

Case 9:   This case reports a 44-year-old female, who sustained flame burns over her chest (Fig. 29.41). Conservative debridement with preservation of the NAC was done in the acute stage. A right breast deformity secondary to scar contractures is later noted (Fig. 29.42). Combined use of tissue expansion and a free flap reconstruction was planned (Fig. 29.43). The scar tissue was excised with preservation of the NAC. The breast mound after contracture release is noted (Fig. 29.44). A free anterior lateral

thigh flap, $25 \times 9 \, cm^2$ in size, based on the descending branch of the lateral femoral artery, in her right thigh was designed (Fig. 29.45). The flap was harvested as a chimeric perforator flap (Figs. 29.46 and 29.47). The donor site was closed primarily (Fig. 29.48). The flap was divided into two segments based on the separated perforators and trimmed according to the size of the defect (Fig. 29.49). The microvascular anastomosis between donor vessels, recipient vessels, and the internal mammary vessels was performed (Fig. 29.50). Follow-up

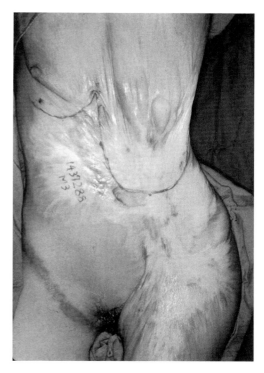

Figure 29.17 Severe scar contracture and resultant under-development of both breasts, especially the left side, of a lady due to flame burn during childhood.

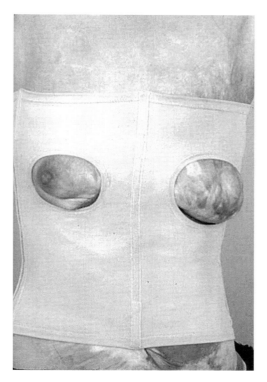

Figure 29.19 Postoperative compression garment was applied to prevent secondary contracture of the graft skin.

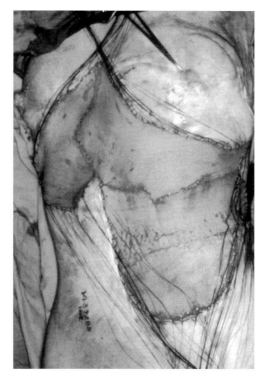

Figure 29.18 Complete release of the scar contracture with preservation of the breast mound was achieved by means of infra-mammary incisions and thick STSG.

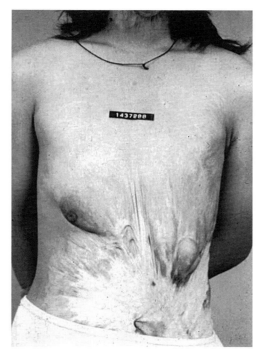

Figure 29.20 Preoperative picture shows severe scar contracture with hypoplasia of both breasts especially the left breast located almost at the abdomen.

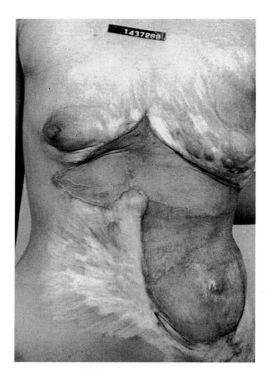

Figure 29.21 Follow-up 1-year later showed satisfactory result. Augmentation mammoplasty was suggested but not accepted because patient thought that it was not necessary.

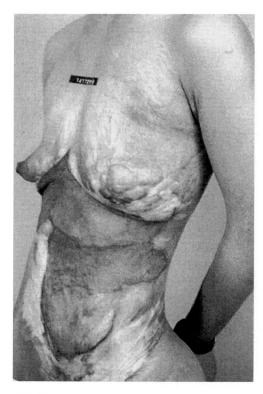

Figure 29.23 Postoperative lateral view shows restoration of original breast mound.

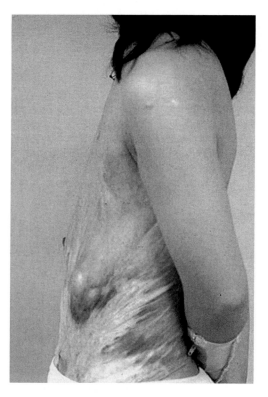

Figure 29.22 Preoperative lateral view shows flat and dislocated breast.

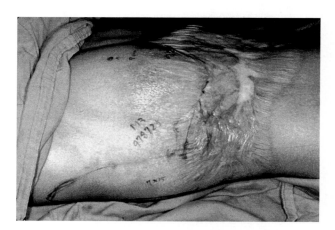

Figure 29.24 A 14-year-old girl with deformity of her right breast due to burn scar contracture received local flap reconstruction. Design of an inferior-based fasciocutaneous flap from right flank is shown in the picture.

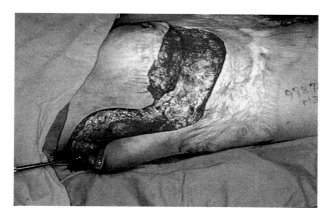

Figure 29.25 The relaxation incision was put along the infra-mammary fold. The contracture was relieved as much as possible and the breast mound was well preserved but not undermined.

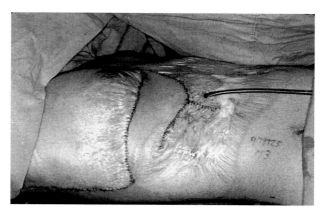

Figure 29.26 Immediate postoperative result of transposition of the fasciocutaneous flap.

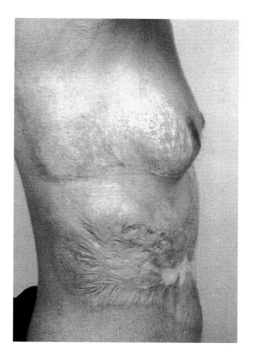

Figure 29.27 Two-year follow-up shows good projection of the right breast from lateral view.

of the patient 8 months later showed a satisfactory aesthetic result (Figs. 29.51 and 29.52).

There are many methods of NAC reconstruction including composite graft for the nipple and skin graft for the areola, tattooing for the areola nipple sharing with the healthy nipple, transposition of the remaining NAC, correction of the malpositioned NAC by transposition of subcutaneous pedicled flap, local flap such as double-bubble technique of Bunchman, wrap around technique of Silversmith, or the skate flap of Pensler (19,30–35,39).

Case 10: A patient with scar contracture over entire chest after a chemical burn with destruction and malposition of the NAC (Fig. 29.53) is reported here. Scar revision and repositioning of the residual nipple was done with satisfactory results (Fig. 29.54).

Case 11: This is another case of a young girl, who sustained burn scar contracture over her chest after scald burns. Most of the scars were removed by tissue expansion leaving the NAC undisturbed before puberty (Fig. 29.55).

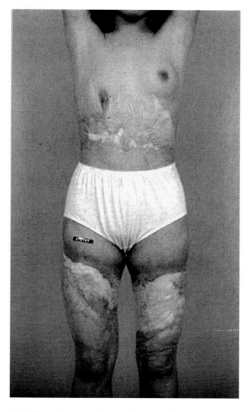

Figure 29.28 Preoperative picture of a patient at puberty showing marked distortion of the right breast. It looks like hypoplasia.

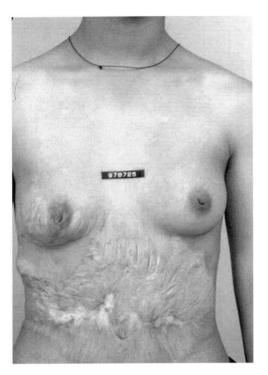

Figure 29.29   After reconstruction with local flap, the breast development seems rather symmetric and the contour satisfactory.

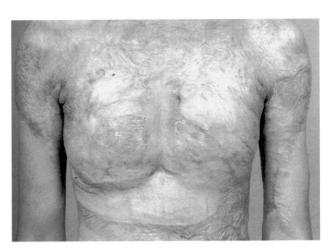

Figure 29.31   Local fasciocutaneous flaps for the inframammary contracture and FTSG for the inframammary area was done before puberty. A 3-year follow-up picture reveals satisfactory breast development.

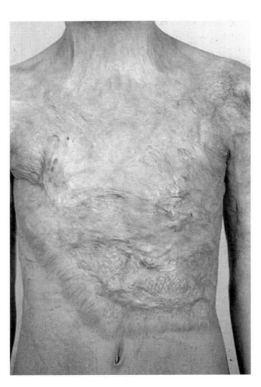

Figure 29.30   Scar tissues over the entire chest with restriction of the development of both breasts.

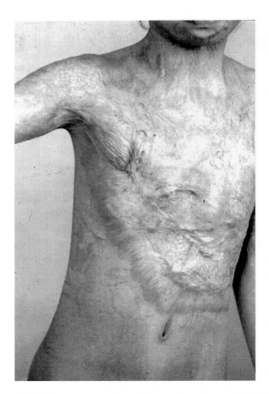

Figure 29.32   Preoperative oblique view shows limitation of breast development.

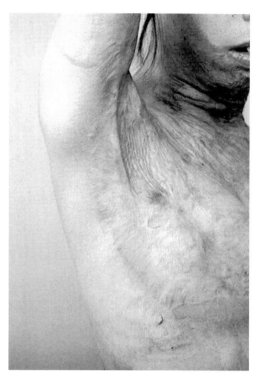

Figure 29.33 Postoperative oblique view shows good development of breasts with minimal donor site scar along the scar margin.

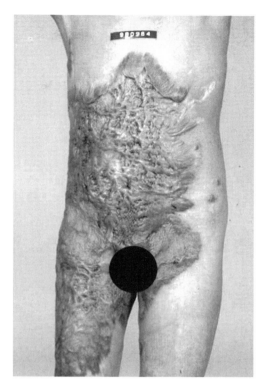

Figure 29.35 Severe scar contracture noted after wound healing.

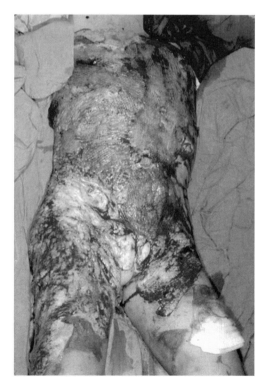

Figure 29.34 Extensive third degree burn over the chest and abdomen of a young girl. Complete escharectomy but careful preservation of the breast mound was done.

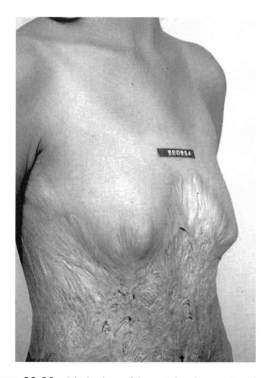

Figure 29.36 Limitation of breast development and caudal retraction of both breasts were noted seven years later.

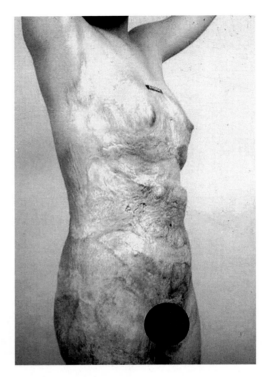

Figure 29.37   The deformities were corrected by local fascio-cutaneous flap reconstruction.

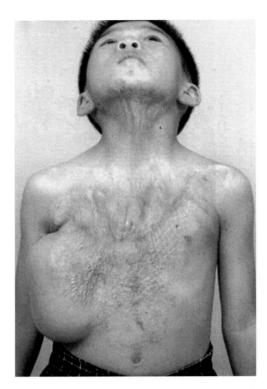

Figure 29.39   Most of the scar tissues were removed by tissue expansion technique step by step.

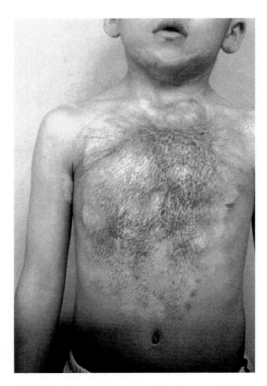

Figure 29.38   Scar contracture of the chest and abdomen with kyphosis noted in a young boy after scald burn.

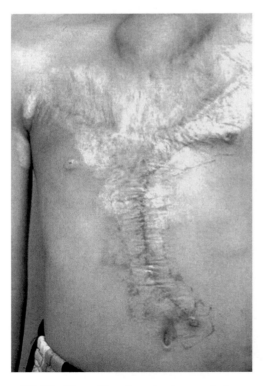

Figure 29.40   The relieved contracture and the corrected kyphosis. The nipples were also preserved after reconstruction.

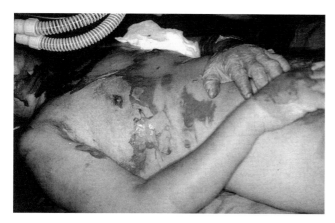

Figure 29.41 A 44-year-old female suffering from flame burn over the chest and upper limbs. Conservative debridement with preservation of the right nipple and breast mound was done in the acute stage.

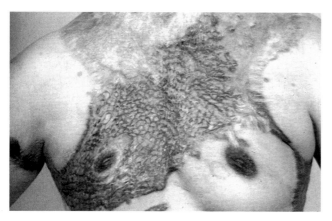

Figure 29.42 Deformity of the right breast due to scar contracture was noted later although breast mound was preserved as much as possible initially.

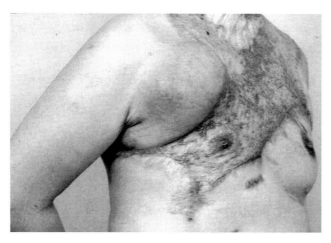

Figure 29.43 The scar tissue around the breasts were excised step by step by means of tissue expansion technique 1 year later.

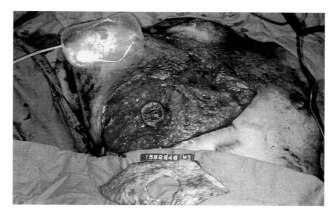

Figure 29.44 The thick scar tissue was removed and revealed that the breast mound still existed after contracture was relieved. The NAC was preserved and put onto the correct position.

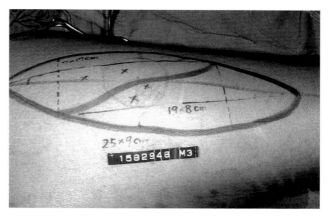

Figure 29.45 A free anterior lateral thigh flap, 25×9 cm^2 in size, designed as a chimeric flap based on two perforators in the patient's right thigh was done.

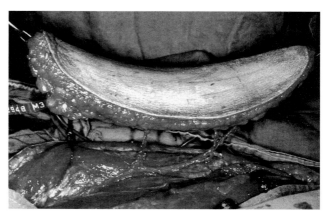

Figure 29.46 The flap was elevated and the perforators can be seen clearly.

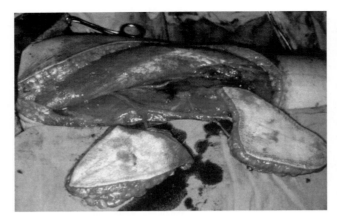

Figure 29.47 The flap was trimmed according to the defect area and properly arranged in good direction.

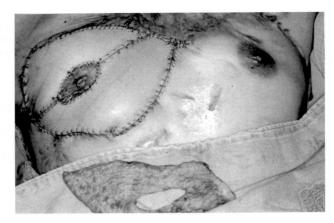

Figure 29.50 Immediate postoperative result of free flap reconstruction.

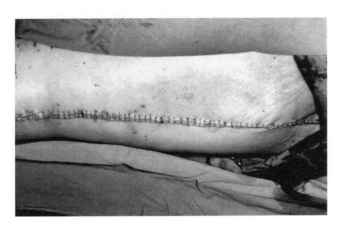

Figure 29.48 The donor site was closed primarily.

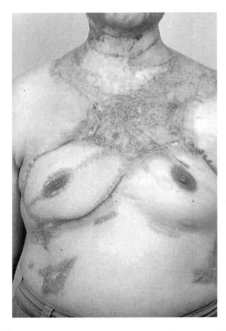

Figure 29.51 Follow-up 6 months later shows good aesthetic breast contour. The patient was satisfactory.

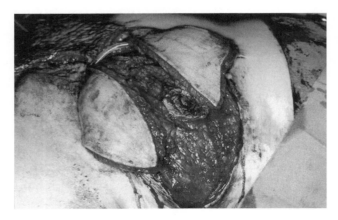

Figure 29.49 Microvascular anastomosis between descending branch of lateral femoral vessels and internal mammary vessels.

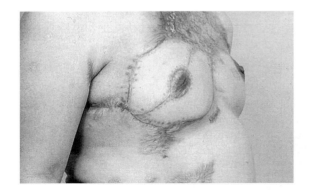

Figure 29.52 The oblique view compared to Fig. 29.43 shows much improvement.

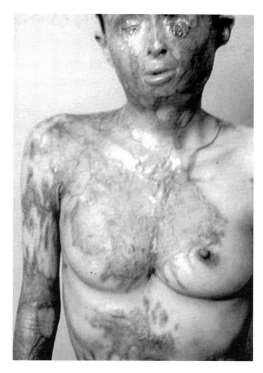

Figure 29.53 Scar contracture of the breasts after a chemical burn in a lady's chest. The ring nipple was destroyed.

The NAC was transposed to proper location during advancement of the expanded skin. After the breasts were well developed, the NAC in both breasts looked rather symmetric (Fig. 29.56).

IV. INTRAOPERATIVE CONSIDERATIONS

Any burn injury involving the chest of a girl or a young female patient should be carefully managed considering

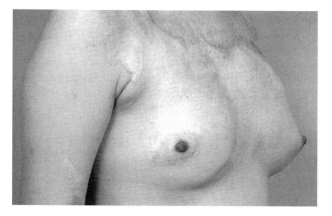

Figure 29.55 Transposition of the NAC was done before puberty for a 17-year-old girl who sustained a scald burn in childhood when the scar tissues were replaced by expanded skin.

the ongoing development of the breasts. Conservative debridement with preservation of the breast buds for further breast development is recommended by many authors (3–6). McCauley et al. (6) reviewed 28 female patients with burns to the anterior chest wall involving NAC and found that in spite of significant thermal injury, all patients developed breasts. The key point is careful tangential excision to the viable tissue and preservation of the underlying tissue as much as possible if surgery is necessary. Even in the full-thickness burns to lactating breasts, surgical tangential excision was delayed (5). This principle is also advocated by other authors and noted in our own experience (Figs. 29.7, 29.8, 29.12, 29.30, and 29.31).

It is clear that different problems occur between childhood and early adulthood in female patients who have sustained thermal burns over the anterior chest wall. The main concern, however, is the status of breast development. In the adult group, the most frequent causes of burn injury

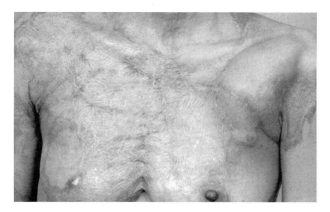

Figure 29.54 Scar revision and transposition of the remaining nipple was done with acceptable results.

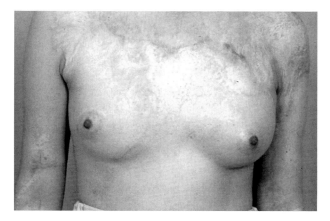

Figure 29.56 The final results of reconstruction were satisfactory.

are chemical injuries or flame burns. The most common problems are scar contractures with distortion or asymmetry of the breasts (Figs. 29.13, 29.42, and 29.53). The most important reconstructive procedure utilized is the release of these scar contractures by excision of the burn scars. The well-developed breast mounds usually still exist even in third degree burns (Figs. 29.14 and 29.44) (14). However, scar replacement using skin graft, tissue expanders, or flaps is sometimes needed (Figs. 29.14, 29.44, and 29.47).

The most frequent cases of burn injury in children are those due to scald injuries and flame burns. The most common problem is scar contracture over the chest. In pediatric female patients, underdevelopment or even aplasia of the breasts may subsequently occur. In this group, for mild postburn breast deformities, scar release by V-Y- or Z-plasty before puberty may provide enough release for breast development (Figs. 29.2, 29.6, 29.10, and 29.12). Scar release by skin graft or by transposition of local flaps such as fasciocutaneous flap is sometimes needed in this group (Figs. 29.26 and 29.31). For severe postburn deformities with underdeveloped mammary glands, breast reconstruction can proceed if the surface area of the breast is restored by means of tissue expansion and a breast prosthesis is substituted for the absent parenchyma (21,22). The myocutaneous flaps such as latissimus dorsi (LD) or transabdominal myocutaneous (TRAM) flap are frequently used for severe destruction of the breasts either in young girls or adult groups (18,36). NAC reconstruction always needs later reconstruction in this situation. This means that more careful initial management of the burn wound and early scar release before adolescence is needed for the child with thermal burns in the anterior chest.

V. PITFALLS

Considering the reconstruction principles, first of all, complete release of the scar contracture cannot be overemphasized (15,19). Usually the incision line is placed in the inframammary fold from the flank to the sternum leaving the breast tissue intact without any undermining (Figs. 29.18, 29.25, and 29.44). Successful resurfacing of the defect using skin graft, local flaps such as slide-swing plasty or fasciocutaneous flap, and expanded skin nearby should be achieved for restoring the breast contour (Figs. 29.14, 29.21, 29.26, 29.31, 29.39, and 29.55) (17,24). Good immobilization of graft skin can be achieved by means of a tie-over dressing, avoiding circulation compromise in flap surgery by proper design (by keeping the length-to-base ratio at 3:1 for fasciocutaneous flap). Careful elevation of the flap to include the fascia, and

secured vessels anastomosis in free tissue transfer should be kept in mind to achieve good results (Fig. 29.18).

The second important principle is delayed reconstruction of the NAC because the definite position of the NAC usually cannot be ensured until full development of the breast and final stage of the reconstruction. Besides, unreliable blood supply of the local flap for NAC reconstruction usually exists if the initial burn injury involves the dermis (15). Pigments used in the tattooing technique for the areola in burn breast reconstruction may fade away later, possibly because the injured dermis cannot keep the pigments longer and hence the technique is not advised by some authors (30). It is better to arrange the NAC reconstruction in the last procedure, if possible, for burn breast reconstruction after scar maturation and contour restoration.

The third key point is not to do any harm. Injury to the sensory nerves toward the breast tissue should be avoided when reconstructive procedure is performed around the lateral chest (4).

VI. NURSING ISSUES

Acute stage wound care for the burn chest is the same as for other thermal burns. The nurses may find that the necrotic tissues around the NAC are not removed after debridement. This may reflect a policy of conservative treatment of surgeons. Therefore, bedside debridement during dressing changes is not performed.

The patient should acquire a full understanding of the methods available for reconstruction of the breast and NAC (4). Informed consent and explanation should be given preoperatively. When reconstruction is carried out on a lactating breast, care must be taken not to let the wound become contaminated by lactation. Tie-over bolsters are used to ensure skin graft adherence. The dressing should be kept clean and dry in the subsequent postoperative days to avoid infection.

When flaps are used for reconstruction, the circulation must be monitored frequently, especially in the first two postoperative days. The appearance of the flap, capillary refill, surface temperature, and transcutaneous oxygen levels should be recorded frequently in the first 24 h postoperatively. One should bear in mind that the development of a hematoma is a frequent cause of skin graft or flap failure. Consequently, a drainage system, either penrose or vacuum drain, should be kept effective. When an implant, such as tissue expander or breast prosthesis is used, perioperative antibiotics are usually recommended. The importance of postoperative pressure therapy for skin grafts or a specially designed device to maintain the breast contour and control of chest deformities should be provided for all patients (40).

VII. REHABILITATION ISSUES

The tie-over bolster dressings are kept in place for 6 or 7 days. After removal of the dressings, a plaster-of-Paris slab is suggested for application to the grafted area and for the breast to maintain its shape and contour (38). A device consisting of a Plastizote molded two-piece body jacket which incorporates a full neck and chin conformer was recommended by Becker to control chest deformities including kyphosis due to burn scarring (40). This device can also be used in the postreconstructive stage.

Custom-made compression garment worn for 6–12 months after breast release is recommended by most plastic surgeons and physical or occupational therapists. Custom-made openings in pressure garments allow for nipple and breast mound projection. Silicone inserts placed in the concave area help scar maturation after reconstruction (Fig. 29.19) (19,41,42). Postoperative splinting combined with regular exercise is recommended by many authors for the prevention of disfigurement and for maintaining range of motion (43–45).

VIII. LONG-TERM OUTCOME

From 1982 to 2000 there were 37 female patients suffering from burn injury with breast deformity and received surgical reconstruction at Linkou Burn Center in Chang Gung Memorial Hospital. The age at injury ranged from 2 months to 50 years with an average of 16.6 years. Among this group, there were 19 children (51.4%) under the age of 12. The remaining 18 patients were adults (48.6%) with a mean age of 31.7 years. In the adult group, 50% of the patients sustained chemical burns. In children, scald burns were the most common cause of injury. The most common method for correction of the resulting defects was the use of Z-plasties, although skin grafts, tissue expansion, fasciocutaneous flaps, and myocutaneous flaps were also used for reconstruction. The use of local tissue dominated this process. For NAC reconstruction also, Z-plasties were the most frequently used method. In children, all the breast mounds were restored after various kinds of reconstructive procedures. Four patients with NAC destruction or distortion due to previous burn injury received transposition of residual NAC showing acceptable results. Two patients with total destruction of the NAC did not receive further reconstruction. Among those patients who received fasciocutaneous flap reconstruction, only one had partial flap tip necrosis. No other serious complication occurred in this group. In the adult group, all patients regained breast mound after reconstruction. Two patients had marked hypoplasia of the breast even after total release of the scar contracture. Three patients with NAC involvement also were satisfied by means of local cutaneous flap reconstruction or transposition of residual NAC. There were also no serious complications in this group.

There are some long-term follow-up noted (Figs. 29.12, 29.23, 29.31, and 29.37). Breast development and contour restoration can be satisfactory if the timing and modality of reconstructive procedures can be done properly.

Consequently, several conclusions can be drawn. Satisfactory aesthetic results for burns, chest and breast deformity reconstruction can be obtained by means of following principles: (1) conservative treatment in the acute stage; (2) prevention of postburn deformity; (3) complete scar release with as much preservation of breast mounds as possible; and (4) aesthetic reconstruction for established deformity in chronic stage using skin grafts, local flaps, free flaps, tissue expansion and transposition, or composite grafts for the NAC. It is especially worthwhile to perform reconstruction for any female with a burned breast deformity.

REFERENCES

1. Luce EA. Electrical injuries. In: McCarthy, ed. Plastic Surgery. Philadelphia: W.B. Saunders, 1990:814–830.
2. Lees VC, Frame JD. Electrical burns. In: Settle JAD, ed. Principles and Practice of Burns Management. New York: Churchill Livingstone, 1996:369–376.
3. Garner WL, Smith DJ. Reconstruction of burns of the trunk and breast. Clin Plast Surg 1992; 19:683–691.
4. Salisbury RE, Bevin AG. Atlas of Reconstructive Burn Surgery. Philadelphia: W.B. Saunders, 1981.
5. Al-Qattan MM, Zuker RM. Management of acute burns of the female pediatric breast: delayed tangential excision versus spontaneous eschar separation. Ann Plast Surg 1994; 33:66–67.
6. McCauley RL, Beraja V, Rutan RL, Huang TT, Abston S, Rutan TC, Robson MC. Longitudinal assessment of breast development in adolescent female patients with burns involving the nipple-areolar complex. Plast Reconstr Surg 1989; 83:676–780.
7. Giele HP, Nguyen H, Wood F, Crocker AD. Management of full thickness burns to lactating breasts. Burns 1994; 20:278–280.
8. Garner WL, Smith DJ. Reconstruction of burn deformities of the extremities and trunk. In: Cohen M, ed. Mastery of Plastic and Reconstructive. Boston: Little Brown Co., 1994:429–440.
9. Achauer BM, VanderKam VM. Burn reconstruction. In: Achauer BM, ed. Plastic Surgery, Indications, Operations and Outcomes. St. Louis: Mosby, 2000:425–446.
10. Kumar P, Varma R. Immediate reconstruction of chest and abdominal wall defect following high voltage electrical injury. Burns 1994; 20:557–559.
11. Capar M, Karatas O, Gozel B, Oztan Y. Anterior chest wall reconstruction with cervicohumeral flap. Ann Plast Surg 2000; 44:114–115.

12. Escudero-Nafs FJ, Rabanal-Suarez F, Leiva-Oliva RM. Costal chondritis following very deep flame burns involving the chest wall. Burns 1989; 15:394–396.

13. Ono I, Tateshita T. Reconstruction of a full thickness defect of the chest wall caused by friction burn using a combined myocutaneous flap of teres major and latissimus dorsi muscles. Burns 2001; 27:283–288.

14. Kunert P, Schneider W, Flory J. Principles and procedures in female breast reconstruction in the young child's burn injury. Aesth Plast Surg 1988; 12:101–106.

15. Achauer BM. Reconstruction of the burned breast and abdomen. In: Achauer BM, ed. Burn Reconstruction. New York: Thieme Medical Publishers, 1991:148–164.

16. Hyakusoku H, Okubo M, Fumiiri M. Combination of the square flap method and the dermal sling to correct flat or inverted nipples. Aesth Plast Surg 1988; 12:107–109.

17. Schrudde J, Beinhoff U. Covering defects in the breast region by the slide-swing plasty. Aesth Plast Surg 1989; 13:41–46.

18. Bishop JB, Fisher J, Bostwick J. The burned female breast. Ann Plast Surg 1980; 4:25–30.

19. MacLennan SE, Wells MD, Neale HW. Reconstruction of the burned breast. Clin Plast Surg 2000; 27:113–119.

20. Marks MW, Argenta LC, Thornton JW. Burn management: the role of tissue expansion. Clin Plast Surg 1987; 14:543–548.

21. Versaci AD, Balkovich ME, Goldstein SA. Breast reconstruction by tissue expansion for congenital and burn deformities. Ann Plast Surg 1986; 16:20–31.

22. Slator RC, Wilson GR, Sharpe DT (with discussion by Neale HW and Kurtzman LC). Postburn breast reconstruction: tissue expansion prior to contracture release. Plast Reconstr Surg 1992; 90:668–674.

23. Yamamoto Y, Yokoyama T, Minakawa H, Sugihara T. Use of the expanded skin flap in esthetic reconstruction of postburn deformity. J Burn Care Rehabil 1996; 17:397–401.

24. Still J, Craft-Coffman B, Law E. Use of pedicled flaps and tissue expanders to reconstruct burn scars of the skin of the anterior abdomen and chest. Ann Plast Surg 1998; 40:226–228.

25. Ohmori S. Correction of burn deformities using free flap transfer. J Trauma 1982; 22:104–111.

26. Yang JY, Tsai FC, Chana JD, Chuang SS, Chang SY, Huang WC. Use of thin free anteriolateral thigh flaps combined with cervicoplasty for reconstruction of postburn anterior cervical contracture. Plast Reconstr Surg 2002; 110:39–46.

27. Jones GE, Nahai F, Bostwick J III. Microsurgical techniques in breast reconstruction. In: Bostwick J III, ed. Plastic and Reconstructive Breast Surgery. St. Louis: QMP, 2000:1147–1251.

28. Stuffer M, Papp CH. Reconstruction of large scar areas with controlled tissue expansion combined with fasciocutaneous flaps. Burns 1991; 17:166–169.

29. Guan WX, Jin YT, Cao HP. Reconstruction of postburn female breast deformity. Ann Plast Surg 1988; 21:65–69.

30. Pensler JM, Haab RL, Parry SW. Reconstruction of the burned nipple–areola complex. Plast Reconstr Surg 1986; 78:480–484.

31. Becker HB. Nipple–areola reconstruction using intradermal tattoo. Plast Reconstr Surg 1986; 81:450–453.

32. Bhatty MA, Berry RB. Nipple–areola reconstruction by tattooing and nipple sharing. Br J Plast Reconstr Surg 1997; 50:331–334.

33. van Straalen WR, van Trier AJM, Groenevelt F. Correction of the postburn malpositioned nipple–areola complex by transposition of subcutaneous pedicled flaps. Br J Plast Surg 2000; 53:406–409.

34. Bunchman HH, Larson DL, Huang TT, Lewis SR. Nipple and areola reconstruction in the burned breast. Plast Reconstr Surg 1974; 54:531–536.

35. Silversmith PE. Nipple reconstruction by quadripod flaps. Plast Reconstr Surg 1983; 72:422.

36. Ozgur F, Gokalan I, Erk Y, Kecik A. Reconstruction of postburn breast deformities. Burns 1992; 18:504–509.

37. Neale HW, Smith GL, Gregory RO, MacMillan BG. Breast reconstruction in the burned adolescent female (An 11-year, 157-patient experience). Plast Reconstr Surg 1982; 70:718–724.

38. Sawhney CP. The correction of post-burn contractures of the breast. Br J Plast Surg 1977; 30:291–294.

39. Neale HW, Kurtzman LC. Reconstruction of the burned breast and abdomen. In: Achauer BM, ed. Burn Reconstruction. New York: Thieme Medical Publishers, 1991:148–164.

40. Becker BE. Hypertrophic burn scarring: control of chest deformities with a new device. Arch Phys Med Rehabil 1980; 61:187–189.

41. Cooper R, Hall S. Occupational therapy and physiotherapy. In: Settle JAD, ed. Principles and Practice of Burns Management. New York: Churchill Livingstone, 1996:453–464.

42. Cooper R, Fenton OM. Disfigurement and disablement. In: Settle JAD, ed. Principles and Practice of Burns Management. New York: Churchill Livingstone, 1996.

43. Leman CJ. Splints and accessories following burn reconstruction. Clin Plast Surg 1992; 19:721–731.

44. Evans EB, Alvarado MI, Ott S, McElroy K. Prevention and treatment of deformity in burned patients. In: Herndon DN, ed. Total Burn Care. London: W.B. Saunders, 1996:443–454.

45. Jordan RB, Daher J, Wasil K. Splints and scar management for acute and reconstructive burn care. Clin Plast Surg 2000; 27:71–85.

30

Reconstruction of Truncal Burns

NELSON SARTO PICCOLO

Instituto Nelson Picolo and Pronto Socorro para Queimaduras, Goiânia, Goiás, Brazil

I. INTRODUCTION

As the trunk is usually covered by clothing on most everyday activities, it is proportionally less injured than the exposed areas of the body. Although clothing may act as a protective barrier against certain types of burn accidents, that is, against cooking gas explosion, it may also be a "complicating" item when it gets soaked with a hot or a chemical agent, or when caught on fire. In these situations, the chances of a deeper burn are increased. This may result in a larger incidence of burn scar sequelae in this region of the body (Fig. 30.1). Excision and grafting has been widely accepted as the treatment of choice for full-thickness burns (1). Although some patients will not seek reconstruction of grafted areas, removal of scar tissue, previously grafted or not, is a very common desire among our patients.

Reconstruction of truncal burns may face restrictive scars around the axillae, base of the neck, and upper extremities, as well as in relatively vast areas of scar tissue around the thorax and abdomen. Functional reconstruction is a priority in all areas of the body, and improvement of shoulder and neck movement can be achieved with truncal procedures alone or combined with more caudal or cephalad procedures. Flat areas of scar tissue, which result in no retraction, may be progressively removed after complete maturation.

In the case of female patients, the tissue damage will be more significant, if the breast or the area of future breast development is injured and subsequently scarred. Assurance that reconstructive procedures can, and will, be done is a must for psychological comfort and to improve compliance with pressure garments and physiotherapy. Procedures around these areas of the trunk usually have to be started early. As the breast bud starts to grow, multiple procedures may be required until development is complete.

Absence of landmark anatomic structures as a result of a deep burn involving the nipple areola complex (NAC) is of significance to both sexes. The same is true for the umbilical scar. The acute burn surgeon will not usually remove these areas upon excising burn lesions, but deep burns may result in their loss regardless of the acute careful surgical technique. Enforcement of proper timing of reconstruction may be difficult and sometimes painful for the surgeon and the patient, who may wish for earlier reconstructive procedures [Fig. 30.2(A–C)]. In our country, patients of both sexes will usually ask to

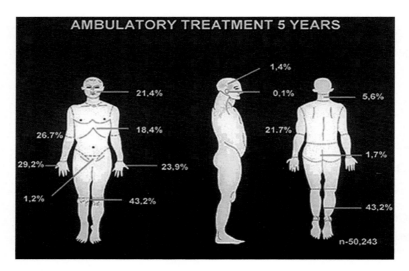

Figure 30.1   Incident of burn lesions according to body region—truncal burns = 18.4% (in a sample of 50,243 burns).

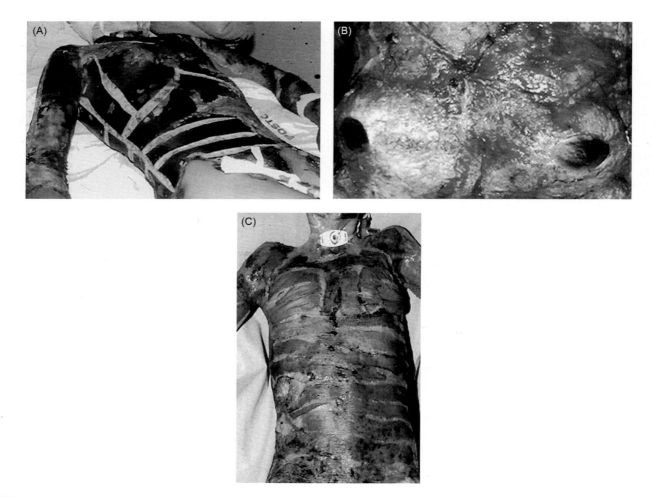

Figure 30.2   (A) Patient with full-thickness burn to the entire trunk and upper extremities. (B) Same patient postexcision, with the attempt of preserving the location of the nipple areola complex (NAC). (C) Same patient, after complete loss of the NAC, and sheet grafting.

reconstruct the upper portion of the trunk first. These areas are commonly exposed daily. Most female patients will agree that "return to femininity," as some will say, can be greatly improved with early reconstruction of the anterior upper thorax.

Since the main goal of any procedure is to obtain a good result, the surgeon, of course, will accommodate the patients wishes, as long as they are realistic and within his armamentarium of surgical options.

II. PREOPERATIVE EVALUATION

As in any other surgical procedure, planning for the operations will require a thorough preoperative assessment to identify functional deficits as well as aesthetic concerns. A complete patient evaluation may include being seen not only by the surgeon but also by the psychologist, the physiotherapist, and the occupational therapist. After these visits, the patient's wishes are needs are prioritized and the reconstructive procedures planned accordingly. The surgical plan is then widely discussed with the patient and/or the patient's family. Very frequently, the patient will initially present with a severe functional complaint. As the treatment plan is outlined, he or she will demonstrate the desire to reconstruct areas for a esthetical reasons. Functional procedures, as a rule, are performed first [Fig. 30.3(A–C)]. One must always realize that most patients with severe burn scar contractures may not only have difficulties with everyday life activities, like brushing their teeth or putting their shoes on, etc. but also have severe psychological difficulties coping with their new appearance and a new different self. An honest and straightforward evaluation may help in the planning

of realistic reconstruction options. However, the surgeon in charge will have to consider all aspects of recovery, if the patient is to benefit from the treatment (2).

If the patient is a child, this task is even more difficult. There may be a lot of guilt involved, with parents reacting in a very wide spectrum of attitudes. Overprotection is the rule, but rejection can also happen. Both will impair adequate preoperative care, such as physiotherapy and the use of pressure garments. This can lead to the blurring of proposed treatment options and postoperative management issues. Strong psychological support and/or treatment may be necessary for several months after the wound has healed (3). After deciding upon the elected procedure and operation dates, the entire team should be briefed about the proposed treatment and become acquainted with the patient. Thus, when the child is admitted, adequate care will be provided. Knowing the patient's case may be influential in the immediate postoperative care, when the difference between inadequate and adequate positioning may signify the success of the surgical procedure.

III. SURGICAL OPTIONS

As any other pathology that requires surgical treatment, burn sequelae to the trunk are present in such a varied spectrum of sizes and shapes that one must evaluate each case as a different case, and the options for treatment must be chosen accordingly.

Closure of the acute wound may be done with meshed or sheet grafting, artificial or bioengineered skin substitutes or even with local or distant flaps. Contraction will usually occur across scar tissue, but it may also occur in

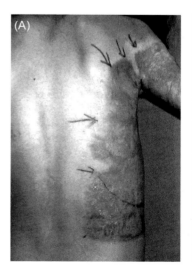 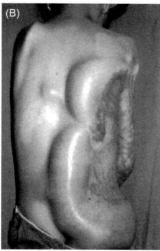 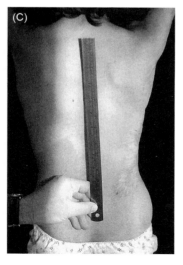

Figure 30.3 (A) Patient with truncal sequelae and severe restriction of shoulder range of motion. (B) Same patient being expanded. (C) Same patient, 1-year follow-up postadvancement of expanded tissue, with significant functional and aesthetical result.

grafted wounds. Alternatively, scar tissue may connect to healthy skin, with subcutaneous scar tissue cords or bands sometimes present in the anterior chest linked to the upper extremities. This may result in impaired movement from the shoulders and upper arms (4,5).

The functional deficits are usually treated first, although the most frequent reason for these are contractures, significant tissue deficits may occur; there may also be a lack of adequate skin donor sites for correction of the problem. Incisional release and resurfacing with grafts on Z-plasties are frequently performed as curative procedures for contracture bands in the upper lateral thorax and base of the neck. Another frequently available option are rotation flaps of lateral posterior thorax tissue for treatment of posterior axillary retraction.

If the patient presents with normal tissue in the periphery of the defect, or if he accepts more than one procedure to gain the proposed result, the treatment of choice, in our opinion, will be normal tissue expansion and advancement. Yet, there is already enough evidence that suggests that future treatment may consist of the replacement of scar tissue by artificial skin. Tissue expansion has been widely used all over the world to treat burn scars. The implants now come in various shapes and sizes, and the learning curve is relatively short, usually with the surgeon understanding the benefits and the incidence of complications when still relatively inexperienced. The best results are achieved when the scar tissue is already mature and the more pliable tissue chosen to be expanded is around the defect (6) [Fig. 30.4(A and B)]. Expansion may also be used as a way of "expanding" donor area skin or to save possible scarring in distant virgin donor areas. The periphery of the sequelae is expanded, and full-thickness skin is removed, with "reattachment" of the residual expanded skin to the defect, without any local cosmetic loss. There is minimal to no donor site morbidity as seen with contractures treated by incision and full-thickness skin grafts. Composite tissue expansion is also a possibility, with muscles, nerves, and vessels all being included in the expansion process, when the defect presents with more than just the absence of normal skin.

IV. INTRAOPERATIVE CONSIDERATIONS

Since burn scars and scar contractures of the trunk may involve one or both sides, and the back, most patients are treated under general anesthesia. Adequate positioning is imperative if the surgeon is rotating a flap or advancing local tissue. The surgeon must be aware of local tissue resistance to advancement and repositioning on the surgical table. Improper positioning can result in advert traction at the suture line or at the base of the flap, when the patient is placed back into the supine position in the immediate postoperative period.

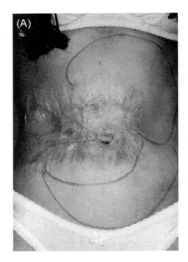

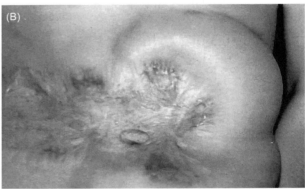

Figure 30.4 (A) Preoperative planning for placement of expander for partial removal of abdominal scar. (B) Expanders in place, matching the defect.

Preoperative planning should always include careful planning of incisions and noting that if flap rotation is necessary, suture lines will be placed in natural skin lines or creases to diminish the incidence of unsightly surgical scars.

V. PITFALLS

The expected results for the surgical technique are presented for the patient or for the patient's family. The occurrence of complications must also be discussed. The experienced surgeon will choose established techniques with which he has acquaintance, so he may expeditiously treat any complications related to the procedure. Modesty upon scar removal may be the single most important factor upon doing these procedures along major joints and round structures, like the lateral region of the trunk, where tension on the advanced flap may be more geometrically demanding. The surgeon must be prepared to act acutely if complications develop, in order to minimize

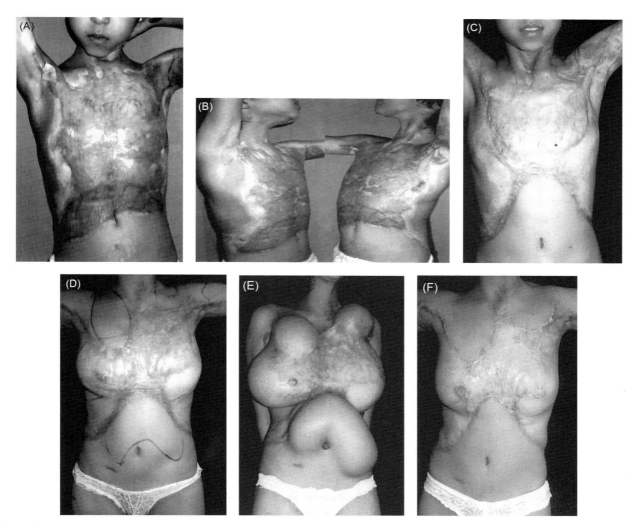

Figure 30.5 (A) Patient 1 year after severe burn to the anterior trunk. (B) Same patient, lateral views. (C) Same patient, after the first expansion. (D) Same patient, after the second expansion. (E) Same patient, on her third expansion. (F) Same patient, after the third expansion.

the chance of total failure. Surgical planning based on inadequate judgment may be the cause of incomplete or unsatisfactory results. A though evaluation of the patient with a comprehensive interview will clarify any doubts there may be about the proposed procedure. Burn patients who seek reconstruction may deal with disfigurement in several different ways. Consequently, information about the technique and disclosure about previous results in similar but unidentified cases may inform the patient or the patient's family about expected results and possible complications (7).

VI. NURSING ISSUES

The burn team members will be completely informed about each patient's case, so they can play their role accordingly,

complementing the success of the procedure with the recommended postoperative care. Knowledge about the performed procedure and how the care should be provided after surgery is paramount to attain the proposed goal. As positioning is very important in most truncal reconstruction cases, the Physiotherapist/Occupational Therapist (PT/OT) group will work together with the nursing staff to guarantee this aspect of postoperative care.

VII. REHABILITATION ISSUES

As in the acute burn care, the physiotherapist's and the occupational therapist's work will contribute to the postoperation rehabilitation of the patient. All procedures are explained in detail and the issues to treatment of compliance are identified as it relates to the expected outcome.

Planning of subsequent procedures is based on the functional gain perceived by the therapists. These professionals will then communicate to the reconstructive team that the patient is ready for the next intervention. In purely aesthetic procedures of scar removal, the use of pressure garments and orthotics is also influential in the final result.

VIII. LONG-TERM OUTCOME

Outcome is determined by a series of factors. Although the reconstructive procedure is only one of them, the surgeon should involve the entire burn team in the patient's treatment. Staged procedures are usually the rule in burn reconstruction. There may be several areas that require simultaneous treatment. Sequential surgical planning should also include the patient's wishes in a realistic manner. Thus, he or she can note that the progress is already being achieved by the initial procedures. In some cases, reconstructive procedures may have to be delayed until full development has been achieved [Fig. 30.5(A–F)].

In some functional cases with major contractures, there may be an actual "gain" of scar tissue area, as the release in performed. Information about the expected result and the changes to be expected with the scar red area will diminish anxiety. Long term evaluation of actual results, can also be anticipated. The planning of future operations for removal of scar tissue may then be assessed (8). The patient must be aware of the importance of the use of pressure garments after each stage of reconstruction to achieve the best results with decreased changes of scar hypertrophy at the suture line of advanced flaps or even partial or complete scar removal.

IX. CONCLUSION

Although the trunk is only injured in about one-fifth of the burn accidents, it is a very frequent site for reconstructive procedures. Thorough and comprehensive planning will insure a larger number of satisfactory results. Unless, a severe functional deficit is present, an operation should only be performed after complete hypertrophic scar maturation. In addition, there must be a complete evaluation by the burn team, which includes the surgeon, physical and occupational therapists, and, if necessary, a psychologist. There must be a continuum of supportive treatment from the acute phase of injury though reconstruction, with long-term planning disclosed as soon as possible. Obtaining the patient's cooperation and "enrolment" into the stages of the treatment is probably the single most important factor in all aspects of burn care.

REFERENCES

1. Still JM, Law EJ. Primary excision of the burn wound. Clin Plast Surg 2000; 27(1):23–47.
2. Fauerbach JA. Barriers to employment among working-aged patients with major burn injury. J Burn Care Rehabil 2001; 22(1):32–34.
3. Moss BF, Everett JJ, Patterson DR. Psychologic support and apin management of the burn patient. In: Richard RL, Staley MJ, eds. Burn Care and Rehabilitation—Principles and Practice. Philadelphia: F.A. Davis Company, 1994.
4. Férnadez-Palocios J, Bayón PB, Sánchez OC, Duque OG. Multilevel release of an extended postburn contracture. Burns 2002; 28(5):490–493.
5. Ono I, Tateshita T. Reconstruction of a full-thickness defect of the chest wall caused by friction burn using a combined myocutaneous flap of teres major and latissimus dorsi muscles. Burns 2001; 27(3):283–288.
6. Youm T, Margiott M, Kasabian A, Karp N. Complications of tissue expansion in a public hospital. Ann Plast Surg 1999; 42(4):396–401.
7. Pisarski GP, Mertens D, Warden GD, Neale HW. Tissue expander complications in the pediatric burn patient. Plast Reconstr Surg 1998; 102(4):1008–1012.
8. Berton RR. Applying what burn survivors have to say to future therapeutic interventions. Burns 1997; 23(1):50–54.

31

Reconstruction of the Perineum and Genitalia

LAWRENCE J. GOTTLIEB
University of Chicago, Chicago, Illinois, USA

MARK A. GREVIOUS
University of Illinois, Chicago, Illinois, USA

I. INTRODUCTION

Burn injury of the genitalia and perineum, like burns of the face, hands, and feet, may result in physical and psychosocial scars and dysfunction out of proportion to the percentage of total body surface area injured (TBSA). Hence, the American Burn Association classifies these burns as major burns. Recovery from perineal burns is a difficult physical and mental challenge. The physical pain that wound care entails is obvious to the most casual observer. Likewise, the psychologic consequences of these injuries should not be overlooked and cannot be overemphasized. The repetitive invasion of the patients' most personal anatomic region tends to erode their sense of modesty as well as self-respect. Fear of sexual dysfunction or unattractiveness may cause depression, increasing the likelihood of the patient's fear of dysfunction coming to fruition. In fact, 25% of all adult burn patients experience a loss of libido or orgasmic dysfunction (1). Direct injury to the genitalia increases the number of patients who have sexual dysfunction to a significantly higher level.

Most burns of the genitalia and perineum are superficial flame or scald injuries. Isolated burn injuries to the genitalia and perineum are infrequent and usually the result of a child spilling hot food or liquid on themselves (Fig. 31.1). These burns are usually partial-thickness injuries. Deep perineal burns are usually associated with either large TBSA flame burns or immersion injury. Rarely, high-voltage electrical injuries cause devastating injuries to this area. Most of the severe genital injuries occur in males, for the anatomy of the female genitalia does not leave it as vulnerable to significant injury. The best treatment of any burn scar deformity is prevention by appropriate care of the acute injury. The management of burns of the genitalia and perineum can be especially challenging to the burn care team. The high bacterial load endogenous to the region as well as its unique anatomy necessitates meticulous and knowledgeable pre- and postoperative care.

II. ACUTE CARE

Although certain qualities of the perineum and genitalia require special care, wound management in this region is similar to that in other areas of the body. Minimization

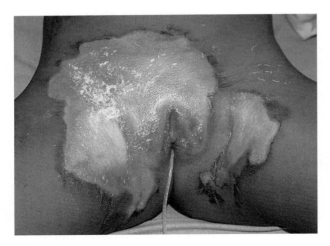

Figure 31.1 Scald burn secondary to hot liquid spill.

of scars and deformity requires adherence to burn wound management principles.

Superficial burns are most efficiently managed non-operatively with topical antimicrobials, maintaining bacteriologic balance ($<10^5$ organisms/g of tissue), while epithelialization occurs. Moderately deep partial-thickness injuries are more likely to heal with unfavorable scars, therefore consideration should be given to early closure with a biologic dressing (Fig. 31.2). Small deep wounds of the perineum and buttocks should also be treated with topical antimicrobials, taking advantage of the fact that perineal wounds tend to rapidly contract and close rapidly by secondary intention. Larger deep wounds are

treated with tangential excision and immediate split-thickness skin graft coverage. The grafts may be meshed to accommodate the irregular contour of the region, but should not be expanded if possible. The perioperative management of the grafts (whether done acutely or during reconstruction) is crucial. The grafts require a well-vascularized wound bed in bacteriologic balance, stabilization with sutures, staples, or fibrin glue, and prevention of postoperative shearing. Nylon mesh secured over the graft may help to prevent shearing. If there is adequate uninjured skin surrounding the wound a vacuum assisted closure (VAC) device may be placed over the graft to assist in stabilization. Postoperatively, legs should be positioned in abduction for wounds that traverse the groin crease.

Concerns regarding contamination by stool is unnecessary and unwarranted if the wound bed is devoid of nonviable tissue, well vascularized, and adequately dressed. A diverting colostomy is unnecessary in most cases.

Treatment of burns of the penis is similar in many respects to that of hand burns. Superficial burns may be treated with topical antimicrobials or biologic dressings. Deep circumferential burns of the penis should be decompressed via escharotomy when vascular compromise is suspected (Fig. 31.3). Tangential excision and grafting should be performed when the patient is hemodynamically

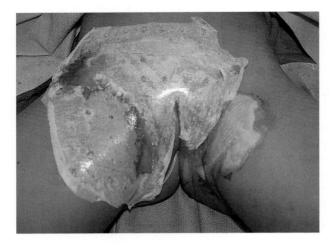

Figure 31.2 Burn injury debrided with a combination of manual dermabrasion and tangential excision. Mons area and labia majora closed with synthetic biologic dressing (Biobrane); right thigh required grafting. The graft was secured with fibrin glue (Tisseal) and the Biobrane was secured with tissue adhesive (Indermil).

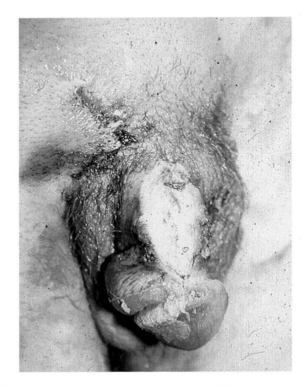

Figure 31.3 Escharotomy of circumferential burn of the penis secondary to an electrical injury.

able to tolerate the procedure. Although meshed grafts are frequently used in the rest of the perineum, nonmeshed grafts are preferred on the penis in order to obtain a superior aesthetic result. If possible, efforts should be made to salvage the superficial fascia (Dartos) of the penis with its rich venous network. This loose areolar layer is analogous to the areolar layer on the dorsum of the hand. If it is preserved, there is little problem with distal swelling, wound contraction, and subsequent contracture following grafting. With more limited wounds or scars, the unique laxity of penile skin enables up to one-quarter of the circumference of the penis to be excised and closed primarily [Fig. 31.4(B)].

Empiric circumcision, discarding nonburned foreskin, should never be done because this skin may be important for acute closure or for subsequent reconstruction. Acute swelling of the foreskin may require a dorsal (or ventral) slit for decompression and access to the glans. Deep burns of the uncircumcised penis usually spare the inner surface of the prepuce. Even with full thickness burns of the rest of the penile skin, a flap of this inner prepuce skin may be used to resurface the debrided penile shaft [Fig. 31.5(A–D)].

Most burns of the scrotum may be treated with debridement of eschar and application of topical antimicrobials. Relatively large wounds will rapidly contract with almost imperceptible scars. Occasionally, grafting is required for full-thickness loss of large areas. In the event of testicular exposure, the testicles should be sutured together for stability and covered with split-thickness skin grafts. Alternatively, if the medial thigh skin is uninjured, the testicles may be temporarily buried under the thigh skin.

Deforming intrinsic contractures of the penis, scrotum, or vulva is rare in superficial injuries; yet extrinsic contractures or webbing across the perineum and groin is a common result of extensive perineal and groin injuries (Fig. 31.6). As in other areas of the body, prevention of contracture is superior to treatment. All patients with groin and perineal wounds should have their lower extremities maintained in abduction. Compression garments and night abduction splinting should be considered for 6 months to 2 years as prophylaxis against contracture formation. Custom foam or elastomer forms may be required under the elastic garments to provide adequate contact with the skin.

III. RECONSTRUCTION

Burn scar deformities of the perineum can be categorized as quantitative or qualitative. Quantitative skin surface area loss is usually due to wound contraction, since most contractures represent a net loss of functional tissue. An example of a more severe quantitative change is loss of all or part of the external genitalia. However, relatively few perineal burn injuries result in major quantitative deformities.

Qualitative skin changes include alterations in texture, pigmentation, moisture, and pliability. These qualitative changes should not be minimized, since problems with sexuality and body image may be produced by these skin alterations. In addition, surface irregularities and dryness may cause the patient to be unable to maintain hygiene and lead to the development of recurrent or persistent skin irritation.

A sympathetic, caring, and understanding burn care team, family, and sexual partner will do much to help these patients accept their qualitative burn scar deformities. Repeated discussion concerning realistic expectations of sexual function, appearance, and reconstructive options is important, beginning early in the acute phase and continuing throughout the reconstruction.

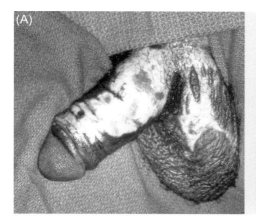 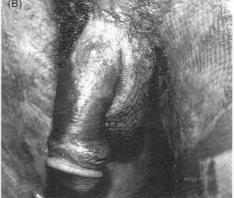

Figure 31.4 (A) Full-thickness burn to dorsum of penis and lateral aspect of scrotum. (B) Distal portion of burn excised and closed primarily. Proximal portion of burn tangentially excised and grafted. Note healing of scrotal burn by contraction.

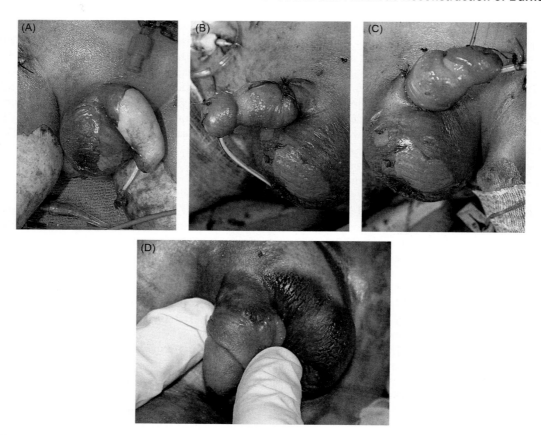

Figure 31.5 (A) Full-thickness scald burn to penis, sparing the inner surface of prepuce. (B and C) After excision of burned shaft and outer prepuce skin, the unburned inner layer of prepuce was used to resurface the shaft. (D) Two weeks postoperative of inner prepuce flap.

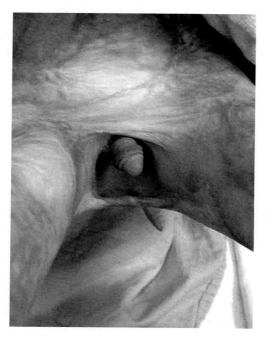

Figure 31.6 Severe webbing of perineum in patient who sustained a 98% burn.

Discussion of surgical intervention of the qualitative and quantitative deformities should include the nature of the deformity, the available options, the realistic expectations of both the patient and the surgeon, and an understanding of the limitations of reconstructive techniques. Patients need to understand that scars cannot be erased. The goal is to exchange an unacceptable scar for a more acceptable one.

The reconstruction of qualitative deformities is perhaps the most difficult challenge in reconstructive surgery. These deformities may not impair function, as such, but instead damage self-image. For example, many perineal scald burns in children are the result of child neglect or abuse. The presence of a "ring sign," which is pathognomonic of abuse, brands these patients for life (Fig. 31.7). The scar is a constant painful reminder of the initial trauma and its alteration of body image. Qualitative reconstruction attempts to restore the altered body image.

Successful intervention for qualitative deformities generally entails resurfacing the entire burn scar area. The desired result may be difficult to obtain because of the presence of limited normal adjacent skin, unacceptable donor

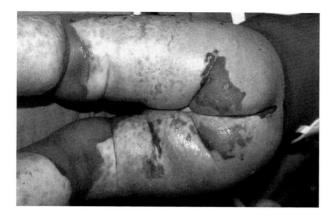

Figure 31.7 "Ring sign." Area of buttock not burned due to the child being forcibly held against the bottom of the tub. This burn distribution is pathognomonic of child abuse.

deformities from available flap or full-thickness graft sites, and the inability of split-thickness grafts to accomplish the desired goals. When the undesirable scar is not extensive and is adjacent to adequate normal skin, tissue expansion is a reasonable way to obtain qualitatively normal skin with little or no donor site deformity. However, expanders in the perineal region (especially in burn patients) tend to have an inordinate amount of complications from infection and erosion (2). In addition, it is mechanically difficult for a patient to tolerate the "bulge" of an expander in the perineum, which interferes with walking, sitting, and normal daily activities. Despite these limitations, when expansion techniques are successful they usually produce satisfactory results. An alternative to expansion of adjacent flaps is expansion of distant flaps or donor sites for full-thickness grafts. This allows for large, good quality full-thickness skin grafts with minimal donor site morbidity.

Correction of quantitative deformities is frequently straightforward even when the deformity is severe. The goals and expectations of both physician and patient are more easily accomplished. Tightness, webbing, and distortion of the external genitalia are all due to a relative lack of skin. Vulvar injuries with subsequent webbing may compromise normal sexual activity and cause difficulty with urination. Webbing can be corrected with any one of the many ways available to lengthen a line. If there is adjacent, relatively pliable skin, then one of the transposition (Z-plasty) or advancement (V-Y) techniques may be used [Fig. 31.8(B)]. This works best if uninjured skin can be interposed to "break up" the scar contracture. When normal adjacent skin is not available and the contracture is totally surrounded by inelastic scarred skin, geometric flaps alone rarely accomplish the goals of complete release. Frequently, additional skin grafts are required to close residual open areas if a full contracture release is to be obtained. Severe contractures can only be released by incising (or excising) the contracting scar band (Fig. 31.9). These large defects require resurfacing with grafts or flaps. Contractures will invariably recur if the resultant defect following release is closed with split-thickness skin grafts. If flaps or full thickness grafts are not available, use of a dermal substitute (such as Integra) should be considered.

The ideal time for contracture release is after active contraction is complete and maximum scar maturation has occurred. This usually requires at least 6 months and even up to 2 years after injury. Occasionally, early contracture release may need to be performed because of severe functional disability.

Intrinsic contractures of the penis may result from injury and subsequent scarring of Dartos fascia, Buck's fascia, the tunica albuginea, or the corpora itself. The

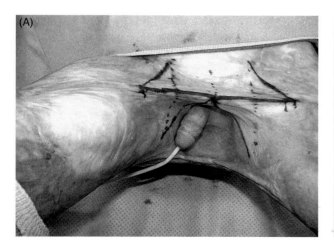
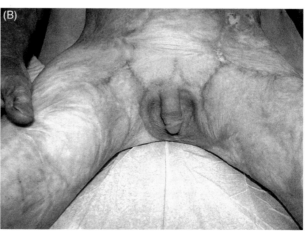

Figure 31.8 (A) Double opposing Z-plasty designed on groin web contracture. (B) Flaps of double opposing Z-plasty transposed to release contracture.

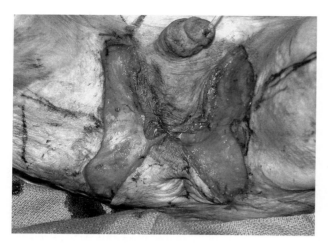

Figure 31.9 Large open wound after incisional release of posterior contracture.

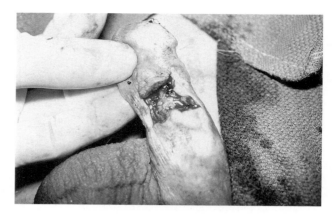

Figure 31.11 Scar released by incision allowing penis to straighten. The resultant defect was closed with a full-thickness skin graft.

resultant scar bends the penis during erection (3) (Fig. 31.10). Treatment is similar to that of secondary hypospadias repairs or Peyronie's disease (4). The basic principle is to release the scar tissue by surgical incision (Fig. 31.11) or, in selected cases, excision. The reconstruction depends on the layer injured. If it is the superficial fascia (along with the overlying skin), then transposition flaps or skin grafts are adequate. If the contracture is due to an injury or deficiency of Buck's fascia or the tunica albuginea, then a dermal graft may be necessary to reconstruct this layer (5). Dermal grafts need to be covered by Byars' flaps or a local flap, depending on the extent of scarring. A Nesbit tuck procedure of the tunica on the convex side of a penile bend may be helpful in some patients with lateral bending (6).

Simple extrinsic contractures of the penis may lend themselves to Z-plasty or surgical release and grafting. In more severe cases the entire penis may be buried

beneath a mass of scar, appearing severely foreshortened or absent. These cases are usually the result of deep partial-thickness burns in children that were allowed to heal secondarily. The penis retracts into the pubic fat and the skin becomes tethered proximally. The loose areola layer is usually intact but may need to be released due to secondary shortening. After aggressive surgical release there is almost always a large raw surface area of the penile shaft (Fig. 31.12). This should be grafted and dressed with a compressive dressing, maintaining its released length.

When scarring involves the urethral meatus, stricture occurs. In mild cases, the patient or parents can be taught to dilate the meatus with an appropriately sized catheter. In more severe cases, Z-plasty or other interdigitation of adjacent skin into the constricting band is necessary. Distal ventral urethral loss secondary to deep burns and/or pressure from Foley catheters is corrected using

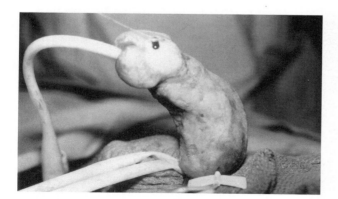

Figure 31.10 Intraoperative artificial erection. After applying Penrose tourniquet to base of penis, saline is injected into corpus with a 23-gauge butterfly catheter.

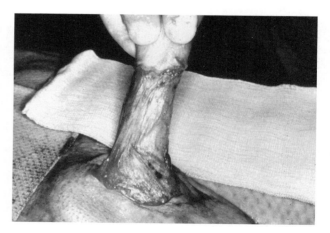

Figure 31.12 Released penis requiring skin graft to entire shaft.

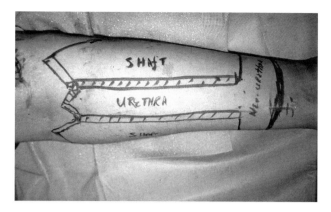

Figure 31.13 Neurosensory radial forearm free flap marked on forearm.

the principles of distal hypospadias repairs (7). Modifications are necessary, depending on the availability of foreskin and the amount of adjacent scarring.

Complete loss of the penis usually requires the creation of a perineal urethrostomy. Considerations of penile reconstruction should await a closed wound and scar maturation. The first reconstruction of the penis was reported in 1936 (8). The history of total penile reconstruction has paralleled the history of flap development in plastic and reconstructive surgery. The multistaged tube pedicle flap reconstruction has given way to the axial pattern skin flaps and muscle flaps (9–11). These procedures have subsequently yielded to the state-of-the-art neurosensory fasciocutaneous free flap (16). Ideally, the reconstructed phallus should fulfill several criteria to be functionally and psychologically satisfying.

It should be aesthetically acceptable with a shaft of adequate length and simulation of a glans. It should have close to normal tactile and erogenous sensitivity. The girth should be adequate for placement of a prosthesis for sexual function, but not too large to preclude intromission. It should contain a neourethra that has the potential to be anastomosed to the patient's residual native urethra. The patient should be able to stand to void through a meatus in the glans (12).

The reconstructive technique that best fulfills all these criteria is the neurosensory radial forearm flap (Fig. 31.13). By connecting the antebrachial cutaneous nerves of the flap to the native penile or pudendal nerves, this flap offers the possibility of both erogenous and protective sensations. Providing protective sensation minimizes the chance of pressure necrosis from the prosthesis placed for erectile function (13). The main drawback of this flap is the skin grafted forearm donor site (Fig. 31.14). Some burn patients may not be candidates for radial forearm flap penile reconstruction due to injury of both forearms. In this situation, although perhaps less optimal in sensation, girth and quality of urethra, alternative methods of penile reconstruction should be considered (14,15).

REFERENCES

1. Andreason NJ, Norris AS. Long term adjustment and adaptation mechanism in severely burned adults. J Nerv Ment Dis 1972; 154:352–362.
2. Gottlieb LJ, Parsons RW, Krizek TJ. The use of tissue expansion techniques in burn reconstruction. J Burn Care Rehab 1986; 7:234–237.
3. Gittes RF, McLaughlin AP. Injection technique to induce penile erection. Urology 1974; 4:473.
4. Horton CE, Devine CJ Jr. Peyronie's disease. Plast Reconstr Surg 1973; 52:503–510.
5. Devine CJ Jr, Horton CE. Surgical treatment of Peyronie's disease with a dermal graft. J Urol 1974; 111:44.
6. Nesbit RM. Congenital curvature of the phallus: a report of three cases with description of correction operation. J Urol 1965; 93:230–232.
7. McDougal WS, Peterson HD, Pruitt BA, Persky L. The thermally injured perineum. J Urol 1979; 121:320–324.
8. Bogoras NA. Ueber die volle plastiche wieder Herstellung eines zum Koitus fahigen Penis. Zentralbl Chir 1936; 63:1271.
9. Gilles H, Harrison RJ. Congenital absence of the penis. Br J Plast Surg 1948; 1:89.
10. Kaplan L, Wesser D. A rapid method for constructing a functional sensitive penis. Br J Plast Surg 1971; 24:342–344.
11. Hester JR, Hill HL, Jurkiewicz MJ. One-stage reconstruction of the penis. Br J Plast Surg 1978; 31:279–285.

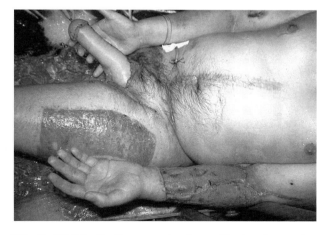

Figure 31.14 Penile reconstruction with its donor sites. Forearm donor site was closed with a skin graft harvested from thigh.

12. Cherup L, Gottlieb LJ, Zachary LS, Levine LA. The sensate functional total phallic reconstruction. Plast Surg Forum 1989; 58:25–27.

13. Levine LA, Zachary LS, Gottlieb LJ. Prosthesis placement after total phallic reconstruction. J Urol 1993; 149:593–598.

14. Shenaq SM, Dinh TA. Total penile and urethral reconstruction with an expanded sensate lateral arm flap: case report. J Reconstr Microsurg 1989; 5(3):245–248.

15. Sadove RC, Sengezer M, McRoberts JW, Wells MD. One-stage total penile reconstruction with a free sensate osteocutaneous fibula flap. Plast Reconstr Surg 1993; 93:1314–1323.

16. Chang T, Hwang W. Forearm flap in one stage reconstruction of the penis. Plast Reconstr Surg 1984; 74:251–258.

32

Management of the Acutely Burned Hand

ROBERT L. SHERIDAN

Shriners Hospital for Children and Massachusetts General Hospital, Boston, Massachusetts, USA

I. INTRODUCTION

Survival after serious burns has improved dramatically over the past 20 years (1). However, despite generally satisfying long-term quality of life, many such patients will have significant lingering physical disability, much of which can be traced to compromised hand function (2). If optimal function is to be recovered after a serious burn, proper acute care of the injured hand is essential.

Before the modern era, hand burns were managed by application of various salves or topical medications while necrotic tissues liquefied (3). With this management, the outcome was a healed wound if the injury was superficial, a closed but distorted hand if the injury was deep dermal, and a chronic open wound if the injury was full thickness. Although early excision of localized deep hand burns was reported 60 years ago, most hand burns were managed with topical antibacterial agents awaiting eschar separation and spontaneous healing until the 1980s, when the improved outcomes with early surgery were reported (4).

II. PREOPERATIVE EVALUATION

A thorough initial evaluation is essential to overall management. Important points of history include the mechanism of injury (particularly to exclude other hand trauma), the nature of the burning agent (including temperature and contact time), and prior hand injuries. A careful physical exam should then be done, even in massively burned patients. Examination should include assessment of wound depth, circumferential components, associated injuries, and soft tissue perfusion. Radiographs are done if indicated by injury mechanism. Injuries of abuse should be suspected with sharply demarcated scalds or deep dorsal contact injuries (Fig. 32.1).

Accurate determination of burn depth can be difficult early after injury. Several diagnostic tools, such as laser doppler, ultrasound, intravenous fluorescein, and indocyanine green have been proposed as aids in diagnosing burn depth, but none are more accurate than the eye of an experienced examiner (5). Differentiation can usually be made between superficial burns, deep dermal or

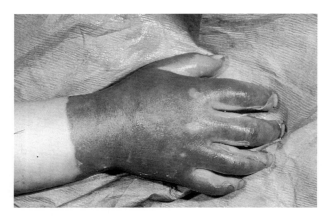

Figure 32.1 Injuries of abuse should be suspected with sharply demarcated scalds, as demonstrated here, or deep dorsal contact injuries.

full-thickness injuries, and injuries involving extensors, joint capsule, or bone. This determination is important as it facilitates prompt operation in those with other than superficial injuries, avoiding the functional problems associated with nonoperative management of deep dermal and full-thickness injuries.

Some hand burns can be reasonably managed in the outpatient setting (6). This management plan should include a daily dressing change with would cleansing, inspection, and passive ranging. Adequate monitoring and follow-up are essential. The costs associated with suboptimal outpatient management, including infection and contractures, make inpatient management cost-effective if adequate outpatient care seems unlikely.

A critical part of the initial care of hand burn is to ensure that soft tissues are well perfused. This is an area in which early surgical intervention can make a tremendous difference to ultimate outcome. Hands at risk for ischemia include those with circumferential or near-circumferential burns, those with very deep burns, and any injuries involving high or intermediate-range voltage. The hand should be dressed so that it can be examined easily, and a specific monitoring plan should be ordered and followed. It is important to look at signs more subtle than the loss of palpable flow in named arteries at the wrist. Mean arterial pressure in the central system is three times higher than capillary pressure, and blood flow may be maintained in these larger vessels when flow in distal soft tissues is impaired. If the hand is warm, soft, and has pulsatile flow detectable by doppler in the palmar arch and digital vessels and a normal transmission pulse oximetry signal at the distal digit, then flow is adequate. As flow is progressively impaired, the hand will become firm, cool, and doppler flow and oximetry signal will be lost. Voluntary motion will become difficult and the hand will assume a clawed position. At this point,

decompression should be performed to prevent otherwise avoidable ischemic injury. Soft tissue pressure measurement $>30 \, cmH_2O$ support the decision to perform escharotomy, but are generally not necessary if serial examinations suggest diminished perfusion.

III. SURGICAL OPTIONS

Should the hand be decompressed and how? Should the wound be grafted? When should the wound be grafted? With what should the wound be closed? What should be done if burns involve joint and bone? These are some of the questions that must be addressed when considering surgical options.

Prompt recognition and correction of impending ischemia secondary to subeschar or intracompartmental edema is essential to a good outcome. As noted earlier, a clear monitoring plan for hands at risk should be set up with the bedside care providers. Once evolving ischemia is suspected, prompt escharotomy and/or fasciotomy is indicated.

Should the wound be grafted? Surgery is indicated for any deep dermal or full-thickness hand burn that will not promptly heal within 3 weeks. Generally, this need is apparent to an experienced examiner within 5 days of injury. The skin of the dorsal hand is much thinner than that of the palmar hand. It is quite common for circumferential hand burns to heal very well over their palmar aspect, yet require grafting on the dorsal surface.

When should the wound be grafted? The patient's overall condition and wound size are important consideration in the decision about operation. When caring for patients with very large burns, priority is given to maximum initial surface area wound excision and closure with skin grafts and the hands are autografted later in the patient's course. Excision and allografting of hand burns while awaiting availability of suitable autograft can be useful in selected patients, but is not necessary if unexcised hands undergo daily ranging and antideformity positioning. There is general agreement that earlier surgery is associated with a better functional result and a decreased need for reconstructive procedures; however, patients with large injuries in whom the hands are definitively closed later in the hospitalization while awaiting autografting. Good outcomes in this setting depend on aggressive daily hand therapy.

Only about 15% of palmar burns require grafting, as the palmar skin is much thicker than the dorsal skin. When the palm is deeply burned and loss of the palmar concavity and range are at risk, the hand is splinted with the palm extended to minimize contracture.

With what should the wound be closed? Practical options include split-thickness autograft, full-thickness autograft, and groin or abdominal flaps. Split-thickness sheet autograft, generally thick, is the optimal cover for most hand burns. Full-thickness grafts are ideally reserved for palmar surface burns, particularly deep wounds of limited extent or reconstructive operations during the acute recovery phase. Groin and abdominal flaps can be very useful when managing isolated fourth-degree injuries, but are rarely needed in other circumstances.

What should be done if the burns are fourth degree, involving tendon, joint, and bone? Is digital amputation indicated? If tissue loss is circumferential, amputation usually is required. However, a common pattern is viable volar tissue with very deep dorsal injury including exposure of burned bone. Many of these digits can be salvaged.

IV. INTRAOPERATIVE CONSIDERATIONS

Surgical treatment of hand burns has become more widely practiced sine the 1970s (3,7). It has become increasingly clear that allowing such injuries to heal over the course of may weeks by contraction will result in very poor long-term results (8). However, the operations need to be performed well and carefully if they are to be effective. Surgical treatment begins with decompression in the face of acute ischemia.

A. Technique of Escharotomy

Escharotomy should be done for decreasing perfusion suggested by decreasing temperature, increasing firmness, decreased capillary filling, and decreasing pulsatile perfusion in the superficial palmar arch and digital vessels as detected by dopper and transmission oximetry. With coagulating electrocautery, longitudinally oriented medial and lateral incisions are made through eschar on the arm and forearm (the former being made anterior to the ulnar styloid to avoid injury to the ulnar nerve), stopping at the metacarpophalangeal joints of the first and fifth digits. Unburned skin or second-degree burn should not be incised as this may result in deformity that will require later treatment [Fig. 32.2(A) and (B)]. The hand is then re-examined for perfusion prior to performing digital escharotomies. Often, blood flow is enhanced adequately by decompression of the arm, making digital escharotomies unnecessary.

The efficacy and safety of digital escharotomies is debated. One study demonstrated a reduced incidence of amputation if digital escharotomies were done on circumferentially burned digits (9). However, particularly in small children, improperly performed finger escharotomies can cause significant injury and are ideally only done by those experienced with this procedure. When

digital perfusion remains marginal or inadequate despite decompression of the arm and forearm, escharotomies of full-thickness burns of the digits should be performed [Fig. 32.2(C)]. Incisions are carefully made with pinpoint electrocautery between the neurovascular bundle and the extensors, avoiding both structures. A single longitudinal incision is made on the radial aspect of the thumb and the ulnar aspect of the digits. This places the incisions on the side of the digit with the least functional importance should the digital nerve be exposed by separation of edematous tissue after escharotomy. The central digital incision can be extended proximally onto the dorsum of the hand between the metacarpals to enhance decompression. Meticulous hemostasis is maintained throughout the procedure and the success of decompression is documented by Doppler examination. Digital escharotomies do not result in injury to the extensor mechanism or digital vessels when properly performed.

Escharotomy can generally de done using aseptic technique at the bedside or in the emergency department. Intubated patients are managed with a brief intravenous anesthetic. Others are treated with conscious sedation supplemented with subeschar injections of local anesthetics. Some patients will require a general anesthetic in the operating room to have this procedure performed properly and humanely, especially if digital escharotomy is needed.

B. Technique of Fasciotomy

Edema within the fascial compartments of the forearm and hand are seen following high-voltage electrical injury or exceptionally deep thermal injury. These procedures should ideally be done in the operating room. Upper-extremity fasciotomy may include volar and dorsal decompression, carpal tunnel release, and dorsal hand fasciotomy. A curvilinear incision is ideal for volar exposure of the compartments of the forearm [Fig. 32.3(A)]. This approach allows one to gain access to all individual muscle bundles in the volar forearm and decompress the carpal tunnel through a contiguous incision, and creates a well-vascularized flap of skin that will maintain coverage over the median nerve at the wrist upon completion of the fasciotomy [Fig. 32.3(B)]. When needed, straight linear incisions are adequate for exposure of the dorsal aspect of the forearm [Fig. 32.3(C)]. Intermetacarpal incisions on the hand allow one to decompress the intrinsic muscles of the hand if this is necessary [Fig. 32.3(D)].

C. Techniques of Excision and Grafting

Deep partial- and full-thickness hand burns generally require layered excision and autografting. These procedures are ideally done after exsanguination of the extremity with

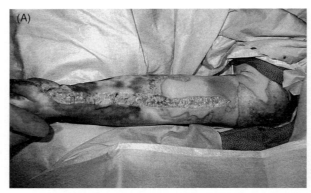

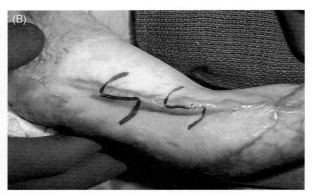

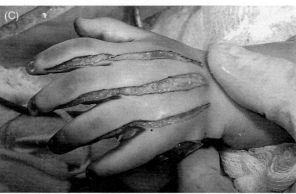

Figure 32.2 (A) When performing escharotomy, unburned skin or second-degree burn should not be incised. (B) This deformity resulting from escharotomy placed in unburned skin required correction (using multiple Z-plasties). (C) When digital perfusion remains marginal or inadequate despite decompression of the arm and forearm, escharotomies of full-thickness burns of the digits should be then performed. Incisions are carefully made with pinpoint electrocautery between the neurovascular bundle and the extensors, avoiding both structures. A single axial incision on the radial aspect of the thumb and the ulnar aspect of the digits is done. The central digital incisions can be extended proximally onto the dorsum of the hand between the metacarpals to enhance decompression.

an elastic wrap and inflation of a pneumatic tourniquet on the arm to decrease blood loss. The excision is done sequentially until a bed of viable tissue is reached. Viable tissue is recognized by a pearly white moist dermis or the presence of bright subcutaneous fat without thrombosed small vessels or extravascular hemoglobin [Fig.32.4(A)]. Recognition of viable tissue in an exsanguinated extremity with a proximal pneumatic tourniquet is an acquired skill that greatly facilitates low blood loss excisions. The hands are then placed in a snug wrap of epinephrine soaked gauze prior to deflation of the pneumatic tourniquet. Definitive hemostasis is secured with judicious use of pinpoint electrocautery after some time is allowed to elapse for spontaneous hemostasis (this is a good time to harvest autograft). Hands are close with sheet autograft, except in the setting of massive injuries, and grafts are secured with interrupted fine absorbable suture. Grafted hands are then covered with a gently compressive gauze wrap and placed in a thermoplastic splint in functional position or may be left open and held in such a splint with hooks glued to the fingernails which are then pulled into the splint by elastic

bands. A compressive gauze dressing seems to be better tolerated by children. The hands are elevated and immobilized for 7 days prior to reinstituting passive and active hand therapy. Skeletal immobilization has been advocated, but thermoplastic splints suffice in most.

D. Techniques to Salvage Length with Fourth-Degree Injury

In the presence of fourth-degree injury, involving underlying extensor mechanism, joint capsule, and bone, management can be more complex and less satisfying. The ultimate outcome is largely dependent on the degree of initial injury, although most patients can be expected to have the ability to perform activities of daily living. Patients with small overall surface area burns are candidates for early debridement with groin or abdominal flap coverage (10). In those with larger injuries, in whom flap coverage is impractical, maintenance of a functional position with splinting and therapy is critically important to an optimal long-term outcome. A common pattern is deep dorsal

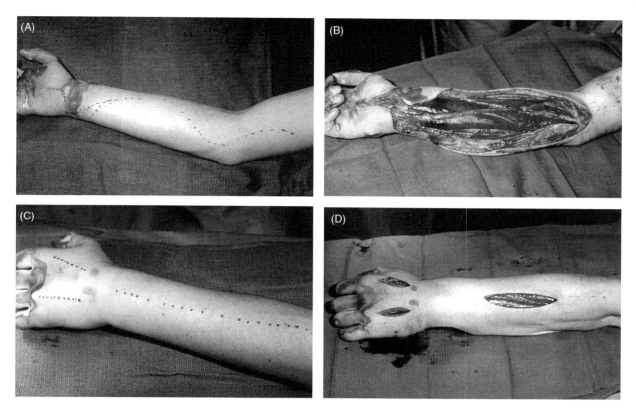

Figure 32.3 (A) A curvilinear incision is ideal for volar exposure of the forearm compartments. (B) This approach allows one to gain access to all individual muscle bundles in the volar forearm, allows one to decompress the carpal tunnel through a contiguous incision, and creates a well-vascularized flap of skin that will maintain coverage over the median nerve at the wrist upon completion of the fasciotomy. (C) On the dorsal aspect of the arm, straight linear incisions provide excellent exposure. (D) Intermetacarpal incisions on the hand allow one to decompress the intrinsic muscles of the hand.

burn with exposure of the proximal interphalangael joints and dorsal phalanges with viable volar tissue. If these wounds are kept moist and clean, and proper position maintained, often the avascular tissue will cover with granulation tissue, which can then be autografted with an acceptable result. Sometimes this process can be facilitated by very carefully debriding off remnants of burned cortical bone [Fig. 32.4(B)]. Autografting is done wherever possible, and exposed joints and bones are allowed to granulate and subsequently are autografted. When autografting is subsequently done, unstable open joints are maintained in a position of function with axially placed Kirchner wires. It is important to prevent desiccation of these wounds with wet dressings or allograft. Joints which remain unstable after coverage is achieved are later fused by open arthrodesis. High priority is placed on maximizing digital length.

E. Palmar Burns

Most palmar burns will heal without surgery, given the thickness of the palmar stratum corneum. Palmar burns that require grafting are usually covered with thick sheet autograft if the defect is large and full-thickness grafts if the defect is small [Fig. 32.5(A)]. Grafts are secured in place with tie-over dressings crafted such that the size of the palmar wound is at a maximum. After 7–10 days, these dressings are removed and passive and active therapy is started. Especially in young children, contractures may evolve over the palm and across the volar metacarpophalangeal and interphalangeal joints. When recalcitrant to therapy, these are ideally addressed with early release and grafting [Fig. 32.5(B)]. Instep grafts have been advocated for aesthetic reasons, but functional results with full-thickness or thick split-thickness grafts are generally excellent [Fig. 32.5(C)].

V. PITFALLS

Common pitfalls in the management of acute hand burns include: (1) inadequate decompression, (2) inadequate ranging and splinting, (3) inadequate excision, (4) inadequate PIP coverage and the burn boutonnière deformity, (5) inadequate early rehabilitation, and (6) inadequate early reconstruction.

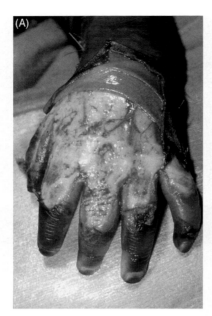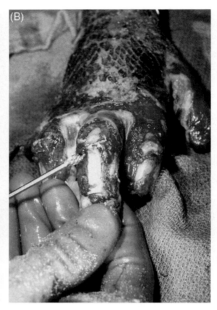

Figure 32.4 (A) Layered excision is done under tourniquet until a bed of viable tissue is reached. Viable tissue is recognized by a pearly white moist dermis or the presence of bright subcutaneous fat without thrombosed small vessels or extravascular hemoglobin. Wounds are closed with sheet autograft. (B) A common pattern of fourth-degree hand burn is deep dorsal burn with exposure of the proximal interphalangeal joints and dorsal phalanges with viable volar tissue. If these wounds are kept moist and clean, and proper position maintained, often the avascular tissue will cover with granulation tissue which can then be autografted with an acceptable result. Sometimes this process can be facilitated by very carefully debriding off remnants of burned cortical bone. Autografting is done wherever possible, and exposed joints and bone are allowed to granulate and subsequently are autografted. When autografting is subsequently done, unstable open joints are maintained in a position of function with axially placed Kirchner wires.

Inadequate decompression occurs when distal ischemia is allowed to progress to the point that irrecoverable soft tissue injury occurs. It is essential to be sensitive to the clinical settings in which this will occur. These include near- or completely circumferential injury, particularly deep injury, and high-voltage injury. In these settings, ischemia is a result of subeschar edema or intracompartmental edema or a combination of both. It is essential to set up a monitoring regimen of hands at risk and to perform prompt escharotomy and/or fasciotomy when distal soft tissue perfusion is compromised.

Inadequate ranging and splinting will result in the "clawed hand" or intrinsic minus deformity, even in the absence of deep hand injury (Fig. 32.6). This deformity, which is difficult to correct, can be prevented by taking each joint through a full range of passive motion each day with resting splinting in the position of function: the metacarpophalangeal joints at 70°–90° of flexion the interphalyangeal joints in extension, the wrist at 20° of extension and the first webspace open. Special attention should be paid to the firth finger, as it is particularly prone to contractures that result in fixed interphalangeal joint flexion and rotation (Fig. 32.7). When established, this can only be corrected operatively.

Inadequate excision is a pitfall in any acute burn operation, as it is the most common reason for graft failure and often results in secondary infection. In the hand, such failures of early closure may compromise the ability to participate in early therapy and possibly compromise long-term outcome or delay full recovery. Inadequate excision is a particular risk as most of these operations are done after inflation of a proximal pneumatic tourniquet. Substantial experience is required to ensure adequate excision of nonviable material using this technique.

Inadequate proximal interphalangeal (PIPJ) coverage is a common problem, particularly in young children, and can lead to the "burn boutonnière" deformity if not recognized and addressed early. This deformity can be very difficult to address subsequently (Fig. 32.8). The skin overlying this joint is thin and there is minimal soft tissue to protect the underlying extensor mechanism. If this is compromised by direct injury or subsequent desiccation and rupture, the collateral bands will migrate volar and the PIPJ will be brought into a position of flexion from which recovery may be impossible. In some case this unfortunate sequence of events can be prevented by ensuring prompt coverage of the PIPJ. If the depth of injury is such that the integrity of the overlying extensor mechanism is threatened, splinting in extension or

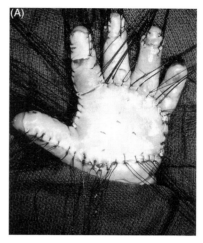

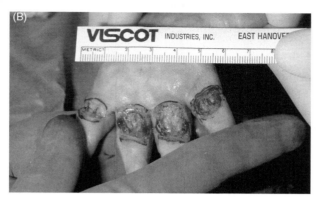

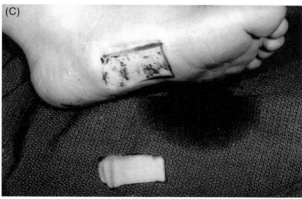

Figure 32.5 (A) Palmar burns that require grafting are usually covered with thick sheet autograft if the defect is large and full-thickness grafts if the defect is smaller. Grafts are secured in place with tie-over dressings. (B) When recalcitrant to therapy, these are ideally addressed with early release and grafting. (C) Instep grafts have been advocated for aesthetic reasons, but functional results with full-thickness or thick split-thickness grafts are generally excellent.

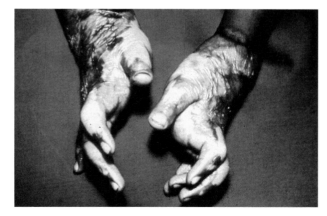

Figure 32.6 Inadequate ranging and splinting will result in the "clawed hand" or intrinsic minus deformity even in the absence of deep hand injury.

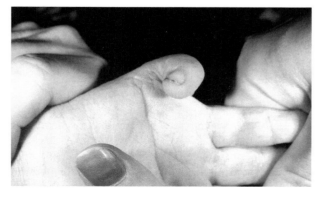

Figure 32.7 Special attention should be paid to the fifth finger, as it is particularly prone to contractures that result in fixed interphalangeal joint flexion and rotation.

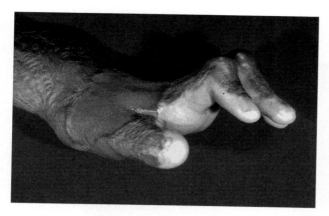

Figure 32.8 Inadequate proximal interphalangeal joint coverage is a common problem, particularly in young children, and can lead to the "burn boutonnière" deformity if not recognized and addressed early. This deformity can be very difficult to address subsequently.

placing and axial Kischner wire across the joint for 2–3 weeks may facilitate healing, with resulting stability. If the overlying extensor mechanism is frankly destroyed, with joint being open, sometimes a partially functional joint can be salvaged by Kischner wire fixation for 2–3 weeks, which may facilitate granulation tissue bridging the open joint which can subsequently be autografted. Such joint need to be closely watched in the weeks and months after recovery for the development of a "burn boutonnière" deformity. Reconstruction of the extensor apparatus in this situation is rarely successful. However, arthrodesis may provide a very functional result.

Close follow-up after initial discharge is essential to ensure that early rehabilitation and reconstruction are adequate. It is quite common for patients to lose range and function after their hand therapy is transferred from the experienced inpatient team to an outpatient therapist who may not be as familiar with burned hands. Monitoring this aspect of recovery is essential to facilitate early intervention.

VI. NURSING CONSIDERATIONS

During initial evaluation, a decision must be made about managing the patient as an inpatient or an outpatient (11). Daily dressing changes with wound inspection and passive ranging by an experienced examiner constitute ideal outpatient management. Patients with small superficial hand burns who have adequate home support and no other significant injuries are good candidates for outpatient management as long as they are able to maintain good follow-up. The complications associated with poor outpatient management, such as infection, contractures, and

pain, make inpatient management the cost-effective alternatives for all other patients.

Most dressing changes are done by nurses. Frequency is debated, but a daily change is generally considered reasonable. These are complex and important activities. The essential aspects of dressing changes are (1) pain and anxiety control, (2) emotional support, (3) would cleansing, (4) wound inspection, (5) passive ranging, (6) choice and application of topical agent, (7) ensuring splint fit, and (8) teaching.

Before any hand dressing can be changed, pain and anxiety must be adequately addressed. This is a complicated issue. The degree of pain and anxiety will vary widely from patient to patient and will vary from day to day in the same patient. Having a clear unit protocol helps a lot, but there is no pharmacologic substitute for patience and a caring manner (12). Dressings should be removed gently and only as fast as the patient can tolerate, after administration of any needed medication.

Even a burn that seems totally mundane to experienced staff is a major issue for the patient. A calm and caring attitude is better than most pain medications. Genuine support and patience are essential. Dressing changes should not be rushed.

Wounds should be gently cleansed of dried topical agent, loose debris, tattered blister remnants, and fibrinous exudate. This should be done gently using a wet technique. There is no place for rough blunt debridement as this will cause unnecessary pain and may disrupt fragile new epithelium, while being ineffective in removing real eschar. Clean intact blisters may be left alone as they will provide excellent pain control while the underlying dermis resurfaces.

After the dressing has been removed, the wound should be inspected for depth and signs suggesting infection. Increased swelling, tenderness, drainage, or malodor should prompt a consultation with the burn team and possible treatment for infection. Digital perfusion should be noted, looking for brisk capillary refill and warm digits. If the burn appears full thickness, the burn team should be consulted, as early surgery, particularly if it is inevitable, may truncate disability and improve functional outcome.

After the wound has been cleansed, it is ideal to take the hand through a range of motion, either by coaching the patient to perform it actively or by passive ranging. This will help to reduce edema and will help to ease rehabilitation when healing is complete. Ideally, this is repeated frequently by co-operative and motivated patients.

After this, a topical agent and a protective dressing should be applied. There is a wide choice or reasonable agents. Topical agents are applied to control pain, decrease vapor loss, prevent desiccation, and slow down bacterial growth. The agent chosen should be based on the experience of the individual practitioner. A protective dressing is then commonly applied, care being taken to prevent constriction. If splints are applied, ensuring proper splint fit is very important. Splints should maintain a proper position (see earlier) without applying undue pressure in any area.

Finally, it is essential that the patient and their family be taught about the burn and its plan of care in a clear and patient way. This may have to be repeated more than once. Taking the time to do this will help to optimize results by enhancing understanding and compliance. It will improve the patient's overall experience and can be a source of genuine satisfaction to the burn care provider.

VII. REHABILITATION ISSUES

Hand therapy is central to an optimal outcome, no mater how good the topical care and surgery (13). During resuscitation and initial stabilization, the hands are elevated to minimize edema and splinted in a functional position. The optimal position is debated, but consensus includes the interphalangeal joints in extension and the metarcarpophalangeal joints at 70°–90° of flexion to maximize collateral ligament length. The wrist is kept at about 20° or 30° of extension and the thumb in a neutral position with the first web space open. Splints must be custom fitted to ensure a proper fit and are placed within 24–48 h after injury. Hands with deep palmar burns are splinted in extension. Even when critically ill, it is advisable to passively range hands twice daily except during periods immediately after grafting. Active therapy is practiced as soon as practical. Continuous passive motion can be useful in selected patients, but an interested occupational therapist is more effective, particularly in children. Progressive active therapy, massage, and compression become increasingly important after the initial phase of healing is complete. Close follow-up in the burn clinic is important to ensure that ongoing therapy is adequate and any needed reconstructive procedures are done in a timely fashion.

It is quite common, especially in growing young children, for function to be compromised within the first one or two postinjury years, by one or more stereotypical hand contractures. It is ideal if these are identified and operated early, to ensure normal development and optimize long-term function. These typical contractures include dorsal web space contractures [Fig. 32.9(A)],

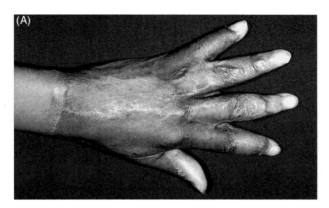
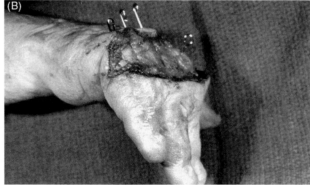
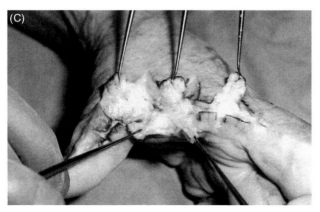

Figure 32.9   (A) Dorsal web space contracture. (B) Dorsal extension contracture. (C) First web space contracture.

dorsal extension contractures [Fig. 32.9(B)], first web space contractures [Fig. 32.9(C)], and digital flexion contractures, particularly of the fifth finger (Fig. 32.7). These deformities can be easily corrected, especially if addressed early. These operations should be done to ensure optimal function.

VIII. LONG-TERM OUTCOMES

There have been three studies published describing the long-term outcomes of serious hand burns. All have documented that acceptable function is achievable in most patients, but that this requires effective surgery and hand therapy.

In a 1985, functional results in 478 adults with 786 burned hands were reported (14). Long-term evaluation showed that early excision and immediate autografting of deep second-degree, mixed second- and third-degree, and third-degree full-thickness hand burns resulted in over 90% acceptable functional results. There were no significant differences in results in patients with superficial second-degree burns treated nonsurgically with early physical therapy compared with results in patients with deep second-degree, mixed second- and third-degree, and third-degree hand burns treated with early excision and grafting. No patient with fourth-degree burns had excellent to good results. Permanent damage was related to the extent of original injury to the extensor tendons and joint capsules.

In a more recent report, long-term functional results in 659 adults with 1047 burned hands were reported (15). The patients were both treated and followed up in a single facility and the injuries were divided into three injury and three functional categories. Injury category I (305 hands/47%) was superficial injuries that required no surgery. Injury category II (309 hands/48%) had deep dermal or full-thickness injuries that required grafting. Injury category III (32 hands/5%) had injuries that involved underlying tendon, joint capsule, and usually bone (fourth-degree injuries). The resulting function was classified using the rehabilitation frame of reference concept in which outcome is based on performance rather than on isolated components of function (16). Functional category A included those hands with normal or near-normal postinjury function. Functional category B hands had abnormal function, but were able to perform activities of daily living, although they might require the assistance of adaptive devices such as padded eating utensil handles. Functional category C hands could not perform activities of daily living even with the assistance of adaptive devices. The authors reported normal function in 97% of those with superficial injuries and 81% of those with deep dermal and full-thickness injuries requiring surgery. Although only 9% of those with injuries involving the extensor mechanism, joint capsule, or bone had normal functional outcomes, 90% were able to independently perform activities of daily living.

There has been only one report of long-term functional outcome in a large cohort of children with serious hand burns. In this study of 495 children with 698 acutely burned hands managed over a 10-year period, normal function was found in 85% of hands after third-degree burn (17). In those children with fourth-degree injuries involving bone, 70% had the ability to perform activities of daily living with the hand. Reconstructive hand surgery was required in 4.4% of second-degree burns, 32% of third-degree burns, and 65% of injuries involving underlying bone and tendon, this need being presumably greater than that in the adults.

Hand function is a central component of the quality of life in those suffering serious burns. These outcome studies have demonstrated that very acceptable functional outcomes are possible in those with serious hand burns, but only if the injuries are managed in a skillful and timely fashion.

REFERENCES

1. Rodeberg DA, Easter AJ, Washam MA, Housinger TA, Greenhalgh DG, Warden GD. Use of a helium-oxygen mixture in the treatment of postextubation stridor in pediatric patients with burns. J Burn Care Rehabil 1995; 16(5):476–480.

2. Moon RE. Treatment of diving emergencies. Crit Care Clin 1999; 15(2):429–456.

3. Braithwaite F. Treatment of dorsal burns of the hand. Br J Plast Surg 1949; 2:1–31.

4. Burke JF, Bondoc CC, Quinby WC Jr, Remensnyder JP. Primary surgical management of the deeply burned hand. Trauma 1976; 16(8):593–598.

5. Heimbach D, Engrav L, Grube B, Marvin J. Burn depth: a review. World J Surg 1992; 16(1):10–15.

6. Coffee T, Yurko L, Fratianne RB. Mixing inpatient with outpatient care: establishing an outpatient clinic on a burn unit. J Burn Care Rehabil 1992; 13(5):587–589.

7. Levine BA, Sirinek KR, Peterson HD, Pruitt BA Jr. Efficacy of tangential excision and immediate autografting of deep second-degree burns of the hand. J Trauma 1979; 19(9):670–673.

8. Goodwin CW, Maguire MS, McManus WF, Pruitt BA Jr. Prospective study of burn wound excision of the hands. J Trauma 1983; 23(6):510–517.

9. Salisbury RE, Taylor JW, Levine NS. Evaluation of digital escharotomy in burned hands. Plast Reconstr Surg 1976; 58(4):440–443.

10. Hanumadass M, Kagan R, Matsuda T. Early coverage of deep hand burns with groin flaps. J Trauma 1987; 27(2):109–114.

11. Mertens DM, Jenkins ME, Warden GD. Outpatient burn management. Nurs Clin North Am 1997; 32(2): 343–364.

12. Sheridan RL, Hinson M, Nackel A, Blaquiere M, Daley W, Querzoli B. Development of a pediatric burn pain and anxiety management program. J Burn Care Rehabil 1997; 18(5):455–459; discussion 453–454.

13. Barillo DJ, Harvey KD, Hobbs CL, Mozingo DW, Cioffi WG, Pruitt BA Jr. Prospective outcome analysis of a protocol for the surgical and rehabilitative management of burns to the hands. Plast Reconstr Surge 1997; 100(6):1442–1451.

14. First W, Ackroyd F, Burke J, Bondoc C. Long-term functional results of selective treatment of hand burns. Am J Surg 1985; 149(4):516–521.

15. Sheridan RL, Hurley J, Smith MA, Ryan CM, Bondoc CC, Quinby WC Jr. The acutely burned hand: management and outcome based on a ten-year experience with 1047 acute hand burns. J Trauma 1995; 38(3):406–411.

16. Dutton R. Rehabilitation frame of reference. In: Hopkins HL, Smith HD, eds. Willard and Spackman's Occupational Therapy. Philadelphia: J.B. Lippincott Co, 1993;79–81.

17. Sheridan RL, Baryza MJ, Pessina MA, O'Neill KM, Cipullo HM, Donelan MB, et al. Acute hand burns in children: management and long-tern outcome based on a 10-year experience with 698 injured hands. Ann Surg 1999; 229(4):558–564.

33

Reconstruction of the Burned Hand

MALACHY E. ASUKU
Ahmadu Bello University Teaching Hospital, Kaduna, Nigeria

ROBERT L. McCAULEY
University of Texas Medical Branch and Shriners Hospital for Children—Galveston Unit, Galveston, Texas, USA

ROCCO C. PIAZZA II
University of Texas Medical Branch School of Medicine, Galveston, Texas, USA

I. INTRODUCTION

Reconstruction of the burned hand is key to the overall functional rehabilitation of the burned patient. Whether the burned hand is an isolated injury or part of a large total body surface area burn, its loss represents a major functional impairment. The American Burn Association recognizes the importance of the burned hand by designating it a major injury (1). In addition, loss of the hand constitutes a 57% loss of function for the whole person (2,3). Thus, successful management of the burned hand is important.

The incidence of hand burn has been extensively reported (4,5). Tredget (4) reported more than 1700 burns during a 10-year period. In patients with a mean total body surface area (TBSA) burn of 15%, 54% of the patients sustained burns to the hand and upper extremity. However, 75% of the burned hands were noted in patients with <20% TBSA burns. Yet, the importance of the severity of hand burn with functional outcome was not addressed until Sheridan et al. (5) reviewed 1047 burned hands. In this classification scheme, patients with category I injuries required no surgical intervention in the management of superficial partial-thickness burns; 97% of these patients demonstrated complete functional return. Patients with category II injuries required skin grafts for closure; 81% of these patients were able to achieve nearly complete functional recovery. Patients with the most severe injuries involving tendons, joints, or bone were assigned to category III; only 9% of patients were noted to have return to normal function (Table 33.1). Thus, it is clear that the initial management of the acute burned hand along with the depth of injury can impact functional outcome.

II. SKIN GRAFTS

It is clear that early closure of the burn wound minimizes edema, decrease pain, and promotes earlier functional rehabilitation. With respect to the hand, the decreased amount of fibrosis with earlier range of motion should decrease the possibility of joint contractures and tendon adhesions. Early closure of burns to the hand is key to the long-term outcome of hand function. The use of meshed grafts vs. sheet grafts for coverage of the burned hand has received some attention. Although no randomized trials exist, it is generally accepted that unexpanded meshed grafts (1:1.5) may have the same functional outcome as sheet grafts (Fig. 33.1). Also of concern has been the use of split-thickness skin grafts (STSG) vs. full-thickness skin grafts (FTSG) to resurface burned hands. Several studies have examined the concept that FTSG are better than STSG. In the acute setting, Schwanholt et al. (6) also showed improved function and a decreased need for reconstructive procedures when FTSGs are used

Table 33.1 Burn Injury and Outcome Categories

Injury Category

I	Second-degree burn that healed without surgery
II	Deep burn that required surgery but did not involve
III	Deep burn involving bone and requiring Kirschner wire fixation

Outcome Category

A	Normal function
B	Abnormal function but able to perform activities of daily living
C	Hand cannot perform activities of daily living, such as feeding and toileting

Source: Reprinted with permission from Sheridan et al. (5).

for the treatment of acute deep palmar burns in children. In reconstruction, Pensler et al. (7) examined the long-term effects of STSG vs. FTSG in the reconstruction of postburn palmar contractures in children. These authors showed that with at least 3-year follow-up, no functional differences were noted between the two groups. Even in cases in which at least 75% of the palmar surface required skin grafting, no functional disparities were noted. It is clear that the thickness of the STSG can have an impact on functional outcome. Although Pensler et al. (7) did not address the issue of graft thickness, Schwanholt et al. (6) compared 0.012–0.015 in. STSG with FTSG. Understandably, grafts of thin to moderate thickness such as these would produce inferior results compared with FTSG. But how do thick STSG (0.20 in.) compare with FTSG? Also, is there a difference in their use in the acutely burned hand vs. their use in reconstructive procedures? These issues have yet to be resolved. The exposure of nerves or tendons in the burned hand constitutes a separate problem. Whether this occurs acutely as in electrical injuries after debridement or after scar releases for severe contractures, skin grafts may not be the best option.

III. SKIN SUBSTITUTES

Inadequate skin coverage or delay in coverage of the burned hand can lead to the development of unstable scars, hypertrophic burn scars, and scar contractures (8). In severe cases, these patients require complete scar excision, placing the metacarpophalangeal joints in flexion and the interphalangeal joints in extension with subsequent resurfacing of the hand. Such interventions are a prelude to physical therapy to restore form and function to the deformed burned hand. Kucan observed that stable and durable skin cover is the first priority in the reconstruction of the burned hand (9). The ability of the hand to withstand the functional demands of everyday life is key. Traditionally, resurfacing of the hand has been guided by the principles of the reconstructive ladder. STSGs are considered before the use of FTSG. When exposure of a nonvascularized bed, nerves, or tendons precludes the use of skin grafts, local uninjured flaps may not be available in the burned hand because of adjacent injury. At the same time, regional and free flaps may be unavailable in patients surviving large TBSA burns. These limitations have stimulated the search for alternative methods of resurfacing in the reconstruction of the burned hand. The use of tissue expansion, to increase donor areas of full-thickness grafts and to improve the availability of flaps while minimizing the donor site morbidity, has received some attention (10). Unfortunately, this technique is not without its own shortcomings. The procedure is a two-stage process that

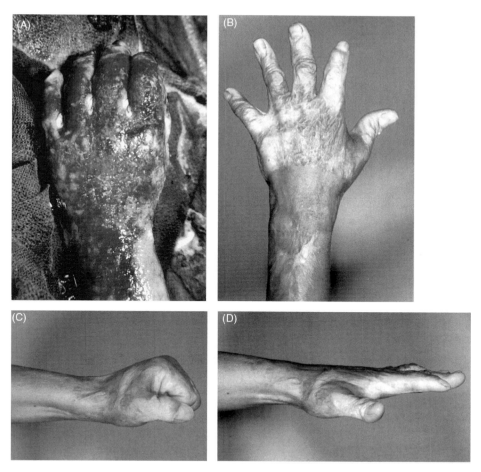

Figure 33.1 (A) Early excision of deep partial-thickness burns of the hand. (B) Result at 6 months after coverage with 1:1.5 unexpanded meshed skin grafts. (C) Excellent flexion noted at 6 months after coverage. (D) Excellent extension noted at 6 months after coverage. [Reprinted from: McCauley RL, Asuku ME. Upper extremity burn reconstruction. In: Mathes S, ed. Plastic Surgery. 2nd ed. Philadelphia: W.B. Saunders (in press).]

requires several months of expansion and may be complicated by problems of infection, exposure, and rupture (10).

Skin substitutes have long been of interest in acute coverage of burn patients. Presently, many products and techniques are available for temporary coverage of burn wounds, but only those methods that offer possibility of permanent wound coverage can be referred to as skin substitutes (11). The ideal skin substitute must possess the physicochemical properties of the skin (Fig. 33.2) (Table 33.2). The use of skin substitutes in upper extremity burns was initially limited to cases in which the lack of skin graft donor sites dictates coverage by other means. Recent clinical reports, however, have suggested that skin substitutes may heal with less scarring than conventional skin grafts. This is a desirable outcome in upper extremity burns. Less scarring may translate into less secondary contractures and fewer indications for reconstruction. Consequently, the last decade has witnessed

anecdotal reports of successes in the use of skin substitutes in burn reconstruction (12,13).

A. Integra®

Integra® was designed by Burke et al. (14). It is a bilaminary acellular matrix consisting of an outer silastic sheet and an inner layer of highly porous structure composed of cross-linked coprecipitate of bovine collagen and chondroitin 6-sulfate derived from shark cartilage. As a skin substitute, the recipient fibroblasts infiltrate the matrix network and synthesize a neo-dermis that is histologically close to normal human dermis while the artificial dermis undergoes biodegradation. Adequate revascularization requires 2–3 weeks, at which time the silastic membrane is removed and replaced by an ultrathin (usually <0.001 in.) epidermal overlay. The resulting coverage is reportedly pliable and nonadherent to deeper structures,

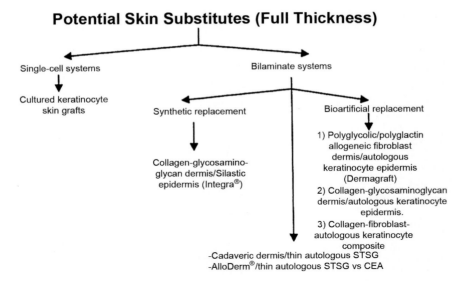

Figure 33.2   Classification of potential skin substitutes. CEA, cultured epithelial autografts; STSG, split-thickness skin grafts. (Modified from Cairns BA, deSerres S, Peterson HD, Meyer AA. Skin replacements: the biotechnological quest for optimal wound closure. Arch Surg 1993; 128:1246–1252. Reprinted with permission.)

while the donor site heals satisfactorily within 1 week (15–18).

In 2001, Dantzer and Braye (12), reported a series of 31 patients who had placed for reconstruction of 39 different sites. Thirty-one of these sites were postburn deformities, with 10 in the upper limb and hands. They emphasized the need to provide a well-vascularized bed with perfect homeostasis for Integra® to take satisfactorily. They noted that the outcome in the reconstruction of the burned hand was excellent as long as complete contracture release with restoration of full range of motion was achieved intraoperatively and an intensive physical therapy program was instituted in the immediate postoperative period. They were particularly impressed by the fact that when it was used over tendons on the

Table 33.2   Properties of Ideal Skin Substitutes

Nonantigenic, nonallergenic, nontoxic, nonirritating
Water vapor transmission similar to that of normal skin
Impermeable to exogenous microorganisms
Prevents proliferation of wound surface flora
Sufficiently thin and pliable to conform to irregular wound surface
Adheres rapidly and permanently to wound surface
Adequate tensile strength to withstand linear and shear stresses
Elastic enough to permit motion of underlying structures
Inner surface structure that permits ingrowth of fibrovascular tissues
Biodegradable
Minimal storage requirements, indefinite shelf life

Source: Modified from Pruitt BA Jr, Levine NS. Characteristics and uses of biologic dressings and skin substitutes. Arch Surg 1984; 19:312.

dorsum of the hand, Integra® provided pliable skin with no adherence to the deeper structures. Other reported advantages of Integra® included immediate availability, simplicity, and reliability. In addition, minimal donor site morbidity is noted with the use of an ultrathin epidermal graft. The disadvantages of use of Integra® for reconstructive surgery include the necessity of two operations, the risk of infection, early detachment of the silastic layer, recurrence of contractures, and cost. They concluded that in light of their preliminary results, Integra® appears to be an alternative to skin grafts and possibly skin flaps in reconstructive surgery.

In the same year, Chou et al. (13) reported the use of Integra® for the reconstruction of burn scar deformities of the upper extremities in 13 severely burned patients. A 2-year follow-up showed increased range of motion in the upper extremity joints, good appearance, and pliable skin using the Vancouver Scar Scale. They advocated the use of Integra® in severely burned patients with insufficient donor sites for full thickness grafts and in whom suitable flaps are not available. Heimbach et al. (15) noted that Integra® which has been available in the United States for life-threatening acute burn care since 1995, has found an "off-label" use in reconstructive surgery. He also noted that Integra® may be as good as an intermediate to thick split-thickness graft. However, Heimbach et al. (15) questioned the use of Integra® in the presence of normal skin. Shakespeare and Shakespeare (19), in a survey of the use of skin substitutes in burn centers in the United Kingdom, found only two units where Integra® was used for the reconstruction of burned patients with satisfactory outcome (19). The survey revealed that the other centers in the United Kingdom were reluctant to use skin substitutes in reconstructive procedures, because clinical evidence supporting such use was still scanty.

B. AlloDerm®

The potential use of allograft donor skin as a permanent skin replacement in full thickness burns is limited by its immunogenic properties. Although allograft skin will routinely take onto a full-thickness wound, it will ultimately be rejected. This immune response to allograft skin is directed primarily against Langhans cells, epidermal cells, endothelial cells, and dermal fibroblasts. The noncellular component of the dermis consisting mainly of intracellular matrix protein and collagen has been shown to be nonimmunogenic (20–22). AlloDerm® is the product of a complex biotechnological process that succeeded in removing the immunogenic cells from the nonimmunogenic dermis of allograft skin, making it possible for it to be used as a permanent skin replacement (22).

AlloDerm® is an acellular allogenic dermal matrix processed from human allograft skin with preservation of the type IV and type V collagen. The final product is devoid of type I and type II major histocompatibility antigens. It is intended to provide a permanent nonimmunogenic template to augment the dermal component of a meshed or sheet split-thickness skin graft when used on a full-thickness wound (21–23). This concept addresses the fact that the degree of scarring and contraction that follow autografting of burn wound with STSGs grafts correlates inversely with the amount of dermis delivered in the graft. Unfortunately, dermal cropping is preferably kept to a minimum to permit repeated harvesting in patients with limited donor sites as a result of massive burns. In addition, harvesting of thicker grafts may result in increased morbidity at the donor site. Unlike Integra®, AlloDerm® allows the successful use of ultrathin autografts that can be applied simultaneously while maximizing the amount of dermis delivered to the burn wound (20,21). Lattari et al. (21), in 1979, reported satisfactory results with the use of Allo-Derm® in acute hand burns. They observed that it permitted early restoration of normal hand function and exhibited excellent elasticity, good pigmentation, and excellent satisfaction with the patients. They concluded, thus, "the high frequency and reproducibility of excellent results with this composite graft, coupled with the reduced trauma and rapid healing of donor sites associated with the ultrathin autografts, has made composite grafting with the use of AlloDerm® their new method of choice for the treatment of full-thickness burns of the hand and feet." A number of authors who advocate the use of AlloDerm® in acute burn care have agreed that its full potential have not yet been realized (21–24). It appears that AlloDerm® may be a viable alternative in the reconstruction of the burned hand. Its ability to immediately support autografts makes it an attractive alternative to Integra®.

IV. RECONSTRUCTION OF THE BURNED HAND

Reconstruction of the burned hand is a challenging problem. Optimal results depend on many factors, including the extent and depth of soft tissue damage, the immediate postburn care, operative intervention, and subsequent physical therapy. Unfortunately, reconstructive surgeons may have control of only one-third of these factors (25). Whitson and Allen (8) summarized the factors that contribute to deformities of the hand as persistent edema, wound infection, poor positioning, prolonged immobilization, and delayed or inadequate skin coverage. Although successful acute management of the burned hand has reduced the need for subsequent reconstruction, burn scar contractures associated with compromised hand functions still occur (26–30). The majority of these cases may be related to the severity of the initial injury. However, some cases may have been prevented by appropriate acute care.

Peacock et al. (31) noted that the need for secondary reconstructive procedures is decreased by proper attention to positioning and ranging of joints during the acute phase of wound care. The success rates of such procedures increase in direct proportion to the degree of motion preserved before reconstruction. Reconstructive goals are easily attained if all the members of the burn team pursue them from the outset. Parry (25) noted that in the delayed evaluation of burned patients, reconstructive goals center on the restoration of function and form. Although many surgeons recognize the difficulties associated with the correction of burn hand deformities, Donelan (32) observed that postburn hand deformities could be confusing to analyze because acute injuries and their methods of treatment vary so widely. In addition, multiple problems can exist in each postburn hand. However, Donelan was able to divide the deformities into three general categories. He commented that all of these might be present in a single hand: soft tissue deformities, joint deformities, and amputations.

A. Soft Tissue Deformities

The soft tissue deformities that commonly occur in the burned hand include unstable scars, hypertrophic scars, and contractures. Brown (33) observed that the difference in the quality between palmar and dorsal skin surfaces of the hand explain the more frequent crippling effects of burns on the dorsal surface as opposed to a palmar surface of the hand. The palmar surface is more protected by the thicker nature of the superficial layer of its epidermis and by the instinctive mechanism of self-protection in which the hands are placed over the face at the time of burning thereby exposing the thin dorsal surface with its sparse subcutaneous tissue. Consequently, most of the interests in burns of the hand and most of the deformities have been noted to occur with dorsal injuries.

1. Scars

Spontaneous healing after deep second-degree burns in which the dermis has been partially destroyed, can result in unstable coverage that is susceptible to recurrent ulcerations and hypertrophic scars. Resurfacing of the burned hand with widely expanded mesh may produce unstable scars. This may ultimately inhibit function. Donelan observed that meshed skin grafts result in permanently abnormal skin texture that does not improve significantly with time. Some authors, however, believe that the use of 1:1.5 unexpanded meshed grafts give satisfactory long-term coverage (34,35). It is known that with expansion of meshed grafts 1:4 and greater, healing in the interstices of the mesh is essentially by secondary intention. This increases the likelihood of both unstable scar function and hypertrophic scar development. Such grafts may fail to provide either the necessary pliability to accommodate the increased range of motion in the multiple joints of the hand or the durability to withstand the stress and strain imposed on the hand by the activities of daily living (ADL).

The healing of superficial partial thickness burns to the hand is usually completed within 2–3 weeks after injury and occurs by re-epithelialization. On the other hand, in deep partial thickness or full thickness burns, healing occurs by secondarily intention. Under such conditions, there is a significant development of granulation tissue, which is a precursor to the development of hypertrophic scars. Magliani et al. (36), in 1979, reported more scar complications in hand burn patients undergoing surgery after 21 days compared with those treated at an earlier stage. Deitch et al. (37), in 1983, noted that a major problem in patients surviving thermal injuries is the development of hypertrophic burn scars. They felt that the most important indicator of hypertrophic scar formation is the time required for the burn to heal. In a series of 100 patients, they observed hypertrophic scar formation in 33% of the patients when the wound healed between 14 and 21 days. Yet, 78% of burn sites that healed after 21 days developed hypertrophic scars. Similarly, Cole et al. (38), in 1992, reported a 79% incidence of hypertrophic scars in patients with deep partial-thickness hand burns who were managed conservatively. All their patients responded to pressure therapy; however, no scarring persisted beyond a mean of 19 months in their series. Hypertrophic scar formation over the dorsum of the hand still occurs despite continuing emphasis on splinting, early

excision and grafting, pressure therapy, and physical therapy.

Parks et al. (39) and Larson et al. (40) popularized the use of pressure garments in the control and prevention of hypertrophic scars. The measures consisted of continuous controlled pressure of the magnitude of 25 mmHg above the capillary pressure, which could be provided by elastic wraps and pressure gloves. These must be worn continuously for several months to be effective in controlling hypertrophic scars. Frequent careful evaluation is necessary to ensure the effectiveness of the program. The patient and family members must be adequately educated about the importance of consistent home care and compliance. Hypertrophic scars are believed to be most responsive to treatment during the first 3–6 months. However, the role of pressure in controlling hypertrophic burn scars came under scrutiny when the use of silicone gel for the same purpose started appearing in the literature (41). Perkins et al. (41) described a patient who rapidly recovered complete active flexion at the metacarpophalangeal joints after application of silicone gel to his dorsal hand scars. They went on to make a number of interesting observations. The mode of action of the silicone gel is unknown. It does not reply on pressure. Over joints, where tight painful scars restrict movement, silicone gel sheets will allow early pain-free movements. When applied over healed skin grafts, silicone gel prevents contraction of the graft. In addition, when applied to advanced hypertrophied scar tissue, the area will soften, thus allowing it to be more easily controlled by pressure therapy. Silicone sheets used alone or in conjunction with accepted pressure and pressure insert techniques allow treatment to be tailored to a patient's needs. Such an option allows a more flexible approach in burn scar management. They concluded that the full potential of silicone gel is probably yet to be realized as newer products are continuously being developed.

2. Correction of Burn Scar Contractures

Achauer et al. (42) noted that surgery on immature hypertrophied scar requires careful consideration because of the possibility of recurrence. It is believed that in many cases the deformity is not usually completely corrected. This group advocated a conservative approach to all such active scars. On the other hand, the mature contracted hypertrophic scar will not respond to conservative measures. Thus, surgical intervention to improve function and appearance becomes necessary. Incisional release and resurfacing with skin grafts may be all that is required (32). Elimination of tension after incisional release can favorably influence the maturity of the residual scar. This decreases the morbidity and complexity of surgery as well as minimizes the requirements for skin graft donor site. Although focal hypertrophic and linear scars can be incised or revised, massive diffuse hypertrophic scars of the hand require complete excision with preservation of as much subcutaneous tissue as possible to be able to provide resurfacing with STSG or FTSG. Elastic compression gloves and splints are usually worn in the postoperative period to prevent recurrence of scar hypertrophy (39,40).

Burn scar contractures are perhaps the most frequent and most frustrating sequela of thermal injuries to the hand. A major contributing factor to the development of contractures correlates with a delay in initiation of appropriate and adequate hand care in the presence of life-threatening issues in patients with large TBSA burns. Unfortunately, stiffness occurs in the burned hand quickly. A week of neglect in the burned hand can lead to malpositioning and distortion that may be difficult to correct (25). Today, even with large TBSA burns, biologic dressings and skin substitutes may assist in the resurfacing of large areas so that the hand can still receive the attention it deserves. In addition, compliance with a postacute care physical therapy program aimed at minimizing scar hypertrophy and contractures plays an equally important role in functional rehabilitation. This is particularly important in children, who may not be able to cooperate with such programs. Although the causes of burn scar contractures are numerous, Larson et al. (40) noted that the burn wound would shorten until it meets an opposing force of at least equal magnitude. In addition, the position of comfort is the position of contracture (40). They further observed that the severity of these effects is directly related to the depth of the initial injury. It suffices to say that contraction within the substance of the scar is a continuing event. The net effect is the consolidation and shortening of the scar resulting in a restrictive scar. This paves the way for the development of contractures. Brown (33) noted that a healed deep partial-thickness burn wound of the dorsum of the hand would almost universally result in the production of hypertrophic scar. Also, secondary contraction of collagen during the remodeling phase produces restrictive scarring in the hand, adding to the deformity (33). Such deformities may be treated clinically by graded traction, serial splinting, and programmed exercises. The timing of these measures is equally important, and any combination may be indicated concurrently or sequentially. Exercise may be effective, but during rest and sleep, some method of positioning and splinting should be used to preserve any function that has been gained (40).

The untreated severely burned hand is susceptible to the development of contractures. Many patients instinctively assume a position that is least painful. Described as the position of comfort, it is diametrically opposed to that of function (33). The position is one of volar flexion at the wrist, hyperextension at the metacarpophalangeal joints, and variable degrees of flexion at the interphalangeal

joints with adduction and extension of the thumb. The transverse metacarpal arch is usually undisturbed at the onset. In fact, in most patients, the initial thermal injury is limited to the skin, with the underlying tendons, joints, and joint capsules being spared. These structures, however, tend to be secondarily affected by prolonged healing. The position of the wrist has been described as one of the key factors in the development of deformity in the burned hand (33). The synergistic effects of extrinsic extensors, resulting in metacarpophalangeal joint extension with wrist flexion, allow laxity of the collateral ligaments in the early stage, and within a short while, these become shortened and contracted, producing the extension deformity that cannot be overcome by the flexor muscles. The transverse intermetacarpal ligaments become shortened and thickened, resulting in loss of the arch. Similarly, the proximal interphalangeal joints assume a position of moderate flexion immediately after burning, and if uninhibited, this progresses to extreme flexion (33). Prevention of the development of this deformity requires splinting of the hand in an anticlaw or "safe" position in the immediate postinjury period. It is, therefore, important that a therapist familiar with burned hands become an active member of the burn team from the outset. Parry (25) emphasized that to achieve the safe position, the interphalangeal joint should be maintained in extension because these joints have no secondary lateral support system if surgical releases are required. Furthermore, the volar plate may become fixed in flexion, increasing the risk of rupture of the central slip of the extensor tendon, resulting in boutonniere deformities. The metacarpophalangeal joints should be placed at 40–70° of flexion to prevent the collateral ligaments from shortening and contracting, as occurs when the joint is extended. The thumb should be abducted and rotated toward the palm to prevent the contraction and fibrosis of its muscles. Finally, the wrist should be at 35° of extension. In severe deformities, maintaining the hand in the safe position may require percutaneous fixation of multiple joints with Kirschner wires for a variable time. McCauley (27) noted that in the correction of severe contractures in children, pinning of the metacarpophalangeal joints for 4–6 weeks resulted in satisfactory outcomes. In adults, however, the fear of joint stiffness calls for caution in deciding the optimal period of immobilization required for the hand.

Burn scar contractures of the hand present a wide spectrum of anatomic distortions and functional disabilities. This makes the development of a universal system of classification difficult and elusive. Such a declassification is necessary since it allows comparison of different treatment modalities and subsequent long-term outcomes from the various centers involved in the complex reconstruction of burned hand. However, burn scar contractures of the hand can be divided into the clinical entities commonly encountered. These are the web space contractures, dorsal contractures, and volar contractures.

3. Dorsal and Volar Contractures

Dorsal contractures of the hand are the most common of all the complications of the burned hand. It is the result of damage to the thin dorsal skin and scant subcutaneous tissue, which offers little protection to the deeper structures. Consequently, these injuries are often deep, resulting in a spectrum of deformities (Figs. 33.3 and 33.4). On the other hand, volar contractures are less common. The relatively thick layer of epidermis, in addition to the reflexive closure of the hand at the time of injury, provides adequate protection for the deeper structures. Deep volar hand injuries, however, can occur after direct contact with flame or a hot object of prolonged duration (Figs. 33.5 and 33.6). Children with poor reflexes and unconscious adults can be susceptible to such injuries.

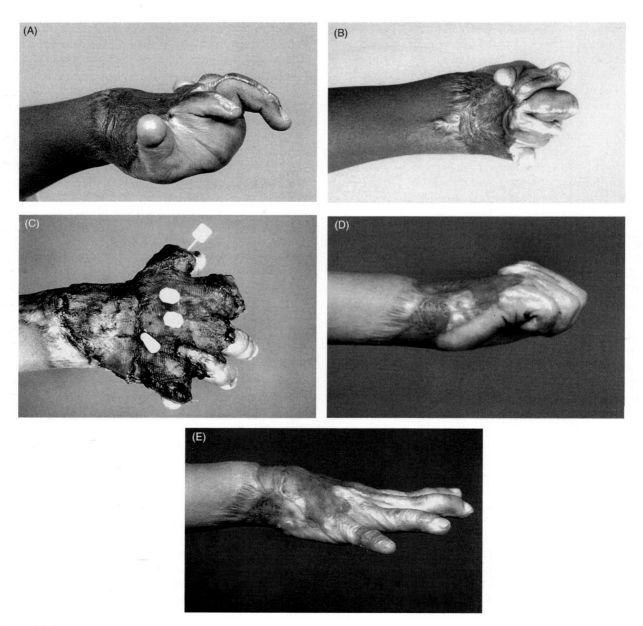

Figure 33.3   (A) Lateral view of neglected burn scar contracture in a 2-year-old. (B) Dorsal view of the same hand. (C) After excisional release, metacarpophalangeal joint immobilization with k-wires and resurfacing with split-thickness sheet graft. (D) Flexion demonstrated at 4 months. (E) Extension demonstrated at 4 months. [Reprinted with permission from McCauley (27).]

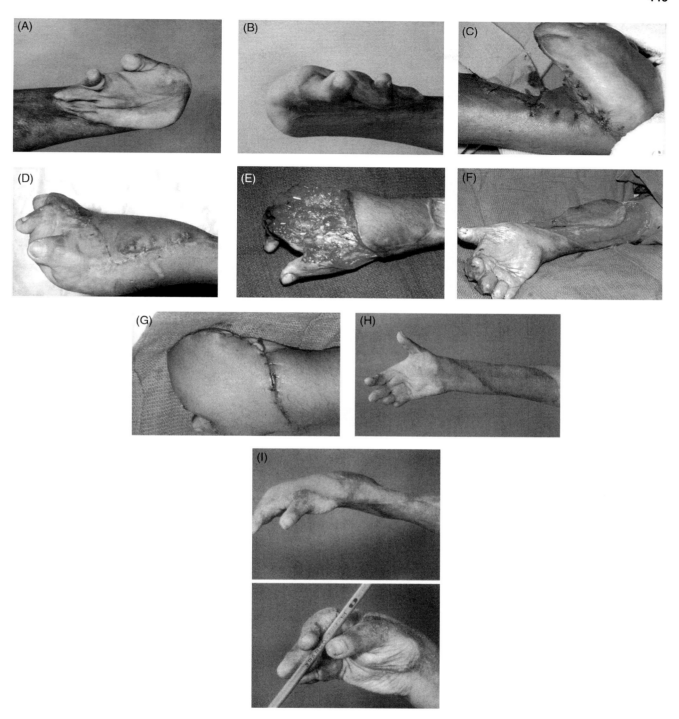

Figure 33.4 (A) Severe dorsal contracture of the right hand (grade IV) in a 13-year-old boy who was burned at 6 months of age. (B) Lateral view showing complete fusion of the entire dorsal of the hand and wrist to the distal portion of the forearm. (C) Release of the wrist contracture and resurfacing with a groin flap. (D) Postoperative appearance after division of the groin flap. (E) Excision of dorsal hand scars with pinning of the metacarpophalangeal joint with k-wires. (F) Elevation of reverse radial artery forearm flap. (G) Fingers are syndactalyzed and the dorsum of the hand resurfaced with the reverse radial artery forearm flap. (H) Appearance of the hand after release of the fingers. (I) Appearance of the hand lateral view of the hand and key pinch noted 6 months after surgery.

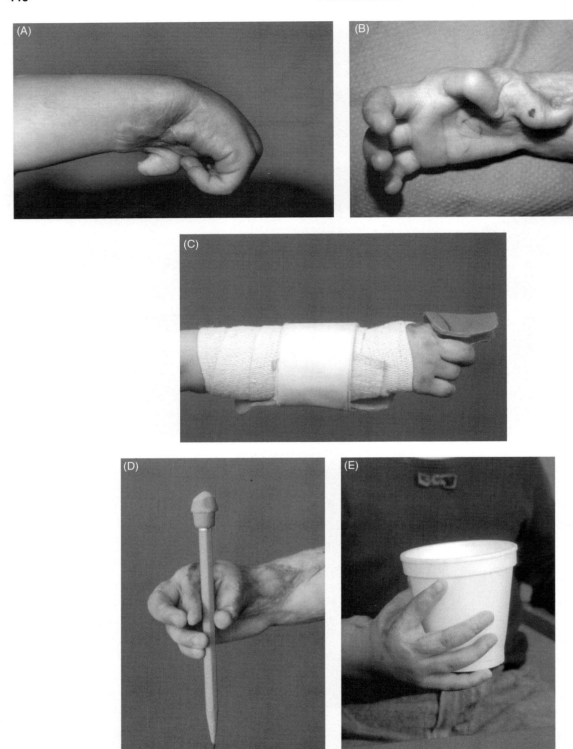

Figure 33.5 (A) Lateral view of severe volar contracture. (B) Volar view showing severe contracture and dislocation of the thumb and index finger. (C) Release of the volar contracture accomplished with split-thickness skin grafts and k-wire fixation of the thumb and index finger followed by splinting. (D) Pinch function demonstrated at 1 year. (E) Grasp function demonstrated at 1 year. [Reprinted from McCauley RL, Asuku ME. Upper extremity burn reconstruction. In: Mathes S, ed. Plastic Surgery. 2nd ed. Philadelphia: W.B. Saunders (in press).]

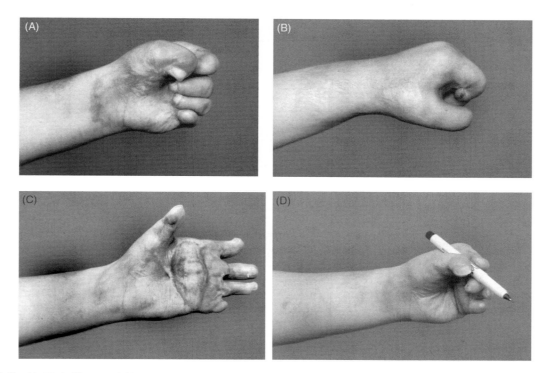

Figure 33.6 (A, B) A 13-year-old boy who stained flame burns to the volar surface of the hand with contracture formation for 7 years. (C) Extension of hand after two operations for release and resurfacing with full-thickness skin grafts. (D) Function after 9 months.

Although the management of such injuries may be controversial, the issue of management both acutely and in the reconstructive phase of care, is still under scrutiny. Pensler et al. (7) favor the use of STSG in palmar burns, whereas Schwanholt et al. (6) are strongly opposed to it, advocating FTSG instead.

McCauley (27) proposed a classification system which correlates the severity of burn scar contractures to hand function (Table 33.3). The grade I and grade II

Table 33.3 Classification of Burn Scar Contractures

Grade I	Symptomatic tightness but no limitation in range of motion, normal architecture
Grade II	Mild decrease in range of motion without significant impact on activities of daily living, no distortion of normal architecture
Grade III	Functional deficit noted, with early changes in normal architecture of hand
Grade IV	Loss of hand function with significant distortion of normal architecture of the hand

Subset classification for Grade III and Grade IV contracture:
  A: Flexion contractures
  B: Extension contractures
  C: Combination of flexion and extension contractures

Source: Reprinted with permission from McCauley (27).

contractures are likely to respond to conservative measures, provided the scars are immature, whereas grade III and grade IV contractures will require surgical intervention to achieve maximum functional outcome. Restoration of function to the grade IV burn scar contractures of the hand is a major undertaking (Fig. 33.4). This group also noted that anatomic restoration of the transverse and longitudinal arches through adequate excisional release is key to satisfactory functional outcome (27). Internal fixation with Kirschner wires to maintain the metacarpophalangeal joints at 70–90° of flexion and the interphalangeal joints at 180° of extension is essential. Resurfacing with thick STSG or FTSG will usually suffice. However, flap coverage will be required in the event of the exposure of joints or tendons (Fig. 33.7). For severe volar contractures, McCauley (27) advocated excisional release and resurfacing with skin grafts or flaps. The metacarpophalangeal joints are kept in extension to maximize the extent of soft tissue release while bolsters are used for immobilization. He reported satisfactory results even in children with the most severe of contractures, concluding that the functional outcome appeared to be maximized with the extended period of Kirschner wire fixation. Donelan (32) observed that timely release of dorsal soft tissue contractures can greatly improve the effect of physical therapy and may prevent the development of permanent joint contractures.

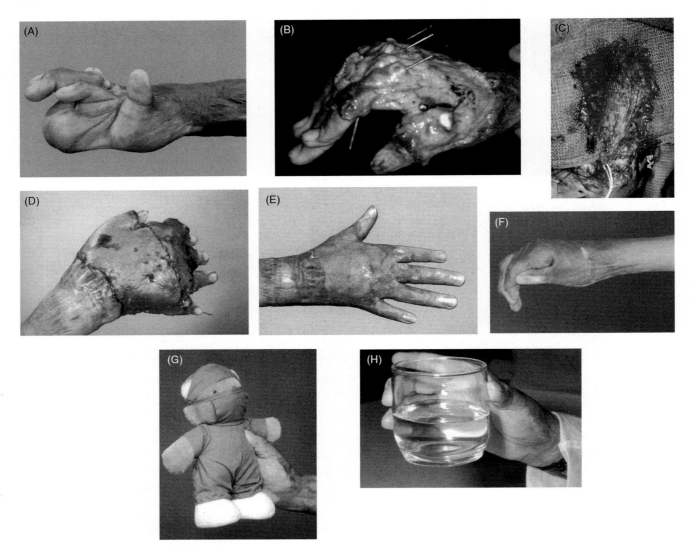

Figure 33.7   (A) Burn scar contracture of the hand of a 12-year-old. Loss of longitudinal and transverse arches as well as subluxation of the metacarpophalangeal joints is noted at 7 years after burn. (B) Excisional release and pinning of the metacarpophalangeal joints at 90°. (C) Elevation of superficial temporoparietal fascial free flap. (D) One week after dorsal resurfacing with superficial temporoparietal fascial free flap and coverage with a split-thickness skin graft. (E) Outcome at 2 months after coverage. (F–H) Functional outcome 4 months after reconstruction. [Reprinted with permission from McCauley (27).]

4.   Web Space Contractures (Adduction Contractures)

Postburn syndactyly or interdigital web contractures are common sequelae of thermal injuries involving the dorsum of the hand and digits (43–45). Groenevelt et al. (43) described syndactyly one of the most common postburn deformities of the hand (43). They previewed 180 burned hands requiring secondary reconstructive surgery. Two hundred and eighty dorsal interdigital contractures distributed unevenly over the four web spaces (Table 33.4). Interdigital web contractures commonly occur as a result of fusion of adjacent burned digits during the healing process. Less commonly, burn syndactyly results from dorsal web scars pulled distally by contraction of healing tissues, leading to dorsal hooding. In

these instances, the deformity is usually only mild to moderate. True postburn syndactyly with varying degrees of fusion of the fingers and complete obliteration of the web space results from dorsal hand burns that extend

Table 33.4   Distribution of Syndactyly and Adduction Contractures

Web I	34%
Web II	24%
Web III	24%
Web IV	18%

Source: Reprinted with permission from Groenevelt et al. (43).

beyond the web space. It is often associated with hyertrophied scarring due to healing over a protected period (32). Krizek et al. (44) observed that despite careful adherence to the basic principles of management of the severely burned hand, webbing may still develop. They proposed that the preservation of web spaces should be incorporated into the basic principles of management of the burned hand. Attention should be directed to spacing between the digits whenever the burned hand is splinted in the safe position. The flexion imposed on the metacarpophalangeal joints places the digits in marked adduction, favoring the development of interdigital webbing. It is, therefore, essential to incorporate spacers between the digits and to encourage frequent abduction. In addition, spreading exercises along with the usual flexion and extension exercises are emphasized (44). When the burn wound of the hand requires operative treatment, the wound should be excised completely and resurfaced with a sheet of graft, avoiding curved uninterrupted lines between the graft and the intact skin around the web space. This can be achieved by placing darts along the line of the skin–graft junction or by bringing normal unburned skin into the web space commisure (44).

5. First Web Space Contractures (Adduction Contractures of the Thumb)

Interdigital contractures can be divided functionally into two groups, first web space contractures and second to fourth web space contractures. Adduction contractures of the first web space can have a significant impact on overall hand function because thumb abduction and opposition are either impaired or lost. Some of the functional deficiencies include loss of grasp and loss of key pinch. Various measures, including skeletal tractions, have been employed in a bid to preserve this important web space (44). When a first web space adduction contracture occurs, it justifies surgical intervention and physical therapy to maintain anatomy and restore function.

Larson et al. (46) observed that if the web space contracture is not mature, the use of pressure might help remodel the wound to overcome the problem. However, for all matured first web space contractures, surgical correction is required. Krizek et al. (44) noted that surgery in these instances is designed to accomplish one of three goals: to break up and add length to a straight line contracture; to re-form the web space by employing local flaps; or for the severely scarred web, to add skin from outside the local area. When the contracture is limited to the leading edge of the web space with adequate adjacent nonscarred tissue, some form of local tissue rearrangement with or without supplemental skin grafts may be all that is required. Krizek et al. (44) noted that the simplest procedure to lengthen the straight-line contracture is the Z-plasty. First described by Horner in 1837 for use in

burned patients, it breaks up the line of the scar and lengthens the scar. Several authors believe that the 60° Z-plasty given optimal results (25,44). When the webbing is over a longer distance, double or multiple Z-plasties side to side or in tandem may give better results because lateral tension is less with two small Z-plasties than with a single large one. The four-flap Z-plasty described by Limberg has been found to increase the net gain in length with satisfactory outcome (47,48). Similarly, the five-flap Z-plasty, which is a combination of double opposed Z-plasties and a Y-V advancement flap, has been used in the release of severe first web space contractures (Fig. 33.8). Other local flaps that have been successfully used in web space contracture releases include the Y-V and the V-M advancement flaps and the dorsally based hourglass flap technique described by Salisbury, Bevin, and Parry (49–51). Krizek et al. (44) observed that the use of local flaps requires meticulous attention to detail in keeping the flaps as short and thick as possible to ensure a better blood supply. When there is a deficiency of tissues, these procedures may have to

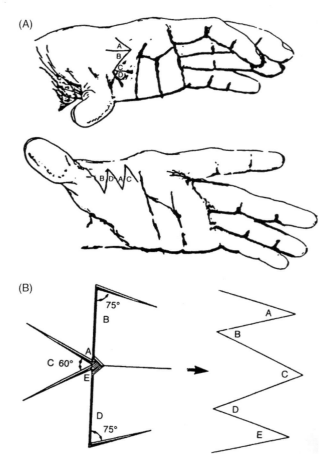

Figure 33.8 Methods for correction of first web space contractures. (A) Four-limb Z-plasty. (B) Five-limb Z-plasty. [Reprinted with permission from Strock et al. (28).]

be combined with supplemental skin grafts. Donelan (32) questioned the rationale of using local flaps where skin grafts have to be used as well. Apparently, it seems to add little to improved function or aesthetics. When the web space contracture is due to extensive dorsal scarring or involvement of both the palmar and dorsal sides of the web space, there is significant deficiency tissue. The introduction of tissue from outside the local area may be necessary to obtain a satisfactory release (32). The important landmarks at surgery are the metacarpophalangeal joints, the proximal interphalangeal joints, and the midpoint between these as the proposed level of the volar edge of the web space. The contracture is then carefully released, preserving the normal slope of the web space. The incisions may extend to normal skin through the full-thickness of the scar to afford complete release. The resulting defect is resurfaced with a thick STSG or a FTSG anchored over bolster dressings with the fingers in abduction and extension. The bolster dressings are usually removed on the fifth to seventh postoperative day for graft inspection. It is advisable to begin aggressive physiotherapy when the skin graft has stabilized. Maintenance of night splints with the thumb in abduction and extension and daytime compressive wraps and gloves with interdigital web space inserts and conformers such as molded silicone elastomer is continued for several months. Donelan (32) observed that skin grafts could provide satisfactory functional and aesthetic results in addition to allowing simultaneous correction of multiple web spaces because the blood supply of adjacent fingers is not compromised. In severe first web space contractures, an adequate release may be compromised by tightness of the underlying adductor pollicis and first dorsal interosseous muscles. A staged release with preservation of muscle function maybe necessary. Some authors have recommended that multiple skin releases with or without skin grafts separated by 6 months or more of intensive physical therapy in order to obtain the desired result (32). In extensive contractures where there is damage to deeper structures, flap coverage of the web space may be the initial procedure.

Spinner (52) described a transpositional flap obtained from the radial side of the index finger for the release of soft tissue adduction contracture of the thumb. The flap donor site is resurfaced with STSGs. They demonstrated satisfactory results with this procedure and concluded that the advantages of the procedure are two-fold. First, local tissue is used, and second, the exposure is excellent for the performance of any other procedures simultaneously. Housinger et al. (53) described the use of a rectangular flap, which they called the goal-post procedure, for the release of first web space adduction contractures in pediatric patients. The rectangular flap is based proximally on the palmar or dorsal surface of the web and is inserted directly into the contracture band. Lateral flaps are then raised along the borders of the post incision and secured to the base of the rectangular flap. A bulky dressing is applied after closure, and physiotherapy is started as early as the second week after surgery. They reported satisfactory results in a series of 31 first web space contractures. There were no wound complications, and none of the patients had redevelopment of contracture in the follow-up period that averaged 20 months.

On occasion, the restoration of the first web space has required the use of distant flaps. Beasley (54) noted that the most widely used design is a superiorly based random flap from the contralateral epigastrium, which is shaped like a parallelogram folded at the point of maximum distance between the first and second metacarpals to provide palmar and dorsal triangles of tissue. A variety of other random flaps from the trunk and contralateral arm have also been used. Although rarely indicated, the possibility of designing and tailoring free flaps to meet specific circumstances must always be kept in mind.

6. Second to Fourth Web Space Contractures

Although interdigital contractures of the second to fourth web spaces may be disfiguring, unless they are extensive, the impact on function may be relatively minimal (Fig. 33.9). However, the presence of interdigital pockets, the inability to wear gloves and difficulties in maintenance of good hygiene may constitute an indication for surgical correction of these problems (45). In addition, many patients will seek surgical correction for aesthetic reasons. Although the principles of surgical correction are similar to those for first web space adduction contractures, the recurrence rate may be higher. Mancoll et al. (55), in a series of 38 patients who underwent surgical correction of web space contractures, reported the use of local flaps in 57%, split-thickness grafts in 24%, full-thickness grafts in 8%, and a combination of local flaps and skin grafts in 11% of the patients. In this series, best results were obtained with the use of local flaps, which had a recurrence rate of 64% during a follow-up period that spanned 1–18 years (mean, 7 years). The multiplicity of approaches and techniques for correction web space contractures is perhaps a reflection of the fact that none is infallible. Flexibility may, therefore, continue to be the key in this area of surgical uncertainty.

B. Joint Deformities

The joints of the hand may be affected in deep thermal injuries either directly by the effect of heat or secondarily by complications of ischemic changes, infection, or the persistence of contracted inflexible scars over the joints (56). The management of the resultant postburn joint

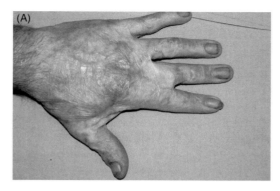 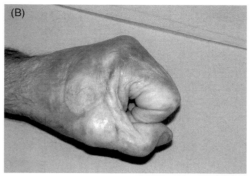

Figure 33.9 (A) Dorsal view of second to fourth web space contractures; note that the first web space is spared. (B) Hand function preserved despite web space contracture. [Reprinted from: McCauley RL, Asuku ME. Upper extremity burn reconstruction. In: Mathes S, ed. Plastic Surgery. 2nd ed. Philadelphia: W.B. Saunders (in press).]

deformities requires a thorough preoperative evaluation, including active and passive range of motion measurements and triplanar radiography, as a prelude to successful therapeutic interventions.

1. Metacarpophalangeal Joint

Thermal injury to the dorsum of the hand can progress to affect the metacarpophalangeal joints, leading to severe compromise in hand function (57). Extension and hyperextension contractures due to scarring of the dorsal skin, extensor mechanism, or joint capsule are the most debilitating complications occurring at this joint (57).

Graham et al. (57) proposed a classification system for the evaluation of metacarpophalangeal joint extension contractures in the burned hand based on the limitation of passive flexion a the joint with the wrist joint maximally extended to eliminate the effect of tenodesis (57). The classification, devised to reflect burn severity and anatomic involvement, is aimed at directing surgical intervention and assessing postoperative results (Fig. 33.10). By this classification, type I deformity is one in which at least 30° of flexion is preserved at the metacarpophalangeal joint; scarring here is limited to the dorsal skin and is described as the dermodesis effect. Type II deformity demonstrates <30° of flexion at the metacarpophalangeal

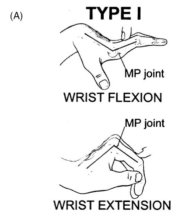

Type I contracture. With wrist flexion, passive MP flexion is less than 30 degrees. With wrist extension, passive MP flexion is greater than 30 degrees. Scarring limited to skin.

Adapted from: Graham TJ, Stern PJ, True SM. Classification and treatment of postburn metacarpophalangeal joint extension contractures in children. J Hand Surg 15A, 3:450-456, 1990.

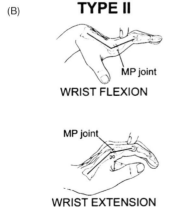

Type II contracture. With wrist flexion, MP flexion severely limited. With wrist extension, MP passive flexion less than 30 degrees. In addition to dermal contracture, deeped structures such as MP joint capsule are scarred.

Adapted from: Graham TJ, Stern PJ, True SM. Classification and treatment of postburn metacarpophalangeal joint extension contractures in children. J Hand Surg 15A, 3:450-456, 1990.

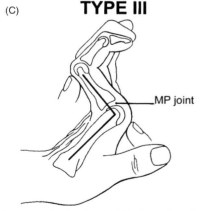

Type III contracture. MP joint fixed regardless of wrist position. MP joint is dislocated and often has articular incongruity.

Adapted from: Graham TJ, Stern PJ, True SM. Classification and treatment of postburn metacarpophalangeal joint extension contractures in children. J Hand Surg 15A, 3:450-456, 1990.

Figure 33.10 (A) Type I metacarpophalangeal joint contracture. (B) Type II metacarpophalangeal joint contracture. (C) Type III metacarpophalangeal joint contracture. [Reprinted with permission from Graham et al. (57).]

joint. Here scarring typically involves the skin, dorsal apparatus, dorsal capsule, and collateral ligaments. In the type III deformity, passive flexion >30° of hyperextension at the metacarpophalangeal joint cannot be attained regardless of wrist position. These hands may reveal extensive dorsal scarring, atrophy of the intrinsic hand muscle, and joint incongruity with dorsal subluxation or dislocation at the metacarpophalangeal joint.

Surgical management of type I deformity may require only a release of the scarred skin and resurfacing with thick STSG or FTSG. The joint, itself, appears to be preserved. Type II deformity, however, requires not only release of the skin on the dorsum of the hand but also release of the deeper tissues with simultaneous capsulotomies. Flap coverage is indicated when the resultant bed is unsuitable for resurfacing with skin grafts. It is desirable to achieve metacarpophalangeal joint flexion of 90°, intraoperatively, and to maintain this by means of external splints or K-wire fixation. In the type III deformity, the joint is severely affected with limited range of motion and narrowing of the joint space on radiographic examination. The role of joint reconstruction is therefore limited. Arthrodesis of the joint may offer the best option for improving function. Ideally, arthrodesis of the metacarpophalangeal joints is performed at an angle of 10–45° of flexion (Table 33.5). In severe cases in which multiple joints are involved, the final therapeutic option may be amputation of the digit. Graham et al. (57) reported a series consisting of 278 surgically treated postburn metacarpophalangeal joint extension contractures. Forty-seven percent were type I deformities. Within this group, 95% had satisfactory improvement in range of motion after surgical intervention. Of the 34% that were type II deformities, 73% had satisfactory outcome. In type III deformities (19%), only 47% had satisfactory surgical outcome. Their armamentarium of reconstructive procedures included dorsal scar releases and coverage with skin grafts, capsulotomies, arthrodesis, and digital amputations. They concluded that with this classification as well as radiographic analysis guiding the choice of

Table 33.5 Recommended Angles for Arthrodesis

	MCP	PIP/IP	DIP
Thumb	10–20	10–20	N/A
Index	20–30	25–35	5–15
Middle	25–35	30–40	5–15
Ring	30–40	35–45	5–15
Little	35–45	40–50	5–15

Note: A range is given because the exact angle of fusion will depend on the individual hand with digit length and expected function. MCP, metacarpophalangeal; PIP/IP, proximal interphalangeal/interphalangeal; DIP, distal interphalangeal.
Source: Reprinted with permission from: Smith MA, Spence RJ. Burns of the hand and upper limb: a review. Burns 1998; 24:493–505.

reconstructive procedure, the potential for satisfactory results could be optimized.

2. Proximal Interphalangeal Joint

The proximal interphalangeal joint may be the most frequently affected deep structure in the burned hand (56,58). Most proximal interphalangeal joint contractures are usually flexion contractures. In dorsal burns, the overlying central slip may be destroyed by direct thermal injury or secondary to edema and constricting scar. This results in a boutonniere deformity. The flexion deformity may also arise from scar contracture of the palmar digital skin. Ulnar nerve palsy arising from heterotopic ossification at the elbow or from an electrical burn injury may also produce proximal interphalangeal joint flexion deformities (45). Stern et al. (59) classified these deformities due to flexion contracture of the palmar digital skin into three categories based on location and severity. In this classification, type I contractures are limited to the skin. In type II contractures, additional capsular shortening exists, requiring a capsulotomy for complete release. Type III contractures have accompanying narrowing of the joint space and articular incongruity, requiring bone shortening or arthrodesis to improve function. The classification also correlated directly with the outcome of surgical treatment. The poorest results are more commonly associated with type III contractures.

Proximal interphalangeal flexion contractures arising from the destruction of the dorsal skin and extensor tendon are most formidable deformities seen in these joints (60). Groenevelt and Schoorl (60) noted that when deeper structures of the dorsum of the hand are involved primarily by thermal injury or by subsequent infection, the most affected area is the proximal interphalangeal joint. This is because the thin overlying skin and scanty subcutaneous tissue confer little protection to the structures of the joint. In addition, metacarpophalangeal joint hyperextension contractures, can lead to flexion at the proximal interphalangeal joint as a result of the effect of tenodesis. Prolonged immobilization of the proximal interphaleangeal joint in flexion during the acute burn period is potentially detrimental. Acute therapy is usually limited to maintaining the proximal interphalangeal joint in extension through external splinting or K-wire fixation. This minimizes tension on the central slip of the extensor tendon and the transverse retinacular ligaments (32). This approach is successful in preserving proximal interphalangeal joint function in mild cases. However, the more severe cases go on to develop early postburn boutonnière deformities, with a fraction progressing to the highly debilitating chronic postburn boutonnière deformities.

Larson et al. (56), observed that the early postburn boutonnière deformity responds satisfactorily to splinting (56). They, therefore, advocated splinting for early cases even if the joint is exposed with the central part of the dorsal hood destroyed. They also noted that splinting might allow the open areas to fill in with scar tissue. Groenevelt and Schoorl (60) supported Larson et al.'s observation but made the distinction between early cases and long-standing boutonnière deformities (60). For the patients with a long-standing or chronic bountonnière deformity, there is rupture of the central slip and the transverse ligaments have given way with volar subluxation of the lateral bands. Here, surgical correction is required. The potential for reconstruction is deemed slim, however, because of the myriad of problems accompanying the deformity. These include the scarred poor quality skin overlying the dorsum of the joint, the damaged articular surfaces of the joint, and the contractures of the capsuloligamentous structures that preclude a delicate and sophisticated reconstruction (32,60). Elliot (61) observed that reconstruction of the proximal interphalangeal joint extensor mechanism in the context of a postburn boutonnière deformity is difficult and rarely successful. Consequently, he recommended arthrodesis. However, reconstructive procedures may be offered to a select few in whom the dorsal tissues are of good quality, the articular surfaces are undamaged, and full passive range of motion is restored through preoperative physical therapy. Groenevelt and Schoorl (60) observed that the reconstructive procedure consists of two parts, correction of the deformity and repair of the extensor mechanism. Correction of the deformity involves freeing the lateral bands from their volar attachment and placing them in their normal positions. A capsulotomy to release the collateral ligaments and occasionally a release of the volar plate may be required. The extensor mechanism is repaired by reattachment of the central slip to restore extension of the middle phalanx and to provide a stabilizing action of the middle phalanx during finger flexion (62). This can be achieved through tendon advancement procedures, depending on the availability and state of the proximal and distal stumps of the central slip (51,63,64). The lateral bands, flexor tendons, or free tendon grafts could also be used in repair of the central slip (63,65–67). Larson et al. (56), in 1970, described the use of free tendon grafts through four short midlateral incisions in place of the popular dorsal approach. This approach avoided postoperative wound breakdown, which can occur with the dorsal approach. They obtained satisfactory results with the approach and concluded that some chronic boutonniere deformities can be corrected satisfactorily by avoidance of dorsal incisions and use of free tendon grafts. Clearly, there are a number of methods to address the correction of boutonnière deformities. However, a mobile joint is crucial in the use of splinting, lateral band transposition or the use of tendon grafts to correct this problem (Fig. 33.11) (Table 33.6). The use of prosthetic implants for joint replacement in the management of these injuries is still in a stage of infancy. Groenevelt and Schoorl have reported the use of resection implant arthroplasty with the Swanson prosthesis on two occasions for postburn bountonnière deformities with ankylosed joints (43,60). They readily admit, however, that the functional outcome with use of the joint prostheses was disappointing in spite of good skin coverage and sufficient extensor mechanisms.

3. Distal Interphalangeal Joint

Deep dorsal burns over the distal interphalangeal joint can lead to rupture or weakening of the extensor tendon at its insertion into the base of the distal phalanx (43). The resultant defect is a mallet finger. If this is associated with hyperextension at the proximal interphalangeal joint, a swan-neck deformity is possible. The articular surfaces of the distal interphalangeal joints can be completely destroyed in these deformities with no residual motion (32,43). Surgical correction by wedge excision arthrodesis in a functional position is often the only option for functional rehabilitation. Digital amputations might have to be considered. A stiff, malpositioned, and painful digit, particularly on the ulnar boarder of the hand, is only a nuisance to the overall function and appearance of the hand.

(A)

(B)

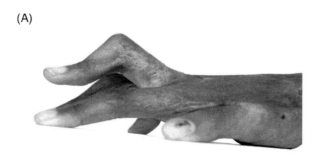
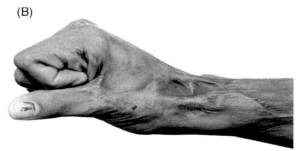

Figure 33.11 (A) Postburn boutonnière deformities of the middle and fifth fingers. (B) Demonstrating joint flexibility, which makes this deformity suitable for surgical correction. [Reprinted from: McCauley RL, Asuku ME. Upper extremity burn reconstruction. In: Mathes S, ed. Plastic Surgery. 2nd ed. Philadelphia: W.B. Saunders (in press).]

Table 33.6 Methods for Correction of Boutonniere Deformities

I. Splinting
II. Lateral band transposition
III. Tendon grafts
IV. Arthrodesis

C. Amputations

Digital losses after vascular compromise can result from severe thermal injuries to the hand. It is crucial that the vascular status of the digit be assessed early in the acute phase of injury. Maneuvers aimed at improving the circulation of the digits such as the elimination of edema, escharotomies, and fasciotomies are important in preserving perfusion to the digits. When the postburn deformed hand is characterized by digital losses, it constitutes a major problem to the reconstructive hand surgeon. The most severe of such injuries result in multiple digital amputations producing a paddle hand. On occasion, with the resultant scars, the remaining phalanges may be hidden and malpositioned. Radiographic examination is therefore essential in the assessment of the patient and is a useful tool in decision-making (32).

In reconstruction of the digits, the thumb and index finger are the most important. Because the thumb accounts for 40–50% of the total function of the hand, it is usually the first to be addressed (68). Diminished thumb function represents a severe handicap to the patient, and this is made worse if the remaining portion of the hand is compromised by heavy scarring, contractures, joint stiffness, and shortened digits (69,70). Ward et al. (71) noted that the absence of the thumb in severe burns poses reconstructive problems not seen in other types of trauma. They observed that there is usually loss of additional digits as well as soft tissue injury to the remainder of the hand. It is believed that the potential for flap loss is markedly increased when local flaps are elevated acutely in scarred and skin-grafted areas. In addition, scar contractures across joints and web spaces are usually present. Burn scars on the trunk may decrease the amount of donor sites available for the use of pedicled flaps. When both hands are involved, the problem is compounded. The goal of reconstruction is to restore adequate thumb function. Adequate thumb function requires the presence of a tactile digit capable of being opposed to at least one other digit or in the hand. The level of amputation, the degree of function, and the status of the remainder of the hand will determine the most suitable reconstructive procedure. The objective of thumb–index finger reconstruction is to provide lateral pinch or key pinch. Of concern are the issues of length, strength, stability, sensibility,

and mobility (72). The methods of reconstructing the thumb range in complexity from first web space releases to the technically complex microvascular toe to thumb transfer (25). The choice of reconstruction of those must be governed by its ability to maximize functional return.

On occasion, the burned hand may be so extensively damaged that reconstruction may not be considered. Yet, such drastic decisions are rarely considered even in the most devastatingly deformed cases. In such cases, amputation and fitting of prosthesis may offer overall improvement. This recommendation, however, requires the most careful consideration for the patient. Factors such as age, sex, vocation and avocation, hand dominance, and status of the contralateral hand must be carefully analyzed (54). When the need for amputation is limited to the digits, consideration must be given to any amputation for improvement of overall functional and aesthetic outcome.

1. Phalangization

Described by Huguier, phalangealization is one of the earliest techniques of thumb reconstruction (72). It is indicated in the severely burned hand with multiple proximal digit loss resulting in the paddle or mitten hand. The goal of thumb reconstruction is to achieve gross pinch between the first ray and the reachable remaining ulnar portion of the hand (72). The procedure consists of first web space deepening, transfer of the adductor pollicis tendon more proximally on the thumb metacarpal shaft, and excision of the index metacarpal shaft. The procedure minimizes the risk of flap elevation and extensive dissections in areas of deep scarring. The result is an apparent increase in thumb length and an increase in the width and depth of the web space. It is a one-stage operation capable of producing excellent functional results as well as an acceptable aesthetic outcome. This technique, however, often produces insufficient thumb length made worse if there is concomitant contracture of the web space. It has generally been replaced by pollicization procedures, which in such a severely burned hand may simply be a second to first metacarpal transfer.

2. Pollicization

Littler (73) popularized the advancement pollicization after World War II. It involves the vascularized osteocutaneous transfer of the remnant of the index metacarpal ray onto the thumb metacarpal stump to produce increased length of the thumb with increased functional capabilities. It is indicated when severe thumb and index finger are rendered relatively useless and the two are converted into a single functional thumb. Best results are obtained when a mobile trapeziometacarpal joint exists, thenar musculature remains functional, and good sensibility of the digit to be pollicized remains (68). May et al. (72) also made several technical observations that are important in achieving satisfactory outcome. They noted that in the presence of severe scarring, flap resurfacing of the burned hand carried out as a preliminary procedure would improve soft tissue quality at the time of pollicization. They also noted that proximal identification of the neurovascular structures at the initial stage of dissection would ensure that the palmar skin island selected for transfer with the index metacarpal is accompanied by the appropriate neurovascular structures. They advocated proximal division of the index metacarpal bone to obtain complete mobilization. However, the wrist flexor and extensor tendons as well as the volar neurovascular pedicle should be preserved. Adduction of the thumb ray as well as splitting the common digital nerve to the second web longitudinally allows maximal advancement. They suggested the use of longitudinal Kirschner wire and interosseous wiring to achieve osteosynthesis. The Kirschner wire is removed in 6–8 weeks after boney union is confirmed by X-rays. The newly created web space should be draped with the available flap and resurfaced with a thick STSG. Progressive first web splinting is used to expand the web for at least 6 weeks, and the splint is then worn as a night splint for up to 6 months postoperatively. Several authors have reported satisfactory functional results in terms of range of motion of the reconstructed thumb and two-pointed discrimination. Single-hand prehensions through the assessments of tip and lateral pinch strengths have been shown to improve with advancement pollicization procedures (68–72) (Figs. 33.12 and 33.13).

3. Distraction Lengthening

Matev (74) introduced metacarpal lengthening by use of a distraction device to increase the length of a shortened thumb. The prerequisites for this procedure include the presence of all or most of the metacarpal, a functional trapeziometacarpal joint, functional muscles of the thumb and adequate soft tissue over the thumb and in the web space. Predistraction soft tissue transfer in the form of a flap may be indicated if the thumb is involved in a dense unyielding scar (75). The technique initially involved the insertion of pins above and below the osteotomy site. A subperiosteal transverse osteotomy at the middle third of the first metacarpal is performed. Distraction is started within a week of the operation. The distraction is done at the rate of 1–1.5 mm daily for 25–40 days, depending on the amount of lengthening required. Matev reported obtaining length increment of up to 38 mm in a 12-year-old boy without significant decrease in sensibility and without injury to the remaining open thumb epiphysis (74). However, he observed that for successful outcome, at least most of first metacarpal must be present and skin coverage of the amputation stump should be adequate.

Immobilization begins after cessation of the distraction and is continued until ossification of the interfragmental gap is complete and there is solid fusion of the bone. Stern et al. used this technique in the reconstruction of burn deformed thumb in a 10-year-old boy. They achieved 25 mm of lengthening during 4 weeks of distraction (76,77). Satisfactory functional and aesthetic results were obtained and they concluded that the procedure is simple and effective and does not risk the loss of an adjacent digit.

4. Toe to Thumb Transfer

The development of microsurgical techniques permitted the single-stage transplantation of tissues and added a new dimension to thumb reconstruction. The great toe to thumb free tissue transfer was first performed experimentally by Buncke and clinically by Cobbett (70). Toe to thumb transplantation is indicated for reconstruction of thumb amputations distal to the proximal third of the first metacarpal. It allows replacement of the missing metacarpophalangeal and interphalangeal joints as well as the nail and specialized cutaneous structures of the thumb (70). Preparatory flap transfer to ensure adequate coverage of vital structures and to provide tissue for a pliable thumb web may be required. Toe to thumb transfer can provide excellent aesthetic and functional rehabilitation of the burned hand when pollicization is not possible. It is limited by problems of availability. In patients who have survived large TBSA burns, the feet may be part of the injury. It is otherwise a safe, reliable, and efficient means of thumb reconstruction that offers significant advantages over other techniques. In the words of Buncke, great toes make great thumbs (70). The subsequent introduction of the use of second toe for transfer has made the procedure possible even when the big toes are unsuitable for transfer. Again, it is emphasized that in patients with large TBSA burns, multiple digits of the hands as well as the feet may be involved with severe burn injury. In cases of multiple digital loss along with toe amputations, this method of reconstruction is not possible.

5. Osteoplastic Thumb Reconstruction

This is a multistaged procedure consisting of lengthening of the thumb remnant with a bone graft placed into a tubed pedicle flap. Later restoration of sensation with a neurovascular island transfer wrap completes the reconstruction. It is often bulky, poorly functional, and aesthetically unacceptable. It has therefore largely been abandoned and is mentioned only for historical interest (68).

V. ELECTRICAL BURNS

Burns resulting from the passage of electric current are among the most devastating of injuries (78,79). Although

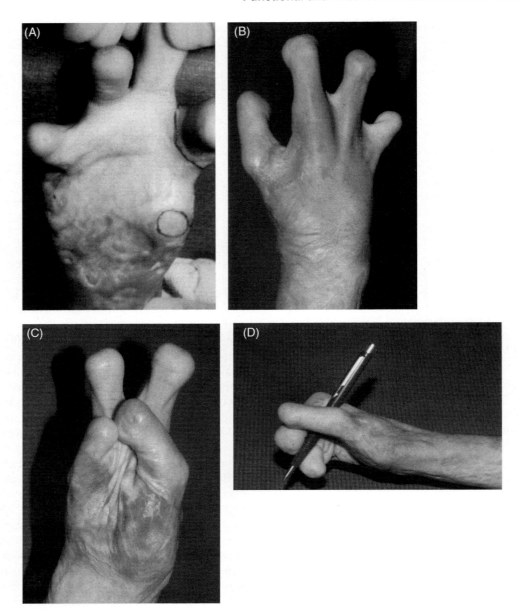

Figure 33.12 (A) A 10-year-old patient with multiple digital amputations. Note loss of thumb. (B) Seven years after first to second metacarpal transfer with growth of amputated stumps and metacarpal transfer. (C) Excellent opposition noted. (D) Functional result also acceptable.

they account for only 3–12% of all burn injuries, electrical burns are associated with multiple complex operative procedures and high amputation rates. Whereas most low-voltage injuries (<1000 V) occur in the home, high-voltage injuries (>1000 V) occur as industrial accidents and are characterized by high morbidity and mortality rates (79). The upper extremity is the most frequently involved region of the body in electrical burn injuries (32,79–84). Most series have reported upper extremity involvement in high-voltage electrical injuries to be as high as 60–80%. This is to be expected because the

hands are usually the entry points in a majority of these injuries that occur as occupational hazards (81,82).

A. Initial Management

Immediate treatment is aimed at resuscitation of the patient and then salvage of the affected limb. The key to the acute management of electrical injuries to the upper extremity is to have a high index of suspicion for potential damage to deeper tissues (32). The initial clinical presentation largely determines the ultimate outcome in the

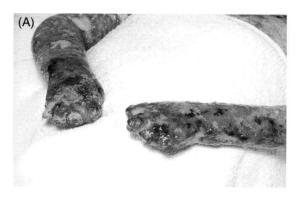
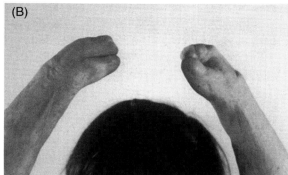
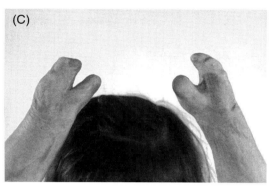

Figure 33.13 (A) A 7-year-old patient with multiple digital amputations. (B) Bilateral metacarpal transfers noted with hands closed. (C) Bilateral metacarpal transfers noted with hands open.

extremity (78,79). The contracted charred extremity with no distal pulses may require amputation and fitting with a prosthesis. In less severe injuries, the ultimate goal is limb salvage to maximize upper extremity function.

Early exploration and debridement is usually carried out to remove necrotic tissue. Hunt et al. (85) observed that escharotomy and fasciotomy in the management of electrical injuries are not only therapeutic but also diagnostic. Carpal tunnel release to minimize median nerve compression is often essential at exploration. Subsequent debridement within a few days after injury may be useful in ensuring complete excision of all devitalized tissues (86). Mann et al. (79) observed that serial debridement has been the historic key to successful management of these injuries. The precise delineation of viable tissue may be difficult to determine during the first 24–72 h (79). They advocate immediate decompression in only a select few who exhibit progressive peripheral nerve dysfunction, clinical manifestation of compartment syndrome, or injury sufficient to cause difficulty in resuscitating the patient. They also suggested that other patients are better served by a more conservative approach. This means delaying the initial operation for a few days until the necrotic tissue can be recognized with subsequent excision and closure of the wound. It is of paramount importance to ensure adequate debridement before closure is pursued.

Technetium Tc99M stannous pyrophosphate scintigraphy has been found to be a useful tool in aiding the diagnosis of focal areas of skeletal muscle necrosis (78,83,87). Yet, it is not a substitute for adequate surgery. In the acute stage, closure with skin grafts to protect vital structures from desiccation may be indicated. However, replacement with flap coverage may subsequently be required as a prelude to reconstruction.

B. Outcome

The outcome of immediate treatment is two-fold. The limbs that have suffered major vascular damage will progress and may require late amputations. On the other hand, other limbs may be deemed salvageable. Yet, in most series the incidence of amputations remain high. Achauer et al. (78) documented a 40% amputation rate in the upper extremity of 22 patients with high-voltage injuries. Salisbury et al. (88) reported an amputation rate of 37% in a series of 76 patients. Mann et al. (79), however, advocated immediate selective compression for high-voltage electrical injuries (79). Their overall amputation rate was reported to be only 10%. Although this is considerably lower than reported rates in most series, 43% of their patients did not require any form of surgery. This suggests that the injuries were less severe.

After severe high-voltage electrical injuries, most salvage limbs suffer variable degrees of deficit that may require reconstruction to maximize hand function. While waiting for reconstruction, these limbs must be adequately managed to prevent progressive disabilities. Neurologic deficits may require physical therapy to maintain muscle bulk and supple joints. The loss of protective sensation is an indication for measures to protect against trauma.

C.   Reconstruction

The general principles of staged reconstruction have remained dependable (78,89). Soft tissue deficits are addressed ahead of nerve repairs, and then tendon and muscle transfers when indicated. Adequate soft tissue cover is a primary concern and often requires the use of flaps. The types of flaps available for coverage of these

injuries are numerous. However, fasciocutaneous flaps are primarily used for reconstruction. The use of free flaps in an extremity that has suffered significant electrical injury calls for the utmost in caution (78). The vascular status of the ulnar and radial arteries needs to be assessed in the event that the hand is surviving on one damaged vessel. Although muscle flaps have been used, the goal of the reconstructive effort should match the necessary soft tissue coverage. Flap coverage allows for later evaluation and deeper reconstruction of vessels, nerves, or tendons. Once coverage is completed, nerve grafts, if indicated, are performed by use of sural nerve cable grafts. In a series of six patients who suffered high-voltage electrical injuries involving the upper extremities, McCauley and Barret (89) reported the use of sural nerve cable grafts of 9–10 cm mean length in repair of the median and ulnar nerves in seven extremities (Fig. 33.14). Soft tissue

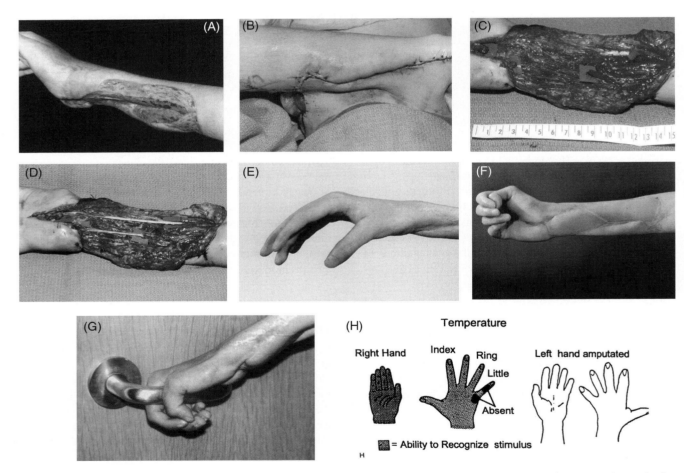

Figure 33.14   (A) A 13-year-old patient with extensive loss of musculature and poor volar surface skin graft coverage 1 month after high-voltage electrical injury. The hand is insensate. (B) Excision of skin graft and coverage with an abdominal flap prior to further reconstruction. (C) Elevation of flap and identification of proximal and distal stumps of the median and ulnar nerves. (D) Reconstruction of the median and ulnar nerves with sural nerve cable grafts. (E) Flexion 1 year after reconstruction. (F) Extension 1 year after reconstruction. (G) Demonstrating hand function 1 year after reconstruction. (H) Analysis of response to temperature changes at 1 year after reconstruction. [Reprinted with permission from McCauley and Barret (89).]

cover was required in five extremities as a prelude to nerve grafting. The outcome was satisfactory as all six patients developed protective sensation within a few months. After nerve repairs, tendon injuries are then addressed. Operations include tendon grafts and tendon transfers. However, supple joints must be considered prerequisites to these procedures. Staged tendon grafts with silicone spacers may also be used successfully. Tendon transfers from a relatively spared compartment may, generally, give better functional outcome (78).

Engrav et al. (90), reported the results of a survey on the outcome of treatment of upper extremity electrical injuries. This group documented the total return of function in 6%, partial return of function in 53%, and no functional return in 28% of the patients (90). They concluded that the potentials for maximizing hand function depend on the degree of initial injury and the salvage efforts instituted in the immediate post injury period. Achauer et al. (78) observed that reconstruction of the severely damaged

hand might take several months and still leave significant loss of strength, agility, and sensitivity. They further noted that rehabilitation for many occupations might be more rapid with amputation and prosthesis. Similarly, McCauley and Barret (89) noted that the neurologic sequelae of high-voltage electrical injuries remain significant, with <6% of adult patients returning to their jobs. Despite this outlook, optimism on the part of the reconstructive team and the patient can yield satisfactory results in even the most severe of these injuries (Fig. 33.15).

VI. CONCLUSION

Reconstruction of the burned hand starts with the acute stage of injury. The elimination of edema, adequate positioning, adequate early resurfacing, and prompt physical therapy are crucial in maintaining hand function (91). The management of the postburn deformities may

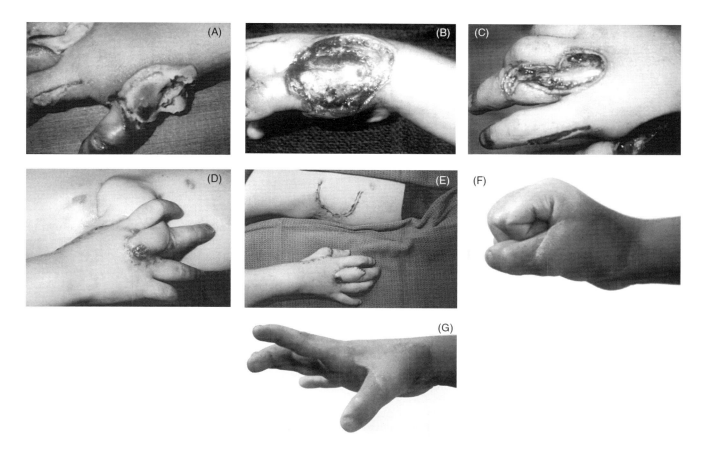

Figure 33.15 (A) Electrical burn with full-thickness burns to the radial aspect of the thumb and dorsal aspect of the third finger. (B) Debridement showing full-thickness injury to the radial aspect of the thumb. (C) Exposure of the extensor tendon and proximal interphalangeal joint. (D) Coverage with a groin flap, split longitudinally to cover both defects. (E) Flap division and insetting. (F) Final outcome, demonstrating flexion. (G) Final outcome, demonstrating extension. [Reprinted from: McCauley RL, Asuku ME. Upper extremity burn reconstruction. In: Mathes S, ed. Plastic Surgery. 2nd ed. Philadelphia: W.B. Saunders (in press).]

require a multidisciplinary approach to address encountered problems. Treatment options must be based on detailed functional assessment and the formulation of realistic goals appropriate for the patient's needs (30,92). The ultimate outcome of treatment is related to function and appearance. It is clear that motivation and optimism are essential in the relationship between the reconstructive team and the patient, a relationship that may span years or decades.

REFERENCES

1. American Burn Association: Guidelines for service standards and severity classifications in the treatment of burn injury. Bull Am Coll Surg 1984; 69:24–29.

2. American Medical Association: Guides to the Evaluation of Permanent Impairment, 4th ed. Chicago: American Medical Association, 1994.

3. Engrav LH, Dutcher KA, Nakamura DY. Rating burn impairment. Clin Plast Surg 1992; 19:569–598.

4. Tredget E. Management of the acutely burned upper extremity. Hand Clin 2000; 16:187–202.

5. Sheridan RL, Hurley J, Smith MA, Ryan CM, Bondoc CC, Quinby WC, Tompking RG, Burke JF. The acutely burned hand: management and outcome based on a ten-year experience with 1047 acute hand burns. J Trauma 1995; 38:406–411.

6. Schwanholt C, Greenbalgh DG, Warden G. A comparison of full-thickness versus split thickness autografts for coverage of deep palmar burns in the very young pediatric patient. J Burn Care Rehabil 1993; 14:29–33.

7. Pensler JM, Stewart R, Lewis SR, Herndon DN. Reconstruction of the burned palm: full-thickness vs. split-thickness skin grafts—long-term followup. Plast Reconstr Surg 1988; 81:46–49.

8. Whitson TC, Allen BD. Management of the burned hand. J Trauma 1971; 11:606.

9. Kucan JO. Burns. In: Russell RC, ed. Hand Surgery. St Louis: Mosby, 2000.

10. Pisarski GP, Mertens D, Warden GD, Neale HW. Tissue expander complications in pediatric burn patient. Plast Reconstr Surg 1998; 102:1008–1012.

11. Hergrueter CA, O'Connor NE. Skin substitutes in supper extremity burns. Hand Clin 1990; 6:239–242.

12. Dantzer E, Braye FM. Reconstructive surgery using an artificial dermis (Integra): results with 39 grafts. Br J Plast Surg 2001; 54:559–664.

13. Chou TD, Chen SL, Lee TW, Chen SG, Cheng TY, Lee CH, Chen TM, Wang HJ. Reconstruction of burn scar of the upper extremities with artificial skin. Plast Reconstr Surg 2001; 108:378–384.

14. Burke JF, Yannas IV, Quinby WC, Bondoc CC, Jung WK. Successful use of physiologically acceptable artificial skin in the treatment of extensive burn injury. Ann Surg 1981; 194:413–428.

15. Heimbach D, Luterman A, Burke J, Cram A, Herndon D, Hunt J, Jordan M, McManus W, Solem L, Warden G,

16. Zawacki B. Artificial dermis for major burns: a multi-center randomized clinical trial. Ann Surg 1988; 208:313–320.

16. Lorenz Ch, Petracic A, Hohl HP, Wessel L, Waag KL. Early wound closure and early reconstruction. Experience with a dermal substitute in a child with 60 percent surface area burn. Burns 1997; 23:505–508.

17. Hunt JA, Moisidis E, Haertsch P. Initial experience in the treatment of post-burn anterior cervical neck contracture. Br J Plast Surg 2000; 53:652–658.

18. Suzuki S, Matsuda K, Maruguchi T, Nishimura Y, Ikada Y. Further applications of "bilayer skin." Br J Plast Surg 1995; 48:222–229.

19. Shakespeare P, Shakespeare V. Survey: use of skin substitute material in UK burns treatment centres. Burns 2002; 28:295–297.

20. Sedmak DD, Orosz CG. The role of vascular endothelial cells in transplantation. Arch Pathol Lab Med 1991; 115:260–265.

21. Lattari V, Jones LM, Varcelotti JR, Latenser BA, Sherman HF, Barrette RR. The use of permanent dermal allograft in full thickness burns of the hand and foot: a report of three cases. J Burn Care Rehabil 1997; 18:147–155.

22. Wainwright DJ. Use of an acellular allograft dermal matrix (Alloderm) in the management of full thickness burns. Burns 1995; 21:243–248.

23. Barret JP, Dziewulski P, McCauley RL, Herndon DN, Desai MH. Dural reconstruction of a class IV calvarial burn with decellularized human dermis. Burns 1999; 25:459–462.

24. Rennekampff HO, Pfau M, Schaller HE. Acellular dermal matrix: immediate or delayed epidermal coverage? Burns 2001; 28:100–101.

25. Parry SW. Reconstruction of the burned hand. Clin Plast Surg 1989; 16:577–586.

26. Robson MC, Smith DJ. Burned hand. In: Jurkiewicz MJ, Krizek TJ, Mathes SJ, Ariyan S, eds. Plastic Surgery: Principles and Practice. St. Louis: Mosby, 1990:781–802.

27. McCauley RL. Reconstruction of the pediatric burned hand. Hand Clin 2000; 16:249–259.

28. Strock LL, McCauley RL, Smith DJ. Reconstruction of the burned hand. In: Herndon DN, ed. Total Burn Care. Philadelphia: W.B. Saunders, 1996:506–514.

29. Mlakar JM, Dougherty WR. Reconstruction of the burned hand. In: Herndon DN, ed. Total Burn Care. 2nd ed. Philadelphia: W.B. Saunders, 2002:628–655.

30. Burns BF, McCauley RL, Murphy FL, Robson MC. Reconstructive management of patients with greater than 80% TBSA burns. Burns 1993; 19:429–433.

31. Peacock EE, Madden JW, Trier WC. Some studies on the treatment of burned hands. Ann Surg 1970; 171:903.

32. Donelan MB. Reconstruction of the burned hand and upper extremity. In: May JW Jr, Littler JW, eds. The Hand. Philadelphia: W.B. Saunders, 1990:5452–5482.

33. Brown HC. Current concept of burn pathology and mechanism of deformity in the burned hand. Orthop Clin North Am 1973; 4:987.

34. Salisbury RE. Acute care of the burned hand. In: McCarthy J, ed. Plastic Surgery. Philadelphia: W.B. Saunders, 1990:5399–5417.

35. Smith MA, Munster AM, Spence RJ. Burns of the hand and upper limb—a review. Burns 1998; 24:493–505.

36. Magliacani G, Bormioli M, Cerutti V. Late results following treatment of deep burns of the hands. Scand J Plast Reconstr Surg 1979; 13:137–139.

37. Deitch EA, Wheelahan TM, Rose MP, Clothier J, Cotter J. Hypertrophic burn scars: analysis of variables. J Trauma 1983; 23:895–898.

38. Cole R, Shakespeare P, Rossi A. Conservative treatment of deep partial thickness hand burns—a long-term audit of outcome. Br J Plast Surg 1992; 45:12–17.

39. Parks DH, Baur PS, Larson DL. Late problems in burns. Clin Plast Surg 1977; 4:547–560.

40. Larson DL, Abston S, Willis B, et al. Contracture and scar formation in the burn patient. Clin Plast Surg 1974; 1:653–666.

41. Perkins K, Davey RB, Wallis KA. Silicone gel: a new treatment for burn scars and contractures. Burns 1982; 9:205–213.

42. Achauer BM, VanderKam VM. Burn reconstruction. In: Auchauer BM, ed. Plastic Surgery: Indications, Operations, and Outcomes, Vol 1. St. Louis: Mosby, 2000:425–446.

43. Groenevelt F, Schoorl R, Hermans RP. Retrospective study of reconstructive surgery of the burned hand. Burns 1985; 11:351–358.

44. Krizek TJ, Robson MC, Flagg SV. Management of burn syndactyly. J Trauma 1974; 14:587–593.

45. Kurtzman LC, Stern PJ. Upper extremity burn contractures. Hand Clin 1990; 6:261–279.

46. Larson DL, Abston S, Evans EB et al. Techniques of decreasing scar formation and contractures in the burned patient. J Trauma 1971; 11:807–823.

47. Limberg AA. Skin plastic and shifting triangular flaps. Leningrad Trauma Inst 1929; 8:62.

48. Wolf RM, Broadbent TR. The four flap Z-plasty. Plast Reconstr Surg 1971; 49:48–51.

49. Ozek C, Cankayali R, Bilkay U, Guner U, Gundogan H, Songu E, Akin Y, Cagdas A. Marjolin's ulcers arising in burn scars. J Burn Care Rehabil 2001; 22:384–389.

50. Upton J. Discussion of correction of postburn syndactyly: an analysis of children with introduction of the V–M plasty and postoperative pressure inserts. Plast Reconstr Surg 1982; 70:353–354.

51. Salisbury RE. Bevin AG. Atlas of Reconstructive Burn Surgery. Philadelphia: W.B. Saunders, 1981.

52. Spinner M. Fashioned transpositional flap for soft tissue adduction contraction of the thumb. Plast Reconstr Surg 1969; 44:345–348.

53. Housinger TA, Ivers B, Warden GD. Release of the first web space with the "goalpost" procedure in pediatric burns. J Burn Care Rehabil 1993; 4:353–355.

54. Beasley RW. Secondary repair of burned hands. Clin Plast Surg 1981; 8:141–162.

55. Mancoll JS, Mlakar JM, McCauley RL. Burn web space contractures—are they just a bad penny. Proc Am Burn Assoc 1996; 28:111.

56. Larson DL, Wofford BH, Evans EB et al. Repair of the boutonnière deformity of the burned hand. J Trauma 1970; 10:481–487.

57. Graham TJ, Stern PJ, True SM. Classification and treatment of post burn metacarpophalangeal joint extension contractures in children. J Hand Surg Am 1990; 15:450–456.

58. Peterson HC, Elton R. Reconstruction of the thermally injured upper extremity. Major Probl Clin Surg 1976; 19:148.

59. Stern PJ, Neale HW, Graham TJ, Warden GD. Classification and treatment of post burn proximal interphalangeal joint flexion contractures in children. J Hand Surg Am 1987; 12:450–457.

60. Groenevelt F, Schoorl R. Reconstructive surgery of the post burn boutonnière deformity. J Hand Surg Br 1986; 11:23–30.

61. Elliot R. Boutonnière deformity. Symposium on the Hand. St. Louis: CV Mosby, 1971:42.

62. Weeks PM. The chronic boutonnière deformity: a method of repair. Plast Reconstr Surg 1967; 40:248–251.

63. Souter WA. The problem of boutonnière deformity. Clin Orthop 1974; 104:116–133.

64. Snow JW. Use of a retrograde tendon flap in repairing a severed extensor tendon in the PIP joint area. Plast Reconstr Surg 1973; 51:555–558.

65. Maisels DO. The middle slip or boutonnière deformity in burned hands. Br J Plast Surg 1965; 18:117–129.

66. Planas J. Buttonhole deformity of the fingers. J Bone Joint Surg Br 1963; 45:424.

67. Matev I. Transposition of the lateral slip of the aponeurosis in treatment of long standing boutonnière deformity of the fingers. Br J Plast Surg 1964; 17:281–286.

68. Kurtzman LC, Stern PJ, Yakuboff KP. Reconstruction of the burned thumb. Hand Clin 1991; 8:107–119.

69. Pohl AL, Larson DL, Lewis SR. Thumb reconstruction of the severely burned hand. Plast Reconstr Surg 1976; 57:320–328.

70. Valauri FA, Buncke HJ. Thumb reconstruction—great toe transfer. Clin Plast Surg 1980; 16:475–489.

71. Ward JW, Pensler JM, Parry SW. Pollicization for thumb reconstruction in severe pediatric hand burns. Plast Reconstr Surg 1985; 76:927–932.

72. May JW, Donelan MB, Toth BA, Wall J. Thumb reconstruction in the burned hand by advancement pollicization of the second ray remnant. J Hand Surg Am 1984; 9:484–489.

73. Littler JW. The neurovascular pedicle method of digital transposition for reconstruction of the thumb. Plast Reconstr Surg 1953; 12:303.

74. Matev IB. Thumb reconstruction in children through metacarpal lengthening. Plast Reconstr Surg 1979; 64:665–669.

75. Matev IB. Gradual elongation of the first metacarpal as a method of thumb reconstruction. In: Stack HG, Bolton H, eds. The Second Hand Club. London: British Society for Surgery of the Hand, 1975:431.

76. Stern PJ, MacMillan BG. Reconstruction of the burned thumb by metacarpal lengthening. Burns 1983; 10:127–130.

77. Stern PJ, Neale HW, Carter W, MacMillan BG. Classification and management of burned thumb contractures in children. Burns 1985; 11:168–174.

78. Achauer B, Applebaum R, VanderKam VM. Electrical burn injury to the upper extremity. Br J Plast Surg 1994; 47:331–340.

79. Mann R, Gibran N, Engrav L, Heimbach D. Is immediate decompression of high voltage electrical injuries to the upper extremity always necessary? J Trauma 1996; 40:584–589.

80. Marshall KA, Fisher JA. Salvage and reconstruction of electrical hand injuries. Am J Surg 1977; 134:385.

81. Skoog T. Electrical injuries. J Trauma 1970; 10:816.

82. Davies MR. Burns causec by electricity: a review of 70 cases. Br J Plast Surg 1959; 11:288.

83. Yakuboff KP, Kurtzman LC, Stern PJ. Acute management of thermal and electrical burns of the upper extremity. Orthop Clin North Am 1992; 23:161–169.

84. Barnard MD, Boswick JA. Electrical injuries of the upper extremity. Rocky Mt Med J 1976; 73:20–24.

85. Hunt JL, McManus WF, Haney WP, Hunt JL, Sato RM, Baxter CR. Acute electrical burns. Arch Surg 1980; 115:434–438.

86. Rouse RG, Dimick AR. Treatment of electrical injury compared to burn injury. J Trauma 1978; 18:43–47.

87. Hunt JL, Lewis S, Parkey R, Baxter C. The use of technetium-99m stannous pyrophosphate scintigraphy to identify muscle damage in acute electrical burns. J Trauma 1979; 19:409–413.

88. Salisbury RE, Hunt JL, Warden GD, Pruitt BA. Management of electrical burns of the upper extremity. Plast Reconstr Surg 1974; 51:648–652.

89. McCauley RL, Barret JP. Electrical injuries. In: Achauer BM, ed. Plastic Surgery: Indications, Operations, and Outcomes. St. Louis: Mosby, 2000:375–385.

90. Engrav LH, Gottlieb JR, Walkinshaw MD. Outcome and treatment of electrical injury with immediate median and ulnar nerve palsy at the wrist; a retrospective review and a survey of members of the American Burn Association. Ann Plast Surg 1990; 25:166–168.

91. Achauer BM. Burn Reconstruction. New York: Thieme, 1991.

92. Mahler D, Benmeir P, Ben Yakar Y, Greber B, Sagi A, Hauben D, Rosenberg L, Sarov B. Treatment of the burned hand: early surgical treatment versus conservative treatment. A comparative study. Burns 1987; 13:45–58.

34

Finger Lengthening of the Burned Hand by Distraction Osteosynthesis

DAVID WAINWRIGHT, DONALD H. PARKS

University of Texas—Houston Medical School, Houston, Texas, USA

I. INTRODUCTION

The hand is commonly involved in thermal injuries, with an incidence of up to 89% of burn patient admissions (1). Sheridan et al. (2) has reported that when tissue destruction is severe (Class C injury—fourth-degree burns), significant functional deficits are observed in >90% of patients. This is particularly true when amputations are necessary. In this situation, very few, if any, reconstructive options are available. Although adaptation to distal, limited amputations is generally satisfactory, more proximal amputations are poorly tolerated, especially if the injury involves the thumb or multiple digits. The effect on pinch and grasp significantly impacts the patient's ability to perform basic acitivites of daily living (ADLs) such as dressing, feeding, and personal hygiene. To address this difficult problem, finger lengthening can serve as an option to improve overall hand function.

II. HISTORY

The development of finger lengthening techniques has primarily focused on the management of congenitally short fingers (especially thumbs) and, to a lesser degree, traumatic amputations. The thumb has enjoyed particular emphasis secondary to its importance to overall hand function, and even construction of a simple, stable post can be very useful.

The approach has been one of either distal augmentation or interpositional distraction. "Pseudolengthening" techniques have also been described, which do not actually produce an increase in length but an increase in "functional length." These include phalangization or simple first webspace deepening techniques. These may also serve as an adjuvant to certain lengthening procedures to increase their effectiveness.

Distal augmentation techniques involve the addition of both bone and soft tissue to the end of the amputated digit and are generally used for very proximal amputations that require greater length or need the function of a digit capable of active motion. This can take the form of techniques where the bone graft and soft tissue flaps for cover are supplied independently (Gilles cocked hat osteoplastic reconstruction toe wrap-around flap) or composite flaps containing all of the required components (osteocutaneous flaps pollicization of an adjacent digit toe to hand transfer) (3–9). Although technically more demanding, the composite flap techniques have the potential for restoring both movement and the most complete and precise sensation. The latter is the most important factor in determining the ultimate use and function of the reconstructed digit.

The Gilles cocked hat technique uses a proximal, volar-based flap of the thumb, which is elevated to surround a free bone graft (generally iliac) that is secured in longitudinal fashion to the bony remnant of the thumb. This is a relatively simple, dependable, one-stage procedure which preserves sensation by using local tissue with the digital nerves intact. There is a limit on the length of bone graft the flap can cover, and the technique is only applicable to reconstruction of the thumb, producing a stable post. Bone graft survival and union can be inconsistent.

Osteoplastic reconstruction involves placement of a pedicled flap (groin, tubed abdominal) around a free bone graft with secondary division of the flap once it has established a blood supply from the hand. Although it has the potential for producing a stable functional post for the thumb, it has the disadvantage of a two-staged procedure and can be overly bulky. Perhaps more importantly, the flap is insensate, diminishing its usefulness, and has generally been combined with a second procedure of a digital neurovascular island flap to provide sensation.

The toe wrap-around technique transfers the skin, nail, pulp, and a variable amount of phalangeal bone from the great toe by microvascular technique to the thumb, often surrounding a free bone graft that provides additional length. It has the advantages of a thumb with good soft tissue bulk, sensation, and cosmesis, and avoids the sacrifice of an entire toe. The microsurgical technique is more demanding and the reconstruction serves as a post only.

Composite techniques can serve as an alternative technique to producing a post or potentially restore a functional digit. A variety of osteocutaneous flaps (rib, radius, iliac crest, scapula, fibula, first metatarsal) are available to the reconstructive surgeon, some of which are applicable to the reconstruction of the thumb. Since the bone is part of the flap and therefore vascularized, bone survival and union are more dependable and successful. It produces a post and, like the osteoplastic technique, has the similar disadvantages of being bulky and insensate. It requires a microsurgical technique and if this is to be used, perhaps a functioning digit would be a better choice.

Pollicization can restore active movement and excellent sensation by transposing an adjacent digit (usually the index) to the thumb for proximal amputation levels. It is particularly useful if there is only an index remnant, as this will salvage use from a digit with suboptimal function. This technique has the added advantage of widening the first webspace.

The toe to hand transfer is the "ultimate composite flap," having the potential for the most precise reconstruction of an amputated digit. The great toe has been used for thumb reconstruction and the second toe has been described for replacing either the thumb or the other digits. This method can restore soft tissue bulk, sensation, active motion, and supplies an intact, mobile joint. It can also provide the best cosmetic result. The procedure is technically demanding and the recipient site must be suitable to accept this transfer. Sacrifice of the great toe may affect the performance of some athletic activities, and some patients dislike the cosmetic result.

While distal augmentation methods attempt to replace the missing bone and soft tissue with additional tissue, interposition techniques focus on the addition of hard tissue and rely on the soft tissue's ability to stretch and expand. This technique was first applied to the lengthening of long bones as described by Codivilla (10) for the lengthening of the lower limb. Interposition techniques in the hand were first described by Matev (11) for the lengthening of a traumatically short thumb. This has also been used for other applications (12,13). An osteotomy was first performed in the bone to be lengthened and the fragments were immediately separated to a specific distance to achieve the desired length. An external fixator was applied which held the fragments in position and permitted further lengthening while new bone developed across the gap. Although this was successful in children, many adults were not capable of forming sufficient osseous tissue across large gaps (>2.5–3.0 cm) and developed a nonunion. Kessler et al. (12) modified this technique to include a bone graft for the adult population or when long distraction gaps were created (13). Manktelow and Wainwright (14) modified the osteotomy design in an effort to obtain primary bone healing and avoid the use of a bone graft. Their step osteotomy was effective; however, this technique required a longer length of residual bone to accommodate the step portion of the osteotomy. Periosteal flaps over the gap section facilitated new bone growth and eventual healing.

To avoid the problems with nonunion experienced when the fragments were immediately distracted, the hand surgeons looked to the orthopedic literature. Putti (15) was the first to propose that lengthening be performed using continuous traction but it is the technical refinements developed by Ilizarov (16,17) which are the basis of most clinical practice today. His technique, often called "callotasis," lengthens the bone after the healing process has been initiated at the osteotomy site. The osteotomy involves the cortex only, preserving the overlying periosteum and the inner endosteum. These undamaged structures are available to participate in the healing process and the generation of new bone. An external fixation device is placed which holds the fracture fragments in their preosteotomy position with no separation at the osteotomy site. There is a 2-week lag period before lengthening begins. This allows new oseous tissue to be formed at the site of injury, forming an early callus. At approximately 2 weeks, lengthening of the bone is initiated. This involves gradual widening of the osteotomy gap by a specific amount each day. Once the desired length is achieved, the external fixation device remains in place to provide immobilization and stability. The interfragmentary gap, now filled with osteoid tissue, is allowed to solidify by calcification.

Application of the Ilizarov technique for hand reconstruction has been described for both congenital and traumatic deformities (13,18–21). In the burn population, this technique has primarily been used for thumb reconstruction to compliment older techniques, although in selected cases it has been applied to other digits (22–24).

III. ETIOLOGY

Shortened digits following burn injury are most commonly a result of a deep fourth-degree injury, necessitating amputations. In children, other mechanisms can be responsible. The burn can retard growth by affecting epiphyseal viability, causing joint destruction, or the restricting effect of a tight scar contracture can modify bone growth.

IV. GOALS

The goal of surgery is not simply to produce a longer finger. In addition to length, finger function, particularly as it applies to the thumb, is dependent on optimizing mobility, sensation, and stability. Therefore, lengthening the finger cannot compromise these other considerations.

Patients with digital amputations will present with specific functional deficits that lengthening of the finger will address. The functions that can be improved by this technique include:

1. improved first webspace opening for holding objects
2. standard pinch
3. key pinch
4. increased security and power of holding large objects.

These particular functions have a corresponding effect on ADLs and other specific tasks. The thumb and index finger are primarily involved with pinch and holding objects in the first webspace while the remaining digits afford security and power to holding larger objects. Feeding and hygiene tasks primarily require a "holding" function while pinch is important for dressing. Although more complex tasks such as buttoning garments and tying shoes are not realistic, holding small (pinch) and large (grasp) objects can be improved.

V. OVERVIEW OF TECHNIQUE

This technique is a modification of a standard distraction osteosynthesis technique used for long bone lengthening. If a sufficient bony remnant exists following digit amputation as a result of burn injury, this procedure can be considered.

There are two important technical aspects that significantly influence the success of this technique. First, ideally a corticotomy, rather than an osteotomy, is performed. This minimizes disruption of the periosteum and the endosteal tissue within the marrow cavity. These structures are therefore available to participate in bone healing with the generation of callus at the corticotomy site.

Second, distraction is delayed by several weeks to allow an early callus to form that contains immature woven bone and more importantly a significant number of osteoprogenitor cells. Therefore, it is actually this healing fracture callus which is lengthened, and so the term "callotasis" (Fig. 34.1). The rate of lengthening is important. Too rapid lengthening may lead to nonunion since the bone forming tissues cannot produce sufficient matrix to fill the gap. In contrast, if distraction is too slow, calcification may occur with early union across the distraction gap, preventing further lengthening.

The standard time course is 2 weeks of stabilization following the corticotomy, gradual, continuous lengthening over 4–6 weeks, followed by a 2–4-week period of stabilization to allow the new bone to calcify and solidify.

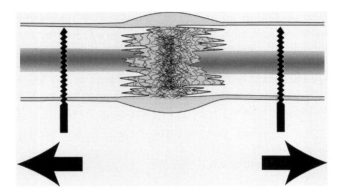

Figure 34.1 Callotasis/callus distraction – callus forms within interfragmentary gap and is lengthened by gradual distraction across the corticotomy site.

VI.   INDICATIONS/CONSIDERATIONS

The decision to reconstruct, and the choice of method to accomplish this, is not a simple one. The patient's needs, desires, the specifics of the injury and anatomic deficit, and the available donor tissues (both local and distant) all have to be considered. This complex decision is particularly true for the thumb, as evidenced by the numerous articles attempting to provide objective criteria and algorithms for determining the most suitable procedure for an individual patient and injury.

A.   Level of Amputation

Not all digital amputation can be managed appropriately with this lengthening technique. Loss of length distal to the mid middle phalanx does not generally require reconstruction since adequate function is usually present at that level of loss. Finger loss at or proximal to the metacarpophalangeal (MCP) joint is generally too severe to permit meaningful reconstruction using a distraction lengthening technique; however, this has been attempted in one case. The majority of our experience has been with amputations at the level of mid-proximal phalanx (Fig. 34.2).

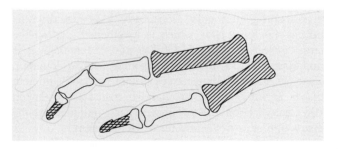

Figure 34.2 Level of amputation – distal amputations do not require reconstruction while very proximal amputation levels will not be adequately managed by distraction lengthening alone.

The thumb is the most important digit for hand function, and preserving its length is critical. Amputations distal to the mid distal phalanx are generally well tolerated. In contrast, when the loss is proximal to the MCP joint, this technique is unlikely to provide a functionally important increase in length and distal augmentation methods should be considered.

Although this technique has recently been applied to traumatic distal phalangeal amputation stumps, the author feels this is unlikely to find application in the burn population (25).

B.   Length of Bone

Sufficient bone must be available to provide room for the placement of the external fixation pins and the osteotomy site. The Mini Hoffman device has two longitudinally oriented pins on either side of the osteotomy. These are 0.5 cm apart and therefore the minimal workable length of the phalangeal remnant is about 1.5 cm.

C.   Number of Digits Injured

Only in exceptional circumstances would one consider lengthening a single shortened digit. Generally, if uninjured or minimally injured digits are present, the patient will adapt to this deficit and the lengthened digits will be ignored, not be used, or possibly get in the way and interfere with function. With isolated finger amputations, alternate approaches should be considered. For example, an isolated index finger amputation at the proximal phalanx may best be managed by ray amputation rather than by lengthening with the uninjured middle finger, assuming the functions of the index. The exception to this single-finger exclusion is when the thumb has been amputated since it contributes substantially to hand function and can provide great benefit when acting simply as a post. The author has generally reserved the distraction lengthening technique for either a shortened thumb or patients with burn amputations of all four fingers.

A relative indication would be an isolated index finger. This may be considered if the third finger is not suitable as a substitute for index function. Since the remaining digits are often injured, lengthening of an isolated index finger may be more appropriate as the number of amputations and severity of associated injury to the other digits increase.

D.   Specific Digits

Since the thumb is such a functionally important digit, lengthening should always be considered. Even as a simple post, the thumb can supply many of the required functions. Lengthening of shortened index and middle fingers can also be helpful since they contribute to standard and key pinch, by acting as posts in combination with the thumb. Lengthening of the ulnar digits is less useful since a "post" will not contribute significantly to grasp, although the "security" and power of holding large objects might be improved. On the ulnar side of the hand, one might consider a secondary wedge osteotomy of a lengthened phalanx to produce an "arthrodesis" in a functional position but the author has not attempted this.

E. Patient Compliance

Patient cooperation is critical for this technique to be successful. The patient is expected to maintain and care for the apparatus during the lengthening period and will be responsible for the day-to-day lengthening. They also must be willing and capable of participating in an intense occupational therapy program following completion of the lengthening process.

F. Timing

This is not a procedure to be considered during the acute phase of burn management. All tissues must be completely matured and there should be no residual hypertrophic scarring or burn contracture of the involved digits.

G. Tissue Condition

Although uninjured skin of the digital remnant is preferable, it is not essential. Stern (22) advocates excising the burn scar and resurfacing the digit, ideally with a flap. The author has not found this to be necessary in all cases as mature scar tissue is capable of stretching. However, if the skin cover is atrophic or unstable and/or little to no soft tissue padding exists over the distal bone, this should be considered. Adequate sensation is crucial so that the patient will and can use the reconstructed digit effectively. Resurfacing with a skin graft or a conventional local flap may diminish this and limit the usefulness of the reconstruction.

The joint proximal to the bone to be lengthened should be stable with an intact ligamentous structure and an acceptable range of motion. In addition, there should be adequately functioning motors, both flexor and extensor, across this joint.

H. Age

Special considerations in the child include the size of the bone structures to be lengthened, and the presence and location of the epiphyseal growth center. The ability of the parents to manage the child's care and comply with the lengthening program also needs to be evaluated.

In the older patient, compliance issues are again important, as they may be unable to tolerate the surgery, distraction, or rehabilitation necessary for the procedure to be successful. Pre-existing problems (e.g., arthritis, trauma) are also more likely to be seen in this population.

VII. CONTRAINDICATIONS

There are a number of clinical situations in which this technique is either not applicable or not advisable. When confronted with an amputation of a single digit, excluding the thumb, lengthening is unlikely to be a benefit and the process involved may ultimately compromise hand function further if the amputated digit interferes with overall hand function. Often a ray amputation may be the best solution in this clinical situation.

Since one of the primary goals of digital lengthening is to restore adequate pinch, amputations on the ulnar side of the hand are less likely to be improved with lengthening since the grasping function of this side of the hand requires effective finger flexion and not simply a static, stable post. Small residual bone fragments cannot be lengthened since there is insufficient bone for placement of the distracting apparatus. Also, amputations proximal to MCP joints generally cannot be lengthened sufficiently to provide an adequate post for pinch. Perhaps most importantly, since the patient needs to participate in the lengthening process and protect the external fixation apparatus, compliance is of paramount importance. If the patient demonstrates an inability to dependably participate in their care, the technique of distraction osteosynthesis of the amputated digit is not an appropriate choice.

VIII. TECHNIQUE

A. Preparation

An aggressive preoperative occupational therapy program is essential to maximize the range of motion of the joint proximal to the bone to be lengthened. In addition, all scar therapy should be completed to include compression therapy and scar release or resurfacing where necessary.

In the thumb, an adduction contracture can exist from muscle shortening and/or scarring as a result of direct thermal injury or inability to maintain the thumb in an abducted position during the acute burn care phase. If a degree of intrinsic tightness exists preoperatively in a digit, it may result in a flexion contracture at the MCP joint proximal to the lengthened bone. Occupational therapy techniques such as passive stretching and dynamic splinting can be used to help rectify these problems. If these measures are unsuccessful, the release of an adductor or an intrinsic muscle will need to be considered.

The patient should be thoroughly educated on the procedure to be undertaken and understand the goals of the reconstruction, their role in the lengthening process, and the need for their strict compliance with postreconstruction therapy.

Anterior-posterior (an X-ray view) and lateral radiographs of the bone to be lengthened are necessary to confirm that adequate length and bone quality are available to perform this procedure. A "mock" surgery can be drawn on the radiograph to confirm this.

B.   Apparatus

The apparatus used by the author is the Hoffman® mini-lengthening and external fixation device (Howmedica, Switzerland) (Fig. 34.3). This technique employs two fixation pins in both the proximal and the distal bone fragments. Although transfixing pins are available, generally threaded, 2.0 mm diameter, self-tapping half pins have been used for distraction lengthening. These are available in a variety of lengths to provide versatility in clinical application.

The pins allow purchase of the lengthening device onto the bone fragments. Although three planes of movement are available with this apparatus, longitudinal lengthening of digits rarely necessitates this feature. Mobility of one of the sliding blocks along the central shaft of the apparatus provides some versatility between pin pairs. A measuring scale from 0 to 25 mm is engraved on the inner shaft of the lengthening device to accurately monitor the lengthening process. Length adjustment of the apparatus is accomplished by rotating and adjusting a nut on one end of the apparatus. There is an additional locking nut at this location to prevent inadvertent movement between adjustment events.

A variety of hand chucks, socket wrenches, and spanners are available for stabilization and adjustment of the apparatus. A drill guide is also available to ensure that

the two pins on each bone fragment are a precise distance apart, so that they can be secured to the pin clamps of the external distraction device.

C.   Surgery

The surgery is performed under either general or block anesthesia and under tourniquet control. The outline of the phalangeal remnant is drawn on the dorsum of the amputated digit and the proposed transverse corticotomy is marked in the center of the phalangeal remnant (Fig. 34.4). A longitudinal line is also drawn perpendicular to the corticotomy line, in the center of the bony fragment. This represents the axis of the pin placement. The proposed pin sites are then marked. The pins are located as far away from the osteotomy site as the length and quality of the bony remnant will permit. The author has found that placement of the pins is much easier if performed prior to the corticotomy. This provides a larger bony fragment to secure while drilling the pin holes and facilitates the accurate placement of the pins along the longitudinal axis of the bone.

Two pins are placed on either side of the corticotomy site in a longitudinal fashion. The first pin to be placed is that furthest away from the corticotomy site. This should be placed as far away from the corticotomy site

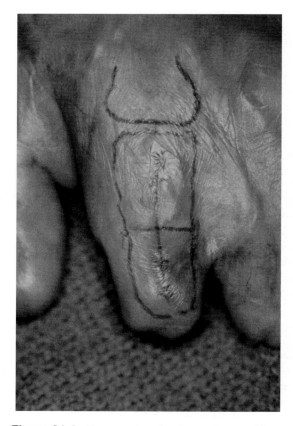

Figure 34.4   Preoperative planning surface markings.

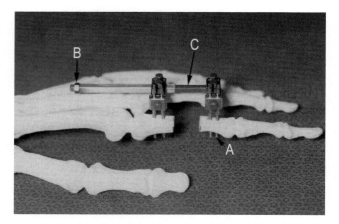

Figure 34.3   Hoffman® mini-lengthening device (A) Distal pin site. (B) Point for distraction wrench. (C) Measurements of distraction length.

as possible but far enough from the end of the bony fragment so that there will be adequate bone for pin purchase and there is no risk of entering the joint. A stab incision is made at the proposed pin location and this is extended down to the bone. Using a fine periosteal elevator, the periosteum is cleared over a small area of bone that is to be drilled. Using a drill guide to protect the skin, a bicortical drill hole is performed using a 1.5 mm drill bit. Care should be taken that this and all subsequent drill holes are placed perpendicular to the dorsal surface of the bone (Fig. 34.5).

Using the special pin insertion hand chuck, a 2.0 mm threaded half pin is placed in this hole. It should be inserted to the entire thickness of bone and one can palpate on the volar surface to feel for the tip as it exits the volar surface of the bone. Once this pin is in place, the two-hole drill guide is placed over this pin. The second hole of the drill guide is placed along the longitudinal axis line and a second 1.5 mm hole is drilled. A second 2.0 mm pin is then inserted at this site. Two pins are then placed by the same technique into the opposite end of the bone fragment.

Once the two fixations pins are placed at either end of the bone fragment, the corticotomy can be performed (Fig. 34.6). It should be noted that in Ilizarov's original description, a corticotomy was performed which preserved the periosteal and endosteal structures for bony generation. Although this is the ideal and should be strived for, it may not be practical. With the small diameter of the phalanx, completely preserving the endosteal structures may not be possible.

An incision is made along the longitudinal axis on the dorsum of the bone. This is taken down to and through the periosteum. A periosteal dissector is then used to separate the periosteum from the phalanx, around its circumference at the proposed corticotomy site. The corticotomy is performed using a small 1 or 2 mm sharp osteotome. This method is more precise and results in less heat and mechanical injury to the surrounding tissues than with the use of powered instruments. This is angulated to the sides, in an attempt to cut the cortical bone only and preserve as much of the internal endosteal tissue as possible. These details minimize the injury to the adjacent tissues and hence, optimize healing. Once the corticotomy is completed, the two ends of the phalangeal fragment should be separated and the surgeon should be able to rotate them slightly in relation to one another. The external apparatus is then applied making sure that the two phalangeal fragments maintain precisely the same orientation that they did preoperatively (Fig. 34.7). The lengthening appliance needs to be positioned, so that it is not protruding unnecessarily and run the risk of damage or hitting it. The latter can cause malalignment of the fragments and also lead to pin loosening. The lengthening apparatus also needs to be positioned, so that it can be accessed easily for subsequent lengthening.

The small dorsal incision is closed and the pin sites wrapped with 0.5 in. antibiotic impregnated gauze. Application of a protective splint completes the procedure.

D. Postoperative Care/Lengthening

The apparatus remains stationary and the wounds permitted to heal over the following 2 weeks. At this stage the repair process has begun at the corticotomy site and early callus has been formed. The apparatus and pins

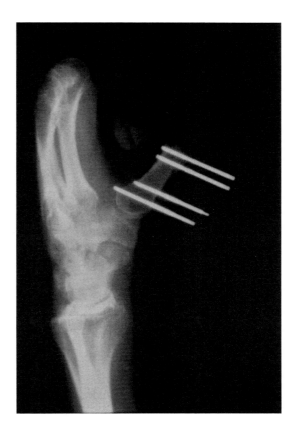

Figure 34.5 Correct pin placement confirmed by X-ray.

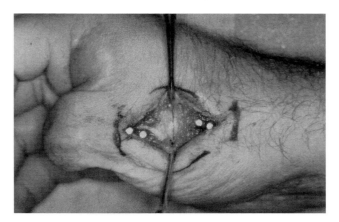

Figure 34.6 Bone exposed for planned corticotomy.

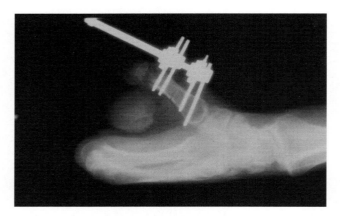

Figure 34.7 External fixation device applied to maintain bone fragments in precorticotomy position.

need to be reinspected to make sure that the longitudinal axis in both the dorsal-volar and the radial-ulnar directions has been preserved. If the two fragments are not aligned correctly, there may be problematic deviation and angulation of the future lengthened bone.

Lengthening is initiated at 2 weeks. This is generally begun at half a turn of the lengthening apparatus (1/2 mm) per day and is soon increased to half a turn twice per day for a total of 1 mm of lengthening per day. This lengthening process is continued until the desired length is achieved, which is generally between 2 and 3 cm. In the authors' experience this usually takes ~1 month (Fig. 34.8).

From this point, the lengthening apparatus takes on the function of an external fixation device. The distracted bony fragments are maintained in position, as stable as possible, to permit new solid bone growth within the distraction gap. Insufficient stabilization can lead to malunion and nonunion. Solidification of the distraction gap generally takes 2–4 weeks.

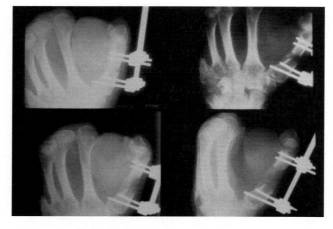

Figure 34.8 Serial X-rays during distraction illustrating gradual lengthening and new bone formation within gap.

E. Removal

At 2–3 weeks, the authors will loosen the external fixator and test the lengthened phalanx for stability. If the distracted bone is deemed solid, the external fixator is removed. This is generally accomplished in the operating room since local anesthesia is inadequate. If it is not solid, the external fixator remains in place for another 2 weeks and the bone is tested again.

Following removal, the finger is protected for another week or two until there is radiographic evidence of bony continuity across the distraction gap. The patient will then be allowed to use the digit in a normal fashion and an aggressive occupational therapy program will be initiated.

IX. MODIFICATIONS

If the digit has been lost with only a small middle phalangeal remnant, lengthening of the intact proximal phalanx can be considered. Since the surgeon is now working at lengthening an entire intact phalanx, the technique is often easier, since a longer length of bone is available. However, in this situation, as the lengthening proceeds there will be inevitable tethering from the long flexor tendons and this may result in flexion contracture across the proximal interphalangeal joint (PIPJ). This can be avoided by stabilizing the PIPJ prior to distraction. Crossed Kirschner wires can be placed across the PIPJ maintaining the middle phalangeal remnant in a neutral position. In this way, some of the distraction forces are more directly applied to the long flexor tendon. This modification is also applicable to the thumb when a small proximal phalangeal remnant is present. Lengthening, in this instance, is performed on the metacarpal.

When only a small proximal phalangeal remnant remains, lengthening of the metacarpal is an option. Once lengthened, the distal metacarpal fragment can be angled volarly, thus creating an "arthrodesis" at an acceptable angle at the MCP joint level. Theoretically, a joint could be transplanted or a joint implant inserted at this site, to provide mobility at this site, but the author has not attempted this.

X. REHABILITATION AND OCCUPATIONAL THERAPY

The rehabilitation of the patient undergoing distraction lengthening of the finger involves two phases. The first phase is during the time the distraction device is in place. Extreme caution must be exercised to protect the external fixation device from trauma to the pin sites since this may result in loosening and/or infection. If excessive forces are generated in a vector that is not parallel to the axis of lengthening, then malalignment will occur. The occupational therapists focus on both the digit being lengthened and the remainder of the hand. They undertake a maintenance program to preserve mobility and function of the adjacent digits and the hand. Active and very gentle passive range of motion exercises can be performed with the lengthened digit(s) within the pain tolerance limit of the patient. Occasionally, the fixation pins may tether the soft tissue structures, especially a tendon, which may produce pain and mechanically block full excursion of the adjacent joints.

Phase 2 of occupational therapy is begun once the external fixation device is removed and a solid bony union is present across the distraction gap. There are two components to this therapy program. First, some tightening of the periarticular structures (ligaments, intrinsic muscles) may have occurred during the lengthening process secondary to immobilization. Once a solid bony union has been achieved, these can be aggressively addressed through a program of active and passive range of motion exercises and possibly dynamic splinting. The aim is a full active and passive range of motion. Webspace tightness may occur necessitating use of static (C-bar) and dynamic splints for the first webspace and soft, custom inserts held in place by a pressure glove for the other webspaces. The second component of occupational therapy at this time is focused on using the lengthened digits for specific functional tasks and ADL. Specifically, this addresses improving pinch function and strength and the ability to hold and manipulate objects in the hand.

XI. ADDITIONAL PROCEDURES

A. Webspace

In instances of a shortened thumb, the first webspace may become tighter as a result of the distal pull on the tissues from the lengthening process. If occupational therapy is unsuccessful, the first webspace may need to be lengthened or deepened. Depending on the severity, release with skin grafts or local tissue rearrangement (four flap Z-plasty), distant flaps, or a second ray amputation may be necessary to optimize the size of the first webspace.

If two adjacent digits are lengthened, the author has observed some distal migration of the webspace skin. In order to maximize individual finger movement it is sometimes necessary to perform a webspace release, using a standard syndactyly reconstruction technique with a dorsal flap and full-thickness skin graft.

B. Intrinsic Release/Tendon Lengthening

Mild adduction contractures of the thumb that were initially missed or clinically insignificant may become more problematic following lengthening and require release.

The inability of the intrinsic hand muscles to lengthen in concert with the bone can result in a flexion contracture at the MCP joint proximal to the lengthened bone and necessitate release.

Occasionally, the flexor tendons will fail to lengthen adequately, thereby causing a flexion contracture. This occurs only when there is a joint distal to the lengthened bone. An example of this is when only a small middle phalangeal fragment is present and distraction osteosynthesis occurs within the proximal phalanx.

XII. COMPLICATIONS

Pin site infection and/or loosening can occur with improper pin insertion technique, inadequate pin care, or trauma to the apparatus while it is in place. A small amount of drainage or minimal loosening might be salvaged with local pin site care and strict immobilization and protection. Otherwise, if significant pin loosening occurs, the procedure will not be successful and needs to be abandoned.

Deviation or malalignment of the distracted bone can occur through inaccurate pin placement and apparatus assembly. Small degrees of malalignment can be adjusted during distraction. Wenner (26) described a case in which a 90° angulation deformity was noted at the osteotomy site 10 days following the initiation of the distraction process. The fragments were realigned in the operating room after a portion of the lengthening was reversed, and held in alignment with a longitudinal smooth K-wire. Further lengthening of the metacarpal proceeded uneventfully with the longitudinal K-wire both preventing further bending and "directing" the direction of subsequent lengthening. Late malunion, occurring once the corticotomy gap has solidified, will require an osteotomy to reposition the bone fragments and benefit from the application of an internal fixation device.

Nonunion is generally a result of either too rapid distraction or failure to adequately immobilize the distracted bone following the completion of lengthening. If identified early, the lengthened digit can be salvaged with immobilization, otherwise secondary bone grafting may be necessary, with or without the added stability of an internal fixation method.

XIII. ADVANTAGES

This technique of distraction osteosynthesis offers certain advantages. It uses local tissue to provide improved function and therefore avoids the necessity of a donor defect. Since the distraction process occurs gradually over a period of time, soft tissue structures can be successfully stretched and lengthened and the pain is generally minimal unless there is movement at the pin site. In addition, since the native neural structures to the digits are preserved, sensation remains intact to the amputation stump. This technique can provide improved function, particularly pinch, and the ability to hold larger objects in the hand. Although this method demands some degree of surgical precision, it is not as technically demanding as the microvascular anastomoses required in toe to hand transfers.

XIV. DISADVANTAGES/LIMITATIONS

This technique is not applicable in all instances of finger amputation, as sufficient bone must be available for the distraction process. There must be a bone fragment of adequate length and quality to achieve reliable, solid purchase of the threaded pins for placement of the distraction apparatus and sufficient room for the corticotomy. There is also a limitation of ~3 cm in overall lengthening. If more ambitious lengthening is attempted, the bone separation may "outstrip" the capacity of the corticotomy gap to ossify and achieve a solid, stable union. In this situation, the gap may require autogenous (nonvascularized) bone graft to facilitate healing. If it is the surgeon's opinion that more than 3 cm length is required to restore satisfactory function, then alternative methods may have to be considered from the outset. This technique simply provides a solid, static post, which relies on adjacent, uninjured joints and tendons for movement. It does not result in increased total active movement of the finger since additional motors and/or joints are not supplied by this method. If additional flexion is necessary for function, then pollicization or a toe to hand procedure is indicated. The lengthening process is prolonged and therefore may run the risk of complications such a malalignment, pin problems, and nonunion. It also requires strict patient cooperation for maintenance of the apparatus and gradual distraction.

XV. RESULTS

This technique can achieve 2–3 cm increased length of an amputated digit. Sensation to the tip is preserved which maximizes the use of the reconstruction. Solid union has been achieved in all cases without use of a bone graft. Pinch and holding objects in the first webspace have been the specific hand functions that are most improved with this method (Figs. 34.9 and 34.10).

XVI. ALTERNATIVES

A. Alternate Lengthening Techniques

There are a number of alternative options for finger lengthening, especially of the thumb. Immediate

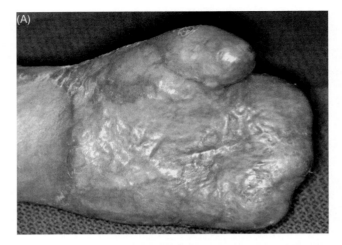

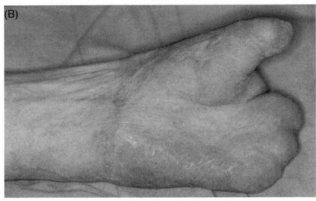

Figure 34.9 (A) Mitten hand with short thumb. (B) Thumb lengthening.

lengthening as described by Matev (27) may be applicable to the pediatric population or short gaps since there would be adequate osteogenic tissue to accomplish bony union. Otherwise, there is a limit in the amount of lengthening that can be achieved with this method and a bone graft is required in the adult. The step osteotomy technique may be possible with larger fragments and be a more dependable technique applicable for older patients, in whom the osteogenic potential of the periosteal and endosteal tissues may not be ideal.

B. Alternate Procedures for Shortened Digits

With amputations proximal to the MCP joint, the technique of distraction lengthening will not be effective, since adequate functional length cannot be achieved with the bone available. Surgical options in this case include creation of a functional post with the Gilles cocked hat, osteoplastic reconstruction, or toe wrap-around procedures or a mobile digit with pollicization or a toe to hand transfer.

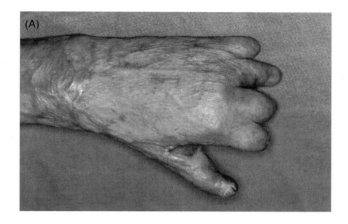

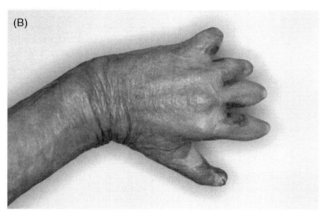

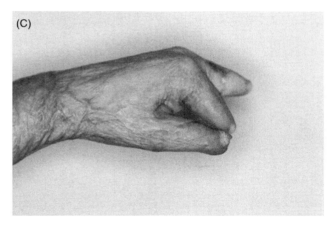

Figure 34.10 (A) Preoperative index–middle finger lengthening. (B) Postoperative index–middle finger lengthening. (C) Key pinch.

XVII. SUMMARY

Distraction osteosynthesis for finger lengthening in burn patients can be an effective tool to improve function in a hand devastated by burn injury. This technique is demanding on both the surgeon and the patient. Although it will not produce normally functioning fingers, it can significantly improve the use of an otherwise nonfunctioning hand to permit the patient to resume some ADLs and restore some degree of normalcy to their life.

REFERENCES

1. Pruitt BA. Burns of the upper extremity. Epidemiology and general considerations. Major Probl Clin Surg 1976; 19:1–15.
2. Sheridan RL, Hurley J, Smith MA, Ryan CM, Bondoc CC, Quinby WC Jr, Tompkins RG, Burke JF. The acutely burned hand: management and outcome based on a ten-year experience with 1047 acute hand burns. J Trauma 1995 Mar. 38(3):406–411.
3. Reid DAC. The Gillies' thumb lengthening operation. Hand 1980; 12(2):123–129.
4. Hughes NC, Moore FT. A preliminary report on the use of a local flap and peg bone graft for lengthening a short thumb. Br J Plast Surg 1950; 3:34.
5. Steichen JB, Weiss APC. Reconstruction of traumatic absence of the thumb by microvascular free tissue transfer from the foot. Hand Clin 1992; 8:17–32.
6. Buck-Gramcko D. Pollicization of the index finger. J Bone Joint Surg 1971; 53:1605.
7. Buck-Gramcko D. Thumb reconstruction by digital transposition. Orthop Clin North Am 1977; 8:329.
8. Cobbett JR. Free digital transfer: report of a case of transfer of a great toe to replace an amputated thumb. J Bone Joint Surg 1969; 51B:677.
9. May JW, Daniel RK. Great toe to hand free tissue transfer. Clin Orthop 1978; 133:140.
10. Codivilla A. On the means of lengthening in the lower limbs the muscles and tissues which are shortened through deformity. Am J Orthop Surg 1905; 2:353–369.
11. Matev IB. Thumb reconstruction after amputation at the metacarpophalangeal joint by bone lengthening. J Bone Joint Surg Am 1970; 52:957–965.
12. Kessler I, Baruch A, Hecht O. Experience with the distraction lengthening of digital rays in congenital anomalies. J Hand Surg 1977; 2:394–401.
13. Paneva-Holevich E, Yankov E. A distraction method for lengthening of the finger metacarpals: a preliminary report. J Hand Surg 1980; 5:160–167.
14. Manktelow RT, Wainwright DJ. A technique of distraction osteosynthesis in the hand. J Hand Surg 1984; 9A(6):858–862.
15. Putti V. The operative lengthening of the femur. J Am Med Assoc 1921; 77:934–935.
16. Ilizarov BA, Shtin VP, Ledyaev VI. The course of reparative regeneration of cortical bone in distraction osteosynthesis under various conditions of fragment fixation. Sksp Khir Anest 1969; 14:3–12.
17. Ilizarov GA. Basic principle of transosseous compression and distraction osteogenesis. Ortop Traumatol Protez 1971; 32:7.
18. Toh S, Marita A, Arai K, Nakashima K, Tsubo K. Distraction lengthening by callotasis in the hand. J Bone Joint Surg Br 2002; 84B(2):205–210.

19. Seitz WH, Froimson AL. Callotasis lengthening in the upper extremity: indications, techniques, and pitfalls. J Hand Surg 1991; 16A(5):932–939.

20. Moy OJ, Peimer CA, Sherwin FS. Reconstruction of traumatic or congenital amputation of the thumb by distraction-lengthening. Hand Clin 1992; 8(1):57–62.

21. Pensler J, Carroll NC, Cheng LF. Distraction osteogenesis in the hand. Plast Reconstr Surg 1998; 102(1):92–95.

22. Stern PJ, Macmillan BG. Reconstruction of the burned thumb by metacarpal lengthening. Burns 1983; 10(2):127–130.

23. Phol AL, Larson DL, Lewis SR. Thumb reconstruction in the severely burned hand. Plast Reconstr Surg 1976; 57:320.

24. May JW, Donelan MB, Toth BA, Wall J. Thumb reconstruction in the burned hand by advancement pollicization of the second ray remnant. J Hand Surg 1984; 9A(4):484–489.

25. Sawaizumi T, Hiromoto I. Lengthening of the amputation stumps of the distal phalanges using the modified Ilizarov method. J Hand Surg 2003; 28A(2):316–322.

26. Wenner SM. Angulation occurring during the distraction lengthening of digits. Orthop Rev 1986; 15(3):110–112.

27. Matev IB. Gradual elongation of the first metacarpal as a method of thumb reconstruction. Proceedings of The Second Hand Club. British Society for Surgery of the Hand, 1975:431.

35

Thumb and Finger Reconstruction by Microvascular Free Tissue Transfer

FU-CHAN WEI, TEWODROS M. GEDEBOU
Chang Gung University and Medical College, Taipei, Taiwan

I. INTRODUCTION

The hand, and its digital extensions represent one of the most important and complex "organs" of the human body. It provides one of the major "senses" and is an invaluable means for sustenance. As the primary structure (besides the foot) with which we directly interact with the external physical world, the hand is prone to injury by various means including burns. Burns of the hand are classified by the American Burn Association as "major", despite its relatively small surface area (3%), in recognition of its central role in human function and appearance.

II. PERTINENT ANATOMY OF THE HAND

Although the anatomy of the hand is complex and is well described elsewhere, relevant anatomy with regards to microsurgical applications in burns is comparatively simpler. The dorsal skin of the digits is thin, flexible and has numerous hair follicles, sebaceous glands, and pigment cells. Resting on a thin layer of subcutaneous tissue, it provides little protective coverage of the underlying extensor mechanism, especially at the level of the proximal interphalangeal joint (PIP), in lieu of maximizing gliding function. In contrast, the skin of the volar aspect of the hand is hairless, unpigmented, and with variable thickness along the axis of each digit. The surface topography includes multiple whorls, arches and ridges designed to maximize grip function and is complemented by underlying retaining ligaments.

The distal digit forms a unique segment beginning distal to the insertion of the sublimis in the fingers or the interphalangeal joint in the thumb. With a stable, adherent nail on the dorsum, volarly it comprises of sensate glaborous pulp skin attached to the underlying distal phalanx by a network of septae. It has the highest neural density of any body surface, due to the presence of Pacinian and Meissner's corpuscles as well as Merkel cell–neurite complexes. The nail maximizes the strong pinch surface area of the finger functions as a platform for the transmission of sensation, and due to its conspicuous location carries significant aesthetic value (1).

Two lateral proper digital arteries provide blood supply to the digits. Located dorsally in relation to the corresponding digital nerves, the proper digital arteries are extensions of the common digital arteries, which in turn branch off the superficial palmar arch. The ulnar and radial arteries contribute to this arch, with the former in dominance in the majority of cases. Multiple veins occur on the dorsal surface of each digit, superficial to the dorsal branches of proper digital arteries and nerves.

Proper function of each digit requires the undisturbed interplay of many critical structures and that of the hand requires interaction between the thumb and fingers. The thumb as the prime digit of the hand exhibits a wide range of circumductal motion at the basal joint, and is required to be opposable, stable, sensible, and of sufficient length (2,3). The index finger with its independent motion and the remaining fingers are important to stabilize objects for manipulation and power grasp. Therefore, pinch, grip, fine motor movement, and sensitive tactile feedback are the basic functions of the hand that require restoration.

III. PATHOPHYSIOLOGY OF THE BURNED HAND

The variable depths of injury from thermal or electrical burns and the anatomic complexity of the hand set the stage for a wide variety of clinical presentations that defy simple classification. Beyond the initial injury, wound healing of the burn goes through different phases correlating with final outcome of the hand. The initial or acute phase is marked by the period of inflammation and ends when epithelialization is complete. During this stage further extension of injury may develop as a result of ischemia due to edema, compartment syndrome, vascular thrombosis, over-zealous debridement and most notably infection (4,5).

After healing of all open wounds and the inflammatory phase has subsided, the burn scar undergoes a period of maturation initially marked by contraction and hypertrophy. Wounds in general usually undergo hypertrophy 3 weeks after injury, peaking at about the third month and stabilizing during the following year. Burn scars, however, undergo significant contraction and cicatrix formation especially if the wound heals by second intention or a thin skin graft used for resurfacing. Hypertrophic wounds overlying areas of motion such as joints develop into extrinsic contractures. The resulting immobilization of the joints over time leads to intrinsic contracture due to fibrosis of underlying ligaments and joint capsules. During this dynamic phase, wound healing may be affected by aggressive physical therapeutic maneuvers.

When maturation ceases, the hard and immobile burn cicatrix becomes a marker for the end-stage burn scar. Physical therapy is futile at this stage, and even surgical intervention yields suboptimal results in restoration of a "normal" digit. The chronic burn wound may develop into a recalcitrant ulcer, and persist for decades becoming a risk factor for malignancy. Another common deformity includes fingers with dorsal burns fixed into the intrinsic minus position (hyperextension of the metacarpophalangeal joint and flexion of the two digital joints) (6–8). Furthermore, if the extensor mechanism has been injured as well, then a Boutonierre deformity results from the volar migration of the lateral bands (6). Another common sequela of burn injury is that of burn syndactyly resulting from the contraction of injured web spaces. Adduction contractures of the thumb are particularly disabling by preventing its opposability, and universally require surgical correction (9). Similarly, flexion contractures of fingers into the palm impede normal function of the entire hand and therefore require early restorative measures (5).

Severe injury to the digits may also lead to structural loss either acutely or secondarily. Fourth degree burns resulting from thermal, electric, or frostbite injuries may lead to acute necrosis of the digits. Secondarily, salvaged but severely injured or poorly managed digits may develop into immobile and deformed posts interfering with the overall function of the hand. If restoration is not possible, then its removal is necessary for improved function and even appearance of the hand. If affecting several digits of the hand, significant disability shall result. The metacarpal hand represents the most severe form with variable loss of digital length as well as number of digits.

IV. GENERAL PRINCIPLES OF MANAGEMENT OF THE BURNED HAND

Outcome of the burned hand is dependent on a complex interplay between the healing process itself as well as therapeutic methods imposed on it. The largest possible impact in the restoration of function of the hand after a burn is during the acute stage. Proper wound care, adequate debridement, prevention of edema and infection, proper resurfacing, correct splinting, and early physical therapy, all play a significant role in the preservation of function. In contrast, improperly managed deep burns to the hand result in detrimental deformities that pose significant challenges to the reconstructive effort. The adequacy of debridement needs to be balanced with the necessity for tissue preservation. Biological dressings can be used and debridement may be undertaken in a staged fashion to allow excisional accuracy without compromising the digit to further injury. When the loss of the digit is inevitable, tissue preservation principles must override the method of amputation to lessen the difficulty of future restorative surgery. Resurfacing is usually accomplished during the acute period with either skin grafts or pedicled flaps such as the groin flap. Local flaps are avoided to prevent further injury to the hand.

Upon healing and entry of the burn wound into the dynamic phase, monitoring for scar hypertrophy, contracture formation, and stability is undertaken and appropriate therapy is directed. Compression garments, silicone gel, and massage may reduce the hypertrophy of burn scars during this period. Physical therapy for improving the range of motion of the joints is an essential ingredient to the functional rehabilitation of the hand.

The end-stage wound with contracture, however, will need release and resurfacing with durable tissue. If the original injury or resultant contracture is relatively minimal, resurfacing can be achieved with thick skin grafts, Z-plasty, or local flaps. If extensive, however, such as adduction contractures of the first web space or dorsal metacarpal extension contractures, then such methods yield suboptimal results. Furthermore, complete structural loss is best reconstructed with toe transfers. For example, loss of the thumb at the level of the proximal phalanx with an adduction contracture will initially require

release and resurfacing of the contracture either with a groin flap. Toe to thumb reconstruction is then undertaken secondarily.

V. INDICATIONS FOR MICROSURGICAL FREE TISSUE TRANSFER RECONSTRUCTION

During the acute stage, truly emergent microsurgical reconstruction is needed only for devascularizing injuries. Emergent restoration of blood supply with vein grafts is imperative in segmental devascularization. In complex cases, a flow-through free flap can be applied to achieve both circulation and coverage requirements (10,11). Exposure of or injury to underlying critical structures requiring resurfacing and conventional flaps are not suitable will also necessitate free tissue transfer. The wound is kept moist with physiological solution wet gauze, edema reduced by elevation, the zone of injury is clearly demarked, and the patient condition optimized prior to undertaking reconstruction. Staged reconstruction with thin free flaps can then be accomplished safely (4,12–14).

After primary healing of all wounds, worsening contractures of the digits unresponsive to physical therapy will require early release and resurfacing with durable tissue to prevent intrinsic contracture formation. Extensive skin defects following adequate release of burn cicatrix contractures are managed by thin free flaps. Similarly, in conditions such as boutonierre deformity of the digit associated with a dorsal burn cicatrix, a thin tendocutaneous free flap can be applied after release.

The most common indication for microsurgical applications, however, is restoration of composite deficiency of digits of the hand. Deformed nail beds, inadequate pulp surfaces, and amputation at various levels of the digit or digits are best reconstituted with "like" tissue transfers from the foot. A variety of clinical presentations exist in this regard. Functional deficit is noted when amputation level is proximal to the midpoint of the proximal phalanx of the finger. Loss of multiple digits imposes even more functional deficit. Both require toe transfers for ideal reconstruction. Reconstruction of the metacarpal hand is dictated according to its classification, with the intent of restoring either triple or pulp-to-pulp pinch for restoration of prehensile function.

VI. EVALUATION BEFORE MICROSURGICAL RECONSTRUCTION

During the acute stage, the extent of the burn injury as well as the vulnerable marginal zone must be recognized early. The search for any early signs that could extend the zone of irreversible injury must be vigilant. The demarcation of viable and nonviable tissue is best evaluated during serial debridement sessions.

Evaluation of the patient presenting during the maturation phase is more focused on a functional basis. The character of the "healed" wound as well as the restrictions it poses to the digits and hand must be recorded in relation to time since injury. Durability of the skin cover must be assessed especially over at-risk areas, such as the dorsal surface overlying the joints of the digits. Photographic or video documentation is a useful addition to a full physical examination and history.

Prior to undertaking any reconstructive effort however, differentiation of the actual disability of the hand from the restrictions the patient faces in his/her life should be made. An overall discussion must include the patient and those supporting him/her so that accurate expectations are understood and focused management plans set forth accordingly. Suitability of microsurgical tissue transfer is determined by evaluating adequacy of recipient as well as donor structures. Vascular supply is assessed by physical examination, Doppler flow, and in rare instances angiography. Most of the microsurgical free tissue transfers can be performed with a two-team approach taking care of donor and recipient sites, simultaneously. However, any doubt regarding suitability of the recipient site requires its exploration prior to free tissue harvest.

VII. OPTIONS IN MICROSURGICAL RECONSTRUCTION

Microsurgical techniques provide a "universal passport" into all areas of the body by transferring a segment of tissue from one part of the body to another. "Excess," and even duplication of various tissues or structures in the human body allow such autotransplantation without significant sacrifice to the donor site. Refinements in surgical technique and knowledge of anatomy continue to add various tissues to the armamentarium of reconstructive surgeons (Table 35.1).

Table 35.1 Flaps Available for Repair of Various Defects of the Hand

Defect requirement	Tissue available
Tendocutaneous	Palmaris longus, DP, TFL
Thin dorsal skin cover	Venous flaps, ALT, RF, LA, DP, MP
Palmar Skin	1st pedal web space, thenar, medial plantar
Flow through coverage	RFF, LA, DP, ALT, venous flaps
Vascularized joints	Metatarsophalangeal joint, PIP joint
Distal or entire digits	Toes

Note: RF, radial forearm; LA, lateral arm; TPF, temporoparietal fascia; TFL, tensor fascia lata; DP, dorsalis pedis; MP, medialis pedis; ALT, anterolateral thigh; PIP, proximal interphalangeal joint.

VIII. GENERAL INTRAOPERATIVE MANAGEMENT OF FREE TISSUE TRANSFER IN BURN HAND RECONSTRUCTION

Although general anesthesia is the norm for free flap reconstruction, regional methods may be applied. Tourniquet applied to involved extremities with 2 h limits, facilitates preparation of donor and recipient sites. In general, a well-coordinated two-team approach allows for the expeditious and safe undertaking of microsurgical reconstruction. The tourniquet can be temporarily released to allow for reperfusion as well as assessment of sufficient vascularity to the donor structures before division. The free tissue is then properly inset and microsurgical anastomosis is undertaken. After re-establishment of adequate vascularity to the transferred tissue, closure of remaining wounds as well as the donor site is completed. Appropriate dressings or splinting allows safe transfer of the patient to the microsurgical intensive care unit.

IX. MICROSURGICAL FREE TISSUE TRANSFER FOR RESURFACING

Loss of dorsal skin of the digits entails replacement with similarly thin tissue that would allow mobility of the finger. Venous flaps taken from the forearm or calf provide the ideal thickness for smaller defects (10,11,13). If multiple digits require dorsal resurfacing, then the radial forearm, dorsalis pedis, lateral arm, pedal first web space, medialis pedis, or anterolateral thigh can provide relatively thin tissue cover. A temporary syndactyly is created, which is divided secondarily in such cases. If the extensor mechanism is also missing due to injury or after release, segmental restoration is accomplished via a tendo-cutaneous free flap. The radial forearm with palmaris longus and the dorsalis pedis with toe extensors are the most commonly used. Venous forearm palmaris longus tendo-cutaneous flaps have also been reported, but are occasionally plagued by venous congestion.

The adduction contracture of the first web space represents one of the more common clinical entities. Excision or release of the burn cicatrix, and on occasion, myotomy of the shortened adductor pollicis is necessary to completely release the contracture. The resultant defect is resurfaced with thin, stable, and durable tissue spacer free flaps as listed earlier (Fig. 35.1). Volar defects pose specific challenges due to the requirement of restoring sensibility and prehensibility as well as providing coverage. Although multiple simple procedures have been described for reconstruction of relatively complex defects of the hand, the ideal method will have to incorporate restoration with "like" tissue that is available from the foot. For

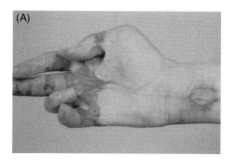 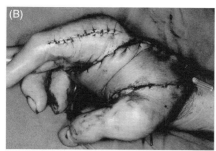 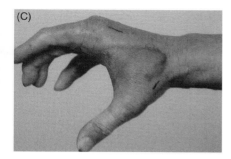

Figure 35.1 (A) Late presentation of a burned right hand resurfaced with skin grafting. The contracture involved the first web space as well as the volar surfaces of the ring and small finger. (B) Immediately after contracture release and resurfacing with a thin lateral arm free flap. (C) Outcome of the hand more than a year following free tissue transfer resulting in excellent return of range of motion of the thumb and fingers.

example, composite or structural deficits of the digits can only be replaced by similar tissue from the toes (Figs. 35.2 and 35.3). The nail, pulp, partial or entire digits, and even combined, adjacent digits are available for transfer (15). A prerequisite for toe transfer, however, is an adequate soft tissue base, which can be provided for by a groin flap (Fig. 35.4).

X. MICROSURGICAL TOE TRANSFER FOR DIGIT RECONSTRUCTION

A. Toe Dissection

1. Marking

A small wedge shaped skin island on the dorsum of the foot is usually designed to facilitate exposure and

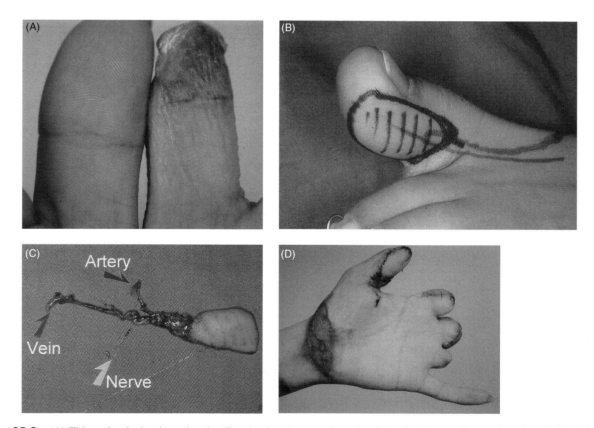

Figure 35.2 (A) This patient's dominant hand suffered a deep burn to the pulp of the thumb as well as to the other digits of the hand. (B) Design of a partial great toe pulp flap. (C) The great toe partial pulp flap after harvest demonstrating pertinent neurovascular structures. (D) Appearance of the thumb 1 week postoperatively with complete flap survival. Given the loss of the middle three digits of the hand, he will undergo finger reconstruction in 1 year.

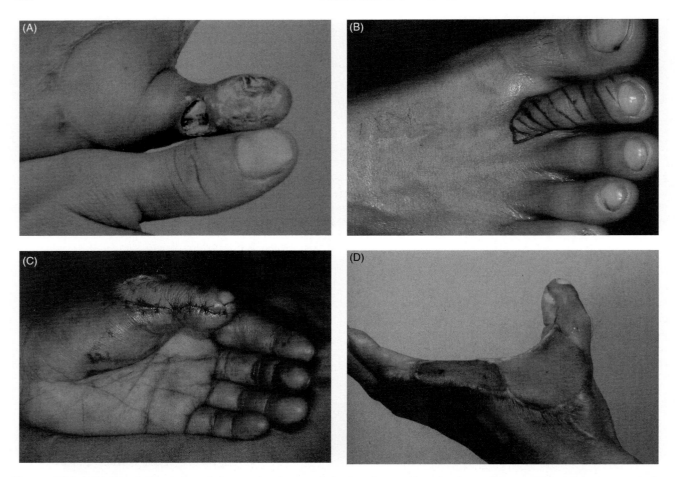

Figure 35.3 (A) Fourth degree burn injury to the dorsum of the thumb as well as the first web space. The patient presented after resurfacing with a groin flap and breakdown of the distal margin. The nail was also obliterated. (B) Designs of a second toe wrap-around flap for dorsal hemicircumferential reconstruction since the volar aspect of the thumb was intact. (C) Immediately following transfer of the second toe wrap-around flap to the thumb. (D) Long-term follow-up of the thumb revealing excellent function and acceptable appearance.

dissection of underlying structures, yet allow primary closure of the donor site.

2. Vascular Pedicle Dissection

Dissection of the vascular pedicle is initiated at the first web space to first identify the junction of the lateral digital artery of the great toe and the medial digital artery of the second. Retrograde dissection is undertaken to delineate arterial anatomy (Fig. 35.5). The first dorsal metatarsal artery (FDMA) is evaluated in comparison to the first plantar metatarsal artery (FPMA). The FDMA is preferred due to its lengthy pedicle and ease of its dissection compared to the FPMA, which disappears in the depths of the foot at the level of the middle of the metatarsal shaft. Veins are plentiful on the dorsal surface and are taken in continuity with the saphenous system at any desired length.

3. Structural Dissection

Dissection of the corresponding nerves is undertaken, isolated, and ends tagged with sutures for later identification. Depending on the length requirement, the digital nerve is lengthened via microscopic fascicular dissection of the common digital nerve. Both flexor tendons, and the extensor tendon are dissected and taken at sufficient length. Osteotomy is carried out at the appropriate level, and the entire donor tissue is left connected only via its blood supply prior to tourniquet release. Of importance, none of the structures are transected at any point prior to determining adequacy of the recipient area as well as any length requirements imposed.

B. Recipient Site Preparation

The digital stump is dissected to allow for coaptation with the harvested toe. The bony stump is cleared of the

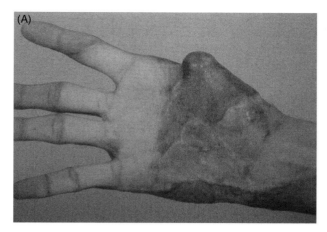

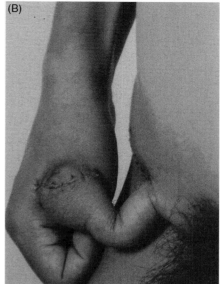

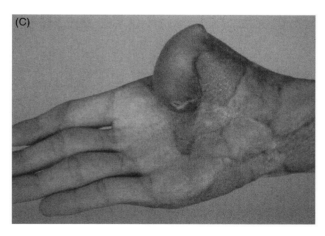

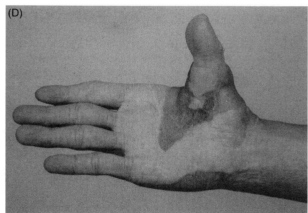

Figure 35.4 (A) Healed burn amputation of the thumb with significant injury to the surrounding tissue. Resurfacing with split-thickness skin graft has resulted in an inadequate soft tissue base as well as a stump contracture. (B) A pedicled groin flap provides sufficient soft-tissue to the thumb stump. (C) A month after the groin flap was inset and carrier portion divided. (D) Long-term follow-up after trimmed great toe transfer resulting in a functional thumb.

surrounding scarred tissue and subperiosteal dissection undertaken for ∼1 cm. If the stump of the recipient finger is >5 mm away from the adjacent joint, interosseus wires are applied ready to accept the toe phalanx. Both digital nerves are dissected, transected proximal to the neuroma where relatively normal fascicular structure is present. The choice of recipient vessels is dependent upon the length and width of the donor vessels and includes the proper or common digital artery, the superficial palmar arch, and the dorsal branch of the radial artery or even the ulnar artery. Sympathectomy is accomplished by extensive adventitiectomy of the arterial wall to prevent spasm especially when anastomosis is planned distal to the superficial palmar arch (16). Usually, veins

are plentiful on the dorsal surface of the hand and if not the vena commitante to the dorsal radial arterial branch should be sufficient. The flexor digitorum profundus and extensor tendons are dissected and transected at appropriate levels to allow for coaptation with the toe equivalents.

C. Completion of Toe Transfer

After completion of dissection of recipient and donor areas, the tourniquet is released for at least 15 min. This period allows sufficient restoration of blood supply to the tissue, but also to control any bleeding areas. Division of the tendons, digital nerves, and vessels are then undertaken, dictated by recipient site requirements (Fig. 35.6).

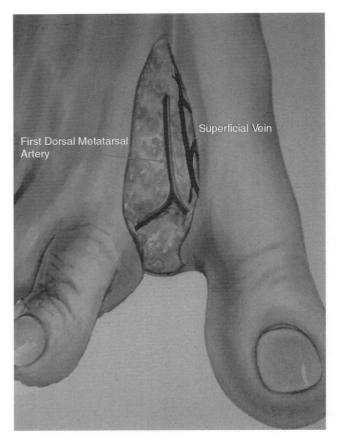

Figure 35.5 Pictorial diagram of the start of the dissection of the great toe. After identification of the digital artery bifurcation in the first web space, retrograde dissection is undertaken to determine dominance between the first dorsal metacarpal artery and the first plantar metacarpal artery.

A specific sequence is followed in completion of the transfer process.

Bone fixation may be achieved by doweling in distal toe to distal digit transfers. The recipient finger phalanx is tapered like a pencil and fit into the medullary cavity of the toe phalanx. If the stump of the recipient finger or toe phalanx is >5 mm from the adjacent joint, fixation is achieved by applying interosseous wiring. Although not

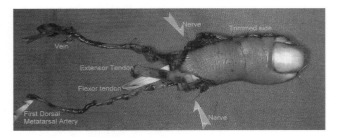

Figure 35.6 Harvest of a trimmed great toe.

rigid, this fixation is stable enough for early passive range of motion exercises. Correction of any improper positioning during the early postoperative period is also possible with wire fixation technique (17,18).

Extensor tendon repair under tension is performed before flexor tendon coaptation with the corresponding tendons of the recipient digit. If a lesser toe is transferred, the extensor tendon is repaired in full extension. To avoid extension lag, the toe is kept in extension with a k-pin through the interphalangeal joint for 3 weeks.

Following completion of osteosynthesis and tendon repair, the nerves are coapted with 10-0 or 11-0 nylon epineurial sutures under the microscope. The artery and vein are anastomosed with 10-0 nylon interrupted sutures and patency as well as distal perfusion checked prior to wound closure.

In all kinds of toe transfers, the donor site should be closed primarily without tension. Weight-bearing ambulation on the foot is postponed until healing of the wound is complete. Although preservation of at least 1 cm of the proximal phalanx of the great toe is crucial for foot function, the lesser toes may be removed at the metatarsal level without significant adverse effect on either function or appearance.

D. Functional and Aesthetic Modifications in Toe Transfers

Aesthetic challenges faced by toe transfers include the size discrepancy between the digits of the foot and hand, lesser toe clawing deformity as well as a bulging interface between donor and stump. At its widest point, the great toe on average is 11–13 mm wider than the thumb (17). The trimmed-toe technique as described by Wei et al. (18) addresses this issue adequately. A longitudinal osteoreductive resection of 4–6 mm of bone is undertaken after raising a hemicircumferential subperiosteal flap including joint capsule and medial collateral ligament (Figs. 35.7– 35.9). This has the added benefit of retaining a medial skin strip that allows avoiding the use of skin grafts to close the donor site after toe harvest. One caveat with this technique, however, is the reduction of about 18° of interphalangeal joint motion, which in the majority of patients does not result in any noticeable functional disturbance (18). Additional reduction of the bulky pulp of the great toe or of the lesser toes is usually undertaken secondarily by a wedge excision at the midline (Fig. 35.10). Discrepancy of the size at the interface between donor and recipient stumps may lead to a noticeable unsightly junction. To minimize such a deformity, four flaps are created on the amputation stump of the recipient, which are undermined sufficiently and thinned. This allows a telescoping effect of the toe over the stump. The neurovascular bundles of the harvested toe are skeletonized to allow

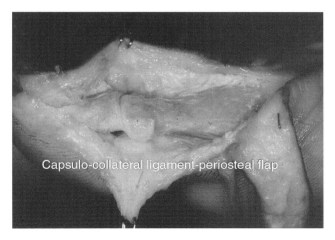

Capsulo-collateral ligament-periosteal flap

Figure 35.7 The interphalangeal joint is exposed by raising a capsulo-collateral ligament-periosteal flap from the dorsal surface of the great toe infero-laterally.

passage through the skin tunnels and primary closure of the recipient site wound. Although the overall appearance of the reconstructed digits is improved significantly by this method, occasionally the need for further debulking develops (Fig. 35.11).

E. Distal Digit Reconstruction with Various Tissues from the Foot

Whereas skin grafts, and local flaps provide coverage, they are unable to restore digital length, nail function, adequate soft tissue padding or functional sensation. Anatomically, the most suitable source for "reproduction" of the distal digit, besides the hand itself, is the foot. If a clean interface exists between healthy and devitalized tissue, reconstruction can be performed while the wound is still

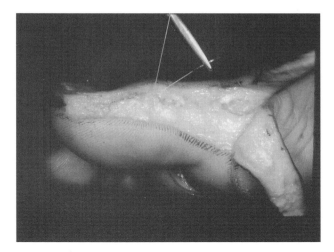

Figure 35.9 The capsulo-collateral ligament-periosteal flap is trimmed and resutured to the dorsal edge in a tight fashion to provide stability to the lateral aspect of the joint.

open. Otherwise, reconstruction is undertaken after the wounds heal.

1. Pulp

Sizable volar defects of the distal digits require restoration of bulky and sensate tissue to allow for proper prehensile function. To this end, glabrous skin from the great toe hemipulp or the first web space of the foot is ideal. Even if adjacent fingers require resurfacing, the pedal first web space can be extended to include the adjacent hemipulps or alternatively the medialis pedis flap can be transferred. The resultant syndactyly is divided 3 weeks later, whereas the donor site is either closed primarily or grafted with skin from the inset of the foot.

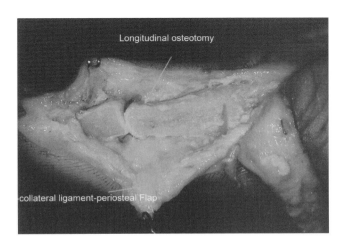

Longitudinal osteotomy

-collateral ligament-periosteal Flap

Figure 35.8 After removal of the lateral one-third of the phalangeal width using an oscillating saw.

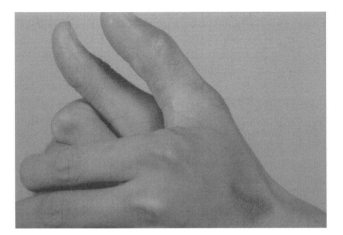

Figure 35.10 Long-term appearance of the trimmed great toe transfer to reconstruct the left thumb in comparison to normal.

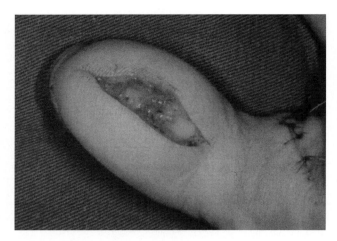

Figure 35.11 After survival of the transferred toe, if the pulp appears too bulky, a longitudinal wedge resection at the midline usually gives an excellent cosmetic outcome.

2. Nail

The absence of the nail complex interferes with function of the finger to moderate extent, however, aesthetic concerns dominate when considering nail transfers from the foot. This can be accomplished by including a minimum of dorsal skin to allow for arterial and venous provisions. Furthermore, the dorsal cortex of the distal phalanx is included to prevent injury to the nail matrix. Shortening the toe may be necessary to allow for primary closure of the wound.

3. Composite

When the burn has led to injury of the distal digit affecting the pulp, skin, and nail, then a similar segment of tissue can be transferred from the toe. The best method for reconstructing a dorsal hemi-circumferential loss of soft tissue and nail of the digit distal to the sublimes insertion with intact skeleton and tendons is the toe wrap-around flap (19,20). To prevent swiveling instability and bone resorption of the fingertip, the distal phalanx of the toe is always included (21).

F. Thumb Reconstruction

Severe burn injury of the thumb resulting in significant structural loss can be reconstructed by four main toe transfer techniques; total great toe, second toe, great toe wrap-around, and trimmed great toe. Each method has its indication to restore a functional and aesthetic thumb yet yield minimal donor site morbidity.

1. The total great toe transfer provides a broad, strong and stable surface area for pinch and grasp, however, lacks precise fine pinch and manipulation. Furthermore, with exception to rare

instances, the great toe is usually much larger than the thumb and therefore cosmetically objectionable (18) (Fig. 35.12).

2. The great toe wrap-around procedure is reserved for patients with thumb amputation distal to the interphalangeal joint or with only soft tissue and nail defects, but intact bone, joint, and tendons. When used in conjunction with an iliac bone graft to reconstruct the entire thumb as originally described, however, problems such as bone fracture, proximal phalangeal resorption and pulp swiveling may arise (21).

3. The trimmed great toe transfer technique involves reduction of both skeleton and soft tissue. It provides an ideal restoration of the thumb with good function and appearance (18). The modest reduction in interphalangeal joint mobility has been an accepted tradeoff for the significant improvement in appearance.

4. The second toe is another option for thumb reconstruction, however, it provides less satisfactory functional and aesthetic match to the thumb because of its relatively small size and claw appearance. It can be reserved for patients who have a sizable second toe or those who object to the sacrifice of their great toes (Fig. 35.13).

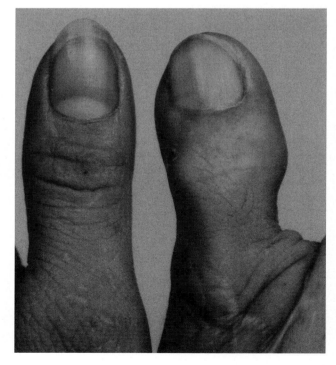

Figure 35.12 Appearance of the total great toe after transfer in contrast to the slimmer normal thumb. Note the wider, bowling pin appearance of the total great toe on the right.

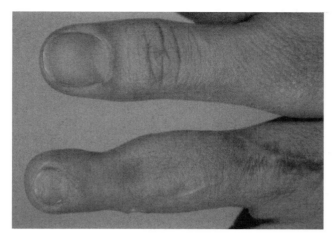

Figure 35.13 Appearance after use of the second toe for thumb reconstruction. It is obviously much smaller than the normal thumb, and is used in cases where the great toe is not available or the patient refuses its loss.

G. Metacarpal Hand Reconstruction

The challenge of reconstructing the hand with missing multiple digits due to burn injury is addressed first by appropriate identification of what is "functionally" missing. For example, if the ring and small fingers are missing, the functional deficit of the hand is minimal unless complex tasks are required. However, the presence of just an index finger requires a thumb as well as another finger for basic triple pinch function. The complexity of the possible clinical presentations of multiple digit injury to the hand is classified with recommended reconstructive methods in Table 35.2.

H. Clinical Experience with Toe Transfers

The microsurgical service at Chang Gung Memorial Hospital in Taiwan has gained significant experience of

toe to hand transfers over the past two decades. During the period of 1984–2001, a total of 1440 cases of microsurgical transfers from the foot to the hand have been undertaken with burn injury as one of the many indications (Table 35.3).

XI. POSTOPERATIVE CARE

Postoperative management is focused on assuring survival of the transferred tissue without neglect of the general care of the patient. This entails maintaining body and flap temperature, fluid balance, hemodynamics, pain control, atraumatic wound care, and above all intensive flap monitoring. Several monitoring methods are available based on the preference or capability of each center. In high volume microsurgical centers such as ours, a microsurgical intensive care unit provides an ideal setting for close and accurate monitoring of transferred tissue based on physical examination and pulse oximetry. Evaluation of skin color, temperature, capillary refill, and turgor by experienced personnel obviates the need for expensive equipment. Re-exploration should be undertaken in a more aggressive manner for any significant change in perfusion characteristics. If it appears that wound closure was too tight, sutures should be removed at bedside and biological dressings applied as needed. Salvage is possible in about 80% of compromised toe transfers in our experience. Patients are usually discharged from the hospital 5 days after surgery.

XII. REHABILITATION

After resurfacing procedures, mobilization is restricted only for the first few days until stable circulation has been established. Physical therapy is then gradually progressed to maximize the range of motion. Pins are

Table 35.2 Classification of the Metacarpal Hand According to Wei et al. (23)

TPE-subtype	Level of finger amputation	Recommendations for reconstruction
1 A	Distal to MCPj	1. Bilateral second toes for amputations distal to the web space 2. Combined second and third toes for amputations proximal to the web space
1 B	Through MCPj with intact MC articular surface	Combined second and third toes (Composite joint transfer)
1 C	Damaged metacarpal articular surface	Combined second and third toes (transmetatarsal transfer)
II	Thumb	
II A	Distal to MCPj with thenar muscles intact	Simultaneous finger and thumb reconstruction
II B	Through or proximal to the MCPj with intact thenar muscles	Same as above
II C	Through or proximal to the MCPj with inadequate thenar muscles	Thumb reconstruction in a second stage after finger reconstruction
II D	Damaged CMCj	As above, but develop immobile thumb post

Note: MCPj, metacarpophalangeal joint; MC, metacarpophalangeal; CMCj, carpometacarpal joint.

Table 35.3 Clinical Experience with Toe to Hand Transfers at Chang Gung Memorial Hospital During the Period 1984–2001

Partial toe		Single toe		Combined toes	
Joint	49	Great Toe	188	2nd/3rd	160
Pulp	109	2nd Toe	774	3rd/4th	3
Wrap-around	116	3rd Toe	37		
		4th Toe	4		

usually removed 3–4 weeks after placement, and splints are utilized for wound protection or maintenance of digital position. For example, if a clawing disposition of a transferred lesser toe is noted, nocturnal extension splints are instituted for up to a year, if necessary (17).

After partial toe transfers, such as the pulp or nail complex, motor rehabilitation is not complex since tendon manipulation is absent. Sensory re-education is the focus of rehabilitation, and training is initiated when the patient is able to perceive 30 cycles/s vibrations from a tuning fork (17). Discrimination of size and shape as well as object identification then becomes the goal of sensory re-education during the late phase.

Total toe transfers on the other hand undergo a five-stage rehabilitation program (17). The therapist for the first 3 days helps observe viability of the flap and gives psychological support to the patient. Starting on day 4 gentle passive range of motion of the joints and more active assistance of uninvolved fingers are undertaken for 3 weeks in order to control edema and prevent joint stiffness. Protective splinting is utilized during this period, and is useful in correction of any problems with maintaining proper axis and rotation. Gentle active exercise is begun during the third stage (week 5–6) in conjunction with the use of a dynamic splint. Scar management and gait training is active during this period as well. As further improvement of the muscle power and range of joint motion is noted during the ensuing week, tasks simulating daily living activities are instituted. After the eighth week, the potential vocational activity of the patient is assessed and additional exercises are recommended based on a complete evaluation of the strength, dexterity, and coordination of the reconstructed digit, in addition to the hand as a whole.

XIII. OUTCOME OF FREE TISSUE TRANSFER IN BURNED HAND

A. Early Period

Results following tissue transplantation during the initial period are primarily based on local factors such as tissue survival and wound healing. Systemic complications are rare. In general free flap survival rates are 95–100%, and

indeed toe transfers are no exception (4,17,22). Although donor site problems are infrequent, open wounds of the foot pose a significant challenge to normal healing.

B. Long-term

In contrast to the initial period, the measure of success of any reconstructive effort involving the hand is the restoration of mobility, strength, sensibility, and appearance in comparison to normal. Following resurfacing procedures, Woo and Seul (5) noted that range of motion improvement for palmar contractions were poor. In contrast, dorsal or first web space resurfacing was associated with significant improvement in range of motion of previously immobile digits. A total range of motion of all joints was 85° on average with improvement recorded in mean grip strength and key pinch in 16 of 18 patients in their series (5). Evaluation of toe transfers on the other hand, is dependent upon the method of reconstruction. In their series of 45 thumb reconstructions, Wei et al. (18) were able to evaluate results in three techniques. Second toe transfer undertaken in 10 patients resulted with an average two-point discrimination of 13 mm, grip strength 60% of normal, and key pinch 40% of normal. The range of motion at the level of the distal interphalangeal joint was 0°–5° and the proximal interphalangeal joint ~25°. The great toe wrap around among 15 patients yielded a two-point discrimination of 12 mm, grip strength 75% of normal, key pinch 80% of normal, and interphalangeal joint motion of 40°. Finally, 20 patients who underwent trimmed great toe transfers resulted with a two-point discrimination of 13 mm, grip strength 66% of normal, key pinch 75% of normal and interphalangeal joint motion of 20° (17). Although, the great toe atrophies by 10–15% within the first 3 years after transfer, it still remains conspicuously large and cosmetically unacceptable (18). The trimmed toe technique provides the most ideal cosmetic appearance compared to all other methods currently available.

C. Donor Site

Donor morbidity following resurfacing procedures is usually minimal and straightforward. Similarly, partial toe transfers such as the nail or pulp is well tolerated. Larger structural toe transfers, however, may result with significant foot deformity or gait problems if proper protocol is not observed during surgery. Whereas the lesser toes may be disarticulated at the metatarsal level without any significant effect on gait and even appearance, the great toe requires a minimum of 1 cm of its proximal phalanx preserved (18). As such the overall function of the foot is maintained, although there may be some impairment in pedal push-off and speed during running or walking on uneven terrain. Incisions on the plantar surface of the foot usually heal very well, although the dorsal foot scar frequently heals with varying degrees of hypertrophy. Improper closure methods may result in wound dehiscence, which result in major problems to the patient due to chronicity and are best avoided.

XIV. CONCLUSION

The hand requires proper functioning digits to play its central role in our daily lives. Given its frequent exposure to the external world, the hand is also subject to various forms of injury including burn injury, which can result in variable depths of injury. Initial management methods by the physician and patient as well as the inherent wound healing characteristics of the patient determine the outcome of the injured hand. The resulting myriad of clinical presentations defies classification, and management of such difficult conditions requires adherence to basic principles. Whereas during the initial periods after injury preservation of tissues and motion is of prime importance, during the late, chronic stages it is that of radical release of cicatricial contractures and accurate restoration. In comparison to existing methods of reconstruction, free tissue transfer is best able to accomplish the goal of restoration by providing a "replica" from the foot of what is missing. In final analysis however, complete restoration of both aesthetic and functional characteristics of the hand is yet to be achieved, therefore our vigilance in searching for better ways to manage these difficult cases should continue unabated.

REFERENCES

1. Zook EG. The perionychium. Clin Plast Surg 1981; 8:21–31.
2. Bunnell S. Physiological reconstruction of a thumb after total loss. Surg Gynecol Obstet 1931; 52:245.
3. Littler JW. On making a thumb. J Hand Surg 1976; 1:35.
4. Asko-Seljavaara S, Pitkänen J, Sundell B. Microvascular free flaps in early reconstruction of burns in the hand and forearm. Scand J Plast Reconstr Surg 1984; 18:139–144.
5. Woo S-H, Seul J-H. Optimizing the correction of severe postburn hand deformities by using aggressive contracture releases and fasciocutaneous free-tissue transfers. Plast Reconstr Surg 2001; 107:1–8.
6. Beasley RW. Secondary repair of burned hands. Hand Clin 1990; 6:319.
7. Kolar J, Vrabek R. Periarticular soft tissue changes as a late consequence of burns. J Bone Joint Surg 1959; 41A:103–111.
8. Salisbury RE. Reconstruction of the burned hand. Clin Plast Surg 2000; 27:65.
9. Krizek TJ, Robson MC, Headley BJ. Management of burn syndactyly. J Trauma 1974; 14:587–593.
10. Wei F-C, Colony LH. Microsurgical reconstruction of opposable digits in mutilating hand injuries. Clin Plast Surg 1989; 16:491.
11. Honda T, et al. The possible applications of a composite skin and subcutaneous vein graft in the replantation of amputated digits. Br J Plast Surg 1984; 37:607–612.
12. Kantarci U, Cepel S, Gurbuz C. Venous free flaps for reconstruction of skin defects of the hand. Microsurgery 1998; 18:166–169.
13. Samson MC, Morris SF, Tweed AE. Dorsalis pedis flap donor site. Plast Reconstr Surg 1998; 102:1549.
14. Woo S-H, Jeong J-H, Seul J-H. Resurfacing relatively large skin defects of the hand using arterialized venous flaps. J Hand Surg (Br) 1996; 21:222.
15. Logan A, Elliot D, Foucher G. Free toe pulp transfer to restore traumatic digital pulp loss. Br J Plast Surg 1985; 38:497.
16. Akizuki T, Harii K, Yamada A. Extremely thinned inferior rectus abdominis free flap. Plast Reconstr Surg 1993; 91:936.
17. Flatt AE. Digital artery sympathectomy. J Hand Surg 1980; 5:550.
18. Wei F-C et al. Microsurgical thumb reconstruction with toe transfer. Plast Reconstr Surg 1992; 93:345.
19. Wei F-C et al. Reconstruction of the thumb with a trimmed-toe transfer technique. Plast Reconstr Surg 1988; 82:506–513.
20. Morrison W, O'Brian MC, Macleod M. Thumb reconstruction with a free neurovascular wrap-around flap from the big toe. J Hand Surg 1980; 5:575.
21. Wei F-C et al. Second toe wrap around flap. Plast Reconstr Surg 1991; 88:837.
22. Leung PC. Problems in toe-to-hand transfers. Ann Acad Med 1983; 12:377.
23. Wei F-C et al. Metacarpal hand: classification and guidelines for microsurgical reconstruction with toe transfer. Plast Reconstr Surg 1997; 29:122.

36

Rehabilitation of the Burned Hand

MICHAEL SERGHIOU, ALEX McLAUGHLIN
Shriners Hospital for Children, Galveston, Texas, USA

I. INTRODUCTION

Burn rehabilitation is a challenging undertaking and in order for it to be successful it requires, among other medical professionals, the expertise of a therapist who progresses the patient along the continuum of care using appropriate interventions.

It is especially critical to manage burn injuries to the hands expeditiously, efficiently, and correctly in order to achieve a positive functional outcome at the completion of the rehabilitative process. Even the most devastating hand burn injury can produce a respectful functional outcome when managed by a knowledgeable interdisciplinary burn team. Selecting the best therapeutic interventions at the correct time prevents hand contractures and deformities which would result in a less desirable functional outcome.

Though burn injuries frequently involve other body surface areas in addition to the hands and affect the patient physically as well as psychologically, this chapter focuses on the management of hand burns and addresses all components of therapy from the emergent phase of recovery to the completion of the rehabilitative process. This chapter provides useful guidance for new and experienced therapists attempting to treat hand burns injuries.

A. Evaluation of the Burned Hand

A comprehensive hand evaluation should be conducted as soon as possible after the injury by an experienced therapist in order to assess the patient's needs and develop a thorough plan of care (1). It is imperative that the therapist performs and documents an accurate physical examination of the patient and gathers all pertinent data needed to develop a quality treatment plan (2–4). A hand evaluation should include the entire upper extremity involved in the assessment and not separate the hand from the wrist, forearm, elbow, and shoulder as the entire extremity works in unison to produce a functional task. Assessing the contralateral uninvolved extremity provides baseline data for developing goals and treatment plans for the patient.

1. History of Present Illness

Gathering as much information from the patient and/or their family about the accident is crucial. First, it is important for the therapist to "paint" a mental picture of how the accident occurred and what caused it (etiology). Any associated injuries such as smoke inhalation, tendon/joint exposure, and fractures should be recorded in the medical record.

2. Medical/Social History

Age, previous level of function, occupation, hand dominance, family support, and other significant social history information may be collected by the therapist in an interview fashion with the patient and/or family (5). During this difficult and stressful time the patient or their family may ask about the patient's future functional level (i.e. returning to previous working environment, pursing a new career, etc.). Any significant past medical history should be documented in the evaluation. All previous operative procedures should be included in the history component of the outpatient evaluation.

3. Wounds

The wound location and depth are relevant to the rehabilitation therapist and require careful assessment. Photographs and diagrams may be used to record the hand wounds. Superficial partial-thickness burn injuries rarely require splinting and exercises begin immediately. Deep partial- and full-thickness injuries need to be positioned correctly to prevent contracture development (6). The location of wounds and their severity may hinder the initiation of exercises during the inflammatory phase of wound healing. During the evaluation process the therapist and physician should determine the most appropriate wound dressing which allows movement and functional use of the hand. Exposed tendons or joints need to be protected through immobilization in order to prevent further injury (7).

4. Edema

Acute edema is a natural response to injury. The inflammatory phase (~0–72 h after injury) is part of the already begun wound healing process (8). In the case of circumferential burn injuries involving the hand, edema may be so severe that an escharotomy may be warranted to prevent ischemia and necrosis of the digits (9,10). During the emergent phase when the edema is acute and pronounced, measurements may be grossly performed. As edema begins to subside and the patient progresses to the acute phase of the recovery process, any persisting edema needs to be assessed and closely monitored. After wound closure, edema in the hand may be assessed utilizing the volumeter technique or by measuring the circumferences of the digits utilizing a tape measure (11–16). Ongoing assessments and accurate documentation of edema would track the patient's progress and guide therapeutic interventions thus preventing further injuries to the hand.

5. Range of Motion

Initially edema, pain, and multiple open areas may significantly affect the patients' ability to move their hand functionally. Baseline goniometric measurements are recorded and used later to track range of motion (ROM) improvement. Later, an in-depth goniometric evaluation should be conducted utilizing a standard methodology in recording all measurements so that communication of findings will be fluent among therapists and physicians (17–20). It is important for the therapist to regularly track active ROM, passive ROM, and total active motion (TAM) in order to make progress projections and develop appropriate plans to ensure optimal outcomes (21,22).

6. Strength

A baseline strength assessment should be performed as soon as the patient's medical status allows. Strength goals are designed based on the patient's probable discharge environment and functional requirements. Initially, a manual muscle test is conducted for the entire upper extremity (17,22,23). Later, a dynamometer and pinch gauge can also be used to assess grip and pinch strength (17,22–28).

7. Soft Tissue Tightness

A thorough physical examination of the hand includes an assessment of soft tissues. Range of motion limitations may be due to ligament, joint, tendon, or skin tightness. Each offending tissue is addressed separately in the treatment plan (4,7,29).

8. Sensation

Sensory re-education of the burned patient who sustained a significant upper extremity burn injury involving the hand poses a challenge to the rehabilitation team. Acutely, a formal evaluation of sensation may not be possible secondary to the presence of wounds, dressings, or nerve injury. As the patient progresses to the acute and rehabilitation phases of recovery, wounds are closed and a thorough sensory evaluation may be performed (30,31). An electrical injury to the upper extremity is often devastating to the sensation of the hand. A thorough sensory test is conducted in these cases in order to track the patient's sensory recovery. One objective way to measure cutaneous sensibility is the use of Semmes–Weistein monofilaments (33–37). Two-point discrimination testing assesses the patient's functional hand sensibility as it relates to the ability to perform fine tasks (38–41). Protective sensation such as heat, cold, and superficial pain such as the pin prick test should also be tested. Skin graft type, depth of wounds, scar hypertrophy, and the stage of scar maturation should be taken into account during the sensory evaluation (42–44). Functional tests

such as the Dellon modification of the Moberg pickup test could be used during sensibility testing (44).

9. Activities of Daily Living

Prior activities of daily living (ADL) status and previous occupation as well as the patient's future vocational goals are documented and considered in developing long-term treatment plans. The patient's current ADL status is assessed including mobility, feeding, grooming, dressing, bathing, toileting, and functional goals are developed that address ADL performance.

Other information that should be gathered during the initial evaluation of the patient includes an inventory of existing splints, inserts, pressure garments, and home exercise programs, which will be addressed later in this chapter.

10. Treatment Plan

Once all the objective components of the evaluation are completed, the patient, his or her family, and the therapist should develop specific meaningful and functional goals that address the patient's needs. A comprehensive plan of care that addresses all the developed goals is then developed. A complete report of the evaluation findings and plan of care should be sent to the patient's physician for review and approval prior to initiating treatment.

The status of the burned hand will continue to change for as long as all scars are active and operative procedures occur. Frequent reassessments are needed as conditions change and short-term goals are met. New goals and plans of care are developed as needed. At the conclusion of treatment, an impairment rating evaluation can be performed to calculate to percentage of permanent functional deficits in the hand (19,45).

II. EDEMA MANAGEMENT

Acute trauma from a burn injury results in edema to the affected area. The deleterious effects of this necessary response to trauma are most obvious in the compact and crowded space of the hand. Superfluous fluid in the hand and fingers is caused by an increase in vascular permeability. This reduces longitudinal freedom of the tendons passing anterior and posterior to the metacarpal phalangeal and interphalangeal joints. Hunter (13) also states that edema causes loss of the transverse and longitudinal hand arches. This posture of "palmar planus" can also be caused by the presence of scar tissue on the dorsal surface of the hand. The resulting pain with movement allows stiffness to develop quickly without proper attention from a rehabilitation therapist.

In order to prevent stiffness after trauma, early motion has been advised by many authors. Movement, when begun early, assists in edema reduction, maintains normal tendon gliding, and normalizes flow of toxic waste out of, and nutrients into, the joint capsule (8,13,46). Exercise can begin almost immediately in extremities having partial-thickness burns. However, full-thickness burns, and deep partial-thickness burns requiring skin grafts must be immobilized for 4–6 days to allow graft adherence. This also applies to burn scar contractures being released in the reconstructive phase.

At the conclusion of the operative procedure the physician applies a bulky compressive dressing. A bolster or small bulky compressive dressing limited to the surgical or injury sight can be used to control bleeding and edema. Care should be taken to maintain separation of the web spaces and the hand should be wrapped to promote the intrinsic plus or fisted position (8,47) (Fig. 36.1). In some cases the surgeon may request a splint to be applied intraoperatively to promote correct positioning of the hand. When a splint is used, it is best applied with minimal dressing on the hand. However, if a large wrap is present, Richard et al. (48) provide a formula that accommodates for a bulky dressing when fabricating a burn resting hand splint. Clinically, excellent results have been observed when splints are applied intraoperatively.

Postoperatively, elevation above the level of the heart cannot be stressed enough to the patient and hospital staff. This can be accomplished with pillows, overhead slings, bedside tables, or arm troughs (Fig. 36.2). Isometric exercise is also helpful in activating the muscle pumping mechanism to remove excess fluid. However, isometric contraction of the intrinsic muscles of the hand is a difficult

concept for many patients to grasp; and should not be part of treatment during postoperative immobilization if contraction of the small hand and forearm muscles cannot occur without associated movement at the wrist and fingers. Graft integrity is more easily preserved when intraoperative splints are used in conjunction with isometric exercise. Young children are not able to cooperate with isometric exercise.

After the bulky bandages are removed by the physician and dressed in a thin antibiotic dressing, the edematous hand and fingers are wrapped in a Coban™ glove (Fig. 36.3). This compressive elastic wrap allows free motion while assisting with edema reduction (49). The wrap is applied to each affected finger distal to proximal. The palm and web spaces should also be wrapped if involved as well. Care should be taken to leave no exposed hand surface where fluid might accumulate.

The first few days after the bulky dressing is removed, elevation should continue. This can be accomplished through the use of arm slings or by simply asking the patient to keep the hand elevated above the heart when walking. Slings are often inefficient because few patients wear them properly due to noncompliance or poor education. When sitting, patients can use pillows or tables to assist with elevation. Moreover, functional activities and intermittent exercise should be incorporated throughout the patient's day. Children are sometimes difficult to engage in play activity due to anxiety related to pain. The importance of a supportive but firm caregiver is very important at this stage. Anxiety is not exclusive to children, however, and a supportive care network is equally important to adults. In cases where pain and anxiety interfere with rehabilitation and daily tasks, consulting pain specialists is helpful.

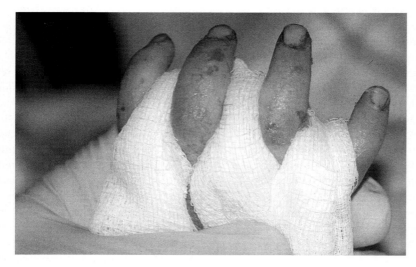

Figure 36.1 Web spaces are separated with gauze and the intrinsic plus splint is being applied intraoperatively.

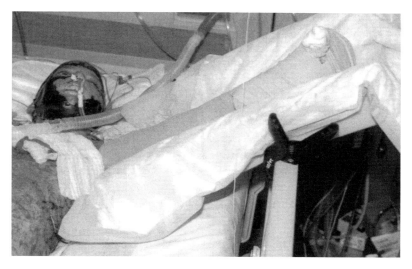

Figure 36.2 Arm troughs may be utilized at the bedside to elevate the grafted extremity above the level of the heart.

Caregivers, patients, and staff can be instructed in gentle retrograde massage. This type of massage, when used prior to exercise or activity is especially helpful in hands with moderate to severe edema. Scarring will begin to form in 2–4 weeks, at this time the skin will tolerate a compression glove. Gloves can be either prefabricated or custom-fit. Custom-fit gloves provide higher compression, but require specialized training for measurement and fitting, and are also more expensive than prefabricated gloves. There are several manufacturers of pressure garments and their products are available throughout the world.

Unfortunately, chronic edema does develop in some cases. Causes are poor patient compliance, delayed referral for therapy, or in the more severe wounds, damage to the lymphatic drainage system of the upper extremity. Most often chronic edema seems to result when two or more of these factors are present. The limited ROM that results will greatly decrease the patient's independence, concurrently increasing the burden of care on the family. Patients such as this require a very aggressive approach using all of the previously mentioned treatment interventions. Sequential intermittent compression pumps have been utilized for burns. Ause-Ellias et al. (50), in a

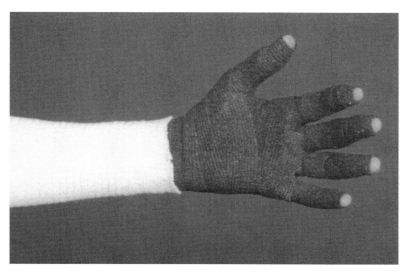

Figure 36.3 Coban™ is wrapped sequentially to provide a thin bandage in which the patient can easily exercise. This prevents edema and protects newly grafted skin from sheer forces.

preliminary study of this modality, reported this modality to be ineffective in reducing hand volume or improving ROM in patients with chronic hand edema. If noncompliance is suspected to be the primary cause of ongoing edema, psychological intervention may be necessary.

III. ANATOMY

The 27 bones of the hand, 28 muscles that insert upon them, various sensory and motor branches of the median, ulnar and radial nerves, and numerous ligamentous connections combine to give us a tool capable of amazing degrees of fine and gross motor movement. A detailed study of this complex anatomy is well beyond the scope of this chapter. Therefore, we will confine ourselves to the practical anatomy that is most often affected by a wound, and how the associated pathology might be addressed through rehabilitation. Those areas include the skin, interphalangeal (IP) joints and metacarpal–phalangeal (MCP) joints, and transverse metacarpal arches.

A mobile dermis layer, which averages <2 mm thick covers the dorsal surface of the hand and fingers (51). This covering is quite thin compared to other regions of the body and leads to several complications in the presence of thermal injury. Take a moment to examine the skin of your own hand. Unless you have experienced trauma, which has resulted in major scarring, you will notice folds of skin over the interphalangeal joints. Now flex the fingers and notice how the skin stretches and unfolds over the dorsum of the joint. At about 60° the skin has to actually lengthen and at maximum flexion a slight resistance to stretch can be felt and blanching at the joint can be observed (52). In the burned hand that has experienced at least a deep partial-thickness burn, scar tissue tightens the normally loose dorsal skin, and can bind it

to the underlying soft tissue. This decreased skin mobility will cause resistance to stretch much earlier than in the hand unaffected by scarring. If the scar is severe, a limitation in range of motion will also occur. This problem is compounded in the pediatric population who often lacks the muscle power necessary to overcome increased resistance. Not to mention the pain that all persons will experience when stretching tightened skin. When left unopposed, scar tissue will result in deformities of the joints that no amount of muscle strength can overcome. Prevention of these contractures is always the best treatment plan. Appropriate splinting and exercise, which will be discussed later in the chapter, when done early and consistently will almost assure that this problem will not occur.

As we go beneath the dorsal palmar skin we find the superficial and supratendinous fascia. Underneath the fascial layers lie the tendons of the extensor pollicis brevis, abductor pollicis longus, extensor carpi radialis longus and brevis, extensor pollicis longus, extensor digitorum, extensor indicis, extensor digiti minimi, and extensor carpi ulnaris. Although any of these tendons could be exposed given a deep enough burn, two stand out as the most commonly damaged. The central slip of the extensor digitorum and the terminal tendon at the distal interphalangeal (DIP) joint are the tendons most commonly damaged in full-thickness burns, either by direct thermal injury, or possibly through ischemia (53,54). Central slip damage, whether partial or total, can upset the intricate forces that balance the hand. Just distal to the insertion of the central tendon lies the triangular ligament. If damage to this ligament occurs a boutonniere deformity can result without proper splinting (55). This deformity occurs because the ineffective triangular ligament allows the lateral bands to fall below the proximal interphalangeal (PIP) joint flexion axis. If damage is isolated to the central tendon an inability to extend the PIP joint occurs

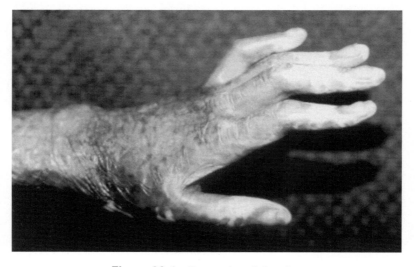

Figure 36.4 Boutonniere deformity.

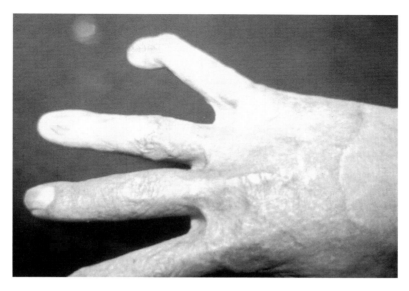

Figure 36.5 Mallet finger.

without the formation of a boutonnière deformity (Fig. 36.4). Rosenthal (56) recommends that conservative treatment of damaged extensor slip and triangular ligament include uninterrupted splinting for 6 weeks followed by 4 weeks of splinting whenever exercise is not occurring. Doyle's (57) review of the literature also recommends 6 weeks of continuous splinting followed by mobilization. Treatment would include digital gutter splinting of the affected fingers in extension for 4–6 weeks.

Exposure of the terminal tendon at its insertion to the distal phalanx also can occur and result in a mallet finger (Fig. 36.5). Treatment would include digital gutter splinting of the affected fingers in slight hyperextension for 6–8 weeks (54,55,57). Honer (58) advocates continuous splinting for 4 weeks followed by 4 weeks of limited flexion during supervised therapy sessions. In the case of terminal tendon damage, the commonly used Stack splints are often ineffective due to the wound dressings required for burn wounds. During this time the affected joint must not be allowed to flex. Percutaneous pinning of the PIP or and DIP joints may also be considered if bulky dressings or noncompliant patients prove splints to be ineffective methods of treatment (Fig. 36.6) (59). Boutonnière and

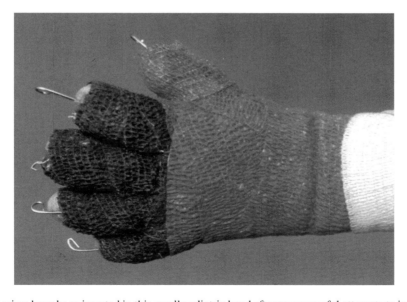

Figure 36.6 Kirschner wires have been inserted in this small pediatric hand after unsuccessful attempts to immobilize the exposed PIP joints with the exposed PIP joints with gutter splints.

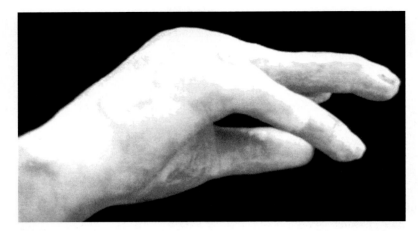

Figure 36.7   Swan-neck deformity occurring due to a damaged transverse retinacular ligament or excessive dorsal scarring.

mallet fingers may also occur when scaring occurs anterior to the joint action. If this is the case treatment is the same as described earlier.

Swan-neck deformities sometimes occur when the transverse retinacular ligament is damaged or when heavy scaring is present posterior to the joint axis of the PIP joint (Fig. 36.7). Salisbury et al. (53) suggest that another cause of this contracture is ischemia to the intrinsic muscles of the hand. These swan-neck deformities seem to be less common than those of the boutonnière type. A posterior digital gutter, or Figure-8 splint is often helpful in preventing these contractures when they are identified early, and should be applied as soon as PIP hyperextension is identified (60).

The MCP joints are often affected by scar tissue on the dorsal aspect of the hand. Hyperextension deformities often occur quickly and are quite difficult to correct if not treated early (Fig. 36.8). When contracture occurs the flexor tendons of the hand are placed at a mechanical disadvantage that makes normal flexion difficult. Also the collateral ligaments shorten along with the long extensor tendons, which serves only to further inhibit flexion. Treatment options include static and dynamic splinting, serial casts, joint mobilizations, strengthening and tendon gliding exercise, and heat modalities (60,61).

IV.   ORTHOTICS

Orthotics are an integral component of physical rehabilitation and their use is vital in achieving positive functional outcomes at the completion of burn hand rehabilitation. Severe burns to the hand may affect structures such as tendons, muscles, joints, nerves, and vessels in addition

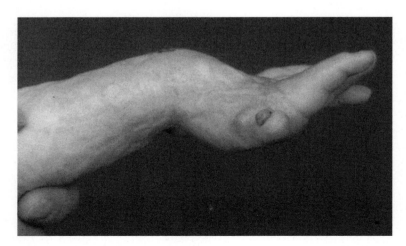

Figure 36.8   Hyperextension deformity at the MCP joint will result in palmar planus significantly compromised mobility if not treated aggressively.

to the destruction of the skin. The rationale for hand splint-ing may include:

- Edema reduction in the emergent phase (0–72 h post injury)
- Functional positioning to allow for movement and performance of ADL
- Protection of new skin grafts or flaps
- Protection of exposed tendons or joints
- Prevention or correction of contractures
- Correction of joint alignment
- Remodeling of scar tissue
- Maintenance or improvement of ROM
- Strengthening of weak muscles by exercising against springs or rubber bands
- Assisting weak or partially innervated muscles to counteract the effects of gravity during function (62–64).

The therapist must be aware of the anatomy and kinesi-ology of the hand as well as the basic mechanical principles of splinting when fabricating a splint (65). Correct use of pressure distribution over a large body surface area, mechan-ical advantage, torque, and rotational forces applied to the splints would prevent pressure points, subluxation, dislo-cation, and other injuries to the joints and surfaces treated. It is imperative that splints are prevented from migrating and shifting to avoid further injury. It is important to recog-nize that once constructed and applied splints should:

- not cause pain
- be functional
- be cosmetically appealing
- easily applied and removed
- be light weight and low profile
- be constructed of perforated materials so that wounds are not occluded

Having all these principles in mind during splint con-struction should help improve the patient's satisfaction and compliance with all orthotics (63,64,66).

No matter how the burn therapist approaches splinting (materials, designs, and application schedules) the goal of burn rehabilitation is to achieve maximum function at the completion of therapy. There are no "cookbook" pro-tocols dictating when to splint, how to splint, how long to splint, and what type of splint to construct. Generally, in burn hand rehabilitation, splinting follows the path of the wound healing phases and the ongoing physical changes of the hand (67).

A. Static Splints for the Burned Hand

Therapists continue to debate whether splints are required immediately after the injury to the hand. In general, a superficial second-degree burn (superficial partial

thickness) to the hand would not require splinting. Move-ment and performance of ADL are recommended immedi-ately. In cases of significant edema presence a burn hand splint may be indicated to position the hand appropriately and aid in reducing edema. Deep burns that result in tendon or joint exposure require immediate splinting and immobilization at all times except in the presence of a therapist. In the case of an electrical burn to the upper extremity where peripheral nerve damage affecting the function of the hand is suspected, the therapist should splint and protect joints to prevent future hand stiffness and deformities (3,8,62,68). Immediately postgrafting a hand splint may be applied to position the hand appropri-ately, protect the graft, and aid in the graft "take".

1. Antideformity Burn Hand Splint

The splint resembles the functional position resting hand splint. It positions the wrist in 0–30° extension, the MCP joints in 70–90° flexion, the interphalangeal joints (proximal and distal) in full extension and the thumb in a combination of carpometacarpal (CMC) joint palmar/radial abduction (68,69) (Fig. 36.9). This splint prevents extension contractures at the MCP joints caused by skin and collateral ligament tightness and flexion contractures of the PIP joints which result from skin and volar plate tightness (64,66). In the case of deep injuries this position must be maintained early on in rehabilitation as it reduces the risk of hand stiffness later in therapy, maintains tissues elongated, and directly relates to the functional use of the hand. The splint should be worn in the cases of deep partial- or full-thickness burn injury, when joints or tendons are exposed, when the hand has suffered peripheral nerve damage and when significant persisting edema in the hand poses a threat for further injury. The splint should be removed for exercises and the perfor-mance of ADL. In the case of tendon or joint exposure the hand should be immobilized at all times to prevent rupture and the splint should only be removed in the pre-sence of a therapist or a hand expert medical personnel (70–72). The schedule of splint application varies from full immobilization, removal for exercises and ADL per-formance, and later application at night only.

2. Resting Pan Extension Splint (Palmar)

Severe circumferential burn injuries to the hand mandate the fabrication of a splint that positions the hand in exten-sion. The resting pan extension splint (Fig. 36.10) pro-vides wrist extension, thumb radial abduction, palmar stretch, MCP joint extension, and interphalangeal joints extension (3,62,68,73,74). All digits are positioned in abduction within the splint to prevent syndactyly of the digits. The range of extension provided should be

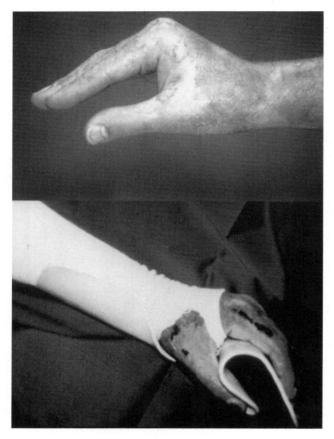

Figure 36.9   The burn hand splint positions the wrist in 0–30° extension, the MCP joints in 70–90° flexion, and IP joints in full extension. The thumb is positioned in combination of CMC joint palmar/radial abduction.

enough to cause blanching of the skin. This splint assists in prevention of palmar contractures, syndactyly of all web spaces, and maintains the excursion of the hand long-flexor musculature. The splint should be altered with the antideformity burn hand splint at set intervals throughout the day. A dorsal resting pan extension splint may be designed to position the hand as described previously and avoid contact with the painful and sensitive volar hand surface (62) (Fig. 36.11).

3.   Sandwich Splint

When the patient's hand is positioned in the antideformity burn hand splint, the interphalangeal joints should be positioned in neutral (0°). In cases where compliance with this splint is an issue (i.e. pediatrics) the interphalangeal joints may flex, which in turn may lead to pressure points on the fingertips and/or flexion contractures at the PIP joints. A sandwich splint may be fabricated to prevent this problem (Fig. 36.12). This splint includes the volar antideformity burn hand splint shell and a dorsal thermoplastic shell, padded with foam and placed over the dorsum of digits 2–5 extending from the proximal phalanges clearing the MCP joints to the fingertips of digits 2–5. In cases where splint migration is an issue, the dorsal component of the splint may extend to the forearm creating the effect of a bivalved cast (62,69,75). The dorsal component of the splint must be padded to prevent pressure points within the splint (Fig. 36.13). Another way to create the sandwich effect is to simply fabricate foam dorsal and volar hand-based shells which sandwich the digits in extension excluding the thumb (75) (Fig. 36.14).

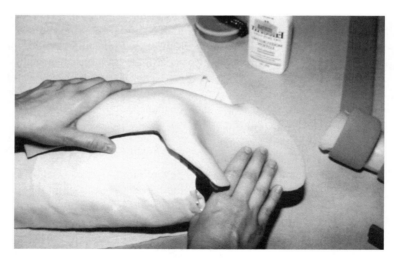

Figure 36.10   The palmar-based resting pan extension splint provides wrist extension, thumb radial abduction, palmar stretch and MCP/IP joint extension.

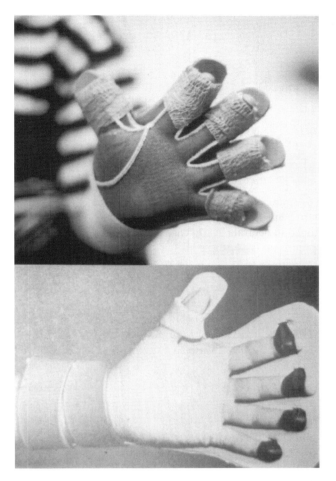

Figure 36.11 A dorsal hand-based resting pan extension splint positions the wrist and digits in extension and avoids contact with the sometimes painful volar hand surface.

4. Digital Gutter Splints

When tendon or joint exposure is present as a result of a deep burn to any of the fingers, a digital gutter splint may be fabricated to immobilize the affected joints in extension until re-epithelialization occurs (72,76,77) (Fig. 36.15). A gutter splint may also be fabricated and serially adjusted to correct a PIP or DIP joint scar contracture. Gutter splints can be constructed as a dorsal, volar, or ulnar digit splint (78–80). A three-point extension splint may also be fabricated to serially correct PIP flexion contractures (81). Digital splints immobilize only the affected joints and allow other fingers to be used in functional tasks.

5. Wrist Splint

In the acute phase of recovery (wound closure/grafting) when exercise and the performance of ADL is encouraged, the therapist may consider fabricating a wrist splint in order to stabilize the wrist and to allow the hand to function properly. The splint is constructed in cases of contractures, neurological impairment, and weakness of the wrist (62,64,68,69,82,83). The design of the wrist splint may vary depending on wound presence, scar location, pain or hypersensitivity. It can be designed as a dorsal or volar splint (Fig. 36.16).

As wound healing continues and scar is formed in a disorganized fashion the therapist needs to assess the need for fabrication of certain specialty splints to counteract the contractile forces exerted onto the hand. Contracting scar, if not attended to, may lead to the development of hand deformities.

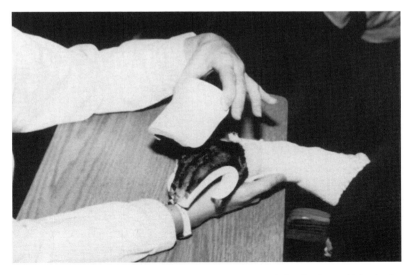

Figure 36.12 A sandwich splint may be fabricated to prevent IP joint flexion within the burn hand splint.

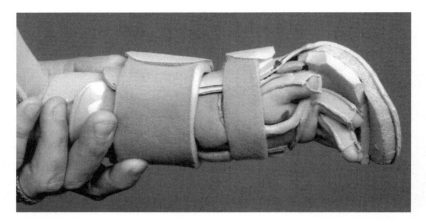

Figure 36.13   To prevent splint migration, the dorsal component of the sandwich splint may be elongated thus creating a splint with two shells resembling a bivalved cast.

6. First Web C-Bar Splint

To prevent first web space syndactyly, a first web C-bar splint is fabricated to maintain the first web opening and functionally position the thumb CMC joint for the performance of opposition and grasp-requiring activities (Fig. 36.17). The splint may be serially adjusted to increase the first web space (62,68,69,84).

7. Thumb Spica Anticupping Splint

Cupping of the palm may occur in cases where the hand has sustained a deep palmar injury (70,85). Scar bands pull the thenar and hypothenar eminence on the volar surface of the hand toward each other creating a "cupping effect" in the hand. The thumb may begin to hyperextend at the MCP joint, which may lead to further injury such as joint subluxation or dislocation in severe cases. A forearm or hand-based thumb spica anticupping

splint may be designed to stretch the palm and position the thumb appropriately for function (Fig. 36.18). A silicone insert may be applied underneath the splint to soften the scar responsible for causing this deformity. The splint is serially adjusted until correction is achieved.

8. Dorsal MCP Block Splint

Severe burn injuries to the dorsum of the hand, if severe, may cause "palmar planus", also referred to as flat palmar arch deformity. As scar causes the hand to contract dorsally, the arches of the palm flatten making it difficult for the patient to flex the hand for grasping (70). A dorsal MCP block splint may be constructed to cup the hand dorsally and serially block the MCP joints into

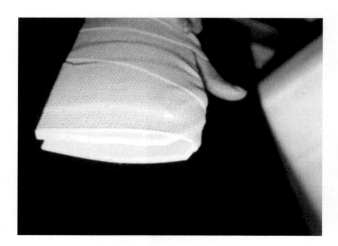

Figure 36.14   A hand sandwich splint may be fabricated utilizing dorsal and volar foam pad components.

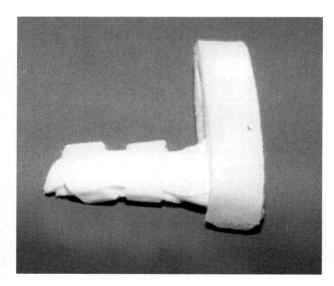

Figure 36.15   Digital gutter splints help immobilize digits in extension and aid in wound healing in cases of tendon/joint exposure.

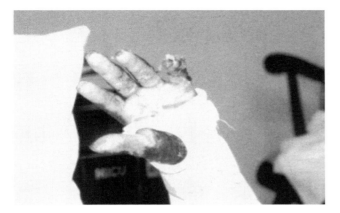

Figure 36.16 A dorsal or volar wrist splint may be fabricated in order to stabilize the wrist and allow the hand to function properly or to correct wrist flexion contractures.

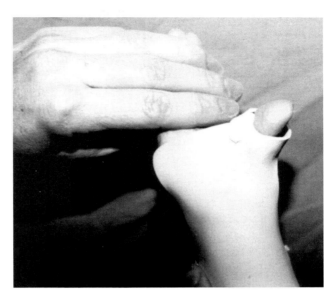

Figure 36.18 A forearm- or hand-based thumb spica that stretches the palm of the hand and positions the thumb in a functional position may be fabricated to prevent the "cupping" of the palm deformity.

flexion (Fig. 36.19). This splint places the hand in a more functional position for grasping. Flattening of the palmar arches may also occur with a claw hand deformity during which the dorsal hand skin becomes tight, the MCP joints hyperextend and the interphalangeal joints flex (8,86). The antideformity burn hand splint described earlier in this chapter may be utilized to appropriately position the claw hand caused by postburn edema.

9. *"Figure 8" Swan-Neck Splint*

Immature contractile scar anterior to the flexion axis of the PIP joint can create an imbalance of forces within the digit's intrinsic and extrinsic muscles resulting in a swan-neck deformity. This deformity presents as hyperextension of the PIP joint and flexion of the DIP joint (87–89). A "Figure-8" swan-neck splint or prefabricated Murphy rings are used to correct mild contractures (8,64,78) [Fig. 36.20(A, B)]. Serial digital casting is used for severe contractures prior to application of Figure 8 or Murphy ring splints. These splints block PIP joint hyperextension and allow PIP flexion during the performance of ADL. They should be worn as prescribed until healing of the involved structures occurs and the contractile scars have matured.

10. *Boutonniere Deformity Digital Gutter Splint*

Severe dorsal hand burns may cause damage to the extensor mechanism, the extensor tendon, and triangular ligament central slip at the level of the PIP joint. The resulting Boutonniere deformity presents as flexion of the PIP joint and hyperextension at the DIP joint (70,88–90). A digital gutter splint will prevent these contractures prior to their occurrence. Three-point extension splints or digital casting may also be used for correcting established contractures. These splints should be worn continuously and removed only in the presence of a therapist for supervised exercise. If the central slip of the extensor is ruptured, then complete immobilization of the PIP

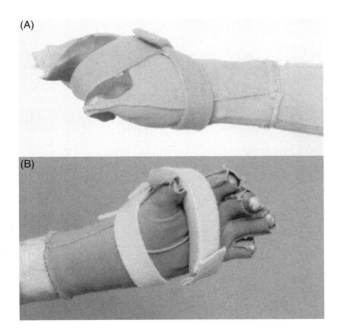

(A)

(B)

Figure 36.17 Web space syndactyly of the first web space may be prevented or corrected with a hard shell (A) of soft shell C-bar (B) that positions the thumb CMC joint in a functional position that allows for opposition and grasping activities.

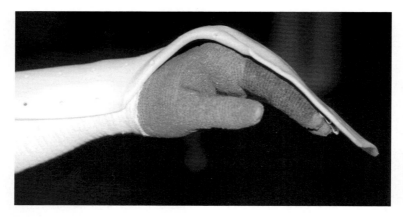

Figure 36.19 A dorsal MCP joint block splint may be constructed to cup the hand dorsally and serially correct MCP joint hyperextension.

joint is prescribed. In cases of tendon rupture complete immobilization of PIP joint during the wound healing phase may lead to the production of strong enough scar resembling a pseudotendon which supports the PIP joint in extension. The therapist should be careful not to disturb or destroy this welcome scar (91).

11. Mallet Deformity Finger Splint

Injury to the extensor tendon over the DIP joint may lead to the development of a mallet deformity which presents as finger drop or flexion of the digit at the DIP joint (8,88,90). If tendon exposure or rupture occurs, the DIP joint is completely immobilized for up to 6–8 weeks in: (A) DIP extension splint gutter volar, and (B) stax splint.

12. "Barrel Splint"

As discussed earlier in this chapter, full-thickness burn injuries to the dorsum of the hand may later lead to MCP

hyperextension contractures (78,92,93) [Fig. 36.21A, B]. A static progressive splint is created by adding a barrel to a dorsal block splints. The "barrel splint" is used to correct MCP joint hyperextension contractures of small difficult to position pediatric hands (94) (Fig. 36.22).

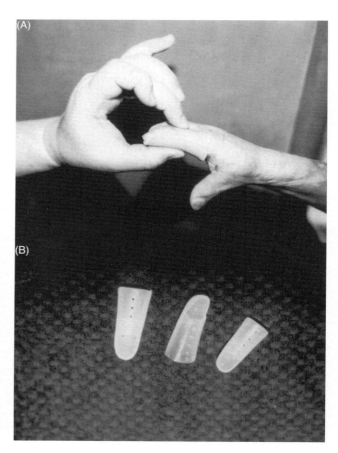

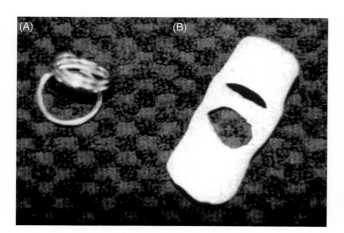

Figure 36.20 A "figure 8" swan-neck splint (A) or prefabricated Murphy rings (B) are used to correct mild swan-neck deformities.

Figure 36.21 If tendon exposure occurs, the DIP joint is completely immobilized for up to 6–8 weeks in an extension utilizing a volar gutter (A) or a Stax splint (B).

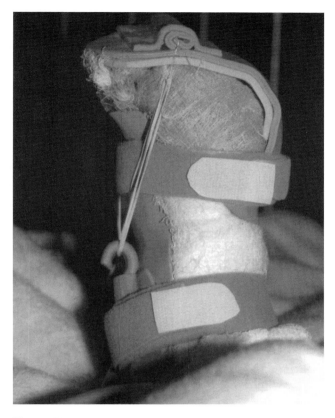

Figure 36.22 The "barrel splint" is used to correct MCP joint hypertension contractures of small difficult to position pediatric hands.

13. Thumb CMC Antideformity Splint

The CMC joint may begin to sublux in cases of deep palmar or dorsal burn injuries when thick immature scar begin to pull the thenar and hypothenar eminence together. A hand-based CMC antideformity splint may be constructed to stabilize the joint in a functional position and allow the thumb to correctly oppose during the performance of ADL (95) (Fig. 36.23).

B. Dynamic Splints for the Burned Hand

Dynamic splints are frequently utilized in burn hand rehabilitation as an adjunct to remodel scar tissue, stretch a tight joint, maintain or increase ROM, and provide for functional hand use during the recovery from a peripheral nerve injury (96,97). Dynamic splints are usually custom made by the burn therapist for the special needs of the patients. However, commercially available prefabricated splints may be utilized with minor adjustments for correct fit (62). Positive functional outcomes of dynamic splinting are increased with proper fit and patient compliance.

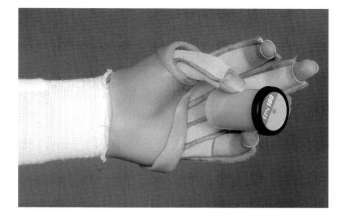

Figure 36.23 A hand-based CMC splint stabilizes the joint in a functional position allowing the thumb to correctly oppose during the performance of ADL.

1. Hand MCP/IP Flexion Splint

Contracting scars on the dorsal surface of the hand may affect hand function and lead to joint tightness and hyperextension deformities. When tightness of the joints and the dorsal skin is detected the therapist may prescribe a flexion splint for the MCP joints (Fig. 36.24) or a composite MCP/IP joint flexion splint (Fig. 36.25). Elastic band traction, monofilament line, and finger slings are attached to a volar forearm based wrist splint to produce MCP joint flexion. PIP joint flexion may be included as well by attaching a hook to the fingernails. To produce PIP flexion, a pulley is created by attaching a D-ring on the distal aspect of the splint. Monofilament is attached to the fingernail hook, threaded through the D-ring and attached proximally with elastic bands. Another D-ring, acting as a tunnel for the monofilament lines to go through, is attached on the volar wrist splint over the proximal palmar crease surface to promote full DIP joint flexion (78,98). In the absence of fingernails, a

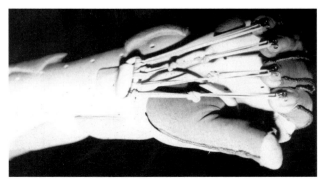

Figure 36.24 A dynamic MCP joint flexion splint may be constructed to stretch the contracted dorsal hand skin surface.

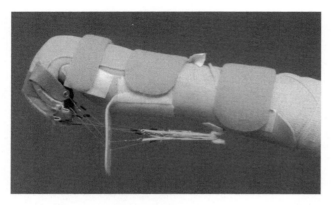

Figure 36.25 A dynamic composite MCP/PIP joint flexion promotes maximum excursion of the extensor tendons and stretches the dorsal hand skin surface.

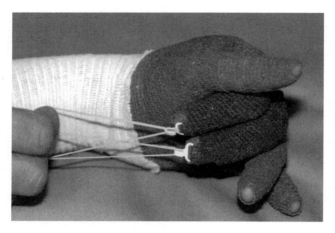

Figure 36.26 A "fingernail Coban hook" may be constructed in the absence of fingernail to aid in achieving a composite finger flexion within a dynamic hand composite flexion splint.

"fingernail coban™ hook" maybe constructed to achieve composite flexion of the hand. A contoured finger hook with a coban™ loop is placed over the nail bed (99). The entire digit is then wrapped with coban securing the fingernail hook to the digit (Fig. 36.26). Due to the volarly placed traction, dynamic flexion splints prevent functional hand use. Dynamic flexion splints are used periodically throughout the day as prescribed and they are removed for exercise and ADL.

Frequent inspections and adjustments of the splints are required to maintain a 90° angle of pull. This angle is important for the prevention of joint compression, distraction, and pressure sores caused by uneven weight distribution over the finger slings. Traction provided by the elastic bands should be between 100 and 300 g and can be measured with a spring tension scale. A flexion glove may be used early in the rehabilitation process for exercise purposes to provide hand flexion vs. a composite one (98,100).

2. Hand MCP/IP Extension Splint

Contracting scar on the volar surface of the hand and fingers may lead to flexion contractures of the MCP and interphalangeal joints. To prevent these disabling contractures, a dorsal forearm based dynamic hand extension splint is fabricated (98,101). A similar splint is fabricated when the burn injury to the upper extremity is complicated with radial nerve injury (78,102). The dynamic MCP extension splint includes the fabrication of a dorsal wrist splint extending to just over the metacarpal heads, a digital extension outrigger, and a thumb MCP extension outrigger attached to the dorsal splint in such a way to allow for the correct angle of pull on all digits (Fig. 36.27). The dynamic traction is provided through

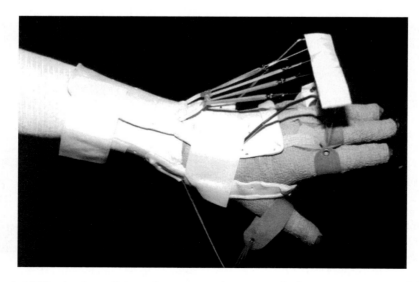

Figure 36.27 A dynamic MCP extension splint may be constructed to prevent flexion scar contractures of the MCP and/or IP joints.

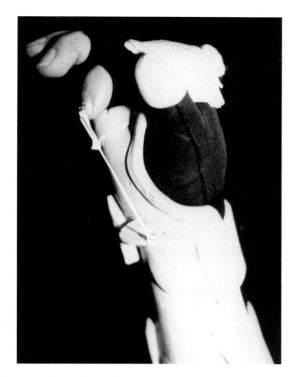

Figure 36.28 Dynamic traction is provided through finger slings or fingernail hooks connected to monofilament line and rubber bands, which in turn connect to a D-ring.

phalanges just above the head of each proximal phalanx (103). The dynamic extension hand splints regardless of their specific intended purpose allow for the functional use of the hand during the performance of ADL.

Devastating burn injuries to the upper extremities may require multiple different splints in the rehabilitative process. Circumferential injuries to the hand would require both flexion and extension splints which in some cases become a burden for the patient to carry around. The "supersplint", includes a forearm based thermoplastic shell with volar and dorsal surfaces (104). Flexion and extension traction is attached, eliminating the requirement for multiple splints (Fig. 36.29).

3. Digital Dynamic Flexion/Extension Splints

Fingers may sustain such severe injury that may require special attention and individual splinting. Contractures to the dorsal or volar surface of the digits may be splinted utilizing custom-made or prefabricated spring loaded splints that correct IP joint contractures (78,101,105). The dynamic tension provided by the spring mechanism must be carefully monitored by the therapist and adjusted as needed to prevent excessive damaging and painful forces exerted on the digits (Fig. 36.30).

C. Serial Casts

Serial casts provide low-load long-duration stress to tightened tissues. Brand (106) popularized the idea of treating leprosy patients with long-standing contractures of the hand. His method used plaster of paris total contact casts to produce "tissue growth". He found cast application without padding prevented cast migration, provided a

finger slings on the proximal phalanges of all digits. The slings are connected to monofilament line and rubber bands which in turn connect to a D-ring on the forearm surface of the splint (Fig. 36.28). If the flexion contractures involve the interphalangeal joints then the dorsal splint is constructed to extend onto the dorsum of the proximal

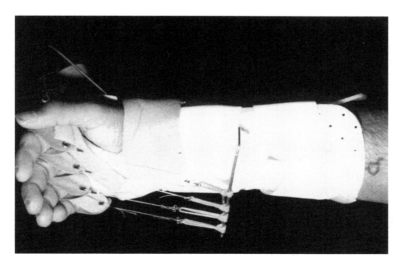

Figure 36.29 The "supersplint" includes a forearm based thermoplastic shell with volar and dorsal surfaces. Flexion and extension traction is attached thus eliminating the requirement for multiple splints.

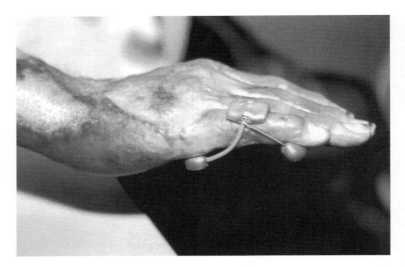

Figure 36.30 Dynamic spring loaded splints may be constructed for individual digits to provide dynamic traction in correcting volar or dorsal scar contractures.

more intimate fit and thus reduced pressure sores. This technique has been adapted and used with both plaster of paris and fiberglass cast tape in burn rehabilitation. Fiberglass may be preferred because a less bulky, lighter, and more durable cast may be fabricated. Clinically, there is no difference between plaster of paris and fiberglass cast tape with regard to pressure sore occurrence. Casts are especially useful in those patients who refuse to or are unable to comply with removable thermoplastic splints. Ridgeway et al. (107) reported success with ankle casting and Bennett et al. (108) have described ROM increases in several joints with serial casting. Bell-Kotroski (109) has also presented her experience with digital cylinder casting to increase ROM of the PIP joint (109) (Fig. 36.31). Moreover, plaster and fiberglass cast tape are less expensive and more accessible than thermoplastic

material in many parts of the world. Recently, Deltacast Polyester conformable Cast Tape™ has become available and shows great potential in children with burns. This material can be univalved and used as a total contact splint (110) (Fig. 36.32). Spellman et al. (111) has reported success using dynamic traction components incorporated into plaster of paris casts (Fig. 36.33).

Serial casts are applied when MCP movement is <30–45° passively. For patients who do not have sensory deficits, casts are applied and changed the next day. If no skin complications are noted a cast is reapplied and changed every 2–7 days. The insensate hand or finger is also a candidate for casts. However, one must have expert technique in application of the device. When considering application of a cast one must carefully assess the skin. The presence of small and medium size wounds are not barriers to using this method; however, they should be clean and free of infection. The casts of these

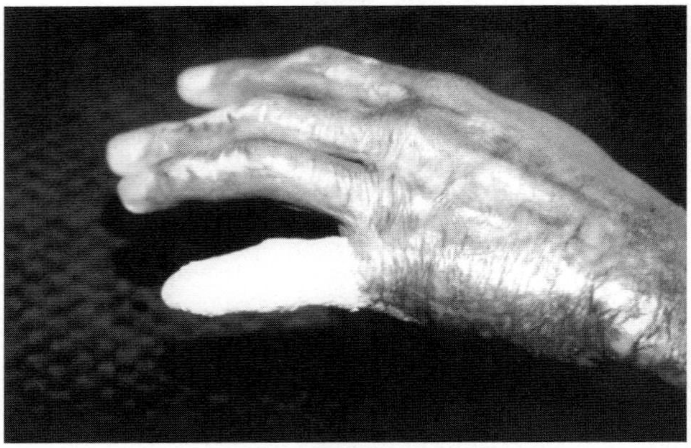

Figure 36.31 Digital cylinder casts can be applied to individual fingers to extend tight PIP and DIP joints that are too tight for conventional thermoplastic or dynamic splinting.

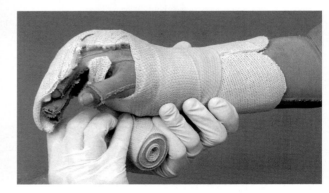

Figure 36.32 A splast, made from Delta Cast Polyester Conformable Cast Tape™ is univalved and applied to the hand.

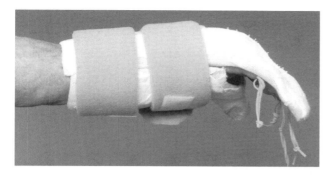

Figure 36.33 Plaster of paris cast with dynamic traction for the fingers.

patients are changed more often (every 1–2 days). Before applying the cast, wounds should be dressed utilizing antibiotic ointments and minimal gauze. Coban® can be applied for pressure to the scars. Pressure garments (custom or prefabricated) should be avoided underneath the casts as they may be damaged or destroyed during cast removal. ROM measurements should be taken before the application of any cast to determine treatment effectiveness.

D. Skeletal Traction and Suspension

Traction and suspension systems reduce the amount of contact between the operated on sites and the patient's bed thus minimizing the risk of graft loss during dressing changes (Fig. 36.34). These systems also allow open management of the grafted wounds postoperatively. ROM can be performed by changing weights to encourage flexion or extension of the elbow. Banjo, halo, and hayrake splints are used in conjunction with elastic bands to suspend fingers in varying positions. The hayrake provides the intrinsic plus positioning (Fig. 36.35). A threaded Steinman pin is inserted through the distal radius. The pin must be strong enough not to bend when weight is applied. There are no reports of damage to either the median nerve or the radial artery when using this method (86).

E. Active Range of Motion

Although splints assist with prevention of contractures, they alone cannot return patients to a functional and productive lifestyle. An exercise program, including active ROM (AROM), passive ROM (PROM) and prolonged stretch, in conjunction with splint wear, is the most efficient way to rehabilitate hand burns. Patients are often hesitant, especially children, to begin movement of the burned extremity. The hand, with its increased sensory awareness, is no exception. Patients and families must be

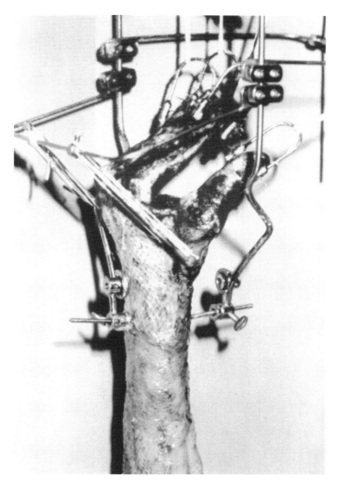

Figure 36.34 Skeletal suspension helps reduce graft loss and edema in the severely burned hand, and assists with proper positioning of the upper extremity.

educated about the positive effects of activity as it relates to strength and bone density. All involved parties must also be aware of the negative effects of prolonged immobilization on soft tissue length.

No discussion of exercise can begin without first addressing the effect of pain associated with thermal injury. No matter how motivated the burn survivor, adequate pain control is necessary to endure the tremendous discomfort associated with these injuries in the acute phase and beyond. Even when pain is diminished, many adults, and most children also experience problems with anxiety that prevent them from receiving full benefit from an exercise program. An interdisciplinary approach, which includes, pharmacy, psychology, psychiatry, nursing, and rehabilitation are often helpful in reducing pain and anxiety (112).

Exercise often begins within the first 24 h after injury. Initially tightness is caused by edema. Activation of the

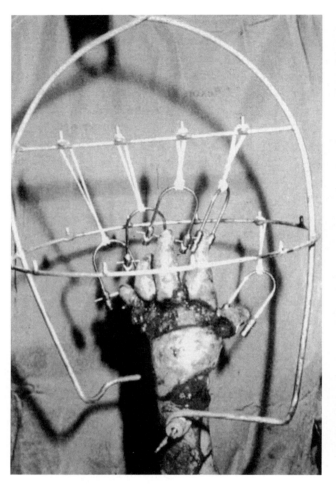

Figure 36.35 A hayrake suspension system provides for intrinsic-plus positioning of the hand while fragile grafts heal. This system also allows for passive movement of the fingers without the need to touch the hand.

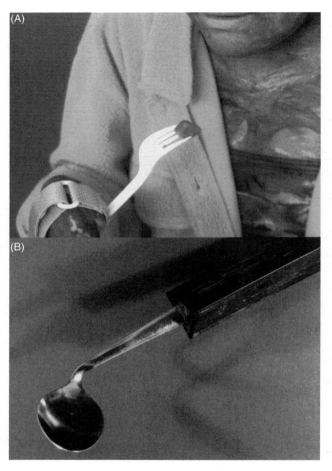

Figure 36.36 A universal cuff (A) or a long-handled spoon (B) are two adaptive devices that are commercially or custom made to assist with feeding.

muscle pump while the hand is elevated above the heart will assist in reducing excess fluid (113). Patients should be encouraged to use as much of their available range as possible and hold the muscle contraction at end range for 3–5 s. Often patients are impressed by the improved range of motion and reduced pain that occurs after several repetitions of this exercise. Independent performance of ADL reduces patient frustration with injury and should be the goal of any exercise program (114). If splints are required they should be removed before meal times, exercise should be performed, and independent feeding encouraged. Utensils and other self-care devices can be adapted as needed to promote independence (Fig. 36.36). The success of any exercise program is judged by improved ADL performance. Few people will follow through with a boring list of exercises if it does not increase their functional independence.

The bulky dressings, present in the emergent and acute phases, decrease the ability to perform fine motor tasks and prevent the use of many strengthening devices. A series of different circumference wooden dowels can be placed in the hand for squeezing exercises (Fig. 36.37). The resistance gives the important proprioceptive feedback necessary to produce strong muscle contractions in the forearm (115). Strong muscles are necessary to overcome the contractile forces, which will be present in the maturation phase of scar healing. As wounds heal and dressings decrease, a greater variety of functional and strengthening activities become available.

Areas requiring skin grafts can continue strengthening during the immobilization phase with isometric exercise. Of course, this is not possible in smaller children or adults who do not possess the cognitive ability to understand and perform this method of strength training. Shear forces produced when isometric contractions result in significant joint movement lead to graft mortality.

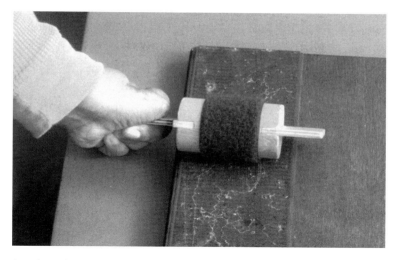

Figure 36.37 Wooden dowels are inexpensive exercise equipment that can be used several times a day for resistance exercise.

Any therapist who knowingly allows graft loss to occur will quickly lose the confidence of the physician who painstakingly performed the operation. Active motion and strengthening can be resumed once graft adherence occurs; usually between 4 and 7 days postoperatively. Sanford and Gore (116) have reported a 95% graft take on skin grafts when using an Unna boot after grafting the hands as an outpatient procedure (116). The Unna boot is removed on the fifth postoperative day and rehabilitation begins.

F. Passive Range of Motion

PROM is beneficial when working with infants, young children, and patients who are unable to cooperate with an active rehabilitation program, such as adults with cognitive impairments. In the acute phase, burns covering large amounts of the body may prevent patients from participating in an effective AROM program. During this time PROM will maintain range of motion, joint elasticity, and provide nutrition to the joint surfaces (114,117,118). Passive motion does not increase muscle strength or decrease edema and should not be used in patients who are able to participate in an active movement program. Covy et al. (119) found continuous passive motion machines, provided results similar to an aggressive active and passive range of motion program. No graft loss occurred when machines were applied to the hand on postoperative day 5. Covey et al. suggest these machines be used when multiple kinetic areas are involved, for patients with decreased cognitive function who cannot participate in AROM, or for patients who refuse and are unwilling to participate in an AROM program.

G. Prolonged Stretch

Prolonged stretch, although a passive movement, does have an important role in treatment of the burned hand. As scars hypertrophy due to an increased and altered extracellular matrix the skin tightens and ROM limitations are noticed (120). Patients who are experiencing limitations in AROM can be moderately stretched for several minutes up to 30 min. To ensure sufficient stretch, mild skin blanching should occur (121). These long-duration stretches provide sufficient time to break the bonds of excess collagen and lengthen skin and other soft tissues. Scar bands that cross more than one joint are stretched concurrently (122). Heat modalities such as hot packs or fluidotherapy are helpful prior to stretching. Combining heat and stretch has been shown to be especially effective (61,123). The hand can be wrapped in a Coban™ fist and dipped in paraffin, or covered with a hot pack (Fig. 36.38). Finally, dynamic and static progressive

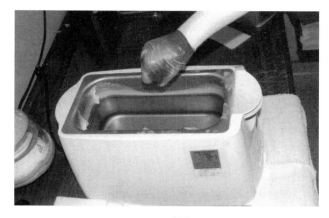

Figure 36.38 Coban™ fist with paraffin.

splints, and serial casts are other ways to provide low-load long-duration stretch. Fingers with limited PIP and DIP ROM due to skin and joint contracture can be progressively stretched using Theraband®, or Coban® (124). Prolonged stretch has been shown to improve ROM in a variety of contractures (125–127). Clinically, the same results have been observed in burn scar contractures of the hand.

Patients often learn substitution patterns to compensate for ROM limitations. Therefore, it is important to include functional and strengthening activities after every stretching session to integrate newly gained range into the patient's movement patterns (128). Functional exercises should focus on basic ADL initially and progress to simulated work situations later. Prolonged stretch can easily be taught to patients and family members and included in the daily home exercise program.

H.   Joint Mobilization and Tendon Gliding

Although the skin of burn survivors is the most obvious source of ROM limitations; several other soft tissues may contribute to tightness after prolonged periods of immobilization or in the presence of well-developed contractures. Collateral ligaments and other periarticular structures at the PIP and DIP joints tighten with extension splinting due to the increase in cross-linking between adjacent collagen fibers (129). The MCP joint is splinted in flexion to prevent collateral ligament tightness. However, noncompliance or severe scarring over the dorsum of the palm can cause hyperextension contractures at this joint. When this deformity occurs, collateral ligaments tighten along with the posterior joint capsule and lumbrical and interossei muscles.

Joint mobilization and joint distraction, designed to lengthen the tightened joint capsule and ligaments are helpful in increasing ROM. Heat modalities can also be implemented to aid in stretching tightened articular tissue (130). At the PIP joint, tight collateral ligaments and oblique retinacular ligaments will also prevent joint flexion. A simple dynamic splint is effective in stretching this joint. Tendon gliding exercises are also useful when trying to gain ROM and prevent peritendinous scar adhesion (131).

I.   Scar Management of the Burned Hand

The desired outcome of any wound as it closes is a flat, soft, and elastic scar. As deep partial- or full-thickness burn hand injuries heal, hypertrophic contractile scars may begin to form ∼8 weeks after wound closure (132,133). Red, raised, and rigid hypertrophic scars are the result of an overabundance of collagen fibers gathered at the injury site to aid in wound healing (134). The

collagen synthesis at the wound exceeds the amount of collagen breakdown (lysis) resulting in a thick nonyielding scar (70,134). Researchers have noted that areas which have undergone skin grafting tend to form less hypertrophic scars than those that have been allowed to heal primarily. Also, scar hypertrophy has been noted to be more prominent at the borders of the grafted areas and the normal skin (134,135). Hand scar management should be initiated early to prevent skin contractures and soft tissue adhesions, which may significantly impair function. Prior to treating hypertrophic scars in the hand the therapist should carefully assess their maturation status and how they may affect function. Their location should be recorded in order to track their progress and the success of therapeutic interventions. Several instruments are available to aid in the assessment of hypertrophic scars (134,136,137).

The therapeutic management of hypertrophic scars continues to be a challenge to the therapists. Even though explaining the process of scar maturation continues to be the focus of researchers, burn hypertrophic scars have been managed clinically through pressure therapy, massage, stretching, and physical agent modalities initiated at different stages in the recovery process (138).

1.   Pressure Therapy

Pressure exerted on hypertrophic scars may be applied in the form of interim or custom garments, inserts, and conforming orthotics.

Pressure Garments

Clinically, pressure garment therapy has been the standard of care for the treatment of hypertrophic scars. However, the efficacy of pressure garments and the amount of pressure needed for therapeutic effect has not yet been objectively demonstrated (139–142).

It has been thought that pressure decreases blood flow to the scar, which, in turn, decreases oxygen within tissues. This decrease results in a balance of collagen synthesis and breakdown (lysis) within scars. Balancing collagen synthesis with breakdown is believed to flatten scar tissue (70,86,135). Pressure therapy in the hands may begin before complete wound closure. Low pressures of ∼10 mmHg may have a positive effect on the remodeling of a scar over time. Continuous pressures >40 mmHg may cause paresthesias and damage tissues (86,133). Average pressure of 25–28 mmHg has been the most accepted by researchers, therapists, and companies fabricating custom pressure garments (134). Self-adherent elastic bandages such as Coban™ may be used initially to control edema and later on to provide pressure to skin grafts postoperatively as well as manage sensitive hypertrophic scars (50). A Coban™ glove although exerting

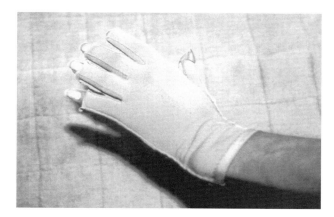

Figure 36.39 Interim hand pressure therapy may include commercially available products such as Isotoner™, spandex, or cotton gloves and finger sleeves.

~10 mmHg pressure when not stretched, may be therapeutic over time (86,134). Application of Coban™ gloves does not interfere with wound dressings and eliminates shearing forces on fragile skin. The Coban™ is applied in a spiral fashion on each digit beginning distally at the fingernail and ending proximally at the head of the MCP joint. The fingertip is exposed to monitor capillary refill. When the Coban™ is applied spirally it should overlap half its width in order to provide equal pressure throughout the finger. When stretched beyond 25% of its elasticity, Coban™ can cause numbness to the fingers. When the Coban™ hand glove is completed, all surfaces of the hand should be covered and no skin should be exposed with composite finger flexion. A small amount of lotion may be applied to the glove to prevent the fingers from sticking together and allow the hand to be used functionally (86). Other forms of interim hand

pressure include commercially available products such as Isotoner™, spandex, or cotton gloves and finger sleeves (70,86) (Fig. 36.39). Interim pressure is introduced first as a form of circumferential pressure to prepare the hand for the next level of care. Once edema subsides and hand sensitivity decreases a custom-made glove is fabricated (Fig. 36.40). The therapist may choose to prescribe a glove with a zipper initially for easy application in preventing excess shearing forces onto the fragile scar. Later, the zipper is discontinued in order to achieve more uniform pressure onto the entire hand surface. Open fingertips should be required in order to provide the patient with the sensory feedback needed to perform ADLs. Pressure gloves should be worn around the clock and removed only for bathing, exercise or wound care. Custom gloves should be monitored closely for good fit and should be replaced every 8–12 weeks depending on wear and tear or growth in the case of children. In cases of deformities in the hand or partial amputation, a positive mold of the hand may be obtained and sent to the garment manufacturer for a custom glove fabrication (143).

Inserts

Because of its unique anatomy and function the hand has very different dorsal and volar surfaces. Palmar arches and the thenar and hypothenar eminence create a concave volar surface which is difficult to manage with pressure garments alone. Also, adequate pressure in the web spaces may be impossible to achieve just with a glove. For these difficult-to-manage surfaces, inserts are used underneath gloves to achieve adequate pressures (86,134,144). Inserts are fabricated from materials available commercially and provide total contact pressure on uneven surfaces. A wide variety of these materials

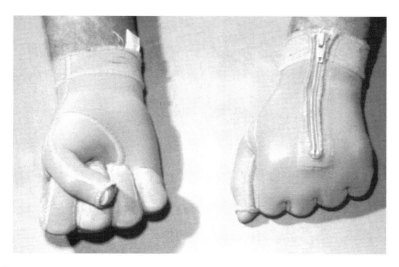

Figure 36.40 Once edema subsides and hand sensitivity decreases, a custom-made glove is fabricated.

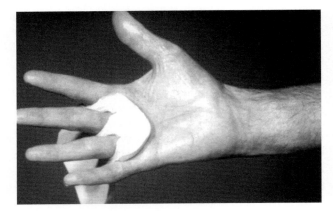

Figure 36.41 (A, B) Initially, in scar management, soft strapping or foam padding material web inserts may be fabricated to prevent or correct syndactyly.

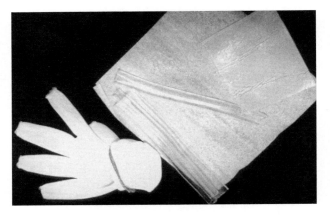

Figure 36.43 Silicone gel inserts are flexible, soft and conform to all hand surfaces.

include foams, silicone gels, silicone elastomers, silastic pads, putties mixed with silicone catalysts, and hard thermoplastic materials. When selecting an insert to be utilized inside the pressure providing glove, the therapist should take into account the stage of the scar maturation. To prevent skin breakdown, initially soft inserts should be utilized. As scars mature, firmer materials can be introduced. Also, it is important to consider the location of the insert application prior to choosing the insert material. Soft, flexible inserts that allow for movement to occur should be used in the palmar surfaces (86).

Soft material inserts: Initially in scar management soft strapping or foam padding material web inserts may be fabricated to prevent or correct syndactyly (144,145) [Fig. 36.41(A, B)]. Roylan® prosthetic foam inserts may be fabricated to fill the concavity on the volar surface of

the hand (Fig. 36.42). This soft, flexible, and expandable insert permits hand flexion for the performance of ADL while providing pressure in the palm of the hand (86,144,146).

Silicone gels: Although the exact mechanism of how silicone affects the burn scar is not well defined, silicone gels appear to be the most widely utilized insert materials in burn rehabilitation (147,148). Because of their flexibility and conformity they may be used on all hand surfaces (Fig. 36.43). Today, silicone gels are available in different sizes and may have one sticky surface which is applied on the scar to avoid insert migration from the treatment surface. These gels even though they are expensive and short-lived, have been clinically observed to depress scar hypertrophy and hydrate the scar thus making it more pliable and yielding (86,144,146).

Silicone elastomer: Liquid elastomer mixed with a catalyst makes a solid yet soft insert for the dorsal or volar surfaces of the hand and its web spaces (Fig. 36.44). Silicone elastomer inserts because of their initial liquid stage

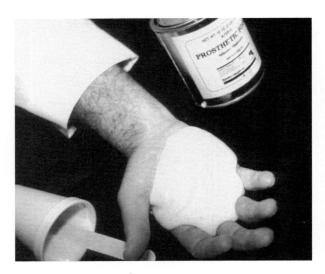

Figure 36.42 Rolyan® prosthetic foam inserts may be fabricated to fill the concavity on the volar surface of the hand.

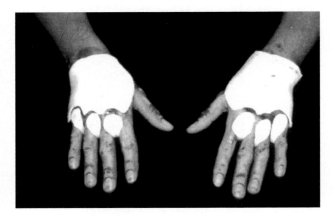

Figure 36.44 Silicone elastomer inserts are custom made to conform greatly to all hand surfaces especially the web spaces.

conform greatly to any anatomical surface and are clinically observed to prevent shrinkage of newly applied skin grafts (86,144,146).

Otoform K™: Several silicone-based putties such as Otoform K™ when mixed with a catalyst result in a semi-rigid insert material which may be utilized in areas such as the dorsum of the hand and the web spaces in the latter stages of scar management when the scars in the hand are not as fragile (86,144) (Fig. 36.45).

Roylan® 50/50 Mix™ elastomer putty: This technology involves mixing two equal size putties to form a semi-rigid insert. Like Otoform K™, this is best used on the dorsum of the hand and web space surfaces in the later stages of scar management (146).

Hard thermoplastic inserts: Conforming splints utilized alone or lined with silicone or other materials may provide adequate pressure needed to depress hypertrophic scars (138). All insert materials must be cleaned frequently and the treated areas must be inspected regularly in order to prevent skin breakdown, scar maceration, or dermatitis. Treatment must be discontinued temporarily when skin irritation occurs. Patients may be allergic to certain

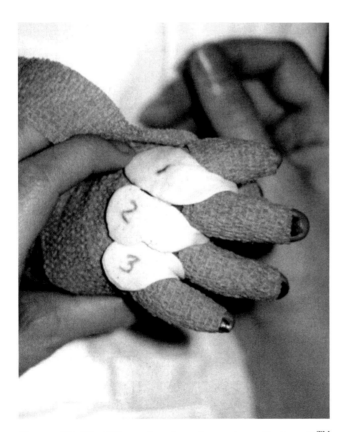

Figure 36.45 Silicone-based putties such as Otoform K™ when mixed with a catalyst result in a semi-rigid insert material, which may be used on the dorsum of the hand or the web spaces during the latter stages of scar management.

insert materials, so in some cases trial and error will show which insert material is best for the patient.

J. Physical Agent Modalities Utilized in Burn Hand Scar Management

Thermal and nonthermal physical agent modalities have been widely utilized as an adjunct to rehabilitation. Even though these modalities are frequently used for a variety of diagnoses, their use in burn rehabilitation remains limited.

Prior to choosing the appropriate modality to manage the burned hand, the hand's unique anatomy must be considered. The structures of the hand are mostly superficial and may respond well to heat that penetrates 1–2 cm beneath the skin. Also, dermal thickness varies from its volar to the dorsal surfaces which allows for structures to be heated at different temperatures (149). A good examination of hand sensation should precede initiation of heat modalities in order to verify the presence of at least protective sensation to prevent further injury to the already compromised hand.

Paraffin wax: One of the most frequently utilized modalities in burn hand management may be paraffin (150). When mixed with mineral oil the temperature of paraffin is lowered to therapeutic levels of 115°F and may heat tissues up to 2 cm subcutaneously via conduction (151). The patient's hand may be stretched into flexion with Coban prior to receiving paraffin. The methods of immersion of dipping of the hand may be utilized after one layer of paraffin wax has covered the hand and has solidified. In the case of a hypersensitive hand paraffin wax may be painted onto the hand or poured in saran wrap creating a paraffin pack which is then wrapped around the hand. Once paraffin is applied to the hand, saran wrap and a towel are applied around it for insulating purposes. This maintains therapeutic heat levels for 12–15 min (114,122,151). The application of paraffin wax on a stretched hand may increase collagen extensibility, may improve skin elasticity, and may increase movement in the hand (152).

Ultrasound: Experimentally, ultrasound has been utilized in burn hand rehabilitation during the wound healing phase and for the management of hypertrophic scars and contractures. Despite several attempts to objectively demonstrate the effects of ultrasound on burn scars thus far studies have been inconclusive and contradictory (70). Theoretically, the benefits of ultrasound are increased circulation, acceleration of wound healing, softening of collagen, increased scar plasticity, decreased pain and muscle spasm, and change in contractile activity of muscles. Clinically, 1 MHz continuous ultrasound at 1.0 W/cm^2 intensity, performed three times weekly onto an approximate 4 × 4 cm^2 surface for 5 min may positively affect scar extensibility and increase joint mobility (153).

Fluidotherapy: The use of this modality may be contraindicated in managing the burn hand acutely as this is a skin-drying physical agent which may further damage the moisture deficient injured skin. It may be utilized later in the rehabilitative phase of recovery when managing the stiff hand with an intact skin surface resulting from an electrical injury to the upper extremity. This convection heat modality allows the therapist and the patient to manipulate the hand while heated in the fluidotherapy machine, thus combining the effects of heat, stretching, and movement.

Other modalities may include hot packs which are in some cases combined with paraffin wax to provide superficial moist heat. Electrical stimulation has been infrequently utilized in burn hand management, however, its efficacy is unsubstantiated (70).

K. Scar Massage

Currently, no objective study clearly and objectively demonstrates how massage may affect hypertrophic burn scars. Limited studies suggest that massage does not affect the vascularity, pliability, and height of burn scars (154). Other studies revealed positive psychological effects of massage therapy for the burned patient related to itching, anxiety, and pain (155,156). Clinically, massage is widely utilized by therapists in managing burn scars (150). Massage may soften or remodel adherent scar tissues by reversing fibrosis, improve blood circulation, and increase joint mobility prior to therapy. Retrograde (pumping) massage should be performed prior to scar massage in order to move any excess fluids away from the hand. Initially, massage may begin as early as 1–2 weeks after wound closure. However, when the scar is still fragile, massage must be performed in a stationary fashion. The therapist performs a nonfriction massage technique by applying gentle stationary pressure on the hand surface treated and mobilizing the blanched skin surface in all directions without friction. No lubrication should be used during this scar massage technique. As the scar continues to mature and is able to withstand shear forces, frictional massage may be introduced. Lubrication may now be used; however, it should not be excessive and movements should be performed slowly in a horizontal, vertical, or circular fashion. If a wound is present, massage and stretching of the scar tissue should be directed toward the wound periphery. This relaxes the surrounding tissues and promotes wound healing. The hand scar tissue may respond better to massage when it is heated and stretched. In addition to manual massage the therapist may provide electrical massage to all hand surfaces including the web spaces. Commercially available electrical massagers with various attachments may be utilized in the clinic or issued to trained patients and their families for home scar management (157). Home massage should be performed at least twice daily for 5–10 min on each treated hand surface. The therapist should frequently inspect the skin integrity to prevent "over massaging" an area and causing skin breakdown or blistering.

V. CAPSULOTOMY

Despite expert hand therapy, contractures of the hand can involve more than tightened skin tissue. Joint capsules and periarticular structures may also be involved and continue to limit ROM after burn scar releases (158). Intraoperative range of motion measurements should be taken of MCP and interphalanged joints. If ROM is not adequate after burn scar release a capsulotomy should be considered.

Rehabilitation should include a pre- and postoperative evaluation which must include AROM, PROM, as well as skin integrity, functional level, and pain tolerance. The preoperative evaluation should also include a strength assessment (159). It is generally accepted that AROM begin within 24–36 h postoperatively (159). However, in the case of a burn scar release and placement of autograft hand therapy must be postponed until grafts are adherent. The therapist's goal during this first phase of treatment is to control edema and maintain proper positioning of joints that have been released.

Once the physician allows ROM to begin the patient must be taught to perform AROM exercises on an hourly basis. Patients must understand that in order to prevent future limitations from scarred skin and joint capsule exercises must be performed religiously. Clinically, splints are helpful in maintaining ROM whenever the patient is not exercising (159). Dynamic splints are helpful in gaining full ROM. Varying heat and prolonged stretch modalities described earlier in this chapter can also be employed if necessary. Strengthening activities begin after edema and pain subside. Limited information has been published on rehabilitation after capsulotomy. However, Gould et al. (160) report between 20° and 30° increases in AROM at the MCP joint (160). Buch (161) also reports an average increase of 30° improvement at the MCP joint, but states that results were significantly less when skin grafts were performed at the same time as capsulotomy (161).

Therapists must use their best clinical judgment when developing a specific treatment plan for the management of these very complex patients. Generally, ROM should begin as soon as possible and basic principles of edema management, prolonged stretch and strengthening should be used.

VI. AMPUTATIONS

Amputations of the fingers occur often in severe burns. However, patients who have mid-proximal phalanx contractures can do quite well with ADLs. It is important with these patients not to lose further length to hypertrophic scar tissue. Care must be taken to maintain the fingers separated at all time to prevent a mitten hand. It is also important to maintain the intrinsic plus position. This is difficult because decreased finger length reduces the lever arm, thereby decreasing splint efficiency. Pinning of the MCP joints in flexion should be considered if splints cannot maintain the desired position. Aesthetic prostheses are available for persons who have lost portions of fingers. These are very realistic but are, for the most part, nonfunctional and expensive.

Prosthetics come in many styles. A consultation with a local prosthetist should be obtained as soon as possible following amputation. The rehabilitation therapist should strengthen the residual limb. Especially the muscles of the shoulder girdle. Most mechanical prostheses require strong shoulder protraction, retraction, and elbow flexion to operate effectively.

VII. SUMMARY

Rehabilitation management of the burned hand can be an overwhelming task, especially in association with other severely injured areas of the body. A team approach, including the physician, nurse, rehabilitation therapist, and family is absolutely necessary for successful outcomes. The physician and therapist must have a comprehensive understanding of hand anatomy, edema prevention, scar formation and maturation, splinting, and the power of low-load long-duration stretch in order to efficiently manage hand burns. Armed with this knowledge, an appropriate treatment plan can be developed to return the patient to a more independent level of function. Nursing staff must be educated to reinforce rehabilitation goals. Most importantly, the family and patient must be involved in and understand the goals of treatment. Without compliance from the patient and support from their loved ones, hand function will certainly be compromised.

REFERENCES

1. Wright PC. Fundamental of acute burn care and physical therapy management. Phys Ther 1984; 64:1217–1231.
2. Aulicino PL. Clinical examination of the hand. In: Hunter J, Mackin E, Callahan A, eds. Rehabilitation of the Hand: Surgery and Therapy. 4th ed. St. Louis: CV Mosby, 1995.
3. Salisbury R, Reeves S, Wright, P. Acute care and rehabilitation of the burned hand. In: Hunter J, Schneider L, Mackin E, Callahan A, eds. Rehabilitation of the Hand: Surgery and Therapy. 3rd ed. St. Louis: CV Mosby, 1990.
4. American Society for Surgery of the Hand. The Hand: Examination and Diagnosis. New York: Churchill Livingstone, 1983.
5. Demling R, LaLonde C. Burn Trauma. New York: Thieme Medical Publishers, 1989.
6. Karaemer MD, Jones T, Deitch EA. Burn contractures: incidence, predisposing factors, and results of surgical therapy. J Burn Care Rehabil 1988; 9:261–265.
7. Adams JC, Hamblem DL. Outline of Orthopaedics. 11th ed. Edinburgh: Churchill Livingstone, 1990.
8. Howell JW. Management of the burned hand. In: Richards RL, Staley MJ, eds. Burn Care and Rehabilitation Principles and Management. Philadelphia: FA Davis Co., 1994:531–575.
9. Dimick AR. Emergency care. In: Hummel RP, ed. Clinical Burn Therapy. Boston: John Wright PSG, 1982.
10. Fess EE. Hand rehabilitation. In: Hopkins HL, Smith HD, eds. Willard and Spackman's Occupational Therapy. 8th ed. Philadelphia: JB Lippincott, 1993.
11. Waylett-Rendall J, Seibly D. A study of the accuracy of a commercially available volumeter. J Hand Ther 1991; 4(1):10–13.
12. King TI II. Circumferential finger measurements utilizing a torque meter to increase reliability. J Hand Ther 1993; 6(1):35–36.
13. Hunter J, Mackin E. Edema: Techniques of evaluation and management. In: Hunter J, Mackin E, Callahan A, eds. Rehabilitation of the Hand: Surgery and Therapy. 4th ed. St. Louis: CV Mosby, 1995.
14. Brand P, Wood H. Hand Volumeter Instruction Sheet. Carville, LA: U.S. Public Health Hospital, 1977.
15. Brand P. Clinical Biomechanics of the Hand. St. Louis: CV Mosby, 1985.
16. Giuliani CA, Perry GA. Factor to consider in the rehabilitation aspect of burn care. Phys Ther 1985; 65:619–623.
17. Kendall FP, McCreary EK, Provance PG. Muscles: Testing and Function. 4th ed. Baltimore: Williams & Wilkins, 1993.
18. Pedretti LW. Evaluation of joint range of motion. In: Pedretti LW, ed. Occupational Therapy: Practice Skills for Physical Dysfunction. 4th ed. St. Louis: CV Mosby, 1996.
19. American Medical Association. Guides to the Evaluation of Permanent Impairment. 4th ed. Chicago: Department of Preventive Medicine and Public Health, 1993.
20. Cambridge-Keeling CA. Range of motion measurement of the hand. In: Hunter J, Mackin E, Callahan A, eds. Rehabilitation of the Hand: Surgery and Therapy. St. Louis: CV Mosby, 1995.
21. Fess EE. Assessment of the upper extremity: instrumentation criteria. Occup Ther Pract 1990; 1(4):1–11.
22. Trombly CA. Evaluation of biomechanical and physiological aspects of motor performance. In: Trombly CA, ed. Occupational Therapy for Physical Dysfunction. Baltimore: Lippincott, Williams & Wilkins, 1997.

23. Pedretti LW. Evaluation of muscle strength. In: Pedretti LW, ed. Occupational Therapy: Practice Skills for Physical Dysfunction. St. Louis: CV Mosby, 1996.

24. Mathiowetz V, Weger K, Volland G, Kashman N. Reliability and validity of grip and pinch strength evaluations. Hand Surg 1984; 9A(2):222–226.

25. Mathiowetz V. Reliability and validity of grip and pinch strength measurements. Crit Rev Phys Rehabil Med 1991; 2(4):201–212.

26. Kuzala EA, Vargo MC. The relationship between elbow position and grip strength. Am J Occup Ther 1992; 46(6):509–512.

27. Mathiowetz V. Grip and pinch strength measurements. In: Amundsen LR, ed. Muscle Strength Testing: Instrumental and Non-Instrumental Systems. New York: Churchill Livingstone, 1990.

28. Bechtal CD. Grip test: use of a dynamometer with adjustable handle spacing. Bone Joint Surg 1954; 36A:820.

29. Kessler RM, Hertlin D. Joint mobilization techniques. In: Kessler RM, Hertling D, eds. Management of Common Musculoskeletal Disorders. New York: Harper and Row, 1983.

30. Bentzel K. Evaluation of sensation. In: Tombly CA, ed. Occupational Therapy for Physical Dysfunction. Baltimore: Lippincott, Williams & Wilkins, 1997.

31. Dunn W. Assessing sensory performance enablers. In: Christiansen C, Baum C, eds. Occupational Therapy: Overcoming Human Performance Deficits. New Jersey: Slack, 1991.

32. Pedretti LW. Evaluation of sensation and treatment of sensory dysfunction. In: Pedretti LW, ed. Occupational Therapy: Practice Skills for Physical Dysfunction. St. Louis: CV Mosby, 1996.

33. Bell-krotioski JA. Light touch–deep pressure testing with Semmes–Weinstein monofilaments. In: Hunter J, Schneider L, Mackin, E, Callahan A, eds. Rehabilitation of the Hand: Surgery and Therapy. St. Louis: CV Mosby, 1990.

34. Bell-Krotoski JA. "Pocket Filaments" and specifications for the Semmes–Weinstein monofilaments. J Hand Ther 1990; 3:26–31.

35. Bell-Krotoski JA, Tomancik E. Repeatability of testing with Semmes–Weinstein monofilaments. J Hand Surg 1987; 12A:155–161.

36. Bowen VL, Criener JS, Jones SV. Threshold of sensation; inter-rater reliability and establishment of normal using the Semmes–Weinstein monofilaments. J Hand Ther 1990; 3:36.

37. Weinstein S. Fifty years of somatosensory research: from the Semmes–Weinstein monofilaments to Weistein enhanced sensory test. J Hand Ther 1993; G:11.

38. Dellon A, Mackinnon S, Crosby P. Reliability of two-point discrimination measurement. J Hand Surg 1987; 12A:693–696.

39. Moberg E. Two point discrimination test. A valuable part of hand surgical rehabilitation, e.g. in tetraplegia. Scand J Rehabil Med 1990; 22:127–134.

40. Dellon A. The moving two-point discrimination test: clinical evaluation of the quickly adapting fiber-receptor system. J Hand Surg 1978; 3:474.

41. Dellon A. Evaluation of Sensibility and Re-education of Sensation in the Hand. Baltimore: Lucas, 1988.

42. Hermanson A, Jonsson CE, Lindblom V. Sensibility after burn injury. Clin Physiol 1986; 6:507.

43. Ward RS, Saffle JR et al. Sensory loss over grafted areas in patients with burns. J Burn Care Rehabil 1989; 10:536–538.

44. Dellon AL. The paper clip: Light hardware to evaluate sensibility in the hand. Contemp Orthop 1979; 1(3):39.

45. Engrav LH, Dutcher KA, Nakamura DY. Rating burn impairment. Clin Plast Surg 1992; 19:569–598.

46. Akeson WH, Amiel D, Woo SL. Immobility effects on synovial joints: the pathomechanics of joint contracture. Biorheology 1980; 17(1–2):95–110.

47. Salisbury RE. Acute care of the burned hand. In: May JW Jr, Littler JW, eds. Plastic Surgery. Philadelphia: WB Saunders, 1990:5399–5417.

48. Richard R, Schall S, Staley M, Miller S. Hand burn splint fabrication for bandage thickness. J Burn Care Rehabil 1994; 15(4):369.

49. Ward RS, Reddy R, Brockary C, Hayes-Lundy C, Mills P. Use of coban self-adherent wrap in management of postburn hand grafts: case report. J Burn Care Rehabil 1994; 15(4):364–369.

50. Ause-Ellias K, Richard R, Miller S, Finley R. The effect of mechanical compression on chronic hand edema after burn injury: a preliminary report. J Burn Care Rehabil 1994; 15(1): 29–33.

51. Goldsmith LA, ed. Biochemistry and Pathology of the Skin. New York: Oxford University Press, 1983:3–63.

52. Brand PW, Hollister AM, Thompson DE. Mechanical resistance. In: Brand PW, Hollister AM, eds. Clinical Mechanics of the Hand. St. Louis: Mosby, 1999:184–232.

53. Salisbury RE, McKeel DW, Mason AD. Ischemic necrosis of the intrinsic muscles of the hand after thermal injury. J Bone Joint Surg 1974; 56:1701–1707.

54. Donnelan MB. Reconstruction of the burned hand and upper extremity. In: McCarthy, ed. Plastic Surgery. Philadelphia: WB Saunders, 1990:452–482.

55. Lovett WL, McCalla M. Management and rehabilitation of extensor tendon injuries. Orthop Clin North Am 1983; 44(4):811–826.

56. Rosenthal EA. The extensor tendons: anatomy and management. In: Hunter J, Mackins G, Callahan A, eds. Rehabilitation of the Hand: Surgery and Therapy. St. Louis: CV Mosby, 1995.

57. Doyle JR. Extensor tendons—acute injuries. In: Green DP, ed. Operative Hand Surgery. New York: Churchill Livingstone, 1993:1925–1954.

58. Honer R. Acute and chrone flexor and extensor mechanism at the distal joint. In: Bowers WH, ed. The Interphalangeal Joints. New York: Churchill Livingstone, 1987:111–117.

59. Royan GM, Mullins PT. Skin necrosis complicating mallet finger splinting and vascularity of the distal interphalangeal joint overlying skin. J Hand Surg 1987; 12A:548.

60. Randall T, Portney L, Harris BA. Effects of mobilization on joint stiffness and active motion of the metacarpal

phalangeal joint. Orthop Sports Phys Ther 1992; 16(1):30–36.

61. Lehmon JF. Effect of tissue temperatures on tendon extensibility. Arch Phys Med Rehabil 1970; 51:481–487.

62. Daugherty MB, Carr-Collins JA. Splinting techniques for the burn patient. In: Richard RL, Staley MJ, eds. Burn Care and Rehabilitation: Principles and Practice. Philadelphia: FA Davis, 1994.

63. Fess EE. Principles and methods of splinting for mobilization of joints. In: Hunter J, Mackins G, Callahan A, eds. Rehabilitation of the Hand: Surgery and Therapy. St. Louis: CV Mosby, 1995.

64. Belkin J, English C, Adler C, Pedrett LN. Hand splinting: principles, practice, and decision making. In: Pedretti LW, ed. Occupational Therapy: Practice Skills for Physical Dysfunction. St. Louis: CV Mosby, 1996.

65. Strickland JW. Anatomy and kinesiology of the hand. In: Fess EE, Philips CA, eds. Hand Splinting: Principles and Methods. St. Louis: CV Mosby, 1987.

66. Fess EE, Philips CA, eds. Hand Splinting: Principles and Methods. St. Louis: CV Mosby, 1987.

67. Rivers EA, Leman-Jordan C. Skin system dysfunction burns. In: Neistadt ME, Crepeau EB, eds. Willard and Spackman's Occupational Therapy. Philadelphia: Lippincott, Williams & Wilkins, 1998.

68. Malick MH, Carr JA. Manual on Management of the Burn Patient: Including Splinting, Mold and Pressure Techniques. Pittsburgh: Harmarville Rehabilitation Center Educational Resource Division, 1982.

69. Walters CJ. Splinting the Burn Patient. Laurel, MD. RAMSCO Publishing Company, 1987.

70. Grigsby-deLinde L, Miles W. Remodeling of scar-tissue in the burned hand. In: Hunter J, Mackin E, Callahan A, eds. Rehabilitation of the Hand: Surgery and Therapy. 4th ed. St. Louis: CV Mosby, 1993.

71. Saffle JR, Schnebly WA. Burn wound care. In: Richard RL, Staley MJ, eds. Burn Care and Rehabilitation: Principles and Practice. Philadelphia: FA Davis, 1994.

72. Pullium GF. Splinting and positioning. In: Fisher SV, Helm PA, eds. Comprehensive Rehabilitation of Burns. Baltimore: Williams and Wilkins, 1984.

73. Fess EE, Philips CA, eds. Patterns in hand splinting: Principles and Methods. 2nd ed. St. Louis: CV Mosby, 1987.

74. Schwanholt C, Daugherty MB, Gaboury T, Warden GD. Splinting the pediatric palmar burn. J Burn Care Rehabil 1992; 13:460–464.

75. Ward RS, Schnebly WA. Have you tried the sandwich splint? A method of preventing hand deformities in children. J Burn Care Rehabil 1989; 10(1):83–85.

76. Fess EE, Philips CA, eds. Splints acting on the fingers. In: Hand Splinting: Principles and Methods. 2nd ed. St. Louis: CV Mosby, 1987.

77. Rivers E et al. The use of individual gutter splints to preserve exposed PIP joints: a case study. American Burn Association Annual Meeting (Abstract), San Francisco, 1984.

78. Wilton JC, ed. Splinting to address the fingers. In: Hand Splinting: Principles of Design and Fabrication. London: WB Saunders, 1997.

79. Benaglia PG, Sartorio F, Franchignoni F. A new thermoplastic splint for proximal interphalangeal joint flexion contractures. J Sports Med Phys Fitness 1999; 39:249–252.

80. Wu S. A belly gutter splint for proximal interphalangeal joint flexion contracture. Am J Occup Ther 1991; 45(9):839–843.

81. Callahan A, McEntee P. Splinting proximal interphalangeal joint flexion contractures: a new design. Am J Occup Ther 1986; 40(6):409–413.

82. Wilton JC, ed. Splinting to address the wrist and hand. In: Hand Splinting: Principles of Design and Fabrication. London: WB Saunders, 1997.

83. Fess EE, Philips CA, eds. Splints acting on the wrist and forearm. In: Hand Splinting: Principles and Methods. 2nd ed. St. Louis: CV Mosby, 1987.

84. Wilton JC, ed. Splinting to address the thumb. In: Hand Splinting: Principles of Design and Fabrication. London: WB Saunders, 1997.

85. Warden CD. The pediatric burn patient: issues in wound management. In: Boots Burn Management Report. Vol. 1. Lincolnshire: Boots Pharmaceuticals, 1991.

86. Serghiou M, Evans EB et al. Comprehensive rehabilitation of the burned patient. In: Herndon DN, ed. Total Burn Care. 2nd ed. London: WB Saunders, 2002.

87. Rosenthal EA. The extensor tendons: anatomy and management. In: Hunter J, Mackin J, Callahan A, eds. Rehabilitation of the Hand: Surgery and Therapy. 4th ed. St. Louis: CV Mosby, 1995.

88. Melvin JL. Rheumatic disease in the adult and child. In: Occupational Therapy and Rehabilitation. 3rd ed. Philadelphia: FA Davis, 1989.

89. Hittle JM, Pedretti LN, Kasch MC. Rheumatoid arthritis. In: Pedretti LW, ed. Occupational Therapy: Practice Skills for Physical Dysfunction. 4th ed. St. Louis: CV Mosby, 1996.

90. Sherif MM, Boswick JA. Postburn proximal interphalangeal joint hyperextension deformity of the fingers. Bull Clin Rev Burn Inj 1985; 3:32–35.

91. Peacock EE Jr. Wound Repair. 3rd ed. Philadelphia: WB Saunders, 1984.

92. Stack HG. A modified splint for mallet fingers. J Hand Surg (Br) 1986; 11:263.

93. Rayan GM, Mullins PT. Skin necrosis complicating mallet finger splinting and vascularity of the distal interphalangeal joint overlying skin. J Hand Surg (am) 1987; 12:549.

94. Farmer S, Serghiou M, Williams G. Adding a barrel to a dorsal block splint to improve metacarpophalangeal joint flexion in the pediatric burned hand. American Burn Association Annual Meeting (Abstract), Chicago, 2002.

95. Colditz JC. The biomechanics of a thumb carpometacarpal immobilization splint: design and fitting. J Hand Ther 2000; 13(3):228–235.

96. Pearson SO. Dynamic splinting. In: Hunter J, Mackin E, Bell-Krotioski J, Shneider L, eds. Rehabilitation of the Hand. 1st ed. St. Louis: CV Mosby, 1978.

97. Fess EE, Philips CA, eds. Exercise and splinting for specific problems. In: Hand Splinting: Principles and Methods. 2nd ed. St. Louis: CV Mosby, 1987.

98. Fess EE, Philips CA, eds. Analysis of splints. In: Hand Splinting: Principles and Methods. 2nd ed. St. Louis: CV Mosby, 1987.

99. Smith and Nephew, Inc. Smith and Nephew Products Catalog. Splinting: Contoured Finger Hooks. USA: Smith and Nephew, Inc., 2002.

100. Otthiers J. A hand glove splint for attachment of dynamic components. J Hand Ther 1995; 8:36–37.

101. Linden CA, Trombly CA. Orthoses: kinds and purposes. In: Trombly CA, ed. Occupational Therapy for Physical Dysfunction. 4th ed. Baltimore: Lippincott Williams & Wilkins, 1997.

102. Reynolds CC. Pre-operative and post-operative management of tendon transfers after radial nerve injury. In: Hunter J, Mackin E, Callahan A, eds. Rehabilitation of the Hand: Surgery and Therapy. 4th ed. St. Louis: CV Mosby, 1995.

103. Hooper RM, North ER. Dynamic interphalangeal extension splint design. Am J Occup Ther 1982; 36(4):257–258.

104. VanStraten O, Sagi A. "Supersplint": a new dynamic combination splint for the burned hand. J Burn Care Rehabil 2000; 21:71–73.

105. Smith and Nephew, Inc. Smith and Nephew Products Catalog: Flexion and Extension Splints. USA: Smith and Nephew, Inc., 2002.

106. Brand PW. The reconstruction of the hand in leprosy. Ann Royal Coll Surg Engl 1952; 11:350.

107. Bennett GB, Helm P, Purdue GF, Hunt JL. Serial casting: a method for treating contractures. J Burn Care Rehabil 1989; 10(6):543–545.

108. Ridgeway CL, Daugherty MB, Warden GD. Serial casting as a technique to correct burn scar contractures: A case report. J Burn Care Rehabil 1991; 12(1):67–72.

109. Bell-Kotroski JA. Plaster cylinder casting for contractures of the interphalangeal joints. In: Hunter JM et al, eds. Rehabilitation of the Hand: Surgery and Therapy. St. Louis: Mosby, 1995:1609–1616.

110. McLaughlin A, Spellman ME, Serghiou M, Evans EB. The "Splast": combining the effects of splinting and casting. [Abstract]. International Society for Burn Injuries, 11th Quadrennial Congress, 2002.

111. Spellman M, Serghiou M, Evans E. "Dynamic serial casting": combining the benefit of movement and stability in the correction of thumb contractures. [Abstract]. American Burn Association, Chicago. J Burn Care Rehabil 2002; 23(2):151.

112. Stoddard FJ, Sheridan RL, Save GN, King BS, King BH, Chedekel DS, Schnitzer JJ, Martyn JA. Treatment of pain in acuity burned children. J Burn Care Rehabil 2002, 23(2):135–156.

113. Howell JN. Management of the acutely burned hand for the non-specialized clinician. Phys Ther 1989; 69(12):1077–1090.

114. Tilley W, McMahon S, Shukalak B. Rehabilitation of the burned upper extremity. Hand Clin 2000; 16(2):303–318.

115. Aagaard P, Simonsen EB, Trolle M, Bangsbo J, Lawsen K. Effects of different strength training regimes on moment and power generation during dynamic knee extension. Eur J Appl Physiol Occup Physiol 1994; 69(5):382–386.

116. Sanford S, Gore D. Unna boot dressings facilitate outpatient skin grafting of hands. J Burn Care Rehabil 1996; 17(4):323–326.

117. Akeson WH et al. Effects of immobilization on joints. Clin Orthop Relat Res 1987; 219:28–37.

118. Enneking WF, Horowitz M. The intra-articular effects of immobilization on the human knee. J Bone Joint Surg 1972; 54A:923.

119. Covy MH, Dutcher K, Marvin JA, Heimbach DM. Efficacy of continuous passive motion devices with hand burns. J Burn Care Rehabil 1988; 9(4):397–400.

120. Scott PG, Ghahary A, Tredget EE. Molecular and cellular basis of hypertrophic scarring. In: Herndon DN, ed. Total Burn Care. Philadelphia: W.B. Saunders, 2002.

121. Ward RS. Physical Rehabilitation in Burn Care and Therapy. Carraugher GJ, ed. St. Louis: Mosby, 1998:293–327.

122. Johnson CL. Physical therapists as scar modifiers. Phys Ther 1984; 64(a):1381–1387.

123. Warren GC, Lehman JF, Koblanski JN. Heat and stretch procedures: an evaluation using rat tail tendon. Arch Phys Med Rehabil 1976; 57:122–126.

124. Hritzo G. Progressive proximal and distal interphalangeal flexion device. J Hand Ther 2001; 146:51–52.

125. Bonutti PM, Windan JE, Ables BA, Miller BG. Static progressive stretch to reestablish elbow range of motion. Clin Orthop Relat Res 1994; 303:128–134.

126. Zander CL. Elbow flexion contractures treated with serial casts and conservative therapy. Am J Hand Surg 1992; 17(4):694–697.

127. Nuismer BA, Ekes AM, Holm MB. The use of low load prolonged stretch devices in rehabilitation programs in the Pacific Northwest. Am J Occup Ther 1997; 51(4):538–542.

128. Kozerefski PM. Exercise and ambulation in the burn patient. In: DiGregorio, ed. Rehabilitation of the Burn Patient. New York: Churchill Livingstone, 1984:58.

129. Akeson WH, Amiel D, Mechanic GL, Woo SL, Harwood AF, Hamer ML. Collagen cross-linking alterations in joint contractures: changes in the reducible cross-linking in periarticular connective tissue after nine weeks of immobilization. Connect Tissue 1977; 5:15–17.

130. Randall T, Portnelf L, Harris BA. Effects of joint mobilization on joint stiffness and active motion of the metacarpal-Phalangeal Joint. J Orthop Sports Phys Ther 1992; 16(1):30–36.

131. Evans RB, Burkhalter WE. A study of the dynamic anatomy of extensor tendons implications for treatment. J Hand Surg 1986; 11A(5):774–779.

132. Abston S. Scar reaction after thermal injury and prevention of scars and contractures. In: Boswick JA Jr, ed. The Art and Science of Burn Care. Aspen System in Tromby 90. Rockville, 1987:846.

133. Reid WH, Evans JH, Naismith RS et al. Hypertrophic scarring and pressure therapy. Burns 1987; 13(suppl):529.

134. Staley MJ, Richard RL. Scar management. In: Richard RL, Staley MJ, eds. Burn Care and Rehabilitation: Principles and Practice. Philadelphia: FA Davis, 1994.

135. Shakespeare PG, Renterghen L. Some observations on the surface structure of collagen in hypertrophic scars. Burns 1985; 11:178–180.

136. Davey RB, Sprod RT, Niel TO. Computerized colour: A technique for the assessment of burn scar hypertrophy. A preliminary report. Burns 1999; 25(3):207–213.

137. Cartotto R, Scott J. The durometer: A new method which evaluates the harness of a burn scar (abstract). American Burn Association Annual Meeting, Chicago, 2002.

138. Ward S. Pressure therapy for the control of hypertrophic scar formation after burn injury. A history and review. J Burn Care Rehabil 1991; 12:257–262.

139. Kealey GP, Jensen KL, Laubenthal KN, Lewis RN. Prospective randomized comparison of two types of pressure therapy garments. J Burn Care Rehabil 1990; 11:334–336.

140. Groce A, McCauley R, Serghiou M, Chinkes D, Herndon D. The effects of high vs. low pressure garments in the control of hypertrophic scar in the burned child: a final report (abstract). American Burn Association Annual Meeting, Boston, 2001.

141. Moore M, Engrav LH, Calderon J. Effectiveness of custom pressure garments in wound management: a prospective trial within wounds and with verified pressure (abstract). American Burn Association Annual Meeting, Las Vegas, 2000.

142. Mann R, Yeong EK, Moore M et al. Do custom fitted pressure garments provide adequate pressure? J Burn Care Rehabil 1997; 18:247–249.

143. Ward S, Schenbly A, Kravitz M et al. Use of positive plaster impressions to facilitate measurement of antiburn scar support gloves for severely burned hands. J Burn Care Rehabil 1989; 10(4):351–353.

144. Carr-Collins JA. Pressure techniques for the prevention of hypertrophic scar. Clin Plast Surg 1992; 19(3):733–743.

145. Smith and Nephew, Inc. Smith and Nephew Products Catalog: Splinting, Padding and Soft Strapping Materials. USA: Smith and Nephew, Inc., 2002.

146. Smith and Nephew, Inc. Smith and Nephew Products Catalog: Rehabilitation Elastomer Products. USA: Smith and Nephew, Inc., 2002.

147. McNee S. The use of silicone gel in the control of hypertrophic scarring. Physiotherapy 1990; 76:194–197.

148. Quinn KJ. Silicone gel in scar treatment. Burns 1987; 13:533–540.

149. Fedorczyk J. The role of physical agents in modulating pain. J Hand Ther 1997; 10:110–121.

150. Serghiou M, Walker K, Baxter C, Partks D, Wainwright D. Therapeutic modalities in burn care (abstract). American Burn Association Annual Meeting, Lake Buena Vista. J Burn Care Rehabil 1999; 2:167.

151. Gross J, Stafford S. Modified method for application of paraffin wax for treatment of burn scar. J Burn Care Rehabil 1984; 5(5):394.

152. Head M, Helm P. Paraffin and sustained stretching in the treatment of burn contractures. Burns 1977; 4:136.

153. Ward S, Hayes-Lundy C, Reddy R et al. Evaluation of topical therapeutic ultrasound to improve response to physical therapy and lessen scar contracture after burn injury. J Burn Care Rehabil 1994; 15:74–77.

154. Patiño U, Novick C, Merlo A et al. Massage in hypertrophic scars. J Burn Care Rehabil 1998; 19:241–249.

155. Field T, Peck M, Krugman S et al. Burn injuries benefit from massage therapy. J Burn Care Rehabil 1998; 19:268–271.

156. Field T, Peck M, Hernandez M et al. Postburn itching, pain and psychological symptoms are reduced with massage therapy. J Burn Care Rehabil 2000; 21:189–193.

157. North Coast Medical. Hand Therapy Catalog. Scar and Massage Care. USA: North Coast Medical, 2001.

158. Stern PJ, Neale MW, Graham JJ et al. Classification on treatment of postburn proximal interphalangeal joint contractures in children. J Hand Surg 1987; 12A:450–457.

159. Cannon NM. Postoperative management of metacarpophalangeal joint capsulectomies. In: Hunter JM et al. Rehabilitation of the Hand Surgery and Therapy. 4th ed. St. Louis: Mosby, 1995:1173–1186.

160. Gould JS et al. Capsulectomy of the metacarpophalangeal and proximal interphalangeal joints. J Hand Surg 1979; 4(5):482–486.

161. Buch VI. Clinical and functional assessment of the hand after metacarpophalangeal capsulotomy. Plast Reconstr Surg 1974; 53(4):452–457.

37

Reconstruction of Burn Deformities of the Lower Extremity

ROBERT L. McCAULEY
University of Texas Medical Branch and Shriners Hospital for Children—Galveston Unit, Galveston, Texas, USA

MALACHY E. ASUKU
Ahmadu Bello University Teaching Hospital, Kaduna, Nigeria

I. OVERALL VIEW OF ACUTE CARE IN LOWER EXTREMITY BURNS: CONCERNS

A. Introduction

According to the Wallace rule of nine, the lower extremities constitute 36% of the total body surface area (TBSA). Using the Lund and Browder charts, this area of the body is 45% in adults and 39% in children (1). Burn injuries to the lower extremities can, therefore, be a major concern either as a result of large TBSA involvement or due to compromise of specialized anatomic and functional units such as the foot (2,3). The American Burn Association, in recognizing the functional importance of the foot, has designated its involvement in burn injury as a major burn requiring inpatient treatment for optimal outcome (2–5). Lower extremities burn injuries, whether occurring in isolation or as part of a more extensive surface area injury can, therefore, significantly affect the overall rehabilitation of the patient (2–6).

B. Special Considerations in Acute Care

Burns to the lower extremities can result from a variety of agents occurring usually under accidental circumstances (2,3). While scald injuries and flame burns often result in superficial and deep partial-thickness burns, contact burns and high-voltage electrical burns will often result in either full-thickness burns or fourth degree burns (5). Less common causes such as chemicals may also produce serious burns to the lower extremities (5). Aside from the depth of the burns, regional characteristics tend to impact on the severity of lower extremity burn injuries

(1–6). First, the edema associated with deep partial- and full-thickness burn injury to the lower extremity is made worse by dependency. Walking, standing, or even sitting with the lower limbs in dependent position without elastic support (such as ace wraps, compression garments, etc.) can lead to increase in hydrostatic pressure resulting in edema in the severely burned limb (1). Edema can enhance inflammation, resulting in pain and a decrease in mobility of the injured parts. These circumstances may result in joint stiffness, which may impair subsequent rehabilitation. In the acute phase of injury, control of edema is best accomplished by elevation of the affected part of the lower extremity in bed. However, one must be cognizant of the attendant dangers of immobilization and hospitalization for such injuries. The goal of management is, therefore, to facilitate early ambulation with supportive stockings (1,5,6).

Second, circumferential injuries resulting in edema in lower extremity burns can lead to the development of compartment syndrome. Elderly patients who may also have antecedent peripheral vascular insufficiency and patients suffering high-voltage electrical injuries are reported to be at increased risk in this regard (1–3). A high index of suspicion is required to embark on a timely evaluation of the neurovascular status of the affected limb in order to determine the need for immediate decompression (1–3). It is important to appreciate the fact that while peroneal nerve palsy may be due to direct injury to the common peroneal nerve at the neck of the fibular, where it runs a relatively superficial course, it may also result from an imminent compartment syndrome. Mani and Charte (1) observed that escharotomies and fasciotomies when indicated should be done early in the resuscitative phase before tissue perfusion is compromised. Although the decision to decompress is often based on clinical features, effective tissue perfusion essentially stops when tissue pressure reaches 40 mmHg (1). While escharotomies can be done at the bedside, fasciotomies require more elaborate preparation for anesthesia and occasionally blood replacement.

The involvement of the lower extremity in high-voltage electrical injuries, however, generates other concerns. The bulky muscles of the thigh may suffer myonecrosis releasing large volumes of breakdown products that may constitute a significant threat to renal function and to the patient (1). The level of threat, however, can be significantly minimized with diligent fluid therapy and timely debridement of nonviable muscle tissue. These patients may eventually require early soft tissue reconstruction in order to close their wounds.

In the past, the technique of wound excision for deep partial- and full-thickness burns was a subject of debate. Surgeons were divided between tangential excisions and fascial excisions (1,6). Proponents of fascial excision argued that such excisions guaranteed complete excision of nonviable tissue and that it is technically easier to perform, and accompanied by lesser requirement for blood transfusions. On the other hand, the proponents of tangential excisions believed that the subcutaneous tissue should be preserved since it has an important role in preventing adhesion of skin grafts to fascia, which is important in the growing child. Furthermore, they observed that the outcome of tangential excision is aesthetically superior to that of fascial excision. However, currently, fascial excisions in the lower extremity have been largely abandoned due to the associated long-term contour deformities as a result of chronic edema, lymphedema, and muscle atrophy (6). Initial concerns over excessive blood loss in tangential excisions are now addressed by meticulous efforts at hemostasis. These include the use of hypotensive anesthesia, the application of tourniquets, the elevation of the limb during surgery, and the use of thrombin and epinephrine on the wound surface (1).

Another problem encountered in lower extremity burns is the paucity of soft tissues over such areas as the tibial tuberosity, the shin, the malleoli, and the toes. These areas are, therefore, more predisposed to deep burns with exposure of tendons, bones, and joints. This is particularly true following electrical burns (2,3). Consequently, these areas may heal in a delayed fashion since they are devoid of the freely mobile soft tissue padding required for any degree of wound contraction to occur. Such areas may require flap coverage in order to obtain satisfactory long-term results.

Fears have been entertained that lower extremity burn wounds may be at increased risk of wound infection with the perineum as a potential source of contamination. This has led to the preference of irrigation of the burned area rather than the immersion that is done during tubbing in some centers (1). Although this fear has remained unsubstantiated, meticulous wound care and appropriate bacterial monitoring as well as the judicious use of topical and systemic antimicrobials should prevent the conversion of partial-thickness wounds to deeper injuries. Superficial partial-thickness burns are, therefore, expected to heal with excellent functional and aesthetic results within 2 weeks (1). On the other hand, deep partial- and full-thickness burns invariably require resurfacing with skin grafts or flaps. Unexpanded sheet grafts are preferred to mesh grafts in resurfacing the lower extremities. However, such an approach is subject to autograft availability since higher priority areas such as the face and hands usually take precedence (2,3).

Traditionally, the lower extremity constitutes the most frequently harvested donor site for autogenous skin grafts. The large and uniform surfaces provided by the thigh make it most suitable as a donor site. Therefore, when the thigh is involved in deep partial- or full-thickness burns, one is not only faced with the problem of covering a large surface but also with the possibility of loss of a quality skin graft donor site. This places a high premium on available donor sites particularly when the injury is part of a large surface area burn. Under such circumstances, other less suitable donor sites such as the back, the buttocks, and the abdomen may have to be utilized and recropping may become necessary. The use of synthetic skin substitutes, cultured autografts, and allografts in burn wound coverage must be seen as attempts at providing more options rather than as alternatives for autogenous skin grafts (1).

Commencement of ambulation following the application of skin grafts to the lower extremity has also been attended by divergent opinions (7–12). However, early ambulation as soon as the grafts have "taken" securely should be the gold standard (6). The grafted lower extremity may require a custom-fitted compression garment and the use of elastic wraps during ambulation to minimize the effect of hydrostatic pressure and edema formation. The use of the Unna Boot® (Dome-Paste Bandage, Mile Inc., West haven, CT) has been acclaimed to solve the problems of blistering and graft separation previously encountered with early ambulation (6,13,14).

Burns of the weight-bearing surface of the foot may be deep enough to require resurfacing despite the limited exposure of the area and the protection provided by the thickened epithelium and the use of footwear. Such deep injuries are commonly encountered as exit wounds in electrical burns or arise from prolonged contact burns in patients with peripheral neuropathies (2,3,6,15,16). The main concern here is over the prospect of obtaining durable coverage. Destruction of the plantar fascia may disrupt the intrinsic mechanism of arch support and mandate long-term orthotic inserts (2,3). There are varied opinions as to the most suitable means of resurfacing the weight-bearing surface of the foot. Split- and full-thickness skin grafts as well as pedicled flaps have all had their moments of glory with each falling short of providing the highly specialized characteristics of the normal plantar skin (16–20). Kucan and co-workers (2,3) noted that a combination of flexibility and durability is required of any tissue used to resurface the sole of the foot and this must be accomplished without excessive tissue bulk that will hinder the use of footwear. The requirement for ideal plantar resurfacing is therefore a durable tissue of moderate volume that will affix tightly to deeper structures resisting shear forces and is capable of attaining protective sensation. This group further observed that split-thickness skin grafts are no less durable than full-thickness skin grafts. Consequently, split-thickness skin grafts continue to be the primary method of coverage for the plantar surface as long as there is adequate supporting subcutaneous tissue.

Another early concern following deep burns of the foot is the tendency to develop shortening of the Archilles tendon (6). Prompt and proper use of splints and casts may be required to maintain the ankle joint in a plantar-grade position while the proper use of footboard may suffice in the nonambulatory patient. However, vigilance and good care of pressure points are required to prevent the development of pressure sores with the use of these appliances (6). The importance of maintaining joint motions particularly in the multijointed ankle and foot in the immediate post injury period cannot be overemphasized. The biomechanics at these joints are highly complex with motions occurring simultaneously in a number of planes during both the weight-bearing and non-weight-bearing phases (2,3). Success at rehabilitation of the burned lower extremity will, therefore, depend on maintaining these joint functions rather than correcting any ensuing deformities.

Finally, the issue of inpatient versus outpatient management of lower extremity burns is one that is frequently debated. Zachary et al. (5) noted that isolated burns of the feet has the distinction of being the most common burn injury to be initially treated on outpatient basis. Yet, many of these patients subsequently require hospitalization due to significant morbidity. They, therefore, suggested that patients with this injury are better served by inpatient care. Lyle et al. (15), in emphasizing the same view, identified cellulitis, hypertrophied scarring, and prolonged hospitalization as possible complications of initial outpatient care of the burned foot (15).

Although the depth of the injury is key to determining the complexity of treatment, effort required in the acute care of the burned lower extremity, control of edema, early tangential excision and resurfacing with skin grafts, appropriate splinting, and early ambulation are fundamental to a successful outcome.

II. RECONSTRUCTION OF THE BURNED LOWER EXTREMITY

Though adequate care in the acute phase of lower extremity burn injuries can significantly minimize the need for reconstructive procedures in later years, less than optimal outcome may occur as a consequence of deep initial injuries. The effects of weight bearing and ambulation as well as growth in patients who have suffered early childhood burns may also contribute to the development of deformities. Varying complexity of reconstructive efforts is, therefore, required in order to obtain the maximum functional potential of the thermally injured or deformed lower extremity. Brou et al. (21) noted that in a survey of 25 patients who survived a mean TBSA burns of 71% (65% full thickness), 27% (136/512) of the total reconstructive needs were in the torso and lower extremities. The principal reconstructive goals for the lower extremity are weight-bearing and unimpeded ambulation. Achieving these goals require the provision of stable and durable skin coverage accompanied by protective sensation and proprioception. The final outcome should not only permit proper shoe fit but also play a role in boosting self-esteem (2,3).

Experience has shown that a sure way to achieving optimal outcome in the reconstruction of the burned patient is through integrated team approach with realistic goals set to meet the individual's needs. According to Kucan and co-workers (2,3) reconstruction of the burned lower extremity may be divided into two phases: (1) early: beginning at admission and extending up to 1 year after injury; and (2) late: commencing after 1 year of injury. In the early phase, reconstructive procedures may be required in the closure of complex wounds as well as in the prevention and correction of early onset functional impairments. The late phase, however, contends with problems of chronic instability of soft tissue coverage, burn scar contractures, contour deformities, growth disturbances in children, and revision of amputation stumps.

A. Early Reconstruction

1. Acute Wound Coverage

Reconstruction for acute wound coverage may be indicated in deep partial-, full-thickness and fourth degree burns in which exposure of underlying structures may present significant wound coverage problems (2,3). These injuries commonly result from high-voltage electrical burns and contact burns typified by the muffler burns commonly seen in motorcycle accidents. Extensive soft tissue losses with exposure of tendons, ligaments, neurovascular trunks, bones, and joint spaces characterize these injuries. Kucan et al. (2,3) observed that skin grafts are inadequate to achieve either short- or long-term reconstructive goals in these injuries. Invariably, composite tissues in the form of flaps are required for closure of such wounds and options will depend to a large extent on the anatomical location of the wound or defect.

The Thigh

The wide circumference of the thigh as well as the abundance of soft tissues allow for excision and primary closure of limited deep burn wounds. When soft tissue loss is extensive, however, the first option lies in the use of adjacent soft tissues as advancement or transpositional flaps to fill up the defect and achieve closure. The nature as well as the location of the defect and recipient bed contributes to determining the tissues best suited for closure. Muscle flaps available for coverage of proximal wounds

include the rectus abdominis, the tensor fascia lata, and the sartorius for smaller defects. In the formidable problem of deep burns of the groin with exposure of the external iliac and femoral vessels, closure requires bulky soft tissues to provide adequate padding and protection. The inferiorly based rectus abdominis muscle flap has been found useful in this reconstruction. More distal defects on the thigh have been reconstructed with the proximally based tensor fascia lata and the vastus medialis transposition muscle flaps (6,22). Additionally, Salisbury and Bevin (22) suggested the use of the distally based sartorius muscle flap for coverage of defects of the distal thigh. They, however, emphasized the need to ascertain the reliability of the distal pedicle in every patient in whom the use of this flap is contemplated.

Currently, the fasciocutaneous flap described by Ponsten (23) and extensively applied to the management of burn injuries by Tolhurst et al. in 1983 (24,25) has become the mainstay in the closure of deep burn wounds in the thigh. The thinness of the fasciocutaneous flap permits one-staged transfer without undue contour deformity and has the added advantage of not compromising functional muscle power (6). Barclay et al. (26), as well as Cormack and Lamberty (27) described the blood supply to these flaps as arising through vessels that pass along the fascial septa between muscle bellies and then fan out at the level of the deep fascia to form a plexus from which blood reaches the skin. The posterior thigh fasciocutaneous flap introduced by Maruyama and Iwahira (28), has been described as versatile in the one-staged closure of deep burn wounds of the posteromedial and posterolateral thigh. This flap, which is distally based, is supplied by a direct branch of the popliteal artery that emerges through the fat between semimembranosus and biceps femoris at the level of the popliteal fossa. Preoperative angiography or Doppler flowmetry is required to provide for safer outcome with the use of the flap. The skin island is designed with its lateral margins situated between the hamstring muscles and can be raised proximally as far as the gluteal crease. The donor site, if <10 cm in width can be closed primarily (28). A similar distally based fasciocutaneous flap is the lower posterolateral thigh flap described by Laitung (29). The flap is supplied by the direct cutaneous branches of the popliteal artery and the lateral superior genicular artery and is also suitable for coverage of deep burn wounds of the anterolateral and posterior thigh (29).

The Knee

Deep burn injuries in the region of the distal thigh and upper leg can be compounded by involvement of the knee joint. When the joint space is exposed, immediate flap closure is required to prevent infection and loss of function. Myocutaneous and muscle flaps are well suited for such closures. Witt and Achauer (6) observed that the advantages of myocutaneous flaps include their ability to obliterate dead spaces by filling up deep cavities and at the same time providing stable skin coverage and good blood supply that accelerates wound healing. However, the donor site deformity that attends to the use of myocutaneous flaps has remained a major drawback. This issue is partly addressed in the use of muscle flaps with split-thickness skin graft in a single or staged procedure.

The gastrocnemius muscle provides by far the most versatile option in the closure of the opened knee joint. While the medial head can be designed to reach the anteromedial aspects of the knee joint, distal thigh, and upper tibia, the lateral head is suitable for closures over the anterolateral aspect of the knee joint and upper tibia (30–32) (Fig. 37.1). The vascular supplies to both heads are relatively consistent. The medial head receives its blood supply from the medial sural artery, a direct branch of the popliteal artery while the supply to the lateral head enters the proximal portion of the deep surface of the muscle just distal to the popliteal crease. Proximal exposure and separation of the two heads of the gastrocnemius muscle and identification of the soleus fascia are essential prelude to distal separation and elevation of either of these flaps.

The major disadvantages in the use of myocutaneous and muscle flaps include the sacrifice of functional muscle and the excessive bulk at the recipient site. The fasciocutaneous flaps, which address these issues, are however only useful where the opened knee joint is not associated with a deep cavity that requires filling. The popliteo-posterior thigh and the lower posterior–lateral thigh fasciocutaneous flaps have both been reportedly used in closure of such superficially opened knee joints. Microsurgical transfer of free flaps provides yet another option for closure of the opened knee joint. Though this option allows the one-stage use of high-quality distant tissues, it has been reserved for more severe cases in which the less complex local options are unavailable.

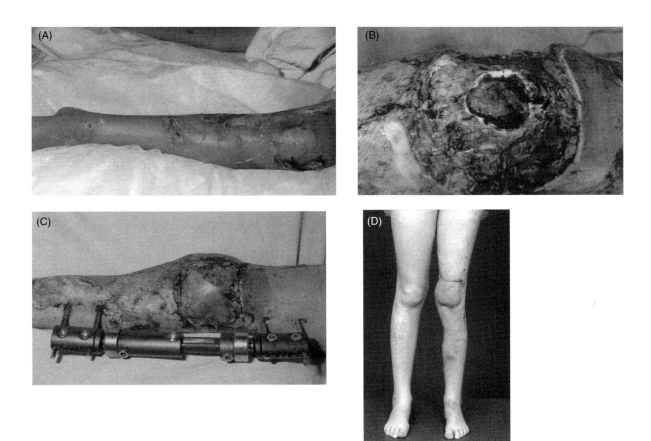

Figure 37.1 (A) Patient with full thickness burn over the left knee after being trapped underneath a car with knee next to muffler. (B) Debridement showing open knee joint. (C) Medial gastrocnemius muscle flap for closure around the knee joint. (D) Final result after closure 1 year later.

The Lower Leg

The distal part of the lower extremity is poorly endowed with myocutaneous flaps for pedicled transfer, particularly for the management of thermal injuries that usually encompass much larger cutaneous areas (2,3). Muscle flaps are therefore the workhorses in the closure of deep burn wounds in this region. Sood et al. (33) observed that the superior third of the lower leg might be reliably covered with the gastrocnemius muscle while the soleus muscle provides a useful flap in the reconstruction of the middle third of the leg. Coverage of wounds in the distal third of the leg is a more daunting task with options limited to the use of the reversed soleus flap or free tissue transfer (33) (Fig. 37.2). Chang et al. (34) and more recently, Sood et al. (33) described the use of the tibialis anterior turnover muscle flap in the coverage of the exposed tibia following severe burns. This flap, which had previously been described for coverage of the tibia following trauma, provides good protection and blood supply to the underlying bone with minimal donor site morbidity (35–37).

Several designs of the fasciocutaneous flaps have also been developed to address specific needs in the leg. In 1985, Moscona et al. (38) introduced the island fasciocutaneous flap of the posterior calf. The design followed the realization that the skin at the base of the fasciocutaneous flap, which can limit rotation and produce local deformity at the pivot point, does not provide vascular support to the distant skin paddle (38). The island fasciocutaneous flap, therefore, allows the use of the required distal skin paddle with improved reach making it suitable for coverage of defects around the knee joint with minimal donor site morbidity. In addition, there is no risk of exposure of vital structures in the popliteal fossa when based over this area as the proximal skin is left in place. Donor site closure, however, often requires the use of skin grafts (Fig. 37.3).

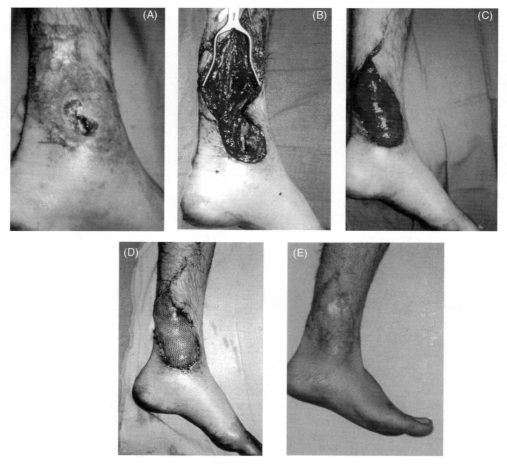

Figure 37.2 (A) A 20-year-old male referred after motorcycle muffler burn over medial aspect of left ankle. Patient referred after failure of skin grafts for closure. (B) Patient noted to have ostsomyelitis requiring extensive debridement of soft tissue and bone. (C) Coverage with a gracilis muscle flap. (D) Coverage of flap with a split thickness skin graft. (E) Appearance 1 year later after treatment of osteomyelitis with stable coverage and full weight bearing.

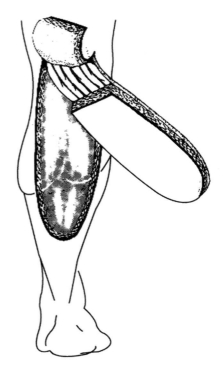

Figure 37.3 The island fasciocutaneous flap—divided into two—proximal random skin flap will cover the popliteal region. The distal flap is transposed to cover the anterolateral part of the knee. [Adapted from Moscona et al. (38).]

The saphenous artery fasciocutaneous flap based on the distal continuation of the saphenous artery onto the lower leg provides a basis for a posteromedial flap, which can be used for closure of adjacent defects (39,40). Similarly, the superficial sural artery fasciocutaneous flap raised along the center of the posterior calf and as far distally as the Achilles tendon, can provide closure for adjacent burn wounds (40). Maruyama et al. (41) introduced the bilobed fasciocutaneous flaps for coverage of defects on the leg (Fig. 37.3). This is intended to improve donor site morbidity by avoiding the use of skin grafts. While this is a useful technique, it may not be suitable for large burn wounds.

More recently, Heymans et al. (42) reported the use of the medial adipofascial flap of the leg for the coverage of full-thickness burns exposing the tibial crest. The saphenous artery and the posterior tibial artery perforators constitute the blood supply to this flap, which can be mobilized to cover the whole length of the tibia. While the donor site is closed primarily, the flap requires coverage with split-thickness skin grafts. The old technique of shaving and overgrafting with thick split-thickness skin grafts to provide good skin protection over exposed tibia still has a place in the reconstruction of the severely burned leg. However, currently dermabrasion has replaced

shaving of epithelial elements. In select cases, this technique may provide better skin durability and obviate the need for flap reconstruction (43).

Hammer et al. (44) as well as a number of other authors have reported satisfactory results with the use of the free latissimus dorsi flap in resurfacing the anterior surface of the lower leg in burn patients. The flap is broad, flat, and can be tailored to fit comfortably into most defects. Other free flaps suitable for resurfacing the burned lower leg include the rectus abdominis, serratus anterior, and the gracilis muscles covered with split-thickness skin grafts (3,6,45).

The Ankle and Achilles Tendon Areas

Closure of deep burn wounds in the ankle and Achilles tendon areas present special difficulties since contour preservation is of utmost importance. Historically, the cross-leg fasciocutaneous flap provided the principal means of closure of such wounds (1). The difficulties associated with this technique, however, ensured the search for better options. This led to the introduction of the relatively thin local fasciocutaneous flaps. Masquelet et al. (46) as well as Clark and Sherman described the lateral supramalleolar fasciocutaneous flap based on the perforating branches of the peroneal artery. The flap is suitable for coverage of the distal Achilles tendon area and ankle defects. Several other similar lateral and posterior calf flaps based on the perforating vessels at the ankle and providing sensate coverage have been described. Their use in burn reconstruction may, however, be limited by the extent of the initial burn injury (48–50).

Today, microvascular free flaps provide the most adequate means of resurfacing deep wounds in the ankle, malleolar, and Achilles tendon areas. The thinner fasciocutaneous and fascial free flaps are most suitable as they preserve the normal contour of the region. The radial forearm free flap, the medial and lateral arm flaps, the temporalis fascial flap, and the scapular flap have all been reported in the literature (3,51–55). These flaps provide satisfactory reconstruction so long as nonviable underlying bony prominences are adequately débrided or decorticated.

The Foot

Fourth degree burns to the foot as may result from electrical injuries are the most likely to present with exposed tendons, ligaments, and joint structures requiring early soft tissue reconstruction. The reconstruction must, however, address the anatomic and functional characteristics of the specific subunits of the foot. Frequently, distant flaps are required as the foot, which is functionally adapted for weight-bearing and ambulation, is provided with scanty and relatively rigid soft tissues. Hitherto, the transfer of distant flaps to the foot was achieved by the cross-leg flap technique first introduced by Hamilton in 1854 (47). The technique, however, is cumbersome and requires multiple stages of surgery. It is associated with high morbidity and frequently results in less than optimal functional and aesthetic outcome. It is not surprising, therefore, that this technique has now been largely abandoned (3,26,56,57). Kucan and co-workers (2,3), however, observed that the cross-leg flap might still be useful in certain rare instances. They, therefore, suggested that the technique should be retained in the repertoire of the burn reconstructive surgeon.

Several thin cutaneous, myocutaneous, and fasciocutaneous regional flaps have since been introduced in the soft tissue reconstruction around the foot. Examples include the extensor digitorum brevis myocutaneous flap, and the medial and lateral plantar fasciocutaneous flaps. These flaps, however, are of limited use in burn reconstruction where the injury tends to affect large and adjacent cutaneous areas (3,58–69). Consequently, the microsurgical transfer of distant tissues has become the gold standard in burn reconstruction around the foot. The technique has enabled the importation of large amounts of perfused, high-quality, and tailored tissue in a single-staged operation. Other advantages include great flexibility of design, shortened hospitalization, and decreased need for postoperative immobilization and physical therapy (2,3,6,70). Free flaps have made significant impact in addressing the difficulties previously encountered in the reconstruction of the weight-bearing sole of the foot (71,72). The transfer of free muscle flaps resurfaced with split-thickness skin grafts has been acclaimed as the most successful in reconstructing the sole of the foot and the heel (1–3,72). Kucan and co-workers (2,3) described the outcome as much more resistant over time to the shearing forces produced by walking. The flaps also attach more precisely to the skeletal framework of the foot maintaining the contour that permits the use of normal footwear. Free muscle flaps may look bulky initially but they shrink over time due to the effect of denervation. This should obviate any need for early debulking or refashioning of a free muscle flap (3). The latissimus dorsi muscle and myocutaneous free flaps seem to be the workhorses in lower extremity burn reconstruction (44,73–76). However, due to considerations for contour preservation, the thinner fasciocutaneous and fascial free flaps have been widely used to resurface the dorsum of the foot, whenever flap coverage is required. The commonly used flaps for this purpose include the radial forearm free flap, the medial and lateral arm flaps, the temporalis fascial flap, and even the omentum (3,51–55).

A major prerequisite in the use of free flaps is the availability of suitable recipient vessels in the vicinity of the wound or defect and yet outside the zone of injury. This requirement may not be readily met in the severely burned lower extremity. However, the concept of using uninjured extremities as free flap carriers to sites with inadequate local recipient vessels has addressed this concern to some extent (77–80). The contralateral limb, where suitable, has been used in lower extremity situations (81–85). In 1991, Lai et al. (81) reported the use of free latissimus dorsi muscle flap in the salvage of a limb that suffered high voltage electrical injury using the contralateral dorsalis pedis pedicle as recipient vessels. Similarly, Yamada et al. (82) reported the use of the cross-leg free rectus abdominis muscle flap for lower limb reconstructions. They described the technique as versatile under difficult and unfavorable conditions.

Free flaps have been monumental in the salvage and reconstruction of extensive burn wounds in the distal lower limb. However, microvascular surgery is most definitely a team effort requiring highly skilled manpower, adequate operating facilities, imaging facilities to map out vascular territories and a sound microsurgical back-up laboratory.

2. Early-Onset Functional Impairment

Reconstructive procedures may also be required in the acute phase of lower extremity burns to prevent or correct the development of rapidly progressing functional impairments as well as contour deformities that may potentially interfere with ambulation and the use of footwear (2,3). Such impairments are often related to problems of burn scar hypertrophy and burn scar contractures and are frequently associated with burns of the dorsum of the foot. Some superficial partial-thickness burns that heal spontaneously can insidiously develop hypertrophic scarring and contracture over subsequent months if not carefully followed. Similarly, when deep partial-thickness burns that should have been excised and grafted is incorrectly diagnosed and allowed to heal over a prolonged period, scar hypertrophy and contractures are bound to develop (1). Despite the reluctance to perform surgery on immature scars, reconstructive procedures may have to be undertaken early when these abnormalities of scarring result in rapidly progressing functional impairments or contour deformities. This is particularly true in children since scar contractures can worsen with time and if uncorrected can eventually result in an alteration in the growth of underlying bones (86).

Hypertrophic Burn Scars

Hypertrophic scarring involving the foot may result in contour distortion severe enough to interfere with the use of footwear and impair ambulation. Isolated burns of the dorsum of the foot tend to result from scalds and grease burns, which may be associated with increased risk of hypertrophic scar formation (5). Furthermore, those resulting from flame burns often occur as part of larger surface area burns so that the burned foot receives attention only after life-threatening issues and higher priority areas have been addressed (5). Deitch et al. (87) noted that a major functional and aesthetic problem in patients surviving thermal injuries is the development of hypertrophic burn scars. They noted that an important factor in the development of hypertrophic scarring is the time required for the burn wound to heal. In a series of 100 patients, they observed hypertrophic scarring in 33% of burn sites when the wound healed between 14 and 21 days and in 78% of burn sites that healed after 21 days.

Larson et al. in 1971 popularized the use of pressure garments in the control and prevention of hypertrophic burn scars (88–90). Although this concept was soon met with controversy, it has remained to this day an adjunct in the control of burn scars. The requirements include the provision of continuous pressure of the magnitude of 25 mmHg above the capillary pressure and long-term use of the garments usually for several months. Frequent careful evaluation is necessary to ensure the effectiveness of the program. The patient and family members must be adequately educated on the importance of consistent home care and compliance. Hypertrophic scars are believed to be most responsive to pressure therapy in the first 3–6 months when they are immature, hard, and often tender. Silicone gel inserts were later found to be equally effective in controlling and preventing the development of hypertrophic burn scars (91). Silicone gel was further reported to soften the matured hypertrophic scar and to decrease shrinkage and contraction of healed skin grafts. Though the mode of action of silicon gel is yet to be completely understood, it certainly does not depend on pressure (91).

Surgical correction is often required for hypertrophic burn scars. Focal and linear hypertrophic scars of unfavorable nature can be excised and the wound primarily closed. However, the broad and unsightly hypertrophic scar with fissures and recurrent cellulitis may be better served by surgical excision and resurfacing with thick split- or full-thickness skin grafts. Splinting in the postgraft period as well as subsequent use of pressure garments may be required in order to prevent recurrence and enhance functional recovery.

Early Burn Scar Contractures

Burn wounds have been shown to exhibit exaggerated wound contraction during healing. The contraction has also been shown to persist within the burn scar tissue particularly where the scar has remained active and hypertrophic (88–90). Over the flexor surfaces of joints, the force of wound contraction may act in unison with contraction of the underlying flexor muscles. The resultant force can be enormous and capable of resulting in the development of contractures (88–90). The hip joint, knee joint, ankle joint, and joints of the forefoot are at risk of developing contractures following severe lower extremity burn injuries.

While early mild to moderate contractures may respond to physical therapy programs, the severe and long-standing contractures invariably require surgical release. The physical therapy programs for early less severe contractures include range of motion exercises and the use of static and dynamic splints (88–90,92–94). Bennett et al. (92) as well as Johnson and Silverberg (93) observed that a fraction of those that fail to respond to these traditional approaches, may respond to serial casting. This technique involves casting the deformity in the closest position toward neutral for the joint. The cast is then changed at least weekly at which time the deformity is progressively corrected. This accomplishes stretching of muscle, tendon, and joint capsules and gradually restores joint function. Splints may be required at the end of the serial casting to maintain the achieved correction. Serial casting is particularly useful in the pediatric age group since the success of the technique does not depend significantly on patient's cooperation (92,93). Bennett et al. (92), however, noted that serial casting is mostly successful in large joints with fewer planes of motion and large lever arms. Serial casting is, therefore, believed to be effective at the knee joint but less effective in the region of the ankle joint and the joints of the forefoot.

Dorsal contractures of the foot are also unlikely to respond to conservative measures. Surgical intervention is reserved for those deformities, which are likely to be unresponsive to conservative measures. Early surgical intervention may be required if the incapacitating late complication of the rocker-bottom deformity is to be avoided (2,3). The quality of the overlying soft tissue scar determines whether a simple incisional release or complete excision and resurfacing is required. Resurfacing with thick split- or full-thickness skin graft will usually suffice. However, when this is less than optimal, flap coverage must be provided. The choice of flap should be based on local conditions of the foot and available donor sites. Physical therapy with splints and range of motion exercises as well as the use of custom-made padded shoes with rigid soles are essentials to obtaining a satisfactory outcome. Although some authors have cautioned against surgery on immature burn scars and contractures on the grounds of high recurrence rates, there are instances when progressive functional impairments may be better served by early surgical intervention (94,95).

B. Late Reconstruction

1. Inadequate Soft Tissue Coverage (Unstable Scars and Chronic Ulcers)

The major potential problem with burn injuries is the tendency to develop poor quality wound healing by secondary intention. This may result in unstable scars capable of interfering with hygiene and function. Spontaneous healing following deep second-degree burns in which the dermis has been partially destroyed results in unstable coverage that is prone to recurrent ulcerations and hypertrophic scarring. The resurfacing of the burned lower extremity with split-thickness skin grafts meshed to a ratio >1:2 may also contribute to subsequent scar instability (89). Furthermore, pressure ulcerations may develop over the trochanteric regions, the malleolar regions, and the heels in patients confined to bed rest either as a result of the severity of their burn injury or due to intercurrent medical conditions.

Chronic ulcerations and unstable scars tend to occur also in relation to contractures where counter-movement is retained and in areas prone to repetitive trauma (2,3). Such areas in the lower extremity include the anterior aspect of the knee joint, the popliteal area, the anterior aspect of the ankle joint, the malleolar and Achilles tendon areas, and the dorsal surfaces of the toes. Under normal circumstances, these areas are provided with thin pliable skin overlying scanty subcutaneous tissues. In the severely burned lower extremity, however, unyielding scars and skin grafts may be incapable of withstanding the tension created in the region. Furthermore, in the region of the foot, skin grafts may fail to provide the required durability to withstand the stress and strain of constant contact with footwear and ambulation. Kucan and co-workers (2,3) observed that split-thickness skin graft coverage of the foot may in the long-term result in hyperkeratosis along the junction of the graft and surrounding skin, fissure formation, ulceration, breakdown, and the development of burn scar contractures. They, however, suggested that split-thickness grafts may be used in early coverage to give the patient and surgeon added time to develop a more adequate reconstructive plan.

Chronic ulcerations are often painful and may impose the additional burden of management of pain, discomfort, and drainage to the rehabilitation of the burn patient (89). Unstable scars can also significantly delay the onset of physical therapy by inhibiting the use of splints and pressure garments. This, in effect, may protract the course of the overall rehabilitation of the burn patient.

The goal of management in patients with unstable scars and chronic ulcers is to obtain stable and durable soft tissue coverage. Meticulous care of pressure areas in patients confined to bed rest will go a long way in preventing this category of ulcerations (6). In most other cases, complete excision or dermabrasion of the poor quality skin and resurfacing with thick split- or full-thickness sheet grafts will usually give satisfactory results. However, certain areas are notorious for recurrent ulcerations and deserve special considerations. These include the anterior aspect of the knee joint and the reconstructed

weight-bearing sole of the foot. Achauer and Vanderkam (94) described the unstable burn scar of the anterior knee as a primary reconstructive problem in which coverage with skin graft may be too thin leading to unstable correction. They advocated over-grafting with a medium to thick split-thickness skin graft or even with a full-thickness graft. While this may suffice in the adult, it may not provide the long-term stable coverage required in the growing child (96). Dhanraj et al. (97) in a review of the management of recalcitrant knee ulcers in pediatric patients observed that excessive longitudinal tension played a contributory role in the etiology of the ulcers. They demonstrated permanent closure of the ulcers when the tension in the lower thigh was eliminated by transverse incisional release and resurfacing with wide sheet split-thickness skin grafts (Fig. 37.4).

Kucan and co-workers (2,3) observed that the unique architecture of the skin and subcutaneous tissues of the sole of the foot is specifically adapted for weight-bearing and cannot be satisfactorily reproduced by available reconstructive techniques. They noted that distant flaps of nonglabrous skin used to resurface the sole of the foot lack the fibrous elements that bind the normal sole to the underlying tissues. The transferred tissue is, therefore, unstable over the underlying bony skeleton and is unable to resist the shear forces during ambulation. In a recent survey of various techniques available for the reconstruction of the sole of the foot, it was noted that the overall incidence of chronic ulceration in fasciocutaneous flaps and skin grafted muscle flaps did not differ significantly. Furthermore, flap sensibility was not different using the two techniques (2,3). The inference, therefore, is that these chronic ulcers are mechanical in origin arising either from untreated osseous abnormalities or from external friction due to poor-fitting footwear (2,3). Meticulous attention to contours while resurfacing the foot should reduce the problems of shoe-fit and frictional ulcers. Kucan and co-workers (2,3) observed that aside from patient selection and postoperative education on the care of the reconstructed foot, the use of custom-made orthotics and padded shoes based on computer-assisted gait analysis are additional factors that enhance long-term successes.

Postburn unstable scars and chronic ulcers in the lower extremity deserve prompt attention particularly having been shown to exhibit an increased risk of malignant transformation. The malignancy, which is described as Marjolin's ulcer, is a squamous cell carcinoma (1,98–102). The exact incidence of malignant degeneration in burn scars is not known, however, it has been estimated that up to 2% of all epidermoid carcinomas of the skin originate in burn scars (98). Aarons et al. (98) and Novick et al. (99) observed a definite predilection for the flexion creases of the extremities. This is collaborated by the report of Ozek et al. (100), who in a series of 40 patients

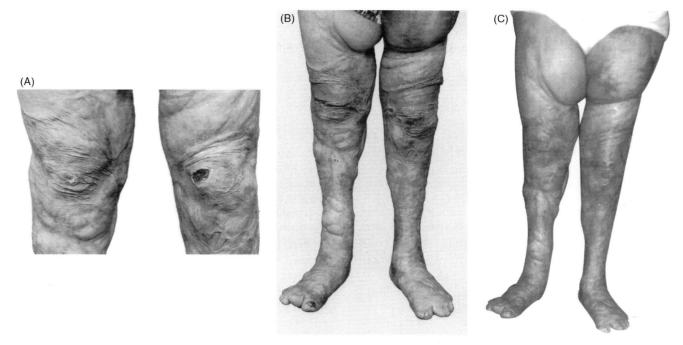

Figure 37.4 (A) A 11-year-old male with bilateral recalcitrant knee ulcers. He had suffered 62% total body surface area burns at the age of one and has had a total of three previous ulcer excisions and grafting to both knees. (B) Four weeks post incisional release and grafting of 160 cm^2 of split thickness skin graft to the left thigh and 120 cm^2 to the right. Both ulcers completely closed. (C) Patient remained ulcer free at 2 years follow-up. [Reprinted with permission from Dhanraj et al. (97).]

with Marjolin's ulcers found >50% of the lesions located in the popliteal region. A latent period of several years to decades of chronic ulcerations in the burn scar may precede malignant degeneration (98–101). Sarma et al. (101) reported the development of Marjolin's ulcer in a 30-year-old below-knee amputation stump following burn injuries. They suggested that the relationship between the burn scar and the chronic irritation from use of an artificial limb over a period of 30 years might have resulted in the malignant transformation.

The diagnosis of Marjolin's ulcer should be based on histological examination of biopsied tissue. Treatment may include wide margin local excision and coverage with split-thickness skin grafts for small lesions. Amputation of the involved extremity may constitute the treatment of choice in advanced cases (98–102). The role of regional lymph node dissection is controversial. Some authors advocate prophylactic node dissection while others advocate node dissection only on the basis of histological grade of the tumor (1,98,103,104). Prognosis is primarily related to the local extent of the disease, its anatomical location, and the presence or absence of regional lymph node metastasis. Investigators in this field agree with the fact that a stable skin coverage following deep thermal injuries can significantly reduce the incidence of burn scar carcinomas (98–100).

2. Burn Scar Contractures

Burn scar contractures are common and frustrating sequelae of thermal injuries (88–90). The depth of the initial injury contributes in no small measures to the development of contractures. The presence of life-threatening issues in patients with large total body surface area burns may correlate to a delay in instituting local wound care with consequence on the quality of healing. In the lower extremities, other factors contributing to the development of postburn contractures include prolonged immobilization and inadequate skin coverage. Additionally, poor compliance with postacute physical therapy programs aimed at minimizing scar hypertrophy and contractures may play a significant role. Larson et al. (88–90) noted that the burn wound has inherent tendency to contract and continues to do so until it meets an opposing force. They further observed that the position of comfort is the position of deformity and that the severity of the deformity may be directly related to the depth of the initial injury (88–90,95). Robson et al. (95) observed that splinting and exercise are important means of providing the required opposing force to halt the development of contractures. Early contractures have been shown to be amenable to positioning, exercise programs, static and dynamic splinting as well as serial casting. In the late and established contractures, however, these measures only serve as adjuncts to surgical release. Peacock et al. (105) observed that the need for secondary reconstructive procedures following burn injuries is decreased by the proper attention to positioning and ranging of joints during the acute phase. They further observed that the success rates of such procedures increase in direct proportion to the degree of motion preserved in these joints before reconstruction.

For the purpose of discussion, it is easier to consider the contractures of individual joints separately. However, this should not underscore the fact that multiple joints may be involved in a single patient with large surface area burns.

Contractures of the Hip Joint

Hip contractures may result from deep burns of the anterior aspect of the upper thigh, the groin, and lower abdomen in children or from poor compliance with an established physical therapy program. The flexion contracture is usually accompanied by some degree of adduction as a result of the slight internal rotation that occurs with flexion at the hip joints. Surgical release may be indicated in all but the very mild and early contractures where splinting and positioning may constitute adequate treatment. Z-plasty and its modifications as well as other local transposition flaps may be effective in breaking-up and correcting contractures resulting from narrow restricting bands. However, the contractures frequently encountered are broad and require more elaborate procedures for correction (106). The contracture is released with an incision parallel to the inguinal ligament through the breadth and thickness of the scarred tissue. It is important to ensure completeness of the release intraoperatively. The resulting defect is resurfaced with thick split- or full-thickness skin grafts depending on availability and surgeon preference. Immobilization in extension is essential in the immediate postoperative period. This may require the use of cross-leg bars in children. Range of motion exercises as well as ambulation should be instituted as soon as the skin grafts take satisfactorily and stability is achieved. Variable periods of splinting may be required in order to prevent recurrence of the contracture. The morbidity associated with the use of skin grafts in the release of these contractures has endeared the prospects of flap coverage to many reconstructive surgeons. In fact, the proponents of flap coverage argue that such difficulties with the use of skin grafts might have contributed to the development of the groin contracture in the first instance (106,107). However, the recent introduction of the vacuum assisted closure (VAC) technique to improve graft-take in difficult contour areas such as the groin may address some of these concerns (108–111).

Flap coverage, however, becomes an absolute necessity in the rare event of exposure of the femoral vessels and nerve during the release of severe groin contractures (106). The large fasciocutaneous flaps popularized by Ponsten (23) have since enjoyed unprecedented fame in burn reconstruction of the lower limb (Fig. 37.5). Described as the "super-flap," the fasciocutaneous flaps are easy and quick to raise, can tolerate a length–breadth ratio of 4:1 and donor defects can usually be closed directly. The flap can be raised in scarred or grafted skin, and yet survive transposition due to its fascial component (106,107). Turley et al. (106) reported the use of the medial fasciocutaneous flap of the thigh for release of post-burn groin contractures. They obtained satisfactory outcome in their series that consisted of four patients with six severe groin contractures. The vascular supply and innervation of the flap had previously been described by Wang et al. (112), who used the same flap laterally for groin reconstruction and medially for vaginal and perineal reconstructions. Another option, which may be less versatile for the release of groin contractures is the antero-medial thigh fasciocutaneous flap described by Hayashi and Maruyama (113). The perfusion of this flap, like the medial thigh flap is nonaxial and is dependent on the extensive vascular communications between the supra fascial and subdermal plexus of the thigh (114).

On rare occasions, the relatively bulky muscle and myocutaneous flaps may better serve the defect resulting from the release of groin contractures. The tensor fascia latae, rectus abdominis, gracilis, and sartorius muscles have been used either as muscle flaps or myocutaneous flaps in such circumstances (115,116). Turley et al. (106) observed that the use of flaps obviate the need for prolonged splinting. Mobilization can be started as early as on the third postoperative day and the patient can be discharged within 10 days of surgery.

Popliteal Contractures

Postburn flexion contractures of the knee joint, also known as popliteal contractures, are perhaps the most frequently encountered in the lower extremity. Yet, they are easily preventable (1). Early surgical intervention as well as early and aggressive physical therapy programs should serve to prevent and reduce the incidence of these contractures. Treatment options for popliteal contractures may correlate with the severity of the contracture as it affects limb function (Table 37.1). Grade I contractures may require no immediate surgical intervention. Functional improvement is expected to follow conservative measures such as use of pressure garments, silicone gel inserts, and moisturizing lotions to soften and increase the pliability of the scars around the knee joint. In grade II contractures there is a demonstrable tightening of the burn scar. Patients exhibit full extension but may require release and lengthening by the use of local transpositional flaps or

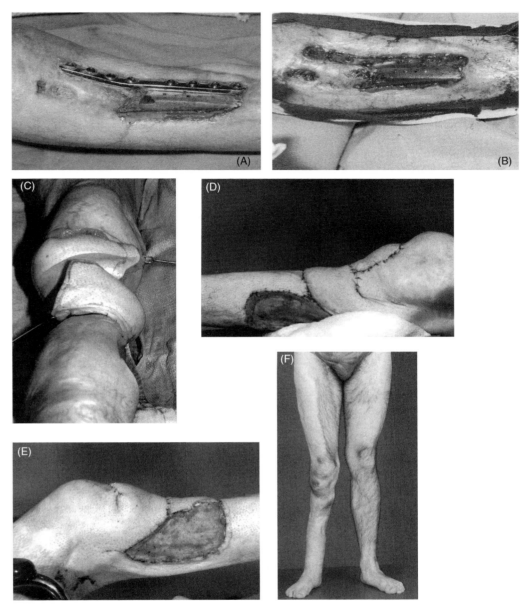

Figure 37.5 (A) A 12-year-old male referred after motor vehicle accident where he sustained an open tibial fracture and arterial repair (femoral–popliteal bypass) to the right lower leg with exposed hardware. (B) Hardware removed and wound subsequently debrided. (C) Bilateral fascio cataneous flaps used to cover the defect over the proximal lower leg. (D) Medial view of flaps and skin grafts used to cover the donor site. (E) Lateral view of flaps and skin grafts used to cover the donor site. (F) Eight-year follow-up with stable wound coverage.

transverse incisional releases across the axis of the joint and resurfacing with thick split- or full-thickness skin grafts. Postoperative immobilization to ensure graft take and subsequent splinting to prevent recurrence may be required. The grade III deformity denotes moderate to severe contracture in which the patient cannot fully extend the leg. This may be complicated by the presence of unstable scars and chronic ulcers due to excessive

stretching of the unyielding coverage. Incisional or excisional release and skin grafting is frequently the first line of therapy with excellent long-term results. Fasciocutaneous and fascial flaps, which are devoid of bulk, may be used as alternatives. Prakash (117) introduced the concept of the central segment expansion method in the release of popliteal burn scar contractures that correspond to the grade III contractures. The technique involves

Table 37.1   Classification of Popliteal Burn Scar Contractures

Grade I	Symptomatic tightness but no limitation in range of motion, normal ambulation is preserved
Grade II	Mild decrease in extension with demonstrable contracting band across the politeal fossa, patient is able to ambulate
Grade III	Moderate to severe contracture with marked decrease in flexion-extension arc, patient is able to ambulate only with a limp
Grade IV	Fixed flexion contracture, patient is unable to stand or ambulate on affected limb

making releasing incisions proximal and distal to the level of the joint, thereby, creating a bipedicle flap over the joint. The defects on either side of the flap are then covered with split-thickness skin grafts. Contraction of the split-thickness skin grafts is expected to result in the slow expansion of the flap.

Extensive contractures may require multiple incisions and therefore multiple bipedicle flaps sandwiched between skin grafts. The authors advocated excision and coverage with the superiorly based medial or lateral fasciocutaneous flap in the presence of unstable scars or chronic ulcers. They, however, extended the concept of flap expansion here too by using narrow flaps such that defects above and below the flap are again resurfaced with skin grafts (118). The disadvantage of this approach however, is that it is staged, protracted and yet to be supported by any long-term follow-up results. More recently, however, Prakash and Mishra (119) reported the use of the posterior calf fascial flap in resurfacing popliteal defects after excision of contractures with unstable scars. They observedthat the advantages of the technique include its reliability since the strong fascia ensures satisfactory graft take thereby preventing recurrence of the contracture. They also noted that harvesting the fascial flap is associated with no functional loss and minimal donor site defect. Robert et al. (120) had previously described the use of the same flap in the reconstruction of traumatic lower extremity defects.

The grade IV contractures, which are fixed flexion contractures, may require more complex reconstructive efforts. The potential problems include shortening and bow stringing of the hamstring tendons, the neurovascular bundles, and anterior dislocation of the knee. There is also the need for large amount of soft tissue for coverage when the contracted structures are released. The goal is to obtain satisfactory extension and subsequent flexion without compromising the perfusion and sensibility of the distal limb (121). Ahmad and Ashraf (121) reported the use of Z-lengthening of contracted hamstring tendons and coverage with the medial gastrocnemius muscle flap. They resorted to the use of additional turn over adipofascial

flap to cover residual lateral defect in one of the very severe cases in their series of five patients with seven severe popliteal contractures. They emphasized the need for postoperative splinting in plaster cast, followed by regular physiotherapy and use of pressure garments in order to achieve complete extension with full range of motion. The presence of bony ankylosis is an indication for osteotomy to remove the bridging bone and restore joint motion. Supracondylar extension osteotomy of the femur has been reported for correction of severe contractures in patients with neurological deficits such as myelomeningocele and cerebral palsy. However, this has not been reported in the correction of postburn contracture deformity (121,122). The use of the Ilizarov external fixator may be extended to the correction of these problems.

Contractures of the Ankle Joint

The postburn contractures encountered at the ankle joint are either in dorsiflexion or in plantarflexion. The dorsiflexion contracture results from deep dorsal burns and usually occurs in concert with extension contractures of the toes due to involvement of the dorsum of the forefoot. A transverse incision across the axis of the ankle joint down to normal subcutaneous tissue may be all that is required to release the isolated dorsiflexion contracture. The defect is then resurfaced with thick split- or full-thickness skin grafts. Postoperative immobilization in slightly overcorrected position is encouraged. Early range of motion exercises as well as use of pressure garments are essential in the restoration of form and function. Correction of severe contractures requires the excision of dense contracted scar, which may result in extensive soft tissue defect and exposure of the extensor tendons. Adequate release may demand certain measures of tenolysis, tenotomies, capsulotomies, and even osteotomies (123). Joint stabilization with Kirschner's wires or insertion of Steinman pins for subsequent skeletal traction may also be required. Following such extensive release procedures, the defect may be resurfaced with thick split- or full-thickness skin grafts (Fig. 37.6). However, where these are inadequate, flap coverage will be required. Local fasciocutaneous flap, such as the lateral supramalleolar fasciocutaneous flap based on the perforating branches of the peroneal artery is a suitable option if available (46,47). However, microsurgical transfer of distant tissues offers the most attractive option in this region. The free radial forearm fasciocutaneous flap, the lateral arm fasciocutaneous flap, and the free temporoparietal fascial flap covered with split skin graft have been used extensively in this reconstruction where contour preservation is a major concern (51,124,125).

The less common plantar flexion contractures at the ankle joint are commonly due to Achilles tendon

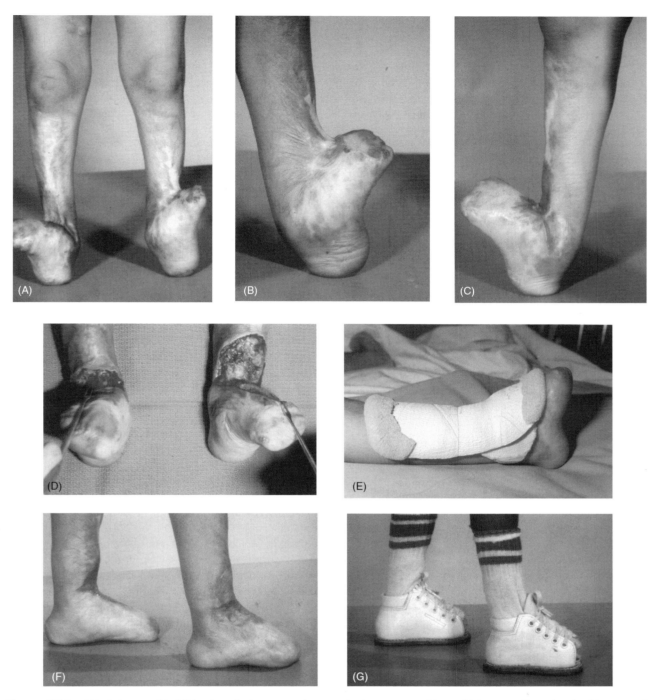

Figure 37.6 (A) A 2-year-old child referred after severe burn to the lower extremities, which were allowed to heal by secondary intention. (B) Close-up of the left foot. (C) Close-up of the right foot. (D) Bilateral release performed with resurfacing with thick split thickness skin grafts. (E) Both feet were splinted after graft take. (F) Three months later both feet in neutral position. (G) Patient shown in first pair of shoes.

shortening where acute care has failed to prevent this complication. The Achilles tendon shortening is a ubiquitous problem in the extensively burned patient with lower extremity involvement (6,93). Uncorrected, the

progressive shortening is capable of resulting in the equinus deformity in which the musculoskeletal structures of the fore foot are secondarily deformed. Surgical correction is directed at tendon lengthening and the more difficult problem of providing suitable coverage. Options for tendon lengthening include the Z-lengthening and skin-strip lengthening techniques. Ideal coverage should provide adequate soft tissue padding to allow healing and subsequent gliding of the tendon. Yet, it must be thin enough to preserve the normal contour of the area in order to permit use of normal footwear (1,6). Local flaps capable of meeting these requirements are difficult to come by. The lateral supramalleolar fasciocutaneous flap has been used for this purpose but again it may not be available in the severely burned lower extremity. Other local flaps that have been used include the inferiorly based de-epithelized turnover flap covered with split skin graft described by Ramakrishnan et al. (126). They reported a series of 35 patients in whom the use of this flap provided satisfactory long-term coverage of the Achilles tendon area (126). Currently, however, microsurgical techniques have allowed satisfactory coverage of these defects with high quality distant tissues. The free fasciocutaneous and fascial flaps are particularly favored to preserve the desired contour. Chicarilli et al. (54) reported the use of a free radial forearm flap in resurfacing the Achilles tendon area utilizing the posterior tibial vessels as recipient vessels. They observed that the flap provided a thin, well-vascularized cutaneous restoration with a satisfactory aesthetic result and low complication rate.

Contractures of the Forefoot

Deep burns of the dorsum of the forefoot frequently result in simple extension contractures of the toes. More severe and extensive dorsal burns, however, may produce the debilitating deformity in which the toes are hyperextended with subluxation or dislocation of the metatarsophalangeal joint. There may be associated loss of the transverse arch resulting in interdigital contractures with over-riding of the toes. This deformity may interfere with normal weight-bearing and ambulation leading to gait abnormalities. It may also inhibit the use of normal footwear (1–6,15). Pap (127) observed that burns of the feet could result in significant morbidity with protracted convalescence and extended absence from work and school. They, therefore, advocated that this injury should be given relatively high priority both in the acute phase and during the reconstructive phase of management. The reconstructive goal is to restore normal anatomy that will permit unimpeded weight-bearing and ambulation as well as allow the use of normal footwear (2,3).

While mild to moderate linear burn scar contractures of the dorsum of the foot may be corrected with Z-plasties and other local transposition flaps, majority of the cases exhibit extensive soft tissue deficiency requiring release and replacement with skin grafts or flaps. The deficiency of soft tissue in the long axis of the foot is frequently addressed by a transverse releasing incision over the

metatarsophalangeal joints extending from the first to the fifth and breaking into fishtails at both ends. Excision of the scar is rarely required as the incision relieves the tension in the scar thereby enhancing subsequent remodeling and flattening of the scar (15). Dissection must be carried down to normal subcutaneous tissue and adequate care taken to protect the extensor tendons and neurovascular structures. On rare occasions, release of severe contractures may require tenotomies of the long extensors and closed capsulotomies of the metatarsophalangeal joints (1). Intermedullary bone fixation with Kirschner's wires may be required to maintain joint position. Resurfacing with thick split- or full-thickness skin graft will usually suffice. Diligent postoperative splinting and use of pressure garments and custom-made shoes with silicone inserts contribute to the overall functional outcome. Despite these measures, however, the recurrence rate has remained high, particularly in the pediatric age group. Waymack et al. (86) reported a 15% recurrence rate within 4 years in a series of 55 children who had 90 reconstructive procedures for the treatment of early burn scar contractures of the feet. They observed that the recurrence rate was influenced by the diligence of postoperative splinting rather than the use of either full- or split-thickness skin grafts. Alison et al. (4), however, observed that the high recurrence rate following release of foot contractures might be related to the concomitant soft tissue deficiency in the transverse metatarsal arch that is often unaddressed (4). They therefore introduced additional incisional release on the dorsum of the foot along its long axis as well as multiple incisions parallel to the plane of the metatarsals into the web spaces as may be required to completely restore the transverse arch of the foot (Figs. 37.7 and 37.8). The latter incisions can in fact be extended to accommodate simultaneous correction of interdigital contractures. In a comparative analysis, Alison et al. (4) observed that the overall recurrence rate in their series of 68 children who had a total of 146 releases for foot contractures was 35.7% when only the longitudinal arch was released and the time interval before recurrence averaged 3.50 ± 0.41 years. However, with the additional release of the transverse arch, the time interval before recurrence averaged 4.29 ± 1.27 years initially and with improvement in execution of the technique, they subsequently recorded no recurrence. Alison et al. (4), however, noted that recurrence was influenced by the expansion ratio of the meshed split-thickness skin grafts used for coverage in the acute phase of management. They found that the time interval between injury and the need for the first surgical release when expansions of 1:2 were used doubled the interval recorded in the use of expansions of 1:4.

Dhanraj et al. (128) documented the efficacy of simultaneous bilateral surgical correction over staged sequential correction of burn scar extension contractures of the foot in patients with bilateral deformities. They observed that

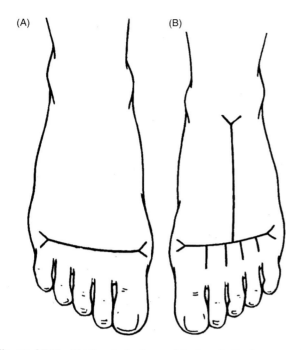

Figure 37.7 (A) Surgical release of the longitudinal metatarsal arch by a perpendicular incision over the metatarsal phalangeal joints. (B) Combined surgical release of both the longitudinal and transverse metatarsal arches. Additional incisions are parallel to the plane of the metatarsals. [Reprinted with permission from Alison et al. (4).]

there is no difference in morbidity between unilateral vs. simultaneous bilateral correction with Kirschner wire fixation.

However, the latter accords the opportunity to correct both contractures early and shortens the overall rehabilitation of the patient. They also noted that recurrence might be as a result of the differential growth of normal tissue vs. adjacent skin grafts in the growing child. They, therefore, recommended simultaneous bilateral correction as well as a close follow-up program in children presenting with bilateral dorsal foot contractures.

Webspace contractures of the toes may accompany both dorsal burns and plantar burns. The associated functional impairment is usually minimal as a result of which surgical correction is rarely undertaken. However, aesthetic concerns as well as repeated fungal infection may compel a patient to request surgical correction. The Z-plasty and its modifications as well as the V-M and the Y-V transposition flaps are favored because they obviate the need for skin grafts (1,6,15). Where these measures prove inadequate, however, routine surgical release, resurfacing with split skin grafts and immobilization with intramedullary pins may become absolutely necessary.

Flexion contractures of the toes frequently follow deep burns of the plantar surface of the foot. The contractures can be corrected by incisional release and resurfacing with split-thickness skin grafts. Postoperative immobilization is, however, difficult and may be accomplished by the

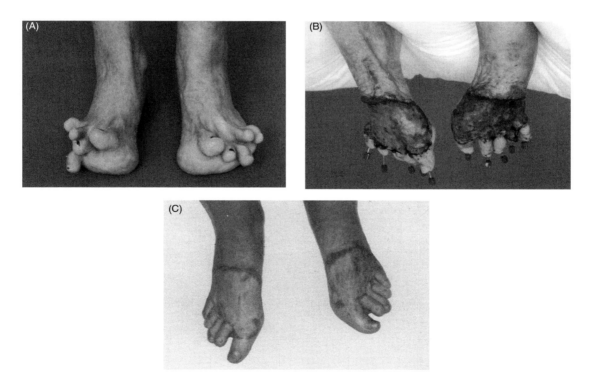

Figure 37.8 (A) A 13-year-old girl referred for reconstruction of her feet: note severe subluxative at the metatarsal joints and loss of the transverse and longitudinal arches of the feet. (B) Correction with split thickness skin grafts and k-wire fixature pins left in place for 6 weeks. (C) Three-month follow-up.

use of stent-type dressings and insertion of intermedullary Kirschner wires in severe cases. Maintenance of the release requires the wearing of shoes 24 h a day preferably with custom-made inserts to prevent recontracture (6). Witt and Achauer (6), however, observed that the correction of these contractures with a variety of local flaps fashioned from the lateral aspect of the toes tend to produce more rapid healing and a more lasting correction. Care must, however, be taken not to compromise weight-bearing surfaces while using such local flaps.

The reconstructive plan for the correction of the multiple deformities that may arise from severe burns of the foot must be based on accurate evaluation and due considerations of the available reconstructive options suited to the individual patient (Fig. 37.9). In severe deformities where orthopedic measures as well as physical therapy expertise are often required, early specialist consultation should help in the formulation of a reconstructive timetable from the outset. The role of an adequately informed physical therapy program in the overall rehabilitation of the patient cannot be overemphasized.

3. Amputations

Lower extremity amputations are occasionally required particularly following high-voltage electrical injuries and deep thermal burns (129). Acikel et al. (130) noted that burn injury constitutes a rare but consistent etiology in lower limb amputations. Although amputation rates ranging from 32% to 60% have been reported for high-voltage electric injuries (131,132), the largest study of major amputations following thermal injuries generally noted an occurrence rate of 1.5% (133). Factors contributing to amputations following burns include extensive involvement of soft tissues and associated open fractures, which are often accompanied by vascular injuries (129). Amputations may also be the consequence of failure to recognize an impending compartment syndrome thereby overlooking the need to perform timely escharotomy or fasciotomy on the lower extremity (2,3). Fortunately, invasive burn wound infection, which was once a leading contributor to lower extremity amputations, have been adequately contained in the last few decades. Amputations

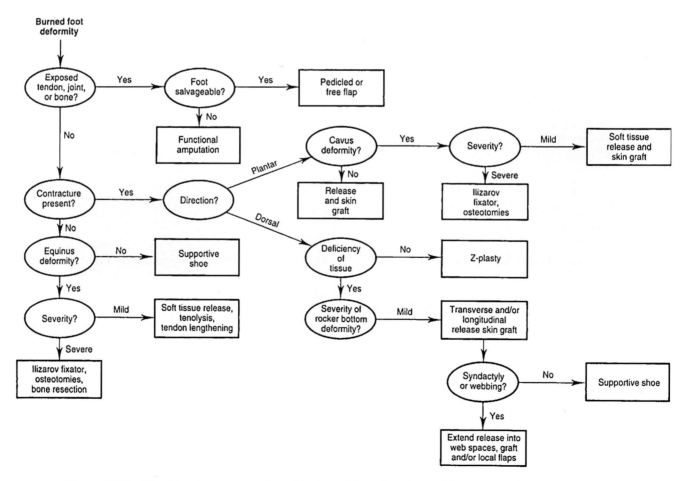

Figure 37.9   Algorithm for reconstruction of the burned foot. [Reprinted with permission from Lyle et al. (15).]

may be required early in the postburn course, occasionally as a life-saving procedure or it may become necessary late in the course of treatment when efforts at limb salvage have failed. Consultations with the orthopedic and vascular surgery teams, physical therapist, and the prosthetist have been found useful when one is faced with the unpleasant prospect of limb amputation. The primary goal of amputation surgery is to salvage as much of the limb length as possible thereby minimizing the functional losses. Efforts must be directed at preserving uninjured tissues, which can aid in achieving stable and durable skin cover at the amputation site so as to minimize the need for future revisions.

Following amputation, physical therapy management is directed at edema reduction, prevention of contractures through positioning and range of motion exercises, stump shaping, both pre- and post-prosthetic fit strengthening exercises of the limb and trunk and gait training (134).

Psychological concerns must be adequately addressed as the fear, anxiety, and guilt associated with burn injury is compounded by the deep sense of limb loss (134). Though the potentials for rehabilitation depend directly on the level of limb loss, patient motivation is equally of paramount importance. Acikel et al. (130) observed that at least 90% of patients with below-knee amputations successfully use prosthesis in contrast to a success rate of <25% for patients with above-knee amputations. They noted that the primary factor is the marked increase in energy required to ambulate with above-knee prosthesis. They concluded that knee function is so critical to prosthetic rehabilitation that every attempt should be made to salvage the knee joint (130). Unfortunately, the paucity of soft tissues at the level of the leg creates a major challenge to obtaining a below-knee amputation with satisfactory stump qualities in a majority of cases. The classic posterior myocutaneous flap has been the most widely used form of coverage for the below-knee amputation stump. However, other options have been used when this flap is unavailable either due to the nature or level of the injury. Yowler et al. (129) described the use of the osteocutaneous pedicle flap of the foot in providing satisfactory below-knee amputation stumps. Other options include the use of the laterally based skin flaps, the combination of anterior and posterior flaps, the posterior muscle flaps covered by laterally based skin flaps and the use of free flaps (135–140). Acikel et al. (130) described the use of gastrocnemius transposition flap covered with thick split-thickness skin graft to secure bilateral below-knee amputations in a patient who had suffered severe thermal injury. With modern prosthetic materials and techniques making it possible for less-than-optimal skin to tolerate the pressures of weight-bearing, more distal amputation levels may be secured with the use of skin grafts (130).

Generally speaking, with concerted team effort and adequate patient motivation, a majority of the thermally injured patients who suffer lower limb losses can be rehabilitated to a level of independence and a good number may be able to eventually return to their preinjury lifestyles (141) (Fig. 37.10).

4. Recent Advances

The last few decades have witnessed a number of technological advancements in the field of both acute and reconstructive burn surgery. Some of these have had direct and others indirect impact on the outlook for lower extremity burn reconstruction.

Vacuum Assisted Closure

The high incidence of late complications and deformities associated with severe lower extremity burns may in part be due to delayed wound healing and poor skin graft-take occasioned by dependency, complex and unfavorable contours, and shearing during ambulation. These problems have resulted in the frequent development of hypertrophic burn scars and scar contractures (1,6,142). The vacuum assisted closure (VAC) device is a modified dressing consisting of a sponge and suction tubing that is secured to the wound with an occlusive dressing. Use of the suction tubing creates a continuous negative-pressure dressing (110). Experimental studies have demonstrated increased oxygen tension, decreased bacterial counts, and increased granulation tissue formation occurring under the negative-pressure system (108,143,144). The technique has also been associated with earlier re-epithelialization and faster healing of burn wounds and has been used to manage complex wounds successfully (145–147). It has been clinically shown to enhance skin graft-take and healing (43,108,110). Blackburn et al. (108) further observed that when the VAC device is used to secure split-thickness skin grafts on rotated muscle flaps, it decreased edema, improved contour conformity, and shortened hospitalization (108). This must be a welcome development to the use of skin grafts on muscle flaps in the reconstruction of the weight-bearing plantar surface of the foot and in securing distal amputation levels. Scherer et al. reported a retrospective study comparing the use of VAC device (n = 34) vs. bolster dressings (n = 27) in securing split-thickness skin grafts in patients with traumatic and thermal tissue losses. They observed that the VAC group required significantly fewer repeated skin grafts (3%) compared to the bolster group (19%) and that no dressing-associated complications occurred in the VAC group. They concluded that though a prospective randomized study is required, the VAC device provides a safe and effective method for securing skin grafts and is associated with improved graft survival (110).

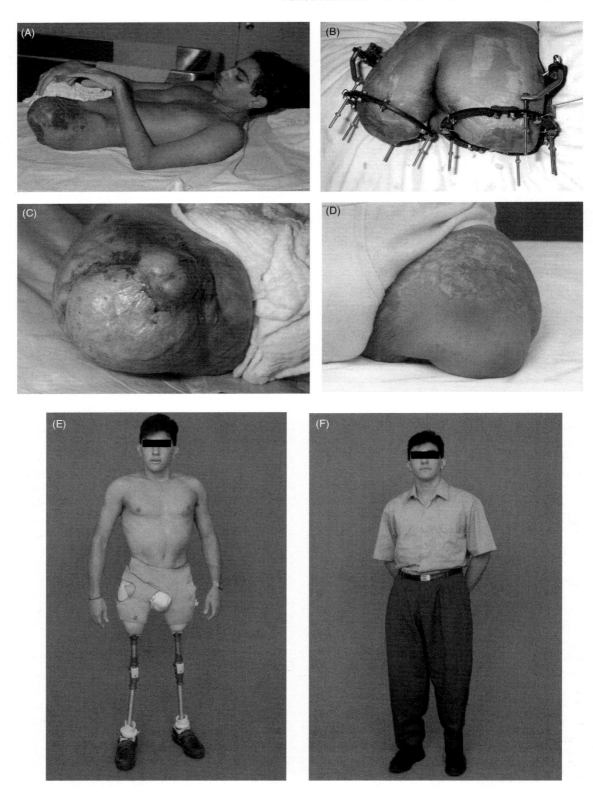

Figure 37.10 (A) A 16-year-old male referred after high bilateral above the knee amputations. Orthopedic surgery services felt that remaining femur was too short for a prosthesis. (B) Once wounds closed, external fixator placed for lower extremity distraction so that patient would be able to wear lower extremity proeteses. (C) Left stump showed erosion of bone through burn scar with distraction. (D) Coverage of left stump with a free latissimus dorsi myocutaneous flap. (E, F) Final result after fitting of prostheses.

The VAC technique is likely to have its greatest role of securing skin grafts in complex contour areas of the lower extremity such as the groin, the popliteal fossa, and around the ankle joints. As this technique becomes widely available, the long-term benefits should include a reduction in the number of burn wounds undergoing protracted healing and consequently a decrease in the incidence of such complications as burn scar hypertrophy and contractures. Furthermore, the technique is potentially useful in reconstructive procedures that require the use of skin grafts to resurface defects created by the release of contractures and the excision of hypertrophied scars, unstable scars, and Marjolin's ulcers. It is expected that the relatively high recurrence rate associated with release of groin and popliteal contractures when resurfaced with skin grafts will be addressed by the VAC technique. This technique, which is undergoing evaluations and modifications in various centers, may find even more use in the comprehensive management of the burned patient. Already, Sposato et al. (109) have introduced a fully portable, battery-operated unit described as the mini-VAC device, which allows for early ambulation, reduces nursing needs and therefore shortens length of hospital stay.

Skin Substitutes

Ever since the introduction of skin substitutes to provide acute coverage in patients suffering life-threatening large surface area burns, its clinical uses have continued to expand beyond this initial concept (148–152). Perhaps the most widely used skin substitutes in present day literature include the bilaminar acellular matrix, Integra® (Marion Laboratory, USA) and the acellular allogeneic dermal transplant, AlloDerm® (LifeCell Corp., The Woodlands, TX) (149,153–156). These materials provide resurfacing for acute burn wounds at an earlier stage than would otherwise have been possible. In fact, even low priority areas such as the lower extremities can now be resurfaced earlier and without necessarily using widely meshed skin grafts. The benefits of this innovation should therefore include a reduction in the incidence of the complications of burns that are in part due to protracted healing occasioned by inadequate and delayed closure of burn wounds (88–90). These complications include unstable scars and chronic ulcers, and burn scar hypertrophy and contractures. Hergrueter and O'Connor (149) observed that recent clinical reports have offered some evidence that skin substitutes may heal with less scarring than conventional skin grafts. This can therefore translate to less secondary contracture and stiffness, a most desirable goal for ambulation and weight-bearing. Early reports on the use of these skin substitutes have shown that they provide durable and stable coverage that is pliable and does not adhere to deeper structures making

them suitable for coverage of areas where mobility of underlying structures is highly desirable such as the dorsum of the hand and foot (148,154–156). Lattari et al. (154) observed that the use of AlloDerm with ultra-thin autogenous split-thickness skin grafts is associated with more rapid healing of the donor site, reduced need for postoperative physical therapy and reduced number and extent of subsequent surgeries for contracture releases and cosmetic repair.

Furthermore, the last decade has witnessed anecdotal reports on successes in the use of skin substitutes in burn reconstruction. Skin substitutes have been used to resurface large defects arising from the release of groin contractures, popliteal contractures, and foot contractures with satisfactory functional and aesthetic outcome (148,155).

Tissue Expansion

Tissue expansion offers many advantages over previous modalities of surgical treatment for burn scars. It allows one to generate sufficient soft tissue to reconstruct defects without unduly creating a new disfiguring donor area. It also obviates the need for transfer of distant tissues, which on occasions may be a major undertaking. Color, tone, texture, thickness, and composition of expanded adjacent skin are aesthetically better matched than grafted skin or tissue transferred from a distance, and it also maintains sensibility (95,157–160). Expansion has, therefore, permitted the elimination of unfavorable burn scars and replacement with adjacent expanded tissue with improved functional and aesthetic outcome (95,158–162). Hudson and Arasteh (157) observed that it is possibly the greatest advance in burn reconstruction in recent times. Gottlieb et al. (159) reported a large series in which tissue expansion techniques were used for the reconstruction of burns scars. They reported satisfactory results in 52%, minor problems in 29%, and significant complications necessitated abandonment of expansion procedures in 19%. They concluded that in the 81% that were successfully managed with expansion, the results were frequently far superior to those possible with available alternative techniques. They noted that the increased vascularity in the expanded tissue ensured safety during transfer and that expansion has decreased the need to resurface flap donor sites with skin grafts.

Unfortunately, however, the narrow circumference of the lower extremity has limited the suitability of tissue expansion in this region where only small-sized expanders can be used. Yet, the risk of extrusion and infection remains unacceptably high. Pitanguy et al. (160) reported a series in which 40 out of a total of 346 expanders used for the treatment of burn sequela in 132 patients were in the lower extremity. They obtained satisfactory outcome in a majority of the patients and reported an overall complication rate of 7.5%. Marks et al. (162) observed that complication rates approaching 35% have been reported in the use of tissue expanders below the level of the knee joint. Reporting a series of 45 patients, they remarked that if patients are selected based on the availability of relatively healthy expandable skin and the principles of expansion followed, complications can be kept to a minimum and successful reconstruction achieved even in the lower extremity.

The Ilizarov External Fixator

Severe and long-standing postburn contractures and deformities of the lower extremity tend to affect tendons, ligaments, joint capsules, and underlying bones. Hitherto, correction of these deformities had entailed major procedures such as tendon elongations, capsulotomies, osteotomies, and bone resections. Coverage of the resultant defect had also demanded the use of flaps, which must invariably be transferred from distant locations. Arthrodesis and amputations had served as last resorts or alternatives to these complex reconstructive procedures (15,163). In the last two decades, however, the Ilizarov external fixator has provided an additional option for the correction of such severe deformities. The morbidity is less and quite often the result is better. Calhoun et al. (163) were first to evaluate the Ilizarov external fixator for use in the correction of chronic burn scar contractures based on their experience with the use of pin fixation for acute burn management and the use of the Ilizarov fixator for correction of other foot deformities. Their result showed that severe lower extremity burn deformities could be successfully treated with the Ilizarov fixator (163). They enumerated the uses and provided details of the use of the fixator in the correction of the ubiquitous postburn equinus deformity obviating the need for Achilles tendon release, elongation, tenolysis or tenotomy. Noting that the fixator could be applied under general, regional or local anesthesia. The frame consists of two tibial–fibular rings, a calcaneal ring and a metatarsal ring secured to the bones with 1.5 mm pins. Correction is achieved by pushing the calcaneus distally while pushing the metatarsals proximally at a rate of 1–2 mm/day. Periodic radiographs were used to assess progress. They observed that correction could take up to 6 weeks after which the limb must be protected in cast for a further period of at least 6 weeks. They further noted that the fixator could be used to distract the calcaneus from the metatarsals in the correction of postburn cavus deformity of the foot without resorting to fascial excisions, mid-foot osteotomies, and the complex resurfacing procedures with flaps.

They also reported the use of the Ilizarov fixator in the correction of severe postburn rocker-bottom deformity to re-create the longitudinal and transverse arches of the foot without resorting to osteotomies and fusion as required by surgical correction. Other uses enumerated include the correction of complex postburn toe dislocations including hallux valgus and varus, which were previously treated with bone resection and amputations. The fixator was also used to lengthen scar tissue by gradual distraction thereby reducing the extent of soft tissue release required to maintain the corrected position. The use of the Ilizarov fixator in combination with other surgical procedures such as tenotomies and tendon elongations to minimize the complexity of surgery and improve outcome in complicated deformities was collaborated by Steinwender et al. (164). They emphasized the fact that such an approach obviates the need for precarious dissection of contracted soft tissue in which muscles, tendons, and neurovascular tissues are interlocked. Calhoun et al. (163) noted that complications with the use of the Ilizarov external fixator in the burned extremity are frequent but manageable. These include pain, infection, nerve and vessel injuries, and technical problems with the device. They, however, observed that adequate preoperative planning is required to minimize the incidence and severity of these complications. They emphasized the need for adequate evaluation and documentation in preparation for the use of the device. Appropriate radiographs are required to establish joint abnormalities such as dislocations, ankylosis, and heterotopic ossifications (163).

Currently, the Ilizarov external fixator is being adapted to correct a wide array of postburn deformities in other parts of the lower extremity and even the upper extremity (165–167). Ullmann et al. (165) in a case report documented the use of the Ilizarov fixator in correcting recurrent postburn fixed flexion contractures (Grade IV) of both knee joints in a noncompliant patient. They noted that the complex and lengthy manipulations required of the Ilizarov technique is justified in patients who cannot comply with the aggressive and demanding physiotherapy that may be required with surgical release. Furthermore, the fixator technique is a viable alternative in patients whose limited donor skin is required for reconstruction of higher priority areas. They further observed that the problems of excessive bulk and scars that accompany distant flap techniques are not seen with the use of the fixator. Latimer et al. (166) reported the use of the Ilizarov external fixator in lengthening below-knee amputation stumps in order to improve prosthetic fit. The Ilizarov external fixator has come to stay as far as the correction of lower extremity burn deformities are concerned. Improvement in the material and technique of the device points at the potential for even wider use in the near future.

REFERENCES

1.   Mani MM, Charte M. Reconstruction of the burned lower extremity. Clin Plast Surg 1992; 19(3):693–703.

2. Kucan JO, Bash D. Reconstruction of the burned foot. Clin Plast Surg 1992; 19(3):705–719.

3. Goldberg DP, Kucan JO, Bash D. Reconstruction of the burned foot. Clin Plast Surg 2000; 27(1):145–161.

4. Alison WE, Moore ML, Reilly DA et al. Reconstruction of foot burn contracture in children. J Burn Care Rehabil 1993; 14:34–38.

5. Zachary LS, Heggers JP, Robson MC et al. Burns of the feet. J Burn Care Rehabil 1987; 8(3):192–194.

6. Witt PD, Achauer BM. Lower extremity. In: Achauer BM, ed. Burn Reconstruction. New York: Thieme Medical Publishers, 1991.

7. Schmitt MA, French L, Kalil PT. How soon is safe? Ambulation of the patient with burns after lower extremity skin grafting. J Burn Care Rehabil 1991; 12:33–37.

8. Bodenham DC, Watson R. The early ambulation of patients with lower limb grafts. Br J Plast Surg 1971; 24:20–22.

9. Johnson CL. Ambulating patients after lower extremity grafting. J Burn Care Rehabil 1984; 5:114–115.

10. Burnsworth B, Krob MJ, Langer-Schnepp M. Immediate ambulation of patients with lower extremity grafts. J Burn Care Rehabil 1992; 13:89–92.

11. Golden PT, Power CG, Skinner JR et al. A technique of lower extremity mesh grafting with early ambulation. Am J Surg 1977; 133:646–647.

12. Sharpe D, Cardoso E, Baheti V. The immediate mobilization of patients with lower limb skin grafts: a clinical report. Br J Plast Surg 1983; 36:105–108.

13. Cox GW, Griswold JA. Outpatient skin grafting of extremity burn wounds with the use of Unna Boot® compression dressings. J Burn Care Rehabil 1993; 14:455–457.

14. Harnar T, Engrav LH, Marvin J et al. Dr Paul Unna's boot and early ambulation after skin grafting the leg: a survey of burn centers and a report of twenty cases. Plast Reconstr Surg 1982; 69:359–360.

15. Lyle WG, Phillips LG, Robson MC. Reconstruction of the foot. In: Herndon DN, ed. Total Burn Care. Philadelphia: W.B. Saunders, 1996, 515–519.

16. Heimburger RA, Marten E, Larson DL et al. Burned feet in children, acute and reconstructive care. Am J Surg 1973; 125:575–579.

17. Brown JB, Cannon B. The repair of surface defects of the foot. Ann Surg 1944; 120:417.

18. Avellan L. Reconstruction of defects in the weight bearing surfaces of the foot. Acta Orthop Scand 1965; 36:340–343.

19. London PS. The burned foot. Br J Surg 1953; 40:293–304.

20. Brown JB, McDowell F. Skin Grafting Of Burns. London: Lippincott, 1943.

21. Brou JA, Robson MC, McCauley RL et al. Inventory of potential reconstructive needs in the patient with burns. J Burn Care Rehabil 1989; 10:555–560.

22. Salisbury RE, Bevin AG. Atlas of reconstructive burn surgery. Philadelphia: W.B. Saunders, 1981:246–249.

23. Ponsten B. The fasciocutaneous flap; its use in soft tissue defects in the lower limb. Br J Plast Surg 1981; 34:215–220.

24. Tolhurst DE. Clinical experience and complications with fasciocutaneous flaps. Scand J Plast Reconstr Surg 1986; 20:75–78.

25. Tolhurst DE, Haeseker B, Zeeman RJ. The development of the fasciocutaneous flap and its clinical applications. Plast Reconstr Surg 1983; 71:597–606.

26. Barclay TL, Sharp DT, Chisholm EM. Cross-leg fasciocutaneous flaps. Plast Reconstr Surg 1983; 72:843–846.

27. Cormack G, Lamberty BG. A classification of fasciocutaneous flaps according to their pattern of vascularization. Br J Plast Surg 1984; 37:80–87.

28. Maruyama Y, Iwahira Y. Popliteo-posterior thigh fasciocutaneous island flap for closure around the knee. Br J Plast Surg 1989; 42:140–143.

29. Laitung JKG. The lower posterolateral thigh flap. Br J Plast Surg 1989; 42:133–139.

30. McCraw JB, Fishman JH, Sharzer LH. The versatile gastrocnemius myocutaneous flap. Plast Reconstr Surg 1978; 62:15–23.

31. McCraw JB, Dibbell DG, Carraway J. Experimental definition of independent myocutaneous vascular territories. Plast Reconstr Surg 1977; 60:341–352.

32. McCraw JB, Dibbell DG, Carraway J. Clinical definition of independent myocutaneous vascular territories. Plast Reconstr Surg 1977; 60:212–220.

33. Sood R, Ranieri J, Murthy V et al. The tibialis anterior muscle flap for full-thickness tibial burns. J Burn Care Rehabil 2003; 24(6):386–391.

34. Chang J, Most D, Hovey LM et al. Tibialis anterior turnover flap coverage of the exposed tibia in a severely burned patient. Burns 1997; 23(1):69–71.

35. Hirschowitz B, Moscona R, Kaufman T et al. External longitudinal splitting of the tibialis anterior muscle for coverage of compound fractures of the middle third of the tibia. Plast Reconstr Surg 1987; 79:407–414.

36. Moller-Larsen F, Petersen NC. Longitudinal split anterior tibial muscle flap with preserved function. Plast Reconstr Surg 1984; 74:398–401.

37. Lo LJ, Chen YR, Weng CJ, Noordhof MS. Use of split anterior tibial muscle flap in treating avulsion of leg associated with tibial exposure. Ann Plast Surg 1993; 31:112–116.

38. Moscona AR, Govrin-Yehudain J, Hirshowitz B. The island fasciocutaneous flap; a new type of flap for defects of the knee. Br J Plast Surg 1985; 38:512–514.

39. Acland RD, Schusterman M, Godina M et al. The saphenous neurovascular free flap. Plast Reconstr Surg 1981; 67:763–774.

40. Walton RL, Bunkis J. The posterior calf fasciocutaneous free flap. Plast Reconstr Surg 1984; 74:76–85.

41. Maruyama Y. Bilobed fasciocutaneous flap. Br J Plast Surg 1985; 38:515–517.

42. Heymans O, Verhelle N, Peters S et al. Use of the medial adipofascial flap of the leg for coverage of full-thickness burns exposing the tibial crest. Burns 2002; 28:674–678.

43. Feller I, Grabb WC. The leg: principles of treatment. In: Feller I, Grabb WC, eds. Reconstruction and Rehabilitation of the Burned Patient. Dexter, MI: Thomson-Shore Inc., 1979:349–361, Chapter XV.

44. Hammer H, Bugyi I, Zellner PR. Soft-tissue reconstruction of the anterior surface of the lower leg in burn patients using a free latissimus dorsi muscle flap. Scand J Plast Reconstr Surg 1986; 20:137–140.

45. Bunkis J, Walton RL, Mathes SJ. The rectus abdominis free flap for lower extremity reconstruction. Ann Plast Surg 1983; 11:373–380.

46. Masquelet MD, Beverage J, Romana C. The lateral supramalleolar flap. Plast Reconstr Surg 1988; 81:74–81.

47. Clark N, Sherman R. Soft-tissue reconstruction of the foot and ankle. Orthop Clin North Am 1993; 24:489–503.

48. Jeng S-F, Wei F-C. Distally based sural island flap for foot reconstruction. Plast Reconstr Surg 1997; 99:744–750.

49. Grabb WC, Argenta LC. The lateral calcaneal artery skin flap. Plast Reconstr Surg 1981; 68:723–730.

50. Rajacic N, Darweesh K, Jayakishnan K et al. The distally based superficial sural flap for reconstruction of the lower leg and foot. Br J Plast Surg 1996; 49:383–389.

51. Raine TJ, Nahai F. Free tissue transfers to the foot. Plast Surg Forum 1984; 7:112.

52. Hollock GG. The radial forearm flap in burn reconstruction. J Burn Care Rehabil 1986; 7:318–322.

53. Hallock GG. Simultaneous bilateral foot reconstruction using a single free radial forearm flap. Plast Reconstr Surg 1987; 80:836–838.

54. Chicarilli ZN, Ariyan S, Cuono CB. Free radial forearm flap versatility for the head and neck and lower extremity. J Reconstr Microsurg 1986; 2:221–228.

55. Goldberg JA, Adkins P, Tsai T-M. Microvascular reconstruction of the foot: weight bearing patterns, gait analysis and long-term follow-up. Plast Reconstr Surg 1993; 92:904–911.

56. Uhm K, Shin KS, Lew J. Crane principle of the cross-leg fasciocutaneous flap: aesthetically pleasing technique for damaged dorsum of foot. Ann plast Surg 1985; 15:257–261.

57. Taylor GA, Hoopson WLG. The cross-foot flap. Plast Reconstr Surg 1975; 55:677–681.

58. Harrison DH, Morgan BDG. The instep island flap to resurface plantar defects. Br J Plast Surg 1981; 34:315–318.

59. Ikuta Y, Murakami T, Yoshioka K et al. Reconstruction of the heel pad by flexor digitorum brevis musculocutaneous flap transfer. Plast Reconstr Surg 1984; 74:86–96.

60. Gibstein L, Abramson D, Sampson C et al. Musculofascial flaps based on the dorsalis pedis vascular pedicle for coverage of the foot and ankle. Ann Plast Surg 1996; 37:152–157.

61. Bostwick J. Reconstruction of the heel pad by muscle transposition and split skin graft. Surg Gynaecol Obstet 1976; 143:973–974.

62. Hartrampf CR, Scheflan M, Bostwick J. The flexor digitorum brevis muscle island pedicle flap: a new dimension in heel reconstruction. Plast Reconstr Surg 1980; 66:264–270.

63. Mathes S, Nahai F. Clinical Applications for Muscle And Musculocutaneous Flaps. St. Louis, MO: CV, Mosby, 1982.

64. Colen LB, Bunke HJ. Neurovascular island flaps from the plantar vessels and nerves for foot reconstruction. Ann Plast Surg 1984; 12(4):327–332.

65. Landi A, Soragni O, Monteleone M. The extensor digitorum brevis muscle island flap for soft tissue loss around the ankle. Plast Reconstr Surg 1985; 75:892–897.

66. Hong G, Steffenes K, Wang FB. Reconstruction of the lower leg and foot with the reverse pedicle posterior tibial fasciocutaneous flap. Br J Plast Surg 1989; 42:515–516.

67. McCraw JB, Furlow LT. The dorsalis pedis arterialized flap: a clinical study. Plast Reconstr Surg 1975; 55:177–185.

68. Shanahan RE, Gingrass RP. Medial plantar sensory flap for coverage of heel defects. Plast Reconstr Surg 1979; 64:295–298.

69. Morrison WA, Crabb DM, O'Brien BM et al. The instep of the foot as a fasciocutaneous flap and as a free flap for heel defects. Plast Reconstr Surg 1983; 72:56–63.

70. Stallings JO, Ban JL, Pandeya NK et al. Secondary burn reconstruction: recent advances with microvascular free flaps, regional flaps, and specialized grafts. Am Surg 1982; 48:505–513.

71. May JW, Halls MJ, Simon SR. Free microvascular muscle flaps with skin graft reconstruction of extensive defects of the feet: a clinical and gait analysis study. Plast Reconstr Surg 1985; 5:627–641.

72. May JW, Rohrich RJ. Foot reconstruction using free microvascular muscle flaps with skin grafts. Clin Plast Surg 1986; 13:681–689.

73. Maxwell GP, Manson PN, Hoopes JE. Experience with thirteen latissimus dorsi myocutaneous free flaps. Plast Reconstr Surg 1979; 64:1–8.

74. Gordon L, Buncke HJ, Albert BS. Free latissimus dorsi muscle flap with split thickness skin graft cover; a report of sixteen cases. Plast Reconstr Surg 1982; 70:173–178.

75. Bailey BN, Godfrey AM. Latissimus dorsi muscle free flaps. Br J Plast Surg 1982; 35:47–52.

76. Dabb RW, Davis RM. Latissimus dorsi free flap in the elderly: an alternative to below-knee amputation. Plast Reconstr Surg 1984; 73:633–640.

77. Taylor GI, Daniel RK. The free flap: composite tissue transfer by vascular anastomosis. Aust NZ J Surg 1973; 43(1):1–3.

78. Sanger JR, Matloub HS, Gosain AK et al. Scalp reconstruction with a prefabricated abdominal flap carried by the radial artery. Plast Reconstr Surg 1992; 89(2):315–319.

79. Brenman SA, Barber WB, Pederson WC et al. Pedicled free flaps: indications in complex reconstruction. Ann Plast Surg 1990; 24:420–426.

80. Mc O'Brien B, Barton RM, Pribaz JJ. The wrist as an immediate free flap carrier for reconstruction of the pelvis: a case report. Br J Plast Surg 1987; 40:427–431.

81. Lai C-S, Lin S-D, Chou C-K et al. Use of a cross-leg free muscle flap to reconstruct an extensive burn wound involving a lower extremity. Burns 1991; 17(6):510–513.

82. Yamada A, Harii K, Ueda K et al. Versatility of the cross-leg free rectus abdominis flap for leg reconstruction under difficult and unfavorable conditions. Plast Reconstr Surg 1995; 95(7):1253–1257.

83. Chen HC, Mosely LH, Tang YB et al. Difficult reconstruction of an extensive injury of the lower extremity with a large cross-leg microvascular composite-tissue flap containing fibula. Plast Reconstr Surg 1989; 83:723–727.

84. Tvrdek M, Pros Z, Nejedly A et al. Free cross leg flap as a method of reconstruction of soft-tissue defects. Acta Chir Plast 1975; 37(1):12–16.

85. Townsend PL. Indications and long-term assessment of 10 cases of cross-leg free DCIA flaps. Ann Plast Surg 1987; 19(3):225–233.

86. Waymack JP, Fidler J, Warden GD. Surgical correction of burn scar contractures of the foot in children. Burns 1988; 14:156–160.

87. Deitch EA, Wheelahan TM, Rose MP et al. Hypertrophic burn scars: analysis of variables. J Trauma 1983; 23:895–898.

88. Larson DL, Abston S, Willis B et al. Contracture and scar formation in the burn patient. Clin Plast Surg 1974; 1(4):653–666.

89. Parks DH, Baur PS, Larson DL. Late problems in burns. Clin Plast Surg 1977; 4(4):547–560.

90. Larson DL, Abston S, Evans EB et al. Techniques of decreasing scar formation and contractures in the burned patient. J Trauma 1971; 11:807–823.

91. Perkins K, Davey RB, Wallis KA. Silicon gel: a new treatment for burns scars and contractures. Burns 1982; 9(3):205–213.

92. Bennett GB, Helm P, Purdue GF et al. Serial casting: a method for treating burn contractures. J Burn Care Rehabil 1989; 10:543–545.

93. Johnson J, Silverberg R. Serial casting of the lower extremity to correct contractures during the acute phase of burn care. Phys Ther 1995; 75:262–266.

94. Achauer BM, Vanderkam VM. Burn reconstruction. In: Achauer BM, ed. Vol. 1. Plastic Surgery; Indications, Operations, and Outcomes. St Louis, MO: Mosby, 2000:425–446, Chapter 29.

95. Robson MC, Barnett RA, Leitch IO et al. Prevention and treatment of postburn scar contracture. World J Surg 1992; 16:87–96.

96. Hirshowitz B, Karev A, Mahler D. Proximal and distal releasing incisions for the treatment of flexion contracture of the popliteal region. Br J Plast Surg 1976; 29:35–37.

97. Dhanraj P, Asuku ME, Oh S, McCauley RL. Management of postburn recalcitrant knee ulcers in pediatric patients. J Burn Care Rehabil 2004; 25(1):129–133.

98. Aarons MS, Lynch JB, Lewis SR. Scar tissue carcinoma: a clinical study with reference to burn scar carcinoma. Ann Surg 1965; 161:170–188.

99. Novick M, Gard DA, Hardy SB, Spira M. Burn scar carcinoma: a review and analysis of 46 cases. J Trauma 1977; 17:809–817.

100. Ozek C, Cankayali R, Ufuk B et al. Marjolin's ulcers arising in burn scars. J Burn Care Rehabil 2001; 22(6):384–389.

101. Sarma D, Weilbaecher TG. Carcinoma arising from burn scar. J Surg Oncol 1985; 29:89–90.

102. Abbas JS, Beecham JE. Burn wound carcinoma: a case report and review of the literature. Burns 1988; 14(3):222–224.

103. Botswick J, Pendergrast WJ, Vasconez LO. Marjolin's ulcer: an immunologically privileged tumor? Plast Reconstr Surg 1975; 57:66–69.

104. Lifeso RM, Bull CA. Squamous cell carcinoma of the extremities. Cancer 1985; 55:2862–2867.

105. Peacock EE, Madden JW, Trier WC. Some studies on the treatment of burned hands. Ann Surg 1970; 171:903.

106. Turley CB, Cutting P, Clarke JA. Medial fasciocutaneous flap of the thigh for release of postburn groin contractures. Br J Plast Surg 1991; 44:36–40.

107. Roberts AHN, Dickson WA. Fasciocutaneous flaps for burn reconstruction: a report of 57 flaps. Br J Plast Surg 1988; 41:150–153.

108. Blackburn JH II, Boemi L, Hall WW et al. Negative pressure dressings as bolster for skin grafts. Ann Plast Surg 1998; 40(5):453–457.

109. Sposato G, Molea G, Di Caprio G et al. Ambulant vacuum-assisted closure of skin-graft dressing in the lower limbs using a portable mini-VAC device. Br J Plast Surg 2001; 54(3):235–237.

110. Scherer LA, Shiver S, Chang M et al. The vacuum assisted closure device: a method of securing skin grafts and improving graft survival. Arch Surg 2002; 137(8):930–934.

111. Webb LX. New techniques in wound management: vacuum-assisted wound closure. J Am Acad Orthop Surg 2002; 10(5):303–311.

112. Wang TN, Whetzel T, Mathes SJ et al. A fasciocutaneous flap for vaginal and perineal reconstruction. Plast Reconstr Surg 1987; 80:95–103.

113. Hayashi A, Maruyama Y. The use of the anteromedial thigh fasciocutaneous flap in the reconstruction of the lower abdomen and inguinal region; a report of two cases. Br J Plast Surg 1988; 41:633–638.

114. Song YG, Chen GZ, Song YL. The free thigh flap: a new free flap concept based on the septo cutaneous artery. Br J Plast Surg 1984; 37:149–159.

115. Bostwick J, Hill HL, Nahai F. Repairs in the lower abdomen, groin, or perineum with myocutaneous or omental flaps. Plast Reconstr Surg 1979; 63:186–194.

116. Gopinath KS, Chandrashekhar M, Kumar MV, Srikant KC. Tensor fasciae latae myocutaneous flaps to reconstruct skin defects after radical inguinal lymphadenectomy. Br J Plast Surg 1988; 41:366–368.

117. Prakash V. A new concept for the management of postburn contractures. Plast Reconstr Surg 2000; 106(1):233–234.

118. Prakash V, Bajaj SP. Flap stretching for management of postburn knee contracture with unstable scar. Plast Reconstr Surg 2001; 108(2):587–588.

119. Prakash V, Mishra A. Use of posterior calf fascial flap: a new concept for the management of knee contracture with unstable scar. Plast Reconstr Surg 2003; 111(1):505.

120. Robert L, Walton W, Matory E et al. The posterior calf fascial free flap. Plast Reconstr Surg 1985; 76:914–924.

121. Ahmad CN, Ashraf DM. Z-lengthening and gastro-cnemius muscle flap in the management of severe postburn flexion contractures of the knee. 1998; 45(1):127–132.

122. Abraham E, Verinder DGR, Sharrard WJW. The treatment of flexion contracture of the knee in myelomeningocele. J Bone Joint Surg Br 1977; 59:433–438.

123. Aydan A. An unusual contracture of the foot caused by a neglected burn wound salvaged by a cross-leg flap. Plast Reconstr Surg 2002; 110(5):1373.

124. Rose EH, Norris MS. The versatile temporoparietal fascial flap: adaptability to a variety of composite defects. Plast Reconstr Surg 1990; 85(2):224–232.

125. Fernandez-Palacios J, DeArmas DF, Deniz HV et al. Radial free flaps in plantar burns. Burns 1996; 22:242–245.

126. Ramakrishnan KM, Ch M, Jayaramoan V et al. Deep-ithelialized turnover flaps in burns. Plast Reconstr Surg 1988; 82:262–266.

127. Pap AS. Hot metal burns of the feet in foundry workers. J Occup Med 1966; 8:537.

128. Dhanraj P, Faro O, Phillips LG, McCauley RL. Burn scar contractures of the feet: efficacy of bilateral simultaneous surgical correction. Burns 2002; 28(8):814–819.

129. Yowler CJ, Patterson BM, Brandt CP et al. Osteocutaneous pedicle flap of the foot for the salvage of below-knee amputation level after burn injury. J Burn Care Rehabil 2001; 22:21–25.

130. Acikel C, Peker F, Akmaz I et al. Muscle transposition and skin grafting for salvage of below-knee amputation level after bilateral lower extremity thermal injury. Burns 2001; 27:849–852.

131. DiVincenti FC, Moncrief JA, Pruitt BA Jr. Electrical injuries; a review of 65 cases. J Trauma 1967; 9:497–507.

132. Haberal M. Electrical burns; a five-year experience. J Trauma 1986; 26:103–109.

133. Yowler CJ, Mozingo DW, Ryan JB et al. Factors contributing to delayed extremity amputation in burn patients. J Trauma 1998; 45:522–526.

134. Ward RS, Hayes-Lundy C, Schnebly WA et al. Rehabilitation of burn patients with concomitant limb amputation: case reports. Burns 1990; 16(5):390–392.

135. Patterson BM, Smith AA, Holdren AM et al. Osteocutaneous pedicle flap of the foot for salvage of below-knee amputation level after lower extremity injury. J Trauma 2000; 48:767–772.

136. Ruckley CV, Stonebridge PA, Prescott RJ. Skewflap versus long posterior flap in below-knee amputations; multicenter trial. J Vasc Surg 1991; 13:423–427.

137. Kaufman JL. Alternative methods for below-knee amputation; reappraisal of the Kendrick procedure. J Am Coll Surg 1995; 181:511–516.

138. Catre MG, Lieberman IH. Laterally based skin flap for below-knee amputation; case report. J Trauma 1997; 43:869–871.

139. Gallico GG, Ehrlichman RJ, Jupiter J et al. Free flaps to preserve below-knee amputation stumps: long-term evaluation. Plast Reconstr Surg 1987; 79:871–877.

140. Kasabian AK, Colen SR, Shaw WW et al. The role of microvascular free flap in salvaging below-knee amputation stumps: a review of 22 cases. J Trauma 1991; 31:495–501.

141. Prasad JK, Bowden ML, McDonald K et al. Rehabilitation of burned patients with above knee amputations. Burns 1990; 16(4):297–301.

142. Heimbach DM, Engrav LH. The lower extremities. In: Surgical Management of the Burned Wound. New York: Raven Press, 1984.

143. Morykwas MJ, Argenta LC, Shelton-Brown El et al. Vacuum-assisted closure: a new method for wound control and treatment: animal studies and basic foundation. Ann Plast Surg 1997; 38:553–562.

144. Argenta LC, Morykwas MJ. Vacuum-assisted closure: a new method for wound control and treatment: clinical experience. Ann Plast Surg 1997; 38:563–576.

145. Genecov DG, Schneider AM, Morykwas MJ et al. A controlled subatmospheric pressure dressing increases the rate of skin graft donor site reepithelialization. Ann Plast Surg 1998; 40:219–225.

146. Deva AK, Buckland GH, Fisher E et al. Topical negative pressure in wound management. Med J Aust 2000; 173:128–131.

147. Elwood ET, Bolitho DG. Negative-pressure dressings in the treatment of hidradenitis suppurativa. Ann Plast Surg 2001; 46:49–51.

148. Trong-Duo C, Shao-Ling C, Tz-Wen L et al. Reconstruction of the upper extremities with artificial skin. Plast Reconstr Surg 2001; 108(2):378–384.

149. Hergrueter CA, O'Connor NE. Skin substitutes in upper extremity burns. Hand Clinics 1990; 6(2):239–242.

150. Cairns BA, deSerres S, Peterson HD et al. Skin replacements: The biotechnological quest for optimal wound closure. Arch Surg 1993; 128:1246–1252.

151. Burke JF, Yannas IV, Quinby WC et al. Successful use of physiologically acceptable artificial skin in the treatment of extensive burn injury. Ann Surg 1981; 194:413–428.

152. Pruitt BA Jr, Levine NS. Characteristics and uses of biologic dressings and skin substitutes. Arch Surg 1984; 119:312–322.

153. Heimbach D, Luterman A, Burke J et al. Artificial dermis for major burns: a multi-center randomized clinical trial. Ann Surg 1988; 208:313–320.

154. Lattari V, Jones LM, Varcelotti JR et al. The use of a permanent dermal allograft in full thickness burns of the hand and foot: a report of three cases. J Burn Care Rehabil 1997; 18(2):147–155.

155. Dantzer E, Braye FM. Reconstructive surgery using an artificial dermis (Integra®): results with 39 grafts. Br J Plast Surg 2001; 54:659–664.

156. Fitton AR, Drew P, Dickson WA. The use of bi-laminate artificial skin substitute (Integra®) in acute resurfacing of burns: an early experience. Br J Plast Surg 2001; 54:208–212.

157. Hudson DA, Arasteh E. Serial tissue expansion for reconstruction of burns of the head and neck. Burns 2001; 27(5):481–487.

158. Argenta LC, Marks MW. Tissue expansion. In: Georgiade GS, Georgiade NG, Reifkohl R, Barwick WJ, eds. Textbook of Plastic, Reconstructive and Maxillofacial Surgery. 2nd ed. Baltimore, MD: Williams and Wilkins, 1992:103–113.

159. Gottlieb LJ, Parsons RW, Krizek TJ. The use of tissue expansion techniques in burn reconstruction. J Burn Care Rehabil 1986; 7:234–237.

160. Pitanguy I, Gontijo de Amorin NF, Radwanski HN et al. Repeated expansion in burn sequela. Burns 2002; 28(5):494–499.

161. Teiji T, Ira M, Katsuyuki A et al. Molecular basis for tissue expansion: clinical implications for the surgeon. Plast Reconstr Surg 1998; 102(1):247–258.
162. Marks MW, Argenta LC, Thornton JW. Burn management: the role of tissue expansion. Clin Plast Surg 1987; 14(3):543–548.
163. Calhoun JH, Evans EB, Herndon DN. Techniques for the management of burns contractures with the Ilizarov fixator. Clin Orthop Relat Res 1992; 280:117–124.
164. Steinwender G, Saraph V, Zwick EB et al. Complex foot deformities associated with soft tissue scarring in children. J Foot Ankle Surg 2001; 40(1):42–49.
165. Ullmann Y, Lerner A, Ramon Y et al. A new approach to deal with post burn knee contracture. Burns 2003; 29(3):284–286.
166. Latimer DH, Dahners LE, Bynum DK. Lengthening of below-knee amputation stumps using the Ilizarov technique. J Orthop Trauma 1990; 4:411–414.
167. Madhuri V, Dhanraj P. Correction of post burns contracture of the wrist with Ilizarov method. Burns 1998; 24:576–578.

38

Reconstruction of Burn Scar Contractures of Feet

PREMA DHANRAJ
Christian Medical College & Hospital, Vellore, Tamil Nadu, India

MALACHY E. ASUKU
Ahmadu Bello University Teaching Hospital, Kaduna, Nigeria

ROBERT L. McCAULEY
University of Texas Medical Branch and Shriners Hospital for Children—Galveston Unit, Galveston, Texas, USA

I. INTRODUCTION

The survival of patients with major thermal injuries has drastically increased in recent years (1). As our ability to save patients lives increases, the concept of total rehabilitation becomes of paramount importance. Burns to the ankle and foot represent some of the most challenging problem in acute wound care, subsequent rehabilitation and reconstruction. Children who sustain large total body surface area (TBSA) burns with involvement of the lower extremity frequently sustain injuries of the dorsum of the feet. Burns of the feet are a very small proportion of the TBSA. Although, it has not been given importance by many surgeons, in patients with large TBSA burns, it continues to cause a major source of morbidity leading to gait disturbances, growth abnormalities, improper shoe fit, and recurrent ulcerations (2). Furthermore, the formation of hypertrophic scars and burn scar contractures can devastate rehabilitation efforts (3). Thus, these injuries are categorized by the American Burn Association as major burns and require careful in-hospital treatment to avoid complications (4).

Currently, great emphasis is given to proper positioning and splinting to maintain mobility during the acute and reconstructive phases of care. In spite of this, scarring and contractures may persist. In part, this is due to the lower priority given to the foot burns when it is associated with larger burns. Also, the inherent contractile nature of scar formation and, in children, growth may accentuate the development of deformities (5). These factors combine to increase contractures leading to both functional and aesthetic problems.

The lower extremity is important for static support of the trunk and ambulation. Burn scar contractures not only affect gait, but in very severe cases, may even preclude standing. The human gait pattern is extensively discussed by various authors (6,7). Goldberg et al. (7) studied the gait patterns in human and classified gait as normal, minor gain abnormality and major gain abnormality. Minor gait abnormality was defined as any insignificant acquired alteration in either stance or swing phase of either the injured or uninjured leg. A major gain abnormality was defined as an alteration that grossly affects the gait pattern of either leg. Prevention of contractures is of utmost importance to prevent permanent skeletal and functional deformity. The reconstructive goals for this region are ambulation and weight bearing. This requires durable stable skin coverage, protective sensation, and anatomic alignment. Clearly, the challenge in any reconstructive procedure to the feet is to provide an outcome where ambulation and weight bearing is painless and as normal as possible.

Although burns of the foot may have received less attention, the importance of the foot cannot be overlooked and the defects that may occur following thermal injury may produce serious functional impairment. The types of thermal injuries affecting the foot are flame, scalds, contact, chemical, and electrical. Even, frostbite also produces severe foot injuries (8). Foot burns may present a solitary injury or part of an extended injury. Treatment, both early and long term, depend on the location of the burn, the extent of the injury as well as associated life-threatening problems. In many cases, limitations of available local tissue may restrict the options available for both acute coverage and reconstruction.

Burn scar contractures of the foot can cause significant morbidity, especially in children. Severe contractures may be very common in developing countries due to poor resources and decreased compliance (9). In addition, there is increased morbidity that results from the multiple operations to reconstruct the foot. The natural tendency of scars to contract combined with the normal growth of a child may accelerate the deformity (10). Also, foot burns can lead to the most troublesome joint contractures when positioning is less than optimal posture.

The standard for reconstruction for burn scar contractures of the feet is restoring the anatomy to normal, then obtaining soft tissue coverage. The timing of

reconstruction has been questioned. Waymack et al. (10) supported early release of contractures to prevent growth abnormalities. Robson et al. (11) suggested possible postponement of reconstruction until scar tissue matures. Yet regardless of these issues, most agree that if the deformity is progressive or causing a significant functional deficit, reconstruction should be initiated. Achieving optimal results for reconstruction depends in many ways on the successful management during the acute phase of injury. Proper splinting, elevation, avoidance of edema, along with physiotherapy and early surgical intervention helps to reduce the need for late reconstructive procedures. In children, release of these contractures and resurfacing the dorsum of the foot with think split-thickness skin grafts appears to be adequate. However, these contractures have been reported to recur in 15–20% of the patients. Since the mean time to recurrence is more that 2 years, these recurrences are probably related to growth as opposed to failure of the skin grafts (12). Waymack et al. (10) noted that recurrent of contractures requiring further surgery is probably due to the growth spurt seen in young children. These tend to worsen with time. Scar tissues cannot grow at the same rate as that of normal skin. Clearly, the prevention of contraction is of utmost importance. However, once contractures occur, it should be reconstructed as early as possible to prevent skeletal and functional deformities.

II. ANATOMY OF THE FOOT

Anatomy of the foot is defined as that area extending distal to the superior aspect of lateral and medial malleoli. The various subunits are dorsal surface, plantar surface, and the ankle. The skin over the dorsum of the foot in thin and supple to permit gliding movement of the underlying tendons. The skin over the sole of the foot is firmly fixed to the deeper structures. The plantar fascia along with the tarsal bones is very important to stabilize the arch of the foot. Destruction of this fascia will disrupt the arch support (13).

The relationship between the anatomy and function is unique in the foot. The weight bearing properties of the foot, as well as the particular characteristics of the soft tissue without intervening muscle between the skeletal element in the skin, can make coverage of foot injuries a very difficult and complex problem. Minor alteration in the normal anatomy can lead to significant dysfunction. The thinness of the skin, the superficial location of the tendons, the high ratio of tendinous bony and ligamentous structures to fatty and muscle tissue make reconstruction more difficult. The foot permits both rigid and flexible ranges of motion that enables us to work. This motion is highly complex and occurs in several planes. The human foot supports the body when standing and provides a smooth functional interface between body and ground during gait. This depends on a complex interaction of small bones, pain free motion of small joints and an intact sensate soft tissue envelope (14–16).

III. CLASSIFICATION OF BURN SCAR CONTRACTURES

A. Dorsal Burn Scar Contractures

Blood supply of the dorsum of the foot is mainly by the dorsalis pedis artery. The nerve supply is from the superficial peroneal nerve, which supplies the dorsum of the foot, and the deep peroneal nerve, which supplies the first web space. The sural nerve supplies the lateral aspect of the foot (Fig. 38.1). The skin of the dorsum of the foot is thin and loosely connected to the underlying fascia. The tendons in this region are located superficially. Burns of the dorsum of the foot can result in distortion of the skin. The skin is very thin and offers less resistance to contraction compared to the think skin of the sole. Dorsal contractures result in tissue shortening, often with enough force to cause hyperextension of toes and subluxation or dislocation of the metatarsophalangeal joint. The metatarsal heads become prominent on the plantar surface (Fig. 38.2). The long flexors of the toes result in flexion at the interphalangeal joints. The accompanying shortening in the transverse axis often results in narrowing of the forefoot with overriding of the toes. This type of deformity occurs either due to the burn wound, which healed spontaneously or from the previous grafted areas.

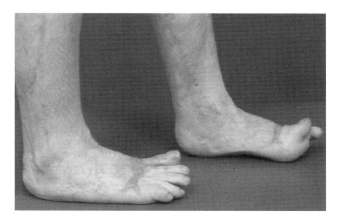

Figure 38.2 Burn scar contractures of the feet with significant dorsal subluxation of the toes on the left.

Inversion contractures of the foot result from contracting bands that extend from the leg to the foot on the medial side pulling the foot into inversion. Eversion contractures of the foot occurs when the contracting band from the leg to the foot is on the lateral side pulling the foot into eversion leading to callous formation and painful gait. This results in an acquired talus deformity where the scar contractures pull skin into dorsiflexion with eversion of the foot and shortening of the calf muscles (Fig. 38.3).

Webbing between the toes is a result of contractures. These dorsal web contractures can occur in burns of the forefoot resulting in overriding the deviation of toes. This is managed with release and skin grafting or Y-V advancement flaps, Z-plasty or V-Y flaps. Skin grafts and local flaps have proven to be satisfactory for reconstructing almost all burn scars of the foot in children. Heimburger et al. (17)

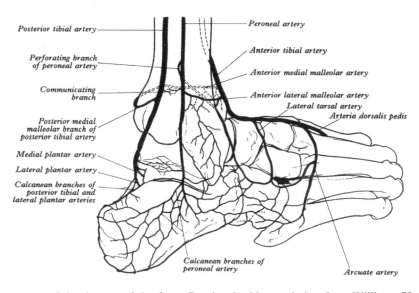

Figure 38.1 Arterial anatomy of the dorsum of the foot. (Reprinted with permission from Williams PL, Warwick R, Dyson M, Bannister L, eds. Gray's Anatomy. 37th ed. New York: Churchill Livingstone, 1989.)

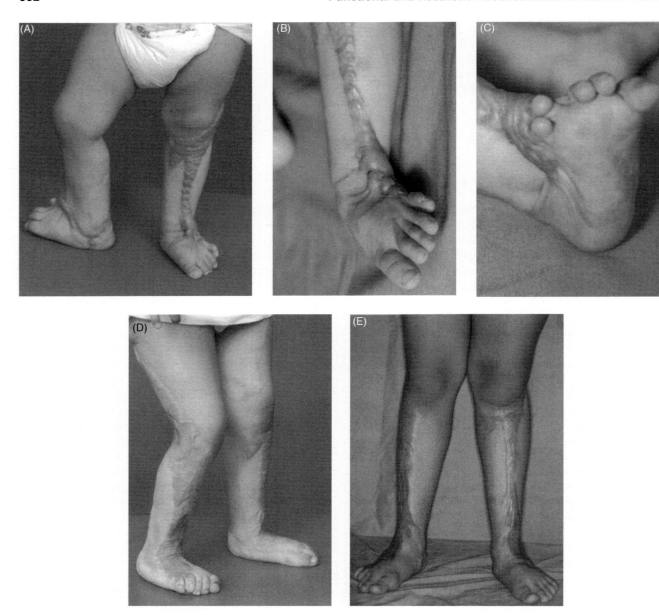

Figure 38.3   (A) A 10-month-old infant with burns to the dorsal surfaces of both feet with eversion of both feet secondary to scar contractures. (B) Close-up of left foot showing contracture and foot eversion. (C) Close-up of right foot showing eversion and fusion of outer
aspect of the dorsum of the foot to the lower leg. (D) Two-year follow-up after release of contractures and resurfacing with thick split-
thickness skin grafts. (E) Four-year follow-up after initial procedures. One and a half years after second release of both feet during growth
period.

have found that skeletal traction through the distal phalanx
of each digit may facilitate better graft take.

B.   Plantar Surface Burn Scar Contractures

Blood supply of the plantar surface is by both the medial
and lateral plantar arteries. The lateral plantar artery is
larger than the medial plantar artery (Fig. 38.4). The
plantar arch is formed by the deep plantar branch of the

dorsalis pedis artery and the distal plantar artery. The
nerve supply of the plantar surface is by the plantar
nerves, which consists of medial calcaneal nerve, which
supplies the heel area, medial plantar, and lateral plantar
nerves. The skin on the plantar surface is very thick and
firmly held on to the underlying fascia by the fibrous
septa. The plantar fascia consists of strong fibrous layers
that are oriented in longitudinal, vertical, and transverse
direction. It extends from the calcaneal region to attach

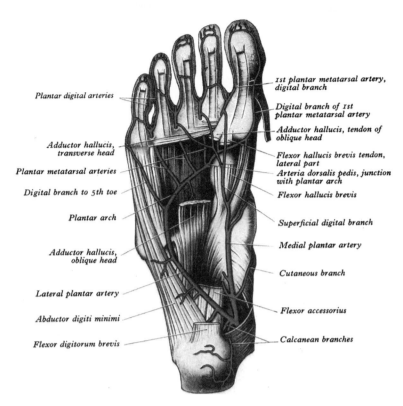

Plantar digital arteries

Adductor hallucis, transverse head

Plantar metatarsal arteries

Digital branch to 5th toe

Plantar arch

Adductor hallucis, oblique head

Lateral plantar artery

Abductor digiti minimi

Flexor digitorum brevis

1st plantar metatarsal artery, digital branch

Digital branch of 1st plantar metatarsal artery

Adductor hallucis, tendon of oblique head

Flexor hallucis brevis tendon, lateral part

Arteria dorsalis pedis, junction with plantar arch

Flexor hallucis brevis

Superficial digital branch

Medial plantar artery

Cutaneous branch

Flexor accessorius

Calcanean branches

Figure 38.4 Blood supply to the plantar surface of the foot. (Reprinted with permission from Williams PL, Warwick R, Dyson M, Bannister L, eds. Gray's Anatomy. 37th ed. New York: Churchill Livingstone, 1989.)

to the plantar aspect of the proximal phalanges. The weight-bearing plantar surface is a challenging area to achieve soft tissue coverage. Preservation of its sensation is important for maintaining a stable weight-bearing surface. The most common type of burns affecting the sole is electrical exit burn. Although, contact burns, which occur, can produce significant injury, the other types of burns are infrequent. This may be due to limited exposure, the thick layer of the skin and/or protective effect of the ground and the footwear (Fig. 38.5). Burns to the plantar surface of the foot rarely lead to full thickness injury. However, if full thickness injuries involve the plantar fascia, the arch support is disrupted and we now have a reconstructive challenge.

An important feature of the foot is the longitudinal and transverse arch. Destruction of these arches occurs in severe burn scar contractures that can cause a decrease in the width and length of the foot. Definitive closure of full-thickness plantar wounds as early as possible is essential to achieve full rehabilitation.

C. Joint Deformity

Equina varus deformities occur when scar tissue following burns results in flexion contractures at the tibiotarsal joint with heel cord shortening. Later standing scar results in capsular contractures and eventually joint deformities causing subluxations and dislocations (17). The joint assumes abnormal positions due to burn scars. The changes in bone morphology includes ankle in equines position with inversion in the hindfoot and equines varus of the forefoot. Treatment of heel cord shortening is by tenolysis of Achillis tendon, tendon lengthening, or tenotomy. The established equinus deformity of the ankle is corrected by calcaneal traction or Ilizarov apparatus. Equino varus deformity can be prevented if ankles are maintained in neutral position by using either static splints or skeletal traction (18). Ulceration of the skin and pressure necrosis are common complications following the use of splints. Consequently, not only is positioning important but also padding. Larson et al. (6) have found skeletal traction uniquely useful in the surgical treatment of burn scars in extremities because of the force of the contracting scar and the fragility of the surrounding skin. The other methods of correcting this deformity have been described in detail by various authors using the Ilizarov (19). To facilitate the use of this apparatus, the joint capsule is released primarily and the soft tissue contracture is gradually released by using distraction devices. This also permits elongation of the skin, the blood vessels, and the nerves.

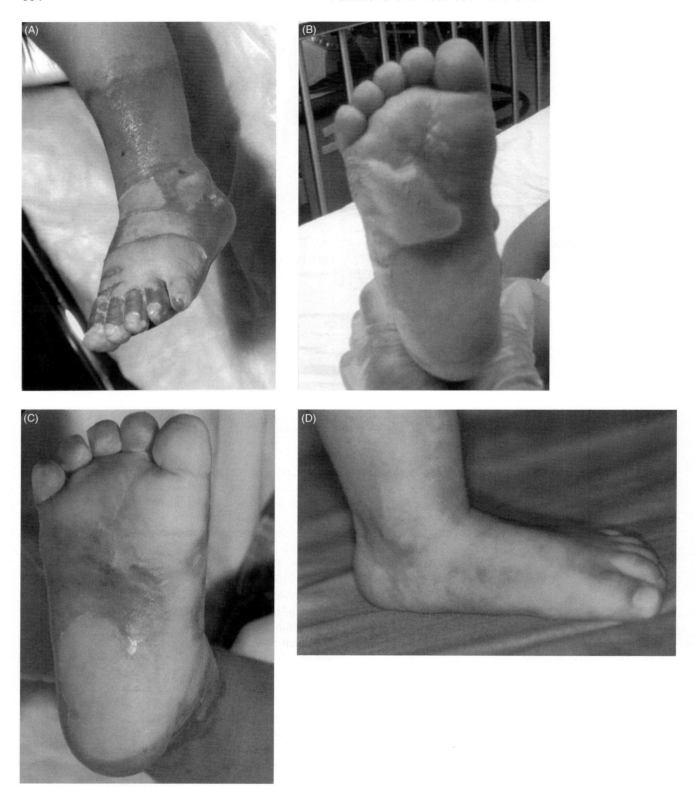

Figure 38.5 (A) Two-year-old child with dorsal scald burns. (B) Blistering also noted on planter surface. (C) Five days later, plantar burn shows only superficial partial thickness injury. (D) Full weight-bearing without surgery within 2 months.

Rocker bottom foot is seen in patients with burns involving the dorsal and plantar surfaces resulting in talus aligning with calcaneum as midfoot and forefoot are pulled into dorsiflexion resulting in rocker bottom foot. This is characterized by extensor tendon shortening, dislocation and subluxation of phalanges and complete reversal of the plantar arch. Early release and skin grafting, transosseous pinning, and long-term pressure support can minimize the deformity (20).

Acquired vertical talus deformity is due to the pull of scar contractures with dorsiflexion and eversion of the foot to the shortening of the calf muscles. Early correction of the contractures either by multiple Z-plasties, skin grafts or flaps, and lengthening of tendo calcaneus may avoid such complications, Jackson et al. (5) pointed out that there was an interactable tendency for the foot to be drawn into eversion, inversion, and valgus positions by the burn scar contractures. It was also found out that the position of the scar contracture in most cases suggests that the scarring is responsible for the deformity. Silk and Wainwright (21) believed the condition to be due to disparity of growth between the muscles and bones of the leg and that if there was no undue soft tissue tension they would grow normally. The problem, therefore, seemed to be one of shortness of the musculotendinous unit due to scar contracture. Patterson et al. (22) also considered that it was the tight soft tissue that produced the bone and joint abnormalities.

IV. TREATMENT

A. Nonsurgical

When the contracture is minimal, either simple skin traction or Steinmann pins have been used for correction. Although, this form of treatment alone, is not applicable to most of the constractures seen in the burn patients. However, skeletal traction in combination with surgical releases has been useful. Serial wedging can be used in conditions where the soft tissue release is limited by either the tendons or muscles. This method allows the tissues to gradually stretch the soft tissues before surgical procedures are attempted (12).

B. Surgical

Split-thickness skin grafts continue to be the primary method of coverage in reconstruction of the dorsal foot burns when the underlying tendons are not exposed. In conditions where the tendons are exposed, if it is a small area, then debridement is sufficient to allow for the development of granulation tissue. Then the use of split-thickness grafts will allow closure. One must bear in mind the fact that skin grafts will not take on bare bone,

cartilage or tendon. Dorsal burns can result in extensive tissue deficiency and require release and resurfacing with skin grafts, both in the longitudinal and transverse plane. Alison et al. (23) noted that when only the longitudinal arch was released the overall recurrence rate was found to be much higher than when release of both longitudinal and transverse arches were performed. The release of both arches also resulted in more natural appearing feet. A transverse incision across the dorsum of the foot is performed proximal to the fifth metatarsal joint. This maneuver releases longitudinal arch. The transverse arch is released by making parallel releases to the plane of the metatarsals, usually in line with the web spaces. If syndactyly is present, then the incisions are carried into the web spaces. K-wire fixations may be necessary to assure correct positioning of the metatarsophalangeal joints. Postoperatively, elevation, and splints are continued until graft take is insured. Ambulation is started with non-weight-bearing, initially, and gradually progressed to full weight bearing. Silicone conformers and pressure garments are fitted and worn continuously until the skin grafts mature (Fig. 38.6).

Severe contractures of the dorsum may require joint capsule releases and/or Kirchner wire in order to maintain position. These pins are placed through the distal phalanx of each toe at the time of contracture release and grafting and left in place for 4–6 weeks. More severe contractures affecting the bone and tendons can be corrected by the Ilizarov external fixator, serial splinting, or casting.

Waymack et al. (10) have suggested early release of contractures to prevent growth abnormalities. Postoperative immobilization has proven to be responsible for superior results. Recurrence rate of contraction has been shown to be 11% in patients with immobilization when compared to a 30% recurrence rate and graft loss in patients with no immobilization postoperatively. This study has shown that splinting is crucial in the postoperative period. Dhanraj et al. (24) elevated the efficacy of bilateral simultaneous surgical release of the burn scar contractures, as compared to unilateral correction of burn scar contractures of the feet. This study showed no statistical difference in terms of mortality, recurrence of contractures, the number of reconstructive procedures or the length of hospital stay. Consequently, patients with contractures of both feet should undergo simultaneous correction. Several authors have advocated early ambulation in both the acute and reconstructive stages of care for patients with burn to the feet (25–27). Plantar contractures are rare. This is due to the fact that full-thickness burns to the plantar surface of the feet are uncommon. However, split thickness grafts have proven to be satisfactory, even on the weight bearing portions of the foot, where the loss is primarily skin with an intact subcutaneous tissue (28). Harrison and Morgan noted that resurfacing the

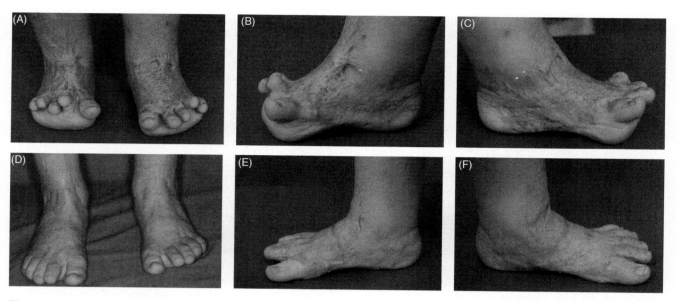

Figure 38.6   (A) A 5-year-old male with severe burn scar contractures of both feet. (B) Lateral view of right foot showing severe sub-luxation at the metatarsophalangeal joint. (C) Lateral view of left foot. (D) Nine months after simultaneous bilateral release of the contractures and resurfacing with skin grafts. (E/F) Right and left lateral postoperative views.

sole of the foot with skin grafts to be unsatisfactory, as most patients avoided weight bearing on a resurfaced area (29). The unique multidirectional fibrous septa of the skin and subcutaneous tissue of the sole also reduces flexibility. As a result, flaps are preferred rather than grafts. Hidalgo and Shaw (30) give importance to preservation of sensation for maintaining a stable weight bearing surface. However, Kucan and Bash (31) found that long-term follow-up of gait analysis of patients who have undergone resurfacing of the weight-bearing area of the foot with skin grafts or flaps had no significant difference among the various treatment modalities. Lister (28) recommended the use of skin grafts to provide sensation to the reconstructed heel.

Reconstruction of the foot using local tissue is limited by the available skin. However, local random pattern flaps have been used for coverage of small defects. Dorsal foot burns with exposed tendon and deeper structures require vascularized coverage using free tissue transfer. Fasciocutaneous flaps are preferred over muscle flaps because of their ability to properly contour. Alternatively, a number of free tissue transfers have been described for the closure of defects of the foot (32,33).

Plantar burn injuries pose a different challenge. Often tissues from non-weight-bearing areas are used to transfer tissue to weight-bearing areas, such as the instep flap. This flap is ideal when the area to be covered is small (34). The specialized characteristic of the skin in combination with relatively poor circulation of the skin in this area limits availability and mobility of nearby tissue (Fig. 38.7). Although many types of flaps have been described, they

all lack the normal plantar skin with its unique fibrous septa (35,36). Heel defects, although rare, can be covered by using medial plantar flaps based on medial plantar artery. These flaps can be rotated to cover heel defects (37). Local subfascial flaps, muscle flaps (i.e., the abductor hallucis, flexor digitorum brevis and abductor digiti minimi muscles) can also be used to cover small heel defects (38,39). The ideal reconstruction for injuries on the plantar surface should be aimed at providing protective and sensate cover (40).

When the injury prevents the use of local flaps, regional or distant flaps can be used. Random pattern flaps like de-epithelized turn over flap advocated by Ramakrishnan et al. (41) are useful. De-epdithelized turn over flap provide a single flap cover in burns with full thickness defects. The advantage is that it can be raised either superiorly or inferiorly based on the site. The defect is débrided into a rectangular shape. The width of the defect must be equal to the base of the flap with twice the length. The hinge should be located about one-third of the distance from the edge of the defect. When this flap is raised along with the deep fascia the increased vascular supply provides a better bed for skin grafts (Fig. 38.8). Several fasciocutaneous flaps have been described for coverage of foot defects. The lateral supramalleolar flap, the sural artery flap, the lateral calcaneal artery flap, as well as the reverse dorsalis pedis flap and reverse first dorsal metatarsal artery flap have been described (42). Based on the three major arteries, the peroneal, anterior tibial, and the posterior tibial artery reverse flow flaps are available for soft tissue defects of the foot. The advantage of using

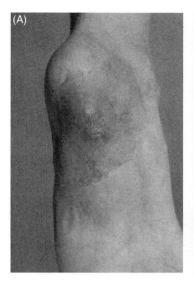
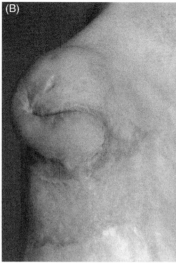
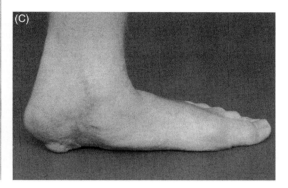

Figure 38.7 (A) A 12-year-old male referred because of tenderness over bony prominence on plantar surface of foot. (B) Delayed bipedicled skin flap from instep used to resurface the defect with follow-up 5 year later. Patient is completely asymptomatic with full weight-bearing. (C) Lateral view.

these flaps is that it is a safe single procedure and does not require immobilization on a long-term basis (43–46). Muscle flaps, like distally based abductor digiti minimi muscle flap and the extensor digitorum brevis are most useful for the Achilles region and is based on the dorsalis pedis artery pedicle (47,48). One must keep in mind that flaps never form a normal sole.

Cross-leg flaps are rapidly fading from use. When burn injury prevented the use of regional flaps, then cross-leg flaps have been used in past. Although rarely used in the modern era, they certainly formed an important part of the armanentarium for recconstructive surgeons (49–51). Free flaps, when all other options are not possible, microsurgical flaps definitely have a place in the reconstruction of the complex foot injuries. The flexibility of design, the transfer of composite tissues and the increased vascularity make it a useful alternative for reconstructing the burn foot. Various free flaps have been used for the foot depending on the type of injury and the tissues that need to be replaced. The more commonly used fasciocutanteous flaps are radial forearm flap, and the scapular flap (52) (Fig. 38.9). The commonly used muscle flaps are rectus abdominis, latissimus dorsi muscle, serratus anterior, and gracilis muscle. However, these tissues tend to be bulky and may prevent the wearing of normal shoes. Many authors prefer the use of microvascular free flaps for plantar surface (53–58). The advances in microsurgical technique has made it possible for reconstruction of extensive plantar defects which can provide protective sensation to the weight bearing surfaces of the foot by using sensory free flaps. Free flaps offer great flexibility of design and ability to obliterate deep spaces. Scapular flaps and deltopectoral flaps provide good support, especially when donor site deformity is inconspicuous. Chang et al. (59,60) have demonstrated sensory reinnervation in microsurgical reconstruction of the heel.

C. Amputation

Appropriate treatment of extensive foot defects is complex. Despite careful treatment, some patients inevitably require amputation. In determining the level of amputation, one must consider the optimal site for prosthetic fitting. The primary goal should be to salvage as much of the foot as possible to minimize functional loss. If the injury is severe resulting in either gangrene or life-threatening infection, then amputation may be the only choice (61).

V. PHYSIOTHERAPY AND SPLINTING

In the management of foot burns, proper positioning is a critical step in the prevention of joint deformities. The detrimental effects of poor positioning and contracture can result in multiple deformities. Following reconstruction with skin grafts, there is an urgent need for immediate and aggressive physiotherapy programs (62). Ambulation is resumed 1 week postoperatively after application of Ace wraps to prevent shearing of the skin grafts. Following discharge from the hospital, these patients are advised of graft care and regular use of splints to prevent further contractures.

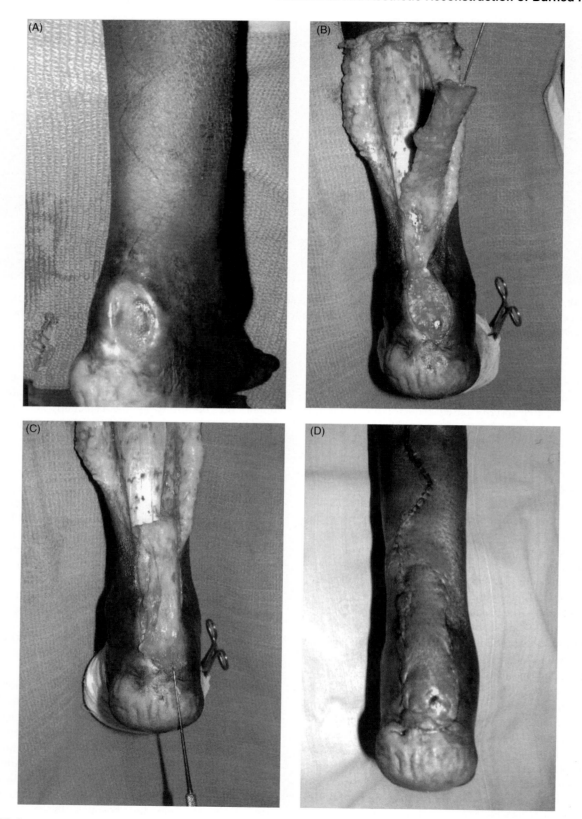

Figure 38.8   (A) A young patient with open wound in heal region. (B) Inferiorly based adipofascial flap raised. (C) Flap turned over to cover the defect. (D) Split-thickness skin graft placed on top of the turnover flap.

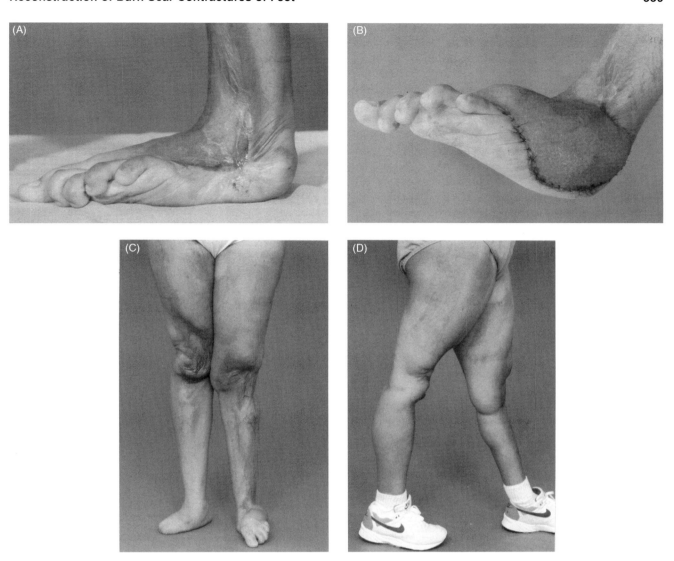

Figure 38.9 (A) A 15-year-old female sustained burns as an infant, now complaining of tenderness of left foot scar, which has frequent ulcerations. (B) Dorsum of the flat plantar surface and ankle resurfaced with a parascapular flap. (C) Frontal view of healed flap. (D) Comfortable wearing of shoes.

Initially, elasitc bandage support is provided for all patients with grafts to prevent increased hydrostatic pressure and graft loss while ambulating. Eventually, all patients are provided with custom-made pressure garments, silicone inserts, footplates, and orthopedic shoes (63). This shoe protects and supports the foot and relieves painful areas from abnormal pressure. Various shoe correctors like footpads, metatarsal bars, and foot and arch supports are often used in combination for comfortable support. Rayatt et al. (64) have used custom-made thermoplastic boot splints for the treatment of burn contractures of the feet in children following surgical release. Application of the Unna boot by Baiba et al. and Harnar et al. (65) has resulted in rapid functional recovery. The

use of splints for 6–9 months is helpful in the preventation of further contractures. The various types of splinting are thermoplastic, dynamic, silicone boots, orthopedic shoes, foot plates, and CASH shoes to maintain a neutral position and high top boots with supporting metatarsal bars. They are utilized to maintain the surgically corrected position.

VI. PITFALLS

Obviously, burns of the foot increase morbidity. Despite the best care, the magnitude of the original burn may warrant further operations, or even amputations. Prolonged weight bearing with abnormal loading on the joints can result in subluxation and joint dislocation. The pitfalls of surgical intervention include graft loss, joint pain, and incomplete correction of the initial problem. Unsuccessful surgery often delays definitive treatment. It not only reduces the physical activity, but many also experience foot pain, hyperkeratosis and ulcerations (66). Over enthusiastic attempts at full correction may result in damage to the neurovascular bundels. Loss of flaps may increase the size of the defect causing more complex problems. Recontractures in children are common. Inattentive care in postoperative splinting can lead to pressure sores and joint stiffness.

VII. NURSING ISSUES

Skin grafts to the lower limb require special nursing care. It is imperative to make sure that the limb is elevated postoperatively to reduce edema and subsequent graft failure. Proper positioning of the splint is checked to avoid pressure sores. After graft take, dressing changes and the use of silicone conformers and splints must be taught prior to discharge. The use of metatarsal bars at night to keep the feet in plantar flexion is helpful in the prevention of subsequent contractures. Ultimately, however, the type of coverage used in the correction of dorsal contractures, that is, skin grafts vs. flaps may be the ultimate determinant of success.

VIII. REHABILITATION ISSUES

Survival following extensive burn injury is no longer the only goal of successful treatment. Advances in the management of acute burns have resulted in survival of patients with 90% TBSA. This has resulted in new challenges for the rehabilitation team in order to achieve maximum functional recovery. The active planning of rehabilitation begins with the acute management and continues as long as satisfactory improvement is achieved (67,68). However, attention should be given not only to the physical well-being of the patient, but also focus on both psychological and social needs.

Physiotherapists and occupational therapists continue to work with the range of motion and muscle tone by providing daily exercise. With burns, there is a need for immediate and aggressive initiation of a rehabilitation program. The wound itself, as well as compliance can affect the outcome of an aggressive physical therapy program. Current means for the prevention of additional deformities are positioning with splints, exercise to maintain range of joint motion and the use of compression garments.

IX. LONG-TERM GOALS

Although foot burns form a small components of the TBSA, they require a high ranking on the priority list. Burns of the foot can result in disabling sequelae, which can produce chronic, lifelong problems. In the reconstruction of these patients, all surgical efforts should be made to overcome severe deformities by restoring the bony foot anatomy to normal. Second, providing sensate cover enables the patient to function normally. Third, care is taken to avoid recurrent ulceration by providing a stable well-padded cover. The unique architecture of the sole skin and subcutaneous tissue, which is adapted for weight bearing, cannot be reproduced. The transferred tissue does not have the ability to resist the shearing force produced during normal ambulation. Studies have been shown that irrespective of proper padding, ulcers can still occur due to bony abnormalities of poorly fitting footwear. Yet, even with out best efforts, patients alter their gait and weight-bearing load on reconstructed areas resulting in an abnormal gait.

X. CONCLUSION

The ankle and the foot are specialized structures for maintaining stability. In order to have proper function, these structures must be stable and capable of bearing weight. The need for late reconstruction depends in large part on the severity of injury and the quality of acute care. Priority should be given to burns of the foot, as early coverage will allow earlier ambulation and rehabilitation (69). Large soft tissue defects present a major reconstructive problem. Skin loss without exposure of the deeper structure can always be covered with skin grafts. However, deeper injuries exposing tendons and bones are best managed with vascularized flaps.

Small defects can usually be closed by local flaps. Larger defects can be problematic. Microvascular free tissue transfer has simplified this problem. The advantage of muscle flap lies in its vascularity and its ability to withstand infection. However, fasciocutaneous flaps conform to the foot better, making it more acceptable to the reconstructive surgeon. Bony prominences, inadequate soft tissue morbidity, and the need for specilized tissue, eliminate many of the options available. Primary closure may not be possible and skin graft may also not be possible due to exposed bone. This leaves the only option of distant flaps for coverage. Postoperative splinting has been shown to be effective in decreasing recurrence in foot contractures.

Burns to the feet and subsequent contractures continue to be a long-term problem. The severity and extent of the injury along with the nature of the acute care given, dictates the need for reconstruction at a later date. Priority treatment of the foot allows earlier ambulation and rehabilitation. However, if functional impairment progresses appropriate release of contractures both in the longitudinal and transverse arches and resurfacing with grafts are appropriate. More complex wounds require the use of flaps for closure. The postoperative rehabilitation program is crucial for a successful surgical outcome (70). Consequently, patient compliance is the key to maximizing our outcomes and preventing delayed complications such as recurrence.

REFERENCES

1. Lyle WG, Phillips LG, Robson MC. Reconstruction of the foot. In: Herndon DN, ed. Total Burn Care. Philadelphia: W.B. Saunders, 1996:515–519.
2. Pap AS. Hot metal burns of the feet in laundry workers. J Occup Med 1966; 8:537.
3. Randy SM. Lower extremity reconstruction. In: Achauer BM, Erikson E, eds. Plastic Surgery: Indication, Operation and Outcome. Vol. 32. St. Louis: Mosby, 2000:486.
4. Zachary LS, Heggers JP, Robson MC, Smith DJ Jr, Maniker AA, Sachs RJ. Burns of the feet. J Burn Care Rehabil 1987; 8(3):192–194.
5. Jackson D. Acquired vertical talus due to burn contractures, J Bone Joint Surg 1978; 60B(2):215–218.
6. Larson DL, Abston S, Willis B, Dobrkovsky M, Evans EB, Lewis SR. Contracture and scar formation in the burn patients. Clin Plast Surg 1974; 1:653.
7. Goldberg JA, Adkins P, Tsai TM. Microvascular reconstruction of the foot: weight-bearing patterns, gait analysis, and long-term follow up. Plast Reconstr Surg 1993; 92(5):904–911.
8. Knize DM. Cold injury. In: Converse JM, ed. Reconstructive Plastic Surgery. Vol. 1. Philadelphia: W.B. Saunders, 1977:516.
9. Daver BM, Antia NH, Furnas DW. Burns Hand Book of Plastic Surgery for General Surgeons. 2nd ed. Oxford: Oxford University Press.
10. Waymack JP, Fidler J, Warden GD. Surgical correction of burn scar contractures of the foot in children. Burns 1988; 14(2):156–160.
11. Robson MC, Barnett RA, Leitch IOW, Hayward PG. Prevention and treatment of post burn scars and contracture. World J Surg 1992; 6:87.
12. Staley M, Serghiou M. Casting guidelines, tips, and techniques: Proceedings from the 1997 American Burn Association PT/OT Casting Workshop. J Burn Care Rehabil 1998; 19(3):254–260.
13. Lamont JG. Functional anatomy of the lower limb. Clin Plast Surg 1986; 13:571.
14. Perry J. Normal and physiologic gait. In: AAOS of Orthopedics. 2nd ed. St Louis: CV Mosby, 1985.
15. Sammarco GJ. Biomechanics of the foot. In: Nordin M, Frankel VH, eds. Basic Biomechanics of the Musculoskeletal System. 2nd ed. Philadelphia: Lea and Febiger, 1989.
16. Sarrafian SK. Anatomy of the Foot and Ankle. Philadelphia: JB Lippincott, 1983.
17. Heimburger RA, Marten E, Larson DL, Abston S, Lewis SR. Burned feet in children. Am J Surg 1973; 125:575–579.
18. Steinwender G, Saraph V, Zwick EB, Uitz C, Linhart W. Complex foot deformities associated with soft-tissue scarring in children. J Foot Ankle Surg 2001; 40(1):42–49.
19. Evans BE, Larson DL, Abston S, Willis B. Prevention and correction of deformity after severe burns. Surg Clin North Am 1970; 50(6):1361–1376.
20. Koepke GH. Reconstruction of the legs and feet. In: Foot and Ankle. National Institute of Burn Medicine, 1979; 364.
21. Silk FF, Wainwright D. The recognition and treatment of congenital flat foot in infancy. J Bone Joint Surg 1967; 49B:628–633.
22. Patterson WR, Fritz DA, Smith WS. The pathologic anatomy of congenital convex pes valgus. J Bone Joint Surg 1968; 50A:458–466.
23. Alison WE, Moore ML, Reilly DA, Phillips LG, McCauley RL, Robson MC. Reconstruction of the foot burn contractures in children. J Burn Care Rehabil 1993; 14(1):34.
24. Dhanraj P, Owiesy F, Phillips LG, McCauley RL. Burn scar contractures of the feet: efficacy of bilateral simultaneous surgical correction. Burns 2002; 28:814–819.
25. Hallock GG. Simultaneous bilateral foot reconstruction using a single radial forearm flap. Plast Reconstr Surg 1987; 80(6):836–838.
26. Grube BJ, Engrav LH, Heimback DM. Early ambulation and discharge in 100 patients with burns of the foot treated by grafts. J Trauma 1992; 33(5):662–664.
27. Schmitt MA, French L, Kalil ET. How soon is safe? Ambulation of the patient with burns after lower extremity skin grafting. J Burn Care Rehabil 1991; 12:33.
28. Lister GD. Use of an innervated skin graft to provide sensation of the reconstructed heel. Plast Reconstr Surg 1978; 62:157–161.
29. Harrison DH, Morgan BDG. The instep island flap to resurface plantar defects. Br J Plast Surg 1981; 34:315–318.
30. Hidalgo DA, Shaw WW. Reconstruction of foot injuries. Clin Plast Surg 1986; 13(4):663–680.
31. Kucan JO, Bash D. Reconstruction of the burned foot. Clin Plast Surg 1992; 19(3):705–718.
32. Alexander G, Thatte MR, Govilkar PS. Use of type III venous flaps: single-and multistaged procedures. Ann Plast Surg 1995; 35(2):214–219.
33. McCraw JB, Leonard TF. The dorsalis pedis arterialized flap. Plastic Reconstr Surg 1975; 55:177.
34. Palacios FJ, De Armas DF, Hernandez VD, Aguirre MR. Radial free flaps in plantar burns. Burns 1990; 22(3):242–245.
35. Yoshikazu I, Murakami T, Yoshioka K, Tsuge K. Reconstruction of the heel pad by flexor digitorum brevis musculocutaneous flap transfer. Plast Reconstr Surg 1984; (1):86–94.
36. Hidalgo D, Shaw GG. Anatomic basis of plantar flap design. Plast Reconstr Surg 1986; 78(5):627–636.

37. Shanahan RE, Gingrass RP. Medial plantar sensory flap for coverage of heel defects. Plastic Reconstr Surg 1979; 64:295.

38. Reiffel RS, McCarthy JG. Coverage of heel and sole defects: a new subfascial arterialized flap. Plast Reconstr Surg 1980; 66(2):250.

39. Hartrampf CR, Scheflan M, Bostwick J. The flexor digitorum brevis muscle island pedicle flap. A new dimension in heel reconstruction. Plast Reconstr Surg 1980; 66(2):264.

40. Colen BL, Buncke HJ. Neuro vascular island flaps from the plantar vessels and nerves for foot reconstruction. Ann Plast Surg 1984; 12(4):327.

41. Ramakrishnan KM, Jayaraman V, Ramachandran K, Mathivanan T. Deepithelialized turnover flaps in burns. Plast Reconstr Surg 1988; 82(2):262–266.

42. Masquelet AC, Beveridge J, Romana C, Gerber C. The lateral supramalleolar flap. Plast Reconstr Surg 1988; 81(1):74–81.

43. Gibstein LA, Abramson DL, Sampson CE, Pribaz JJ. Musculo fascial flaps based on the dorsalis pedis vascular pedicle for coverage of the foot and ankle. Ann Plast Surg 1996; 37:152.

44. Grabb WC, Argenta LC. The lateral calcaneal artery skin flap (the lateral calcaneal artery, lesser saphenous vein, and sural nerve skin flap). Plast Reconstr Surg 1981; 68(5):723–730.

45. Smith AA, Arons JA, Reyes R, Hegstad SJ. Distal foot coverage with a reverse dorsalis pedis flap. Ann Plast Surg 1995; 34(2):191–199.

46. Hayashi A, Maruyama YU. Reverse first dorsal metatarsal artery flap for reconstruction of the distal foot. Ann Plast Surg 1993; 1:117.

47. Yoshimura Y, Nakajima T, Kami T. Distally based abdutor digiti minimi muscle flap. Ann Plast Surg 1985; 14(4):375.

48. Scheflan M, Nahai F, Hartrampf CR. Surgical management of heel ulcers—a comprehensive approach. Ann Plast Surg 981; 7(5):385.

49. Uhm K, Shin KS, Lew JD. Crane principle of the cross-leg fasciocutaneous flap:aesthetially pleasing technique for damaged dorsum of foot. Ann Plast Surg 1985; 15(3):257–261.

50. Taylor AG, Hopson GWL. The cross foot flap. Plast Reconstr Surg 1975; 55:677.

51. Barclay TL, Sharpe DT, Chisholm EM. Cross leg fasciocutaneous flap. Plast Reconstr Surg 1983; 72(6):843–846.

52. Hallock GG. The fadial forearm flap in burn reconstruction. J Burn Care Rehabil 1986; 7(4):318–322.

53. Bunkis J, Walton RL, Mathes JS. The rectus abdominis free flap for lower extremity reconstruction. Ann Plast Surg 1983; 11(5):373.

54. Milanov NO, Adamyan RT. Functional results of microsurgical reconstruction of plantar defects. Ann Plast Surg 1994; 32(1):52–56.

55. Stevenson TR, Mathes SJ. Management of foot injuries with free-muscle flaps. Plast Reconstr Surg 1986; 78(5):665–669.

56. Stevenson TR, Mathes SJ. Management of foot injuries with free-muscle flaps: Plast Reconstr Surg 1986; 78(5):670–671.

57. Rautio J, Asko-Seljavaara S, Laasonen L, Härmä M. Suitability of the scapular flap for reconstructions of the foot. Plast Reconstr Surg 1990; 85(6):922–928.

58. Noever G, Brüser P, Köhler L. Reconstruction of heel and sole defects by free flaps. Plast Reconstr Surg 1986; 78(3):345–350.

59. Chang KN, De Armond SJ, Buncke HJ. Sensory reinnervation in microsurgical reconstruction of the heel. Plast Reconstr Surg 1986; 78(5):652–663.

60. Chang KN, De Armond SJ, Buncke HJ. Sensory Reinnervation in microsurgical reconstruction of the heel. Plast Reconstr Surg 1986; 78(5):664.

61. May JW, Rohrich RJ. Foot reconstruction using free microvascular muscle flaps with skin grafts. Clin Plast Surg 1986; 13(4):681–689.

62. Petro JA, Salisbury RE. Rehabilitation of burn patient. Clin Plast Surg 1986; 13(1):145–149.

63. Melvin HJ. Shoes and shoe modifications. In: The Foot. National Institute of Burn Medicine, 1979; 267.

64. Rayatt SS, Grew P, Powell BM. A custom-made thermoplastic boot splint for the treatment of burns contractures of the feet in children. Burns 2000; 26:106–108.

65. Harnar T, Engrav LH, Marvin J, Heimbach D, Cain V, Johnson C. Dr. Paul Unna's boot and early ambulation after skin grafting the leg: a survey of burn centers and a report of 20 cases. Plast Reconstr Surg 1982; 69:359–360.

66. Sommerlad BC, McGrouther DA. Resurfacing the sole: long-term follow up and comparsion of techniques. Brit J Plast Surg 1978; 31:107–116.

67. Gore D, Desai M, Herndon DN, Abston S, Evans BE. Comparison of complications during rehabilitation between conservative and early surgical management in thermal burns involving the feet of children and adolescents. J Burn Care Rehabil 1988; 9(1):92–95.

68. Feller I. Reconstruction and Rehabilitation of the Burned Patient. National Institute for Burn Medicine, 1979.

69. Witt PD, Achauer BM. Lower Extremity: Burn Reconstruction. Thieme Medical Publishers Inc., 1991:134.

70. Goldberg DP, Kucan JO, Bash D. Reconstructions of the burned foot. Clin Plast Surg 2000; 27(1):45–161.

39

The Role of External Fixators in the Correction of the Equinovarus Deformities in Burn Patients

JASON H. CALHOUN
University of Missouri–Columbia, Columbia, Missouri, USA

KELLY D. CARMICHAEL
University of Texas Medical Branch, Galveston, Texas, USA

DEBRA BENJAMIN
Shriners Hospital for Children, Galveston, Texas, USA

I. INTRODUCTION

Burns of the feet are classified as a major burn injury by the American Burn Association and the American College of Surgeons and should be referred to burn centers for specialized care and treatment (1). The feet, farthest away from the heart and the oxygenated blood from the lungs, are at risk of slower healing and a longer period for scar maturation. The feet are also at risk for increased swelling and inflammation as the normal tissue support surrounding the lymphatics in the area has changed with the burn injury and thus may be less successful working against gravity.

Burn scars have long been, and continue to be, a disabling complication of burn injury. They not only cause cosmetic disfigurement, but also adversely affect functional outcome. The burn wound scar, or muscle and bone loss from the initial injury, can lead to muscle shortening and bone structure abnormalities resulting in foot deformities. Burn scars of the feet can lead to deformities that compromise ambulation and prevent the independence of mobility.

II. ACUTE MANAGEMENT OF FOOT BURNS

When diagnosing the depth of burn involving the feet, the characteristics will be similar to those of burn injuries on other areas of the body. The feet do, however, have a unique quality of skin coverage. The skin on the plantar side of the foot normally has a thick dermis and epidermis, which often protects this portion of the foot from a deeper injury. In contrast, the dorsal foot tends to have less subcutaneous tissue and may result in deeper burn injuries that may require grafting. If grafting of the dorsal foot is required, it should be done as early as possible to decrease a local inflammatory response and reduce scarring and contracture formation. If the foot receives only a superficial burn injury, it may be treated on an outpatient basis. The patient should be instructed to keep his feet elevated above the heart to decrease edema and be educated to watch for signs of infection and cellulitus. The patient should also be evaluated for risks of circulation problems and level of compliance for elevating his feet. If the physician has any concerns, the patient should be hospitalized for 24–72 h for observation and treatment.

Passive and active range of motion exercises should begin immediately with superficial burn injuries, and within 5–7 days after grafting is performed. Early splinting of the burned foot is necessary to maintain proper position. Foot burns that involve the ankle area are prone to develop an inverted plantar flexion. This is a common complication seen with foot and ankle burns. Proper positioning can be accomplished with footboards or foot and lower leg splints that place the foot at a 90° angle to the leg. With ambulation, it is important to provide the foot and leg with proper support. Ace wraps or support hose are helpful during early recovery to provide support to the ankle, to provide pressure to the burn scars, and to improve circulation to an area distant from the heart at risk of venous stasis. After edema and swelling resolve, the patient should be fitted with snug supportive shoes. Silicone inserts may be needed to provide pressure to specific areas of the foot. Even after ambulation has begun, it is important to maintain foot position with splints when the patient is at rest or sleeping.

A. Scarring and Deformities

The burned foot is an area of the body at greatest risk of scarring with major deformities. Because of the shape and various curvatures in the foot, it is difficult to maintain even pressure for scar control. The requirements of movement for ambulation continually force flexion of the toes upward without an equal force of the toes toward extension. As scar forms over the dorsum of the foot, scar contraction occurs, which pulls the toes up even more. Burns around the back of the ankle can lead to scarring and contractures of the skin causing shortening of the Achilles tendon which produces a plantar flexion of the foot. This scar tissue can also bind the tendons and even trap bones and joints to cause major deformities. These deformities can lead to significant pain and mobility difficulties for the patient.

Bone deformities of the burned foot have been classified as simple and complex. This is based on associated deformities, musculoskeletal function, and the difficulty associated with correction. Simple deformities are unidirectional in nature and have relatively normal bone and soft tissue. They include equinus, cavus, and toe dislocations. These are fairly easy to correct and maintain. Complex deformities include varus or valgus angulations, the rocker bottom foot, bone abnormalities, and contractures due to muscle loss. These deformities are more difficult to correct and maintain (2).

Toe deformities and dislocations, which are the gross hyperextension and subluxation of the toes, are the most common (3). Simple dorsal toe dislocation in burned patients is due to dorsal soft tissue contracture. Although functional mobility is usually adequate, toe contractures often cause problems with shoe fit and chronic friction ulcerations. More complex toe deformities include hallux varus and valgus, or metatarsal and phalangeal bone abnormalities.

A rocker bottom foot is a deformity caused by a dorsal burn scar contracture or overcorrection of the forefoot for an equines deformity. Rocker bottom is classified as severe when the metatarsal–calcaneal angle is >200°.

A cavus deformity is a contraction of the plantar portion of the foot. It can also occur with an equinus deformity. A cavus is classified as severe when the metatarsal–calcaneal angle is <120°.

Equines deformities, which are a shortening of the Achilles tendon, can be caused by postburn contracture, anterior muscle loss, improper postburn splinting, and tibial growth into a rigid scar. If not too severe, this contracture can often be corrected with the release of the Achilles tendon. Severe equinus (>40°) cannot be corrected with a soft tissue release because of insufficient soft tissue posterior to the ankle. Simple equinovarus involves a single deformity that is in one plane and in one direction. Complex equinovarus, on the other hand, involves more than one type of deformity. Examples of complex equinus contracture cases are equinovarus (an additional medial contraction of the foot) without active dorsiflexors or caves and equinovarus with bone deformities or a nonfunctional ankle joint. Another complex equinus is the equinovulgus (an additional lateral contracture of the foot) (2).

The equinovarus foot deformity makes walking difficult or impossible and can cause ulcers, infections, and other deformities. Prevention and treatment of the equinovarus foot deformity is challenging, particularly in the patient with multiple injuries and systemic problems associated with burns. The equinovarus deformity is prevented though correct positioning of the foot during the acute phase of burn management. Splints, calcaneal traction pins, and physical therapy are ways to control foot position.

All of these methods are used to keep the ankle in the 90° neutral position while preventing inversion. Burn injury, compartment syndrome of the leg and foot, and brain injury can cause loss of muscle control. The peroneals and anterior tibial and toe extensor muscles are frequently affected, leading to weakness in eversion and dorsiflexion. The tricep surae is often spared in peripheral injuries, as its nerves are more proximal and deep posterior. The tricep surae is the most powerful muscle acting across the ankle, so plantar flexion deformity can occur quickly when other muscle groups are weakened and the patient can actively plantar flex. When ambulation begins after an injury, patients often plantar flex or "toe walk," and the plantar flexed position becomes more established, rigid, and extensive. Improper or inadequate bracing during the period of recovery allows for plantar flexion and inversion, thus worsening the equinovarus deformity.

B. Physical Examination

The physical examination of the equinovarus deformity includes an assessment of the position of the ankle, hindfoot, and forefoot. Disability due to foot and ankle position is described in the "Guides to the Evaluation of Permanent Impairment" (4). Impairment due to equinus deformities is graded as follows: mild plantar flexion (10°–19°) is considered 7% whole-person impairment, moderate (20°–29°) is 15%, and severe plantar flexion (>30°) is 21% (Table 39.1). An ankle in fixed plantar flexion will cause difficulty with ambulation. Consequences of ankle equinus include walking with the foot in external rotation, a "vaulting" type gait as the patient jumps over the plantar flexed foot, toe walking, and hyperextension of the knee. The knee is affected by ankle equinus because of the "plantar flexion–knee extension" couple. In normal gait/strength, plantar flexion of the ankle is coupled to knee extension during the gait cycle. Increased plantar flexion or plantar flexion strength will cause a knee hyperextension gait. Weak or insufficient plantar flexion is associated with a crouched knee gait.

Impairment can also include hindfoot varus, which can be graded as mild (10°–19°), moderate (20°–29°), or

Table 39.1 Ankle Impairment Due to Ankylosis in Plantar Flexion or Dorsiflexion

Position	Whole person (lower extremity) [foot] impairment (%)
>20° dorsiflexion	15 (37) [53]
10°–19° dorsiflexion	7 (17) [24]
10°–19° plantar flexion	7 (17) [24]
20°–29° plantar flexion	15 (37) [53]
>30° plantar flexion	21 (52) [74]

Source: From the American Medical Association (1)

severe (>30°). Other forms of impairment can be noted in the hindfoot, calcaneus, and midfoot (internal rotation), forefoot, nerves, muscles, and soft tissue. With all these potential problems, impairment can be up to 50% in a burned lower extremity with an equinovarus deformity; the majority (38%) is due to the equinovarus.

Gait abnormalities should be noted during the physical examination. Other joint abnormalities to quantify are the degree of plantar flexion and varus. Deformities of the calcaneus, midfoot, and forefoot should be noted. Weight-bearing radiographs of the ankle and foot with the knee straight should be taken to aid the evaluation of bone or joint abnormalities. Scarring, with hypertrophy or breakdown, and nerve and muscle function should be noted. Nerve and muscle dysfunction may be the cause of the deformity and may also affect any treatments. Weakness or absence of the peroneal (longus, brevis) and anterior tibial muscles (tibialis anticus, extensor digitorum longus, and extensor hallucis longus) can contribute to the varus. The gastro-soleus muscle is frequently normal, which leads to increased plantar flexion. Functioning toe flexors can also contribute to equinus as well as claw toe. A functioning posterior tibial muscle will contribute to both plantar flexion and varus.

C. Treatment Options

The treatment goal is to prevent contractures with physical therapy and splinting. Mild and moderate contractures may be treated with aggressive physical therapy, splinting and/or casting, or incisional releases of the soft tissue or osteotomies. Severe contractures have been treated with amputations and Ilizarov external fixators.

Equinovarus treatment depends on the severity of the burn and the severity of the deformity. In the acute period equinovarus deformity responds to physical therapy. Skeletal traction through the calcaneus can also be helpful in the patient confined to the bed (Fig. 39.1). In the chronic phase the burn scar is more rigid and is not as responsive to physical therapy and traction.

The severity of the burn will influence treatment. Less severe burns isolated to the lower leg can be treated more aggressively as the first priority. However, more extensive burns are limb- or life-threatening and, appropriately, attention to the lower extremities becomes secondary to keeping the patient or extremity alive. As with impairment rating, it is helpful to "stage" an equinovarus deformity as mild (<15°), moderate (<30°), or severe (>30°). The equinovarus can be further identified as either simple or complex as described earlier. Complex deformities treated with traditional surgeries often require staged corrective surgery. One deformity may be addressed in the first surgery and another deformity in a subsequent surgery. Releases are often combined with subsequent fusions to maintain or further correct deformities.

Mild equinus or equinovarus with functional nerves, muscles, bones, and joints can frequently be corrected with serial casts to the functional position of neutral. Percutaneous Achilles tendon releases (5,6) can be added to casting to correct moderate deformities. Severe equinus or equinovarus deformities with functional tissue can be corrected with the Ilizarov circular external fixator (7) or staged traditional open surgeries. However, in severe deformities, traditional surgeries are often complicated by soft tissue tension and wound-healing problems. The gradual correction obtained by the Ilizarov method was designed to minimize these complications. Complex equinus or equinovarus deformities will require the complicating problem to be addressed after correction has been obtained. With functional nerves and muscles, especially the anterior tibial muscle, the deformity will recur unless very aggressive physical therapy and splints, tendon transfers and releases, or joint arthromeres are used after correction. With bone or joint abnormalities, then, osteotomies and arthrodeses may be needed to achieve and maintain correction. Other deformities such as cavus, calcaneal equines, forefoot and midfoot inversion, and pes planus and rocker bottom may be seen as a simple or complicating deformity with equinovarus.

Contraindications to correction of equinovarus include poor blood supply, chronic irreversible edema, and insensitivity. These contraindications, if severe enough, may indicate amputation of the extremity or, at least,

observation, therapy, splints, and special prosthetics for function.

D. Ilizarov External Fixator

Professor Gavriil Ilizarov developed the Ilizarov external fixation system. It allows precise control of bone segments, including angulation, rotation, translation, lengthening, and shortening. The system encourages tissue regeneration through the principles of distraction histogenesis of bone and soft tissues. The Ilizarov fixator aids in the correction of bone and soft tissue deformities and defects. The Ilizarov and its techniques for use preserve limb function when properly applied. The Ilizarov external fixator is a circular frame consisting of (1) implant-grade stainless steel wires that attach to rings with bolts, buckles, and/or nuts; (2) rods that interconnect the rings; and (3) connection plates, supports, posts, hinges, washers, sockets, and bushings that complete the assembly of the fixator. Special wrenches and wire tensioners are required for proper assembly.

In the 1960s the Ilizarov was used for the treatment of clubfoot and other congenital foot deformities. The Ilizarov was first used in 1988, at the Galveston Shriners Burn Hospital, for the treatment of bone deformities of the foot from severe scar contractures. For treatment of foot deformities caused by burn scar, the Ilizarov frame usually has two tibial–fibular rings, one calcaneal half-ring, and one metatarsal half-ring. The frames are attached to the bone with 1.5 mm pins. There are also a set of

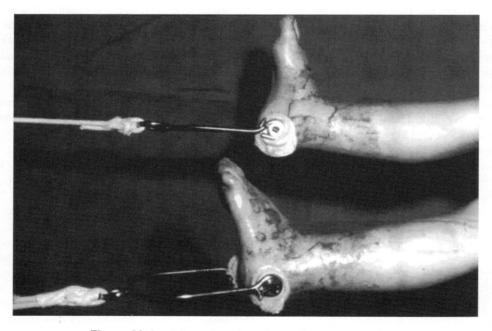

Figure 39.1   Calcaneal traction pins used to prevent equines.

distraction rods connecting the rings together to manipulate the position of the foot over time.

E. Ilizarov Indications and Treatment

The Ilizarov fixator can be used for toe dislocations and also with hallux varus and valgus deformities. This can be accomplished with phalangeal pins connecting to half-rings or outriggers. The bones will be gradually pulled into place as the scarred skin is stretched and lengthened. For the cavus deformity in the midfoot area, the Ilizarov provides correction by distracting the calcaneus and metatarsals in a half-ring frame. The rocker bottom foot can be treated with the Ilizarov with a frame similar to the cavus frame except that a midfoot half-ring frame is pulled dorsally to re-create the arch. A more complex rocker bottom foot may need additional frame pieces and wires (2).

A simple equinus deformity can be treated with an Ilizarov frame consisting of two tibial–fibular rings, one calcaneal half-ring and one metatarsal half-ring. A complex equinus deformity involving a varus or valgus contracture requires a more complex frame to accommodate the additional twisting of the foot. Risks of complications also are increased in this more complex treatment.

F. Operative Technique

The flexible frame can be used for simple, unidirectional deformities and when bony deformities are not present. This frame consists of a tibial ring, one calcaneal half-ring, and one metatarsal half-ring as mentioned earlier [Fig. 39.2(A) and (B)]. The tibial ring is positioned approximately at the junction of the middle and distal third of the leg. It is secured with a single posterolateral to anteromedial wire and three anterior half-pins attached with the Rancho cube system (hybrid technique). The remaining half-rings are connected to bone with 1.5 or 1.8 mm wires (for children and adults, respectively) that are tensioned to 90 kg of force on the half-rings. The calcaneal wire is directed from the medial to lateral side to avoid the medial neurovascular bundle. The wire is located relatively proximally and posteriorly in the calcaneus to prevent wire cutout and increase its biomechanical advantage. The metatarsal pin is directed medial to lateral from the first metatarsal to the fifth metatarsal. Only the first and fifth metatarsals are pinned so that a synostosis does not develop between adjacent metatarsals. Half-rings are connected to the calcaneal and metatarsal wires. The calcaneus half-ring is connected to the tibial ring with threaded distraction rods, and the metatarsal half-ring is connected with threaded compression rods. Calcaneus distraction requires only proximal hinges without distal hinges to allow posterior translation of the calcaneus pin as the calcaneus moves plantarly. Metatarsal

dorsiflexion requires hinges on the metatarsal ring and a rotating post at the tibial ring to allow the metatarsal pin to translate anteriorly as the deformity is corrected. The ankle joint must be distracted before other deformity correction is possible. Distraction is performed at the time of frame placement. In a simple equinus correction, the ankle should be distracted 2–5 mm compared with preoperative radiographs. This limits ankle-joint cartilage compression and midfoot dorsiflexion deformity (rocker bottom deformity). Distraction of the hindfoot must be done in a posteriorly inclined direction. If distraction is performed in a purely axial direction, parallel to the tibia, the talus tends to sublux anteriorly (9).

Depending on the cause of the deformity, tendon transfers or joint fusions may be needed to prevent recurrence. Two technical points of frame application deserve special mention:

1. This unconstrained technique, in which the correction is done around the natural axis of rotation of the joints and soft tissue hinges (10), is more forgiving than a constrained technique, in which correction is through a precisely placed pair of hinges along the defined anatomic axis of the joint. The two keys to the use of an unconstrained technique are that distraction must be applied to the ankle joint before any attempted correction and that posterior hinges are placed proximally on the tibial ring and distally on the metatarsal ring to allow translational movement.

2. Frames for the correction of a simple equinus contracture require much less rigidity than those for bony instability. It has been the authors' experience that frames classically described as equinus frames are also more rigid than is required. A single tibial ring with a single wire and three half-pins (hybrid technique) has proven to be more than adequate proximal fixation. The use of a footplate or connecting bars between the calcaneal and metatarsal half-rings has not been needed for simple equinus correction, but can be added for cavus and midfoot deformities.

G. Post Surgery Care Following Placement of External Fixator

Immediately following surgery, the foot or feet with the Ilizarov(s) should be kept elevated above the level of the heart to reduce swelling and promote circulation. Appropriate pain control should be used for the first few days following surgery, and then Tylenol should be adequate during the weeks of treatment. Pin sites should be cleaned with betadine four times a day for 1 week or until pin sites are dry. After that, pin sites may be cleaned daily with betadine soaked Q-tips. If sites become infected during treatment, the wound should be cultured, and appropriate topical and oral antibiotics should be administered.

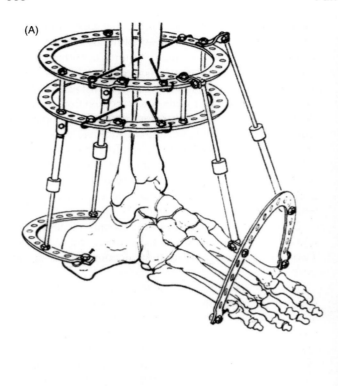

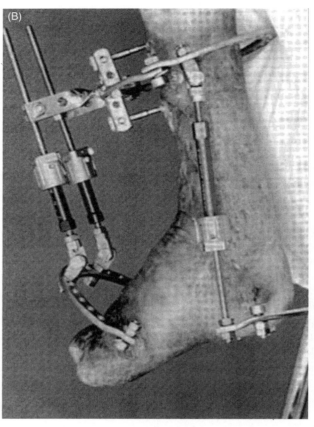

Figure 39.2 (A) Galveston frame for equinus correction. Tibial ring is secure with one wire from the fibula to the tibia. The calcaneal wire and half-ring allow distraction of the calcaneus and ankle joint. The metatarsal and half-ring allow for correction of the equinus. (B) Clinical photograph of the frame. [Adapted from Calhoun et al. (2), used with permission from Elsevier, 1998 (4).]

Postoperatively, deformity correction is started as soon as the patient can tolerate it comfortably, which is usually in 1–3 days. The Ilizarov fixator will begin its extension to stretch the foot into position. The calcaneus is pushed distally and the metatarsals are pulled proximally at a rate of 1–3 mm/day. With a wrench the screws are loosened and/ or tightened as appropriate every 4–6 h, $\sim \frac{1}{4} - \frac{1}{2}$ mm each time. Because the forefoot lever arm (metatarsal pin) is further from the axis of rotation (ankle) than the posterior lever arm (calcaneal pin), a difference in angular correction occurs if all telescoping rods are distracted and compressed at the same rate. Theoretically, it is possible to compensate for this tendency by increasing the rate of dorsiflexion of the metatarsal ring in relation to the distraction of the calcaneal ring. In practice, however, doing so has been unnecessary. The distraction of the calcaneus is the primary driver of correction and the dorsiflexion of the metatarsals is of secondary importance.

Following surgery the patient may begin ambulating as tolerated with crutches or a walker. This process of stretching and repositioning the foot with the Ilizarov can take several weeks. Postoperative radiographs taken at 1, 2, 4,

and 6 weeks are important; they are used to follow deformity correction and to ensure that the ankle remains distracted 2–5 mm without any subluxation. After correcting between 5° and 10° of ankle dorsiflexion, the frame is left in place for 2–6 weeks, depending on the rigidity of the soft tissue.

H. Post-Ilizarov Care

Following successful treatment it is imperative to maintain the newly obtained position of the foot. This can be done after frame removal with a short leg-walking cast, which is typically applied for 6 weeks. Alternatively, an ankle–foot orthosis (AFO) can be constructed with 10° of built-in dorsiflexion that is removed only for range of motion exercises. After cast removal, splints should be made to maintain position and should be worn while at rest for several months after the Ilizarov has been removed. The splints may need to be revised over time with continued wear and with the child's growth as the leg will grow longer, but the scar tissue may stay the same size, leading to a new equinus. Physical therapy is also extremely important to continue to stretch the skin and scar, to develop strength in the muscles of the foot and ankle, and to maintain range of motion. It is important to note that additional surgeries may be needed, especially in children as they continue to grow, to maintain proper position or to prevent reoccurrence.

I. Follow-up Results

A follow-up was performed on all patients who had received treatment with an Ilizarov external fixator. Twenty-seven children had been treated with the Ilizarov for burn scar contractures and bony deformities of the foot, and 36 Ilizarovs were used. Seventy-five percent of these children had an equinus element to their foot deformity. The mean age at the time of Ilizarov treatment was 10 years, with age ranges between 2 and 18 years. The average length of time the Ilizarov was used for treatment was 10.5 weeks. Follow-up was documented on these patients for an average of 3.6 years. During the 10-year period that Ilizarov treatment was reviewed, nine of the patients that had received Ilizarovs needed surgical revisions, and four of the Ilizarovs developed pin-site infections.

Unfortunately, four Ilizarovs had ended treatment prematurely. Two of the Ilizarovs, the physician removed early: two due to infection, and one because the parent requested to have it removed early. Two casts, which are used after the Ilizarov to maintain position, were removed early by the patient at home. One of the early cast removal patients was the same as an early Ilizarov removal patient. Twenty-three or 68% of the feet treated with Ilizarovs had no complications or unplanned occurrences during treatment (11). An example of the Ilizarov treatment course is shown in Fig. 39.3(A–F).

Of the 36 feet treated with Ilizarov external fixators, 56% of the patients had satisfactory results as measured by a gait within normal limits and a deformity of <25° from neutral. Thirty-nine percent of the applications ended in a poor

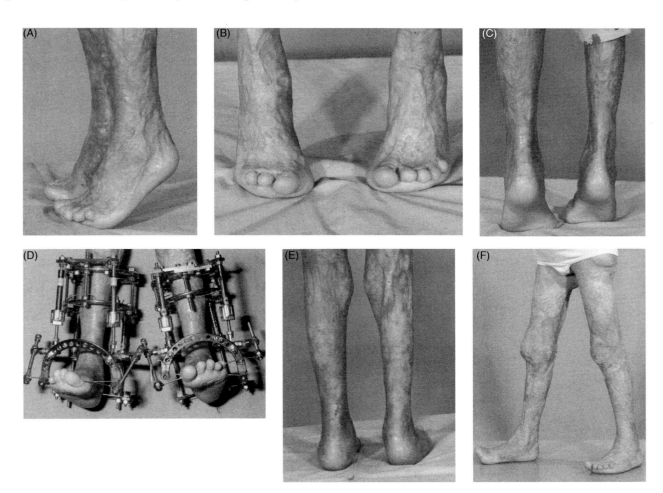

Figure 39.3 (A) Eight-year-old patient before-Ilizarov treatment, demonstrating, severe shortening of the Achilles tendon and equinus deformity with dorsal subluxation of toes. (B and C) Anterior and posterior view of both feet before Ilizarov treatment. (D) Bilateral Ilizarov treatment for correction of foot deformities. (E and G) Posterior and lateral view of feet following Ilizarov lengthening of Achilles tendon. Mild dorsal subluxation of toes still requires attention. (Photos courtesy of Jason Calhoun, MD.)

result, as measured by a return of the original deformity or a deviation of $>25°$ from neutral. Of this group of patients, one required a below-the-knee amputation. Five have had repeated applications. Three of these now have satisfactory results, and one with a bilateral application remained in the poor results group. Three of the patients with poor results have requested no further surgery at this time. This is not necessarily an uncommon request of children with major burn injuries who have gone through years of reconstructive procedures. Three patients with single Ilizarov applications did not return for follow-up.

All patients treated with the Ilizarov had successful results immediately following the removal of the fixator. It was not, however, expected that perfect position would be maintained. Children, especially the very young, have many years to grow, and burn scars do not always stretch as children grow.

Contractures with growth are expected in children, and a reoccurrence of the deformity from foot and leg burn scars is expected. This scenario is thoroughly explained to the child and their families. They are also told that because of growth and future scarring, the Ilizarov may need to be reapplied at a later date.

J. Ilizarov Complications

Complications of the Ilizarov during the treatment phase can include pain, pin-site infections, nerve damage, circulatory damage, the necessity of surgical revision of the Ilizarov fixator, and intolerability of the process causing the patient to request an end to the treatment. Complications after successful treatment are the return of contractures limiting functional mobility. Complications following treatment may be heavily affected by the family dynamics, including the influence of family and patient/family compliance during treatment.

K. Amputation

Amputation may be indicated for severe equinovarus deformities that have contraindications to corrective surgery and for those deformities that are more debilitating than a prosthesis. A below-the-knee prosthesis can be less disabling than a severely burned, contracted, insensate leg. Most patients and their families, however, are very hesitant to allow an amputation unless the benefits are clear and obvious. Long, detailed, compassionate discussions with the patient and their family and caregivers are necessary. No patient with a chronic equinovarus deformity should be taken to the operating room unless all understand the planned surgery, potential complications, duration of fixator placement, pain, and difficulties.

III. SUMMARY

Foot burn deformities in the burned patient are best prevented with early grafting, immediate postburn splinting, and vigorous physical therapy. Treatment of deformity should be aggressive in the weeks and months after the burn injury to prevent and resolve mild and moderate deformities. Equinovarus deformities can also be treated acutely with calcaneal pins. Severe equinovarus deformities can be treated with external fixators and with techniques to prevent recurrence to avoid amputation.

Successful treatment of severe foot contractures in burned children continues to be a problem. Ilizarov external fixators have primarily been used in Galveston, Texas, with the most severe foot deformities and have been used successfully to provide improvement in these patients. Significant failure still exists; however, the alternative for these deformities may include amputation or being wheelchair bound.

REFERENCES

1. Committee on Trauma. Guidelines for the Operation of Burn Units. Resources for Optimal Care of the Injured Patient: 1999. American College of Surgeons, 1998.
2. Calhoun JH, Evans EB, Herndon DN. Techniques for the management of burn contractures with the Ilizarov fixator. Clin Orthop Rel Res 1992; 280:117–124.
3. Lyle WG, Phillips LG, Robson MC. Reconstruction of the foot. In: Herndon DN, ed. Total Burn Care. London: W.B. Saunders Company, 2003:515–519.
4. Cocchiarella L, Andersson GBJ, eds. The Lower Extremities. Guides to the Evaluation of Permanent Impairment. 5th ed. Chicago, IL: American Medical Association Press, 2001:523–564.
5. Hatt RF, Lamphier TA. Triple hemisection: a simplified procedure for lengthening the Achilles tendon. N Engl J Med 1947; 236:166–169.
6. Waters RL, Garland DE. Disorders of the lower extremity in the stroke and head trauma patient. In: Jahss MH, ed. Disorders of the Foot and Ankle. Vol. III. Philadelphia, PA: W.B. Saunders Company, 1991:2084–2085.
7. Thompson DM, Calhoun JH. Advanced techniques in foot and ankle reconstruction. Foot Ankle Clin 2000; 5:417–442.
8. Richards Medical Company. The Ilizarov External Fixator, General Surgical Techniques Brochure. Milan, Italy: Richards Medical Company, Medical Plastic s.r.l. 1989.
9. Cierny G III. Classification and treatment of osteomyelitis. In: Evarts CM, ed. Surgery of the Musculoskeletal System. New York: Churchill Livingstone, 1990:4337–4381.
10. Cierny G III, Cook WG, Mader JT. Ankle arthrodesis in the presence of ongoing sepsis: indications, methods, and results. Orthop Clin North Am 1989; 20:709–721.
11. Benjamin DA, Calhoun J, Evans EB, McCauley RL, Wolf SE, Desai MH, Herndon DN. Ilizarov external fixators for severe foot deformities in pediatric burn patients. J Burn Care Rehabil 1998; 19(1 part 2):s210.

Index

About the Editor

Robert L. McCauley is Professor of Surgery, University of Texas Medical Branch, Galveston; Chief of Plastic and Reconstructive Surgery, Shriners Hospital for Children—Galveston Unit, Galveston, Texas; and Medical Director of the Shriners Burn Hospital Tissue Bank, Galveston, Texas. The author, coauthor, or editor of numerous professional publications, book chapters, and journal articles, Dr. McCauley serves on the editorial board of the *Journal of Trauma*, the *Journal of Burn Care and Rehabilitation*, the international *Journal of Burns*, and the *Journal of the National Medical Association*. He is a Fellow of the American College of Surgeons and a member of the American Society of Plastic Surgeons, the Wound Healing Society, and the American Burn Association, among many other organizations. Dr. McCauley received the M.D. degree (1977) from the Pritzker School of Medicine, University of Chicago, Illinois.